Healing Beyond Blood Sugar

Krishnendu Adhikary · Pradipta Banerjee ·
Krishnendu Ganguly
Editors

Healing Beyond Blood Sugar

A Complete Guide to Managing Diabetes-Related Disabilities

Springer

Editors
Krishnendu Adhikary
Department of Medical Lab Technology
Paramedical College Durgapur
Durgapur, West Bengal, India

Research and Development Cell
Lovely Professional University
Jalandhar, Phagwara, Punjab, India

Krishnendu Ganguly
Department of Medical Lab Technology
Paramedical College Durgapur
Durgapur, West Bengal, India

Pradipta Banerjee
Department of Surgery
University of Pittsburgh
Pittsburgh, PA, USA

ISBN 978-981-95-8945-6 ISBN 978-981-95-8946-3 (eBook)
https://doi.org/10.1007/978-981-95-8946-3

This Springer imprint is published by the registered company Springer Nature Singapore Pte Ltd.
The registered company address is: 152 Beach Road, #21-01/04 Gateway East, Singapore 189721, Singapore

I dedicate this work with deepest love and gratitude to my beloved parents, Ms. Sonali Adhikary *and* Mr. Dipak Adhikary, *My sister* Ms. Barnali Adhikary *and My Wife* Ms. Supriya Adhikary, *whose unconditional support, sacrifices, values, and constant encouragement have been the foundation of my academic journey and personal growth. Their faith in my dreams gave me the strength to persevere through every challenge.*

I also respectfully dedicate this book to my esteemed Ph.D. guides and to all my teachers throughout my life. Their wisdom, mentorship, patience, and scholarly guidance have shaped my scientific thinking, nurtured my curiosity, and inspired my commitment to research and learning.

This work stands as a humble tribute to their lasting influence on my life and career.

Preface

Diabetes mellitus has long been framed through the narrow lens of glycemic control numbers, targets, medications, and metabolic indices. While these remain essential to clinical management, they represent only one dimension of a far more complex and human condition. Across the globe, millions of individuals living with diabetes quietly navigate a second, often under-acknowledged reality: the progressive disabilities and functional limitations that emerge from long-term complications. It is within this overlooked terrain that *Healing Beyond Blood Sugar: A Complete Guide to Managing Diabetes-Related Disabilities* finds its purpose.

This book was conceived from a shared realization among clinicians, researchers, rehabilitation specialists, and educators that diabetes care must evolve beyond glucose monitoring alone. Neuropathy, retinopathy, nephropathy, chronic wounds, cognitive decline, sexual dysfunction, psychological distress, and mobility impairments are not isolated sequelae—they are life-altering conditions that shape independence, dignity, and quality of life. Yet patients and caregivers frequently report fragmented guidance once such complications arise. Traditional diabetes manuals seldom address the lived experience of disability, rehabilitation pathways, or long-term functional adaptation. This volume seeks to bridge that gap.

Organized into fifteen thematically integrated chapters, the book adopts a multidisciplinary and person-centered approach. It begins by expanding the clinical narrative examining the full spectrum of diabetes complications and the mechanisms underlying progressive disability. Subsequent chapters focus on early recognition of functional decline, followed by in-depth explorations of major complication domains: nerve damage, non-healing wounds, visual impairment, renal dysfunction, cognitive and mental health challenges, and musculoskeletal limitations.

Importantly, this work does not remain confined to pathology. Equal emphasis is placed on restoration, adaptation, and empowerment. Dedicated sections explore therapeutic nutrition, rehabilitative exercise, infection control, digital health technologies, assistive devices, and strategies for sustaining independence in daily living. Psychosocial dimensions including stigma, intimacy, caregiver burden, and social participation are addressed with sensitivity, recognizing that healing is as much emotional and societal as it is biological.

A defining strength of this book lies in its interdisciplinary authorship. Contributors span clinical medicine, biomedical sciences, rehabilitation, public health, and allied health professions. This diversity enables a 360-degree perspective blending evidence-based medicine with practical care models, case insights, and culturally responsive strategies. The integration of real-world experiences alongside scientific discourse ensures that the text remains both academically grounded and pragmatically useful.

The intended readership is equally broad yet interconnected. Healthcare professionals will find guidance for multidisciplinary care planning and long-term complication management. Rehabilitation specialists and nurses may use the text to design function-focused interventions. Public health practitioners can draw on its disability-inclusive frameworks. Most importantly, individuals living with diabetes and those who care for them will discover actionable knowledge to preserve mobility, autonomy, and well-being.

As global diabetes prevalence continues to rise alongside aging populations and multimorbidity, the burden of diabetes-related disability will expand in parallel. Health systems must therefore transition from episodic metabolic care to continuous, life-course support models. By foregrounding function, independence, and quality of life, this book aligns with that emerging paradigm.

This volume is not merely a clinical reference; it is an advocacy effort. It calls for recognition of diabetes-related disabilities as a critical public health priority and urges the integration of rehabilitation, psychosocial care, and assistive innovation into mainstream diabetes management.

We extend our sincere appreciation to all chapter contributors, reviewers, and professional collaborators whose scholarship and dedication made this work possible. We are equally grateful to the patients and caregivers whose lived experiences continue to inform, challenge, and inspire advancements in compassionate chronic care.

It is our hope that *Healing Beyond Blood Sugar* will serve as a meaningful resource guiding readers not only in managing complications, but in restoring possibility, resilience, and dignity beyond diagnosis.

Durgapur, India — Krishnendu Adhikary
Pittsburgh, PA, USA — Pradipta Banerjee
Durgapur, India — Krishnendu Ganguly

Acknowledgements

The editors of the book *Healing Beyond Blood Sugar* would like to thank each person who helped with this book in some way, and express their appreciation for the successful completion of this book.

We would like to take this opportunity to sincerely acknowledge and thank the authors and researchers whose expertise and commitment in the area of metabolic health and integrative healing provided the depth and breadth of knowledge contained in this book. This is an immense contribution towards improving knowledge and providing support for those individuals seeking optimal health.

We would also like to personally thank the editorial and production teams at *Springer* for their guidance, input, and constant support during the entire production process for their role in ensuring that the manuscript was completed to an extremely high level of excellence.

Additionally, we would like to acknowledge our universities, research centers, and laboratories for providing encouragement and for providing an environment that enables collaborative intellectual effort and writing.

Last, but certainly not least, we would like to express our deep appreciation to our families, friends, colleagues, and supporters for their patience and continued support throughout the process of producing this book. Without their faith and belief that our work would be successful, we could never have completed the project.

Dr. Krishnendu Adhikary

Contents

1 **Beyond Glucose: Understanding the Full Scope of Diabetes Complications** ... 1
Riya Sarkar, Dibya Pal, Sudipta Kumar Das, Mounir Trabelsi, and Debidas Ghosh

2 **Silent Damage: Recognizing Early Signs of Diabetic Disabilities** ... 33
Shahnaz Alom, Farak Ali, and Bibhuti Bhusan Kakoti

3 **Nerve Under Siege: Managing Diabetic Neuropathy and Pain** ... 69
Shahnaz Alom, Farak Ali, Md. Abubakar, Samiksha Yogi, and Hans Raj Bhat

4 **Non-healing Foot Ulcers in Diabetes: Challenges in Wound Healing and Strategies For Limb Preservation** ... 127
Krishnendu Adhikary, Sumana Roy Chowdhury, Krishnendu Ganguly, and Sabina Yasmin

5 **Eyes on the Future: Preventing Vision Loss and Retinopathy** ... 155
Riya Sarkar, Rajat Kanti Ghosal, Koyel Banerjee, Pradipta Banerjee, and Rajkumar Maiti

6 **When the Kidney Fail: Navigating Nephropathy and Dialysis** ... 185
Arijit Mondal, Ishita Sil, Nirjhar Duttagupta, Suddhasattya Dey, and Sabina Yasmin

7 **The Body-Brain Connection: Cognitive Decline and Mental Health** ... 217
Abhishek Ambawatiya, Ritu Dahiya, Sarasa Meenakshi, Mamta Bishnoi, Sirajudheen Anwar, Krishna Murti, Md. Abubakar, and Nitesh Kumar

8 Movement Matters: Musculoskeletal Disorders and Mobility Solutions 249
Subhankari Prasad Chakraborty and Mokhtar Rejili

9 Breaking the Stigma: Addressing Sexual Dysfunction and Intimacy in Diabetes 265
Dibya Pal, Riya Sarkar, Sangita Das, Mounir Trabelsi, and Debidas Ghosh

10 Food as Medicine: Therapeutic Nutrition for Healing and Function in Diabetic Patients 295
Dipankar Saha, Surajit Majumder, Nirmalya Kumar Sinha, Pradipta Banerjee, and Rajkumar Maiti

11 Infection Control in Diabetes: The Role of Antibiotics and Antiseptics 319
Susmita Chakrabarty, Bangmayee Dash, Sunday Oyedemi, and Shasank Sekhar Swain

12 Digital Healing for Diabetic Disabilities: Tools for Monitoring, Mobility, and Self-Management 345
Krishnendu Adhikary, Krishnendu Ganguly, Monalisha Maity, Priyanka Mahata, and Oyindamola John Samson

13 Assisted Devices and Daily Life Adaptations in Diabetes 371
Ushasi Das, Dhiman Roy, Sudarshan Singh, and Sanchita Mandal

14 The Psychological and Social Impact of Diabetes on Patients' Lives 401
Md Abubakar, Ritu Dahiya, Kanika Goyal, Nitesh Kumar, Irshad Khan, Krishna Murti, and Amita Rai

15 Sustained Approaches to Prevent Recurrence and Support Ongoing Diabetes Health 419
Abhishek Ambawatiya, Kanika Goyal, Ritu Dahiya, Zeeshan Hyderi, Lalit Kumar Singh, Jayahari Srivastava, Nitesh Kumar, and Md Abubakar

Abbreviations

AC	Aadhesive capsulitis
ADL	Activities of daily living
AGEs	Advanced glycation end products
AI	Artificial Intelligence
CTS	Carpal Tunnel Syndrome
DM	Diabetes mellitus
IGF	Iinsulin-like growth factor
LJM	Limited Joint Mobility
MSDs	Musculoskeletal disorders
NSAIDs	Non-steroidal anti-inflammatory drugs
OA	Oosteoarthritis
RAGE	Receptor for advanced glycation end-products
ROM	Range of Motion
SfTf	Stenosing flexor tenosynovitis of the finger

Chapter 1
Beyond Glucose: Understanding the Full Scope of Diabetes Complications

Riya Sarkar, Dibya Pal, Sudipta Kumar Das, Mounir Trabelsi, and Debidas Ghosh

Abstract Diabetes mellitus is a multi-system disorder results of insufficient insulin production, impaired insulin action, or both and defined by consistently enhanced blood glucose level. While glycemic control remains central to diabetes management, the condition is a multifaceted systemic disease with far-reaching effects beyond blood glucose regulation. This chapter explores the broad spectrum of diabetes-related complications that demand a comprehensive and integrated management approach. Diabetes affects various body systems, causing complications such as musculoskeletal problems, heart and kidney diseases, nerve damage, cognitive issues, and mental health disorders. These issues mainly results from long-term elevated blood glucose and insulin resistance, which trigger inflammation, oxidative damage, and harm to blood vessels. The disease also weakens the immune system, increasing vulnerability to infections such as tuberculosis and urinary tract infections. Additionally, diabetes can lead to reproductive challenges including hormone imbalances, erectile dysfunction, menstrual problems, and reduced fertility. Recent advancements in therapeutic approaches and medical technologies including insulin pump

R. Sarkar
Department of Medical Lab Technology, Dr. B. C. Roy Academy of Professional Courses, Formerly Known As Dr. B. C. Roy Engineering College, Durgapur, India

D. Pal
Molecular Medicine, Department of Bio-Medical Laboratory Science and Management, Nutrigenomics and Public Health Research Laboratory, Vidyasagar University, Paschim Medinipur, India

S. K. Das
Department of Biotechnology, Brainware University, Barasat, India

M. Trabelsi
Laboratory of Histology and Cytogenetic, Molecular Biology and Biology of Reproduction, Faculty of Medicine Sousse, University of Sousse Tunisia, Sousse, Tunisia

D. Ghosh (✉)
Debra Thana Sahid Kshudiram Smriti Mahavidyalaya, NAAC 'A' Grade College, Paschim Medinipur, India
e-mail: debidasghosh999@gmail.com

K. Adhikary et al. (eds.), *Healing Beyond Blood Sugar*,
https://doi.org/10.1007/978-981-95-8946-3_1

therapy, renal glucose reuptake inhibitors targeting sodium-glucose co-transporter-2, incretin-based agents that activate glucagon-like peptide-1 receptors, and continuous glucose monitoring systems have significantly improved glycemic regulation and provided enhanced protection for cardiovascular and renal systems in individuals with diabetes. This chapter emphasizes the importance of a holistic approach to diabetes care, incorporating both traditional and emerging strategies to address its complex and systemic nature.

Keywords Hyperglycemia · Microvascular damage · Macrovascular complications · Diabetic retinopathy · Diabetic nephropathy · Peripheral neuropathy · Insulin resistance · SGLT2 inhibitors · GLP-1 agonists

1.1 Introduction

The diabetes epidemic continues to escalate in the world-wide, posing a major public health challenge. Despite strong evidence that lifestyle modification and medical therapy can delay or prevent the onset of type 2 diabetes (T2D), routine integration of these strategies into clinical practice has been limited, and health disparities persist. There are proven strategies to manage blood glucose, cholesterol levels, hypertension, and when implemented promptly, they can help lessen the risk of developing small-vessel damage, nerve disorders, and heart-related complications (Astrup & Finer, 2000). Yet, treatment gaps remain entrenched, especially among vulnerable populations. Diabetes, therefore, is not merely a biomedical issue but often reflects broader social adversity. This is evident in the disproportionate prevalence of T2D among socioeconomically disadvantaged groups (Tatulashvili et al., 2020). For instance, studies among Mexican Americans in Chicago revealed how diabetes is described as an "idiom of distress," linking physical symptoms to psychological and social suffering. These narratives highlight how the disease embodies both the consequences and manifestations of social distress (Brown et al., 2000).

Worldwide, diabetes is rising rapidly and has become a growing health concern. In Europe, both prevalence and incidence are rising sharply, influenced by demographic shifts in age, gender, race, and urbanization, but most significantly by rising obesity rates. From 1995 to 2025, diabetes prevalence in developed countries is projected to grow by 27%, with the absolute number of affected individuals expected to rise by more than 40% (Mauricio et al., 2023). This trend underscores the intertwined relationship between obesity and T2D. While not all obese individuals develop diabetes, excess body weight remains the strongest modifiable risk factor, amplified by sedentary lifestyles, high caloric intake, and diets rich in saturated fats. Genetic predisposition and early dietary exposures may further influence disease onset, though the interplay remains incompletely understood (Brown et al., 2000).

Crucially, intervention studies demonstrate that even modest weight reduction can substantially lower diabetes risk. For example, clinical trials revealed that obese individuals with altered glucose metabolism can avert T2D with as little as a 5%

loss in body weight (Herman & Schillinger, 2023). However, weight management remains underutilized in diabetes care. Many clinics focus primarily on glycemic and lipid control rather than targeting obesity, often relying on costly drug regimens to address complications. This approach neglects the root cause of the disease. To shift outcomes meaningfully, effective weight management strategies must begin at the earliest stages—ideally in individuals with prediabetes or abdominal obesity. The concept of "diabesity," which frames T2D as primarily a consequence of excess body fat, offers a clearer understanding of its etiology and underscores the urgency of preventive and weight-focused interventions (Kahn & Sievenpiper, 2014).

1.2 Pathophysiology of Diabetes Complications

1.2.1 Chronic Hyperglycemia and Systemic Effects

Oxidative Stress (OxS) and Reductive Stress: The body produces too many dangerous chemicals known as reactive oxygen species (ROS) and too much NADH when blood glucose stays persistently elevated over a long duration. This leads to a form of "reductive stress." This interferes with the regular operation of the mitochondria, the cell's energy-producing organelles. Consequently, the body begins to use alternative pathways for digesting glucose, such as the polyol pathway and the production of advanced glycation end products (AGEs). These alterations increase the strain on cells, resulting in tissue damage and endothelial dysfunction, which damage blood vessel linings (Yan, 2014).

AGEs: When glucose level is elevated, glucose can attach to proteins through a non-enzymatic process, giving rise to AGEs. Enhancement of AGEs in tissues over time, causing extracellular matrix proteins to cling to one another, stiffening blood vessels and delaying the body's natural healing process. Furthermore, AGEs attach to a particular receptor known as RAGE, which triggers inflammation and contributes to the problems frequently observed in diabetes (Twarda-Clapa et al., 2022).

Vascular Complications and Endothelial Dysfunction: Chronic hyperglycemia damages the endothelium by reducing nitric oxide (NO) and increasing vasoconstrictors, promoting clotting, and increasing susceptibility to heart disease and cerebrovascular events (Galicia-Garcia et al., 2020).

- **Microvascular problems**: When small blood vessels are damaged by persistent hyperglycemia, microvascular problems result.
- **Retinopathy**: Vision impairment and possible blindness are resulted from damage in retinal blood vessels.
- **Nephropathy**: Proteinuria and gradual renal failure are caused by glomerular injury.

- **Neuropathy**: Pain, tingling, loss of feeling, and autonomic dysfunction are all signs of nerve injury.
- **Inflammatory Pathways**:Chronic high blood glucose activates inflammatory pathways by promoting pro-inflammatory cytokine release and NF-κB signaling, driving both microvascular and macrovascular complications.

Insulin Resistance and Inflammation: Insulin resistance (IR) and chronic inflammation are key drivers of T2D and other metabolic disorders, with each condition reinforcing the other. Research showed that inflammation can initiate IR, while IR, in turn, worsens inflammation (Zhao et al., 2023).

- **Adipose Tissue Inflammation**: In obesity, adipose tissue becomes inflamed and recruits immune cells, particularly macrophages. These cells secrete inflammatory mediators which disrupt the insulin pathway, diminish cellular responsiveness to insulin, and eventually drive the development of insulin resistance.
- **Inflammatory Pathway Activation**:Key signaling pathways, including NF-κB and JNK, become overactivated during inflammation that resulted phosphorylation of insulin receptor substrates (IRS), disrupting downstream signaling and reducing insulin effectiveness (Yung & Giacca, 2020).
- **Insulin Sensitivity and Systemic Inflammation**: Insulin resistance is closely linked with elevated levels of inflammation in the body, which are frequently assessed by indicators such as high-sensitivity C-reactive protein (hsCRP). Indeed, long-term research indicates that increasing hsCRP levels frequently precede the onset of insulin resistance, focusing that inflammation may be a direct cause of it (Stanimirovic et al., 2022; Banjac et al., 2023).

The OxS Pathway and Glycation End Products: Oxidative stress happens when the body's protective antioxidant mechanisms are insufficient to counteract the damaging effects of ROS. Oxidative stress and AGEs play central roles in diabetes and cardiovascular disease (CVD), reinforcing inflammation and tissue damage. During AGE formation, ROS drive lipid peroxidation, generating highly Reactive Carbonyl Species (RCS) such as methylglyoxal. These RCS further react with biomolecules to form more AGEs, creating a feedback loop that amplifies oxidative damage (Jomova et al., 2023).

Diabetes and the Three Ps: The well-known warning indicators of elevated blood glucose are the traditional "3 Ps" of diabetes: polydipsia (excessive thirst), polyuria (frequent urine), and polyphagia (increased appetite). They frequently manifest prior to a formal diagnosis of diabetes, indicating the body's inability to manage consistently high blood glucose level (Best et al., 2021).

- **Three Ps pathophysiology**: Frequent urination, or polyuria, occurs when blood glucose level is too high for the kidneys to reabsorb. Because of its osmotic impact, the excess glucose pulls water with it as it overflows into the urine (glycosuria). Urine volume consequently rises noticeably. Dehydration results from this process, even though it aids in the body's removal of extra glucose. Persistent polyuria is a significant red flag that frequently indicates the need for diabetes assessment and testing.

- **Polydipsia (Excessive Thirst)**: Dehydration brought on by fluid loss from polyuria activates hypothalamic osmoreceptors, which heighten thirst. When people have an insatiable thirst, they frequently drink a lot of water to try to rehydrate.
- **Polyphagia (Increased Hunger)**: Insulin resistance or insufficiency hinders the uptake of glucose by cells, resulting in cellular energy deficits even in the face of elevated blood glucose level. As the body looks for other sources of energy, this sets out hunger signals. Ironically, patients may report feeling more hungry and consuming more food, but this does not help them lose weight or feel less exhausted.

1.2.2 Complications from Macrovascular Disease

Cardiovascular Disease: The risk of CVD is almost doubled by the T2D, making it equivalent to the chance of having experienced a previous heart attack. Furthermore, T2D patients had much greater rates of heart failure and reinfarction following acute coronary syndromes, leading to inferior outcomes. Peripheral arterial disorders, myocardial infarction, stroke, and atherosclerosis are all signs of macrovascular illness that affects the big arteries.

Through mitochondrial overactivity, NADPH oxidase, xanthine oxidase, and uncoupled eNOS, hyperglycemia causes an excess of ROS while impairing antioxidant defenses. Nitric oxide is reduced by ROS to create peroxynitrite ($ONOO^-$), which compromises vascular tone and endothelial cell viability. Atherosclerosis and CVD are caused by poor vasodilation, which is facilitated by chronic endothelial damage (Zhu & Jiang, 2023).

Cerebrovascular Disease: Compared to those without diabetes, the persons with diabetes have a significantly increased risk of stroke—roughly 2.3 times greater for ischemic stroke and 1.6 times higher for hemorrhagic stroke (Mosenzon et al., 2023). Approximately 25% of patients with hemorrhagic stroke and 33% of those with ischemic stroke also have diabetes.

Diabetes causes high blood glucose, aberrant cholesterol, insulin resistance, AGE accumulation, and chronic inflammation, all of which hasten the accumulation of plaque in arteries. The risk of arterial blockages and stroke is increased by these unstable plaques.

Elevated blood glucose level during a stroke exacerbate brain damage, resulting in bigger infarcts, increased swelling, a poor recovery, and a higher mortality risk. This occurs because hyperglycemia exacerbates brain damage and reduces blood flow by promoting inflammation, OxS, blood–brain barrier disruption, excitotoxicity, and metabolic imbalance.

Peripheral Arterial Disease (PAD): A significant vascular consequence of diabetes, PAD is characterized by atherosclerosis-induced leg artery constriction. High blood glucose, insulin resistance, aberrant lipid levels, endothelial dysfunction, and OxS—all of which promote inflammation and plaque accumulation, contribute to diabetes' acceleration of this process.

Critical limb ischemia, slow-healing wounds, intermittent claudication (leg pain when walking), and even amputation are significantly more frequent in diabetic individuals and PAD. Diagnosis is delayed because PAD is frequently overlooked until it is severe because diabetic neuropathy can conceal symptoms. To stop development and enhance results, early detection and thorough management are crucial. This includes healthy lifestyle modifications, antiplatelet therapy, blood pressure, cholesterol management, and appropriate blood glucose control (Signorelli et al., 2020).

Strategies for Risk Stratification and Prevention: When it comes to diabetes, risk stratification aids in identifying those who are most at risk for major vascular problems including heart disease, stroke, or PAD. This entails evaluating biomarkers (HbA1c, lipid profile, hs-CRP), imaging tests (assessment of coronary artery calcium, measurement of carotid artery wall thickness, and ankle-to-arm blood pressure comparison), and conventional risk factors (such as age, months or years of living with diabetes, hypertension, dyslipidemia, smoking, obesity, and family history) (Zakir et al., 2023).

Prevention calls for a multifaceted strategy:

- **Control of blood glucose**: Long-term risk is decreased by keeping blood glucose within a reasonable range, but excessively rigid goals can occasionally increase the risk of hypoglycemia and CVD (Stolar, 2010).
- **Blood pressure control**: Lowering blood pressure below 130/80 mmHg decreases the likelihood of developing heart disease and stroke.
- **Lipid control**: PCSK9 inhibitors, ezetimibe, and statins can reduce atherosclerosis events.
- **Antiplatelet therapy**: For high-risk patients, drugs such as clopidogrel or aspirin are recommended.
- **Lifestyle modifications**: The cornerstones of care continue to be a healthy diet, consistent exercise, giving up smoking, and controlling weight.
- Strong heart-protective benefits have also been demonstrated by more recent medications including SGLT2 inhibitors and GLP-1 receptor agonists, which reduce the incidence of major CVD events and death in high-risk individuals. Reducing the burden of macrovascular disease in diabetics requires early prevention that is customized for each patient.

1.3 Microvascular Complications

Diabetes causes chronic microvascular complications that, if undetected, can lead to irreversible disability. These arise from damage to small vessels (arterioles, capillaries, venules) and primarily affect the retina (retinopathy), kidneys (nephropathy), and nerves (neuropathy).

Diabetic retinopathy (DR): A very common, vision-threatening co-morbidity of diabetes that results in preventable blindness worldwide. Its silent progression damages retinal microvasculature, often without early symptoms, leading to irreversible vision loss if untreated (Koop et al., 2023).

Globally, about one-third of people with diabetes develop retinopathy, and a similar proportion progress to vision-threatening stages like PDR or diabetic macular edema (Lee et al. 2015). In resource-limited countries such as India, rising T2D among youth increases early-onset risk. The resulting vision loss has major socioeconomic impacts on productivity, quality of life, and healthcare costs.

- **Pathophysiology: From Hyperglycemia to Retinal Damage**

The retina is an exceptionally active tissue, requiring a continuous supply of oxygen and nutrient to sustain the complex processes involved in vision. The delicate balance of its microvascular network makes it highly vulnerable to fluctuations in blood glucose and vascular integrity.

1.3.1 Early Changes

- Loss of pericytes (specialized mural cells that support retinal capillaries) is one of the first pathological hallmarks.
- Thickening of the small vessel basement layer restricts the exchange of oxygen and nutrient.
- Microaneurysms, the earliest clinical sign, appear due to weakening of capillary walls.

1.3.2 Metabolic Pathways Driving Damage

- Polyol pathway activation → sorbitol accumulation → osmotic and OxS.
- AGEs → cross-linking of proteins, vascular stiffness, and activation of pro-inflammatory RAGE signaling.
- Protein kinase C (PKC) activation → vascular leakage, altered blood flow, and angiogenesis.
- OxS and mitochondrial dysfunction → endothelial apoptosis and capillary dropout.

- Inflammation and leukostasis → vascular occlusion and ischemia.

1.3.3 Retinal Hypoxia and VEGF Surge

As capillaries close, localized hypoxia develops. This stabilizes HIF-1α (hypoxia-inducible factor), which in turn stimulates VEGF (vascular endothelial growth factor) production. It is a double-edged sword, promotes neovascularization to restore oxygen delivery, but the new vessels are fragile and leaky, leading to hemorrhage and macular edema.

1.3.4 Phases of DR

Non-PDR:

- Early or Mild Stage: Presence of tiny outpouchings of retinal capillaries (microaneurysms) and a few small intraretinalhemorrhages.
- Moderate Stage: Development of soft exudates (cotton-wool spots caused by nerve fiber ischemia), irregularities in retinal veins, and abnormal capillary networks within the retina.
- Severe Stage (defined by the "4–2-1 rule"): Extensive hemorrhages affecting all four retinal quadrants, venous changes seen in at least two quadrants, and intraretinal vascular anomalies visible in one or more quadrants.

PDR:

- Marked by the emergence of fragile newly formed blood vessels on the optic disc or other areas of the retina.
- Carries a significant risk of bleeding into the vitreous and can result in retinal detachment due to fibrous tissue pulling on the retina (Sun & Aiello, 2022).

1.3.5 Diabetic Retinal Macular Edema

This can occur at any stage. Leakage from damaged capillaries leads to retinal thickening at the macula, which governs central vision. This is the predominant reason for vision loss associated with diabetes.

1.3.6 Molecular and Cellular Insights

- **Pericyte apoptosis**: AGEs, OxS, and sorbitol cause pericyte loss, weakening capillaries.
- **Endothelial dysfunction**: Disrupted tight junctions impair the blood–retinal barrier.
- **Basement membrane thickening**: Excess matrix reduces vessel flexibility.
- **Inflammation**: Cytokines (TNF-α, IL-6, ICAM-1) promote leukocyte adhesion and capillary blockage.
- **Neurodegeneration**: Glutamate toxicity and loss of neurotrophic support lead to early visual deficits.
- **Epigenetic changes**: "Metabolic memory" sustains damage despite glucose control, highlighting need for early treatment.

1.3.7 Diagnosis and Screening

- Retinal evaluation using ophthalmoscopy or retinal imaging techniques to visualize vascular and structural changes.
- Optical coherence tomography plays a vital role in identifying fluid accumulation and swelling in the macula. Fluorescein angiography: Identifies areas of ischemia and leakage.
- Screening is recommended annually for people with diabetes, though frequency may vary based on risk and disease duration.

1.3.8 Management Approaches

The management of diabetic retinopathy involves a dual approach that addresses both systemic factors and local ocular disease. Systemic care focuses on maintaining strict glycemic control with a target HbA1c below 7%, along with effective regulation of blood pressure and lipid levels, complemented by lifestyle measures such as balanced nutrition, regular exercises, and smoking cessation to reduce overall risk. At the ocular level, laser photocoagulation remains a key therapy, helping to prevent vision loss by sealing abnormal or leaking vessels and lowering vascular endothelial growth factor (VEGF) activity. In addition, intravitreal therapies are widely used, with anti-VEGF agents including ranibizumab, aflibercept, and bevacizumab regarded as the standard first-choice therapy in diabetic macular edema and proliferative disease, while corticosteroid injections may be considered for patients with inadequate therapeutic response to anti-VEGF agents. In advanced stages where serious sequelae like vitreous hemorrhage or tractional retinal detachment occur, surgical intervention through vitrectomy is often required to preserve vision.

1.3.9 Diabetes Nephropathy

Diabetic nephropathy is a long-term small vessel complication of diabetes, marked by gradual deterioration of kidney function that manifests as albumin in the urine, a steady fall in renal filtration capacity (GFR), and in advanced stages, progression to end-stage renal disease (ESRD) (Samsu, 2021). It is one of the most common causes of chronic kidney disease (CKD) worldwide and accounts for nearly 40–50% of all ESRD cases requiring dialysis or transplantation (Hoogaveen, 2022).

Both major types of diabetes mellitus can lead to DN, although the timeline and clinical patterns may vary. Typically, DN develops after at least 5–10 years of poorly controlled diabetes, but earlier onset is possible in genetically susceptible individuals.

1.3.10 Pathophysiology

The pathophysiology of nephropathy caused by diabetes is multifactorial, involving a complex interplay of metabolic, hemodynamic, oxidative, and inflammatory mechanisms that ultimately produce structural damage in the kidney. Sustained high blood glucose levels promote chemical attachment of glucose to circulating and tissue proteins, resulting in the generation of AGEs. These compounds gradually build up within the glomerular basement layer and the mesangial region, leading to structural thickening, reduced flexibility, and impaired filtration efficiency of the kidney (Jha et al., 2024). The AGEs also bind to specific receptors on endothelial and mesangial cells, triggering OxS as well as NF-κBsignaling, and subsequent cytokine release. Simultaneously, hyperglycemia activates the renin–angiotensin–aldosterone system (RAAS), and angiotensin II increases intraglomerular pressure by dilating the afferent arteriole and constricting the efferent arteriole, resulting in glomerular hypertension and progressive scarring. In addition, excess glucose metabolism through the polyol and hexosamine cascades, PKC activation, and mitochondrial overload generates ROS, which damage endothelial cells, podocytes, and mesangial cells. Inflammatory mediators like TNF-α, IL-6, and especially TGF-β further amplify injury by stimulating extracellular matrix deposition and fibrogenesis. Collectively, these processes manifest as characteristic structural lesions: diffuse and nodular mesangial expansion, basement membrane expansion glomerulus, podocyte loss leading to persistent proteinuria, formation of Kimmelstiel–Wilson nodules that are pathognomonic of nodular glomerulosclerosis, and progressive tubulointerstitial fibrosis that marks advanced disease and correlates strongly with renal functional decline (Dwivedi & Sikarwar, 2024).

1.3.11 Stages of Diabetic Nephropathy (Mogensen's Classification)

Stage 1—Hyperfiltration (Early Diabetes)

- GFR is increased.
- Kidneys are enlarged.
- No clinical proteinuria.

Stage 2—Silent Stage (Structural Changes)

- GBM thickening, mesangial expansion start.
- Normal GFR.
- Albumin excretion still normal.

Stage 3—Incipient Nephropathy (Microalbuminuria)

- Urinary albumin excretion: 30–300 mg/day (microalbuminuria).
- GFR begins to decline.
- This stage is reversible with tight control.

Stage 4—Overt Nephropathy (Macroalbuminuria/Proteinuria)

- Albumin excretion > 300 mg/day.
- Hypertension appears.
- GFR declines progressively.

Stage 5—ESRD

- Severe proteinuria, progressive renal dysfunction or failure.
- GFR less than 15 mL/min/1.73 m^2.
- The individual necessitates dialysis or renal transplantation (Mongensen et al., 1983).

Clinical Features

- **Early stages**: Asymptomatic, detected only by urine tests.
- **Microalbuminuria**: First clinical marker, often accompanied by rising blood pressure.
- **Overt stage**: Frothy urine (due to proteinuria), edema, hypertension, declining renal function.
- **Advanced stage**: Symptoms of CKD—fatigue, anorexia, nausea, pruritus, anemia, electrolyte disturbances.

1.3.12 Diagnostic Criteria

The diagnosis of diabetic nephropathy relies on both laboratory and imaging markers that help in identifying the stage and severity of kidney involvement. One of the most important parameters is urinary albumin excretion, where values below 30 mg/day are considered normal, 30–300 mg/day indicate microalbuminuria, and levels above 300 mg/day are classified as macroalbuminuria, reflecting more advanced disease. Instead of a 24-h urine collection, the spot urine albumin-to-creatinine ratio (ACR) is now preferred for convenience and reliability, with an ACR greater than 30 mg/g regarded as abnormal and suggestive of early renal damage. Serum creatinine levels, along with estimated glomerular filtration rate (eGFR), are routinely assessed to monitor renal function and detect progressive decline. In addition, complementary tests such as lipid profile, glycatedhemoglobin (HbA1c), and regular blood pressure monitoring are essential, as dyslipidemia, poor glycemic control, and hypertension significantly influence the progression of nephropathy. Imaging techniques, particularly renal ultrasonography, may reveal enlarged kidneys during the initial phase of the disease, while shrunken or contracted kidneys are often seen in advanced stages. Although not frequently required in routine practice, kidney biopsy can provide a definitive histological diagnosis, typically demonstrating nodular glomerulosclerosis with the characteristic Kimmelstiel–Wilson nodules, which remain the hallmark lesion of diabetic nephropathy.

1.3.13 Management of Diabetic Nephropathy

The management of said condition focuses on a combination of preventive strategies, lifestyle interventions, and pharmacological measures aimed at slowing disease progression and preserving renal function. Prevention focuses on maintaining tight blood glucose regulation. Lifestyle modifications form the cornerstone of early management, including adherence to a low-salt diet with sodium intake restricted to not more than 2000 mg per day, maintaining an adequate but not excessive protein intake of around 0.8 g/kg/day in CKD patients, weight regulation, smoking cessation, and regular physical activity. Managing blood pressure is key in therapy, and this is usually accomplished with drugs that block the renin–angiotensin system, such as ACE inhibitors (e.g., enalapril) or ARBs (e.g., losartan). These medications are preferred since they both reduce hypertension and protect kidney function by lowering protein excretion, aiming for control below 130/80 mmHg. Glycemic management can be achieved using insulin or oral antidiabetic agents, while SGLT2 inhibitors such as empagliflozin have demonstrated additional renal protective effects. Dyslipidemia is addressed with statin therapy to reduce cardiovascular risk, which is commonly elevated in diabetes patients with kidney disease. In addition to established treatments, several novel therapies are under investigation, including endothelin receptor antagonists, agents targeting TGF-β, and bardoxolone methyl, an antioxidant with potential renoprotective benefits.

1.3.14 Diabetic Neuropathy

It is the most frequent chronic complications of diabetes mellitus, distinguished by cumulative injury to the peripheral and autonomic nervous system due to long-standing hyperglycemia and associated metabolic and vascular insults. It manifests clinically as sensory loss, neuropathic pain, motor weakness, and dysfunction of autonomic systems (cardiovascular, gastrointestinal, genitourinary, sudomotor). It not only impairs quality of life but also increases morbidity through complications such as diabetic foot ulcers, infections, orthostatic hypotension, and silent myocardial ischemia.

1.3.15 Pathophysiology

The pathogenesis of diabetic neuropathy is intricate and multi-mechanistic, driven by chronic hyperglycemia that disrupts both neuronal metabolism and vascular support systems, ultimately leading to axonal degeneration and demyelination. Metabolic disturbances are pivotal, as elevated glucose concentrations enhance flux through the polyol pathway, with aldose reductase mediating its reduction to sorbitol and subsequently fructose. This process induces osmotic imbalance, depletes myo-inositol, and disrupts Na^+/K^+-ATPase function, ultimately leading to reduced nerve conduction velocity. Simultaneously, AGEs accumulate in nerve and vascular proteins, stiffening microvasculature and inducing ischemia, while the hexosamine pathway alters gene transcription critical for nerve integrity and PKC activation disrupts blood flow regulation. These metabolic derangements intensifyOxS, as hyperglycemia drives mitochondrial overproduction of ROS, which damage neuronal DNA, lipids, and proteins, while also impairing Schwann cell function and remyelination. In parallel, diabetic microangiopathy affecting the vasa nervorum causes endothelial dysfunction and basement membrane thickening, compromising oxygen and nutrient delivery and producing chronic ischemia. Inflammatory pathways, mediated by cytokines with NF-κB activation, perpetuate low-grade inflammation that further injures axons and Schwann cells. Together, these processes translate into characteristic structural changes, including distal "dying-back" axonal degeneration, segmental demyelination and remyelination, selective loss of small unmyelinatedfibers responsible for pain and temperature sensation, and fibrotic thickening of endoneurial and perineurial vessels—lesions that underpin the progressive sensory, motor, and autonomic deficits observed in diabetic neuropathy (Yang et al., 2025).

1.3.16 Types of Diabetic Neuropathy

Peripheral Neuropathy

Symmetrical distal polyneuropathy or peripheral neuropathy, which involves sensory, motor, and small autonomic fibers. It typically presents in a characteristic "glove and stocking" distribution of sensory loss, starting distally in the feet and hands and progressing proximally. Patients often complain of burning, tingling, stabbing pain, and numbness, with gradual impairment of vibration, temperature, and pain perception. As the condition advances, motor involvement can cause weakness and muscle wasting, while autonomic fiber damage may contribute to dry skin and altered sweating. The major complications of this form include foot ulceration, recurrent infections, and elevated likelihood of lower-extremity amputation, making early recognition and preventive care essential.

Autonomic Neuropathy

Autonomic neuropathy in diabetes affects involuntary body functions and involves multiple organs, causing a broad range of symptoms. In the cardiovascular system, it causes resting tachycardia, reduced exercise tolerance, orthostatic hypotension, and silent myocardial ischemia. The gastrointestinal system may present with gastroparesis, bloating, constipation, or diarrhea due to impaired motility. Genitourinary involvement includes bladder dysfunction with either retention or incontinence, erectile dysfunction (ED) in men, and retrograde ejaculation. Sudomotor dysfunction results in abnormal sweating patterns such as anhidrosis, which predisposes to dry, cracked skin and secondary infections, or compensatory hyperhidrosis. Additionally, pupillary abnormalities such as impaired light reflex and poor adaptation to dim light further reflect autonomic nerve damage, underscoring the systemic nature and significant morbidity associated with diabetic autonomic neuropathy.

Focal and Multifocal Neuropathies

In diabetes it is typically present as sudden, localized nerve damage affecting either cranial, peripheral, or spinal nerve roots. Cranial mononeuropathies, most often involving the oculomotor nerve, can cause acute diplopia, ptosis, and eye movement abnormalities. Peripheral mononeuropathies may affect individual nerves such as the median, ulnar, or peroneal nerves, leading to focal weakness, sensory loss, or entrapment-like syndromes such as carpal tunnel syndrome. In contrast, radiculopathies or radiculoplexopathies present with painful, asymmetric involvement of lumbar, thoracic, or cervical roots and plexuses, producing radiating aches, fatigue, and loss of muscle mass in the affected region. Although often self-limiting, these forms of diabetic neuropathy can cause significant discomfort and functional impairment.

Proximal Neuropathy (Diabetic Amyotrophy)

Proximal neuropathy, often referred as diabetic amyotrophy, usually affects aged individuals having T2D and is distinguished by the sudden onset of severe pain, weakness, and wasting in the thigh or hip muscles. Patients often struggle with functional activities such as climbing stairs, standing from a seated position, or walking due to marked proximal muscle weakness. The condition is typically asymmetric at onset but may become bilateral over time, and although it can partially improve, recovery is often slow and incomplete, leaving residual disability.

Diagnosis

- Clinical examination: monofilament test (10 g), tuning fork (128 Hz) for vibration, pinprick, temperature sensation, ankle reflex.
- Nerve conduction studies: detect demyelination and axonal loss.
- Quantitative sensory testing (QST): assesses vibration and thermal thresholds.
- Autonomic function tests: heart rate variability, orthostatic BP measurements, gastric emptying studies.

1.3.17 Management of Diabetic Neuropathy

Diabetic neuropathy requires an integrated management plan that combines preventive, supportive, and pharmacological strategies to alleviate symptoms and reduce complications. Preventive and supportive measures primarily involve maintaining optimal glycemic control with a target HbA1c level of less than 7%, alongside lifestyle changes such as smoking cessation, regular workouts, and adherence to a balanced diet to minimize further nerve damage. Patient education and routine foot care are essential components, as they help prevent ulceration, infections, and amputations, which are common consequences of peripheral neuropathy. Pharmacological interventions are directed toward symptom relief, particularly neuropathic pain, where first-line agents include duloxetine, pregabalin, and gabapentin, while tricyclic antidepressants like amitriptyline, as well as topical agents such as capsaicin cream or lidocaine patches, may be considered as alternatives in resistant cases. Management of autonomic dysfunction depends on the affected system; midodrine or fludrocortisone is used for orthostatic hypotension, prokinetic agents such as metoclopramide or domperidone are prescribed for diabetic gastroparesis, and phosphodiesterase-5 inhibitors like sildenafil are recommended for ED. In addition to these established therapies, adjunctive agents including alpha-lipoic acid, antioxidants, and experimental therapies such as nerve growth factors are being explored for their potential neuroprotective effects. Together, these measures aim not only to relieve symptoms but also to preserve quality of life and limit long-term disability in individuals with diabetic neuropathy.

1.4 Emerging and Less Common Complications

While the classical co-morbidities of diabetes like retinopathy, nephropathy, and neuropathy are well recognized, a number of less common yet clinically important conditions are increasingly being documented. These complications often remain underdiagnosed, yet they significantly impair quality of life and can aggravate the disease burden.

1.4.1 Diabetic Dermopathy and Skin Involvement

Skin manifestations are among the earliest external signs of diabetes. Diabetic dermopathy, characterized by hyperpigmented, atrophic, brownish patches, typically over the shins, is the most frequent. The exact cause is not fully understood, but microangiopathy and impaired dermal blood flow are believed to play central roles. Other dermatological presentations include necrobiosislipoidica, acanthosisnigricans, bullous diabeticorum, and recurrent fungal or bacterial infections. Chronic hyperglycemia disrupts collagen turnover, reduces skin elasticity, and alters immune defense, making the skin more prone to delayed wound healing and recurrent ulceration (Naik & Farrukh, 2020).

1.4.2 Musculoskeletal Complications

Diabetes is associated with a spectrum of musculoskeletal disorders that interfere with mobility and daily activities. Limited joint mobility (diabetic cheiroarthropathy) manifests as stiffness of the small joints of the hands, impairing the ability to fully extend the fingers. This is linked to non-enzymatic glycation of collagen, leading to thickening of periarticular connective tissues. Other musculoskeletal problems include frozen shoulder (adhesive capsulitis), Dupuytren's contracture, carpal tunnel syndrome, and diffuse idiopathic skeletal hyperostosis. These disorders arise from a combination of AGE deposition, microvascular ischemia, and low-grade inflammation, resulting in chronic pain, reduced flexibility, and functional disability (Hordon et al., 2017).

1.4.3 Cognitive Decline and Alzheimer's Disease

Growing evidence indicates that diabetes significantly increases the risk of cognitive impairment, dementia, and Alzheimer's disease (Mesarič et al., 2023). Chronic hyperglycemia, insulin resistance, and vascular injury compromise cerebral perfusion and neuronal survival. Impaired insulin signaling in the brain reduces synaptic plasticity, while AGE accumulation and OxSpromote β-amyloid deposition and tau hyperphosphorylation—hallmarks of Alzheimer's pathology. Several studies refer to this overlap as "type 3 diabetes," highlighting the central role of insulin dysfunction in neurodegeneration. Clinically, patients may present with memory deficits, impaired executive function, and reduced attention span, ultimately progressing to dementia in severe cases (Janoutova et al., 2022).

1.4.4 Depression and Mental Health Disorders

Diabetes and mental health are interconnected through a bidirectional relationship. Individuals with diabetes have nearly double the likelihood of onset of depression compared to the common people. The daily demands of glucose monitoring, dietary restrictions, fear of complications, and social stigma contribute to psychological distress. On the biological side, chronic inflammation, altered hypothalamic–pituitary–adrenal (HPA) axis activity, and neurotransmitter imbalances have been implicated. Anxiety disorders, diabetes-related distress, and reduced quality of life are also common. Untreated depression not only worsens glycemic control through poor adherence to therapy but also accelerates the onset of vascular complications, creating a vicious cycle.

1.4.5 Increased Risk of Infections and Immune Dysregulation

Diabetes is a state of immunological vulnerability, where both innate and adaptive immunity are compromised. Neutrophil chemotaxis and phagocytosis are impaired, while glycation of immunoglobulins reduces their effectiveness. Persistent hyperglycemia also provides a nutrient-rich environment that supports microbial growth. Consequently, patients are more susceptible to urinary tract infections, skin and soft tissue infections, candidiasis, pneumonia, and tuberculosis. In severe cases, diabetes predisposes to life-threatening infections such as mucormycosis and diabetic foot sepsis. Moreover, low-grade systemic inflammation in diabetes alters cytokine signaling, leading to a chronic state of immune dysregulation (Erener, 2020).

1.4.6 Diabetes and Reproductive Disorders

Reproductive health is increasingly recognized as being affected by diabetes in both sexes. In men, diabetes contributes to ED, retrograde ejaculation, reduced testosterone levels, and altered spermatogenesis, largely due to OxS and microvascular damage (Zhang et al., 2025). In women, hyperglycemia is linked to menstrual irregularities, polycystic ovarian syndrome (PCOS), reduced fertility, and adverse pregnancy outcomes such as miscarriage, preeclampsia, and congenital anomalies. At the molecular level, insulin resistance and chronic inflammation disrupt gonadal steroidogenesis and impair gamete quality. Gestational diabetes, in particular, poses dual risks, affecting maternal health and predisposing offspring to future metabolic disorders (Basmatzou & Hatziveis, 2016; Pal et al., 2024).

1.5 Impact of Diabetes on Organ Systems

Persistent hyperglycemia, coupled with insulin resistance and lipid abnormalities, exerts a profound impact on multiple organ systems through mechanisms such asOxS, AGE formation, low-grade inflammation, and endothelial dysfunction. Among the organs affected, the liver, gastrointestinal tract, urologic system, and kidneys are particularly vulnerable.

1.5.1 Hepatic Complications: NAFLD and NASH

Diabetes is strongly linked with non-alcoholic fatty liver disease (NAFLD) and its progressive form, non-alcoholic steatohepatitis (NASH). Clinically, patients often remain asymptomatic in the early phase, though hepatic steatosis may be detected by imaging or liver enzymes. Over time, this may leads to fibrosis, cirrhosis, or hepatocellular carcinoma.

Impaired insulin signaling via the IRS-1/PI3K/AKT pathway reduces suppression of gluconeogenesis while paradoxically stimulating lipogenesis through sustained activation of SREBP-1c. This imbalance promotes hepatic triglyceride deposition. Additionally, increased free fatty acid (FFA) flux from insulin-resistant adipose tissue produces toxic intermediates such as diacylglycerol and ceramides, which further inhibit insulin signaling through PKCε activation.

Mitochondrial overload by excess FFAs generates ROS, driving lipid peroxidation, mitochondrial dysfunction, and hepatocyte apoptosis. Injured hepatocytes release DAMPs that activate Kupffer cells and stellate cells via TLR4–NF-κBsignaling, leading to cytokine release (TNF-α, IL-1β) and fibrogenic activity through TGF-β. These cascades promote inflammation and fibrosis, marking the transition from simple steatosis to NASH (Garg et al., 2020).

1.5.2 Gastrointestinal Dysfunction: Gastroparesis and Enteropathy

Gastroparesis

Clinically, diabetic gastroparesis manifests as nausea, vomiting, bloating, early satiety, and unpredictable gastric emptying, typically in long-standing diabetes.

Molecularly, hyperglycemia reduces neuronal NO synthase (nNOS) expression in enteric inhibitory neurons, diminishing NO-mediated relaxation of gastric smooth muscle. In addition, AGEs accumulate within gastric neural and muscular tissues, altering protein function and promoting OxS. Loss of interstitial cells of Cajal (ICC), the gastric pacemakers, linked to impaired c-Kit signaling, further compromises gastric motility. The net effect is delayed gastric emptying.

Enteropathy

Diabetic enteropathy results in diarrhea, constipation, or alternating bowel patterns. Damage to the myenteric plexus by ROS and AGEs disrupts coordinated peristalsis. Hyperglycemia alters aquaporin channel expression in colonic epithelial cells, disturbing fluid balance. NF-κB–driven cytokine release promotes mucosal inflammation, while small intestinal bacterial overgrowth (SIBO) secondary to dysmotility aggravates diarrhea and malabsorption (Maisey, 2016).

1.5.3 Urologic Complications: Bladder Dysfunction and Erectile Dysfunction

Bladder Dysfunction

Clinically, diabetic cystopathy manifests as reduced bladder sensation, incomplete emptying, urinary retention, or overflow incontinence, particularly in older patients with long-standing diabetes. Autonomic neuropathy impairs parasympathetic cholinergic input to the detrusor muscle. Hyperglycemia drives the polyol pathway, leading to sorbitol accumulation and NADPH depletion, which reduces antioxidant defenses and impairs Na^+/K^+-ATPase activity, slowing nerve conduction. Moreover, AGE-mediated collagen cross-linking stiffens the bladder wall, reducing compliance. Microangiopathy compromises vesical perfusion, while OxS diminishes smooth muscle contractility, producing the characteristic atonic bladder.

Erectile Dysfunction (ED)

Erectile dysfunction is a frequent complication in diabetic men, presenting as difficulty in achieving or maintaining erections. Hyperglycemia reduces eNOS activity, limiting NO bioavailability essential for penile vasodilation. Excess ROS scavenges

NO to form peroxynitrite, further impairing vascular relaxation. AGE–RAGE interactions activate NF-κB, leading to upregulation of vasoconstrictors such as endothelin-1. Neuropathy reduces cavernous nerve signaling, while mitochondrial stress in cavernosal smooth muscle promotes apoptosis, reducing tissue compliance. The convergence of these mechanisms underlies the increased prevalence of erectile dysfunction observed in diabetic men (Blair et al., 2022).

Renal Dysfunction

End-stage renal disease is frequently attributed to diabetic nephropathy, which remains a predominant cause worldwide. Clinically, the disease develops in stages, beginning with microalbuminuria and progressing to proteinuria, reduced glomerular filtration rate, and eventual kidney failure. Sustained hyperglycemia promotes non-enzymatic glycation of glomerular basement membrane proteins, producing AGEs that thicken and stiffen the barrier. Binding of AGEs to RAGE receptors on mesangial and endothelial cells activates NF-κB, inducing ROS generation and pro-inflammatory cytokines. Concurrently, excess glucose flux through the polyol pathway depletes NADPH, impairing glutathione regeneration and amplifying oxidative injury. Activation of the hexosamine pathway alters gene expression of profibrotic mediators, while PKC-β signaling increases vascular permeability and mesangial expansion. Hemodynamic changes mediated by the RAAS elevate intraglomerular pressure, accelerating podocyte injury and apoptosis. Angiotensin II further induces TGF-β, stimulating extracellular matrix accumulation and glomerulosclerosis. Progressive tubulointerstitial fibrosis eventually culminates in chronic kidney disease.

1.6 Complications in Specific Populations

Diabetes mellitus affects diverse groups of patients across the lifespan, and the pattern, onset, and severity of complications vary according to diabetes type, age, physiological state, and comorbid conditions. Understanding these population-specific differences is critical for early intervention, targeted screening, and long-term management.

1.6.1 Type 1 vs Type 2 Diabetes: Complication Profiles

Although both types of diabetes predispose to microvascular and macrovascular complications, the timeline and pathophysiology differ considerably:

Type 1 Diabetes

Typically presents in childhood or adolescence with an abrupt onset of insulin deficiency. The duration of hyperglycemia is the key determinant of complications, and risk increases significantly after 10–15 years of disease. Microvascular complications (retinopathy, nephropathy, neuropathy) are more common earlier in life. Cardiovascular disease occurs, but usually later, influenced by the cumulative burden of chronic hyperglycemia and other risk factors. Intensive insulin therapy reduces risk, but poor adherence in youth can accelerate complication onset.

Type 2 Diabetes

The condition may remain silent for several years, and by the time it is detected, many individuals already show early complications. Macrovascular complications (coronary artery disease, stroke-related cerebrovascular disease, peripheral arterial disease) are disproportionately higher due to accompanying insulin resistance, dyslipidemia, obesity, and hypertension. Microvascular complications also occur, but tend to coexist with CVD. The "legacy effect" or "metabolic memory" plays a strong role; early poor glycemic control leads to long-term damage even if glucose control improves later. Thus, type 1 diabetes favors microvascular dominance, while T2D carries a dual burden of microvascular and macrovascular disease, often compounded by comorbidities.

Paediatric and Adolescent Patients

Children and adolescents with diabetes represent a unique challenge due to the interplay of growth, hormonal changes, and psychosocial factors.

Early-Onset Complications

- Although rare in childhood, early signs of microalbuminuria, retinopathy, and neuropathy may appear within 5–10 years of poorly controlled type 1 diabetes.
- Pubertal hormonal surges (growth hormone, sex steroids, cortisol) induce physiological insulin resistance, worsening glycemic control and increasing complication risk (Luk et al., 2025).

Neurocognitive Impact

- Chronic hyperglycemia and recurrent hypoglycemia in young children can impair brain development, memory, and academic performance (Ducat et al., 2015).
- Functional imaging studies reveal structural changes in the hippocampus and prefrontal cortex.

Psychosocial Burden

- Adolescents may experience diabetes burnout, anxiety, and depression, leading to poor treatment adherence.
- Risk-taking behaviors (skipping insulin, erratic diet) exacerbate complications.

Growth and Pubertal Issues

- Poorly controlled diabetes can delay puberty, impair linear growth, and in girls, cause menstrual irregularities.

Overall, in pediatric populations, complications are less advanced than in adults, but metabolic instability during adolescence accelerates long-term risks if glycemic control is not maintained.

1.6.2 Elderly and Frail Populations

With increasing life expectancy, more individuals are living into old age with diabetes, often accompanied by comorbidities such as hypertension, atherosclerosis, renal insufficiency, and dementia. The complication profile in the elderly is distinct:

Cardiovascular Dominance

- Macrovascular complications, particularly myocardial infarction, stroke, and peripheral artery disease, are leading causes of morbidity and mortality.
- Autonomic neuropathy contributes to silent ischemia, making CVD harder to detect.

Cognitive Decline and Dementia

- Diabetes is strongly linked with vascular dementia and Alzheimer's disease.
- Mechanisms include chronic cerebral hypoperfusion, cerebral insulin resistance, and enhanced β-amyloid accumulation.

Frailty and Sarcopenia

- Chronic inflammation and insulin resistance lead to muscle wasting, reduced strength, and impaired mobility.
- Neuropathy and retinopathy further increase risk of falls, fractures, and disability.

Polypharmacy and Hypoglycemia Risk

- Elderly patients often take multiple medications, raising risk of drug-drug interactions.
- Impaired renal clearance and reduced counter-regulatory responses increase the risk of severe hypoglycemia, which can precipitate arrhythmias, falls, and cognitive decline.

Thus, in elderly populations, the emphasis is on functional independence, quality of life, and cardiovascular protection rather than aggressive glycemic targets that increase hypoglycemia risk.

1.6.3 Gestational Diabetes: Postpartum Risk and Long-Term Impact

Although it occurs temporarily during pregnancy, its effects persist well beyond childbirth.

Maternal Complications

- Women with GDM are at increased risk of hypertensive disorders, preeclampsia, cesarean delivery, and future T2D (Khanna & Kumaresan, 2024).
- A significant proportion, roughly 30–50%, of women with GDM develop T2D within a decade following childbirth.
- Long-term cardiovascular risk (coronary artery disease, metabolic syndrome) is elevated due to persistent insulin resistance.

Fetal and Neonatal Complications

- In utero exposure to hyperglycemia leads to macrosomia, neonatal hypoglycemia, respiratory distress, and congenital anomalies.
- Offspring are at higher risk of obesity, impaired glucose tolerance, and early-onset T2D due to epigenetic programming and altered intrauterine environment.
- Maternal hyperglycemia triggers fetalhyperinsulinemia, leading to excess fat deposition and altered growth. Epigenetic changes in genes regulating insulin signaling, adipogenesis, and appetite contribute to long-term transgenerational effects.

Hence, gestational diabetes is not only a short-term pregnancy complication but also a harbinger of chronic metabolic disease for both mother and child, warranting long-term surveillance and preventive Scare.

1.7 Multimorbidity and Diabetes

1.7.1 Interaction with Hypertension, Dyslipidemia, and Obesity

Multimorbidity, which is defined as having two or more chronic diseases at the same time, is thought to affect up to 95% of primary care patients 65 and older. In Southeast Asia, 90 million people suffer from diabetes, and the disease's consequences cause one death every five seconds worldwide. The most prevalent chronic conditions among people with multiple comorbidities are strock, cancer, heart disease and COPD. According to the census, the number of senior citizens in Nepal increased from 1.5 million (6.5%) in 2001 to 2.5 million (8.1%) in 2011 (Bonaventura et al., 2019).

Most people are affected with multimorbidity, but little is known about the patterns of multimorbidity. Our objectives were to identify the various multimorbidity patterns for the individuals with the disease and investigate in contributing factors which are connected with these patterns. In addition to having the largest senior population and the world's fastest aging rate, China is also seeing an affinity with the treatment and burden for the type 2 disorder. Over a million and the number goes higher are currently associated with hypertension (HTN), a major risk of kidney, brain, and heart damage of premature death worldwide (Lee et al., 2020).

For normal cases, clinicians guide more on the relationship between the factors causing risk and its result of treatment. Risk factors such as obesity and hypertension are the main reason for high blood pressure. The time these two conditions coexist, they may work together to increase the likelihood of developing hypertension and its related problems. By learning the complex relationships that exist between obesity, dyslipidemia, and hypertension is essential for effectively preventing and treating these interconnected health issues.

1.7.2 Polypharmacy and Drug-Complication Interactions

Polypharmacy poses a serious health risk to older adults. Comorbidities, inadequate prospective data, and differences in classification have complicated research on polypharmacy, which is linked to several geriatric conditions, including frailty, falls, and cognitive decline. In this study, we discuss many definitions of polypharmacy and emphasize the need for a common definition for future studies. We carefully examine deprescribing and pharmaceutical prescription reduction strategies as a means of reducing the likely negative effects of polypharmacy. In the future, we examine how high-throughput technologies and new analytics, like multiomics profiling, can support polypharmacy research and the development of novel approaches to risk stratification in the precision medicine era.

The aging of the people is known to be the major issue of the twenty-first century. A complex human, social, cultural, economic, and health issue is population aging. Older people are more susceptible to a variety of illnesses due to the physiological changes brought on by aging. Many illnesses are more common in the elderly, which increases drug use and, in turn, the risk of drug-related problems. Deteriorating cardiac efficiency, reduced hepatic and renal function, hemodynamic abnormalities, drug interactions, and over-the-counter medication use all exacerbate the clinical state of the elderly (Palmer et al., 2021).

Health status, health centre characteristics, and geriatric demography are the three main categories into which many risk factors associated with PPH can be separated. According to a number of studies, PPH is more common in older adults. The spread of over-the-counter medications, poor treatment use, medication errors, loose drug usage restrictions, and an increase in incorrect drug prescriptions could all contribute to this. In addition to age, other factors that may influence PPH status include sex, occupation, and medication compliance (Palmer et al., 2021). Elderly polypharmacy is depended upon several factors, such as age, gender, level of education, frequency of medical visits, and the types and severity of illnesses.

People with diabetes and coronary artery disease may take up to six or nine prescriptions, as aging and other illnesses increase the need for medication consumption. Because the patient may be prescribed new medications, hospitalization and multiple medical visits increase the risk of polypharmacy. Patients' poor comprehension and literacy are among the most common causes of polypharmacy. Additionally, in most of the studies, women were more polypharmacy-prone than men (Chowdury & Chakraborty, 2017).

1.7.3 Socioeconomic and Racial Disparities in Complication Burden

Type 2 diabetes prevalence has come with a socioeconomic gradient in high-income countries. However, there is no evidence that socioeconomic status has an impact on diabetic complications. Thus, the goal of this systematic review was to gather data on the risk of challenges for T2D patients according to socioeconomic status. Every nation in the world is seeing an increase in the prevalence of diabetes.

Similarly, the prevalence of diabetes appears to disproportionately affect women in countries like Norway and England, where it has increased with higher attainment. In contrast, trends in educational disparities are generally more favorable in Spain and the United States. In normal case the initiatives, no reduction in health disparities has been observed. Socioeconomic status influences follow-up in T2D patients on several levels, including patient capacities, neighborhood or community support, health-related behaviors, treatment process, and access to care, just like it does for many chronic illnesses. Actually, people with diabetes who are from lower socioeconomic backgrounds are more likely to report problems getting care, such as limited access, high costs, poor health, and increased disability. Healthcare coverage, access, and utilization are still impacted by socioeconomic disparities (Chowdhury & Chakraborty, 2017).

1.8 Prevention, Early Detection, and Management

1.8.1 Role of Glycemic Control and Beyond

A major medical and financial burden on the global health care system, diabetes is a chronic ailment that is getting more and more frequent. Younger age groups have witnessed the highest increase in the prevalence of diabetes. One CVD and other long-term effects of diabetes are substantially to blame for the morbidity and expense. A therapy approach that treats multiple physiological problems, such as hyperglycaemia, dyslipidemia, and hypertension, is important to avert severe consequences. The majority of patients are not fulfilling their treatment objectives, even though two significant intervention trials and a number of observational studies have revealed the advantages of intensive diabetes control. In order to accomplish targets for glucose control, lipids, blood pressure, and other disease indicators, clinicians must actively monitor diabetic patients and alter medication as necessary. However, this issue is growing more and more challenging in today's healthcare (Chowdury & Chakraborty, 2017).

1.8.2 Lifestyle and Behavioral Interventions

Most fatalities worldwide are caused by chronic noncommunicable diseases, which are caused by a confluence of environmental, behavioral, physiological, and genetic variables. Unhealthy food consumption, physical inactivity, alcohol use, and tobacco use are the most prevalent behavioral risk factors for diabetes. Regular exercise, healthy eating, quitting smoking, getting enough sleep, managing weight, and reducing stress are all lifestyle choices that significantly improve health outcomes and manage diabetes (Norris et al., 2004).

1.8.3 Pharmacologic Strategies

The frequency of diabetes has steadily climbed in recent years, also its currently estimated that 415 million populations have the disease. Diabetes raises the risk of both acute and chronic problems, which can significantly affect quality of life and cost the healthcare system money in terms of hospital stays and outpatient visits. Glycaemic controls the risk of microvascular problems of diabetic patients, but it has no effect on macrovascular complications or mortality, as evidenced by the higher residual cardiovascular (CV) risk in diabetics than in non-diabetics. These results support the idea that improving glycaemic management by itself might not be a viable way to lower the death rate from CV disease (Hosseini et al., 2018).

The CV safety and effectiveness of SGLT-2 inhibitors and GLP-1 receptor agonists (GLP-1 RAs) are covered in this narrative review. All GLP-1 RAs significantly decreased HbA1c levels from baseline, however, they were quite variable, varying between 0.3% and 1.9% across the various trials. Despite this, they cannot be directly compared because of variations in research design and participant populations.

1.8.4 Multidisciplinary Care Models

It has long been recognized that managing calls for the multidisciplinary team approach that incorporates behavioral modifications, exercise, nutrition, and insulin administration. A multidisciplinary team, however, is often unavailable to patients with T2D. Most people with T2D in developing countries are treated by a general practitioner in a primary level health center, or by an internist or family practice physician. Understanding the perceived barriers, attitudes, enablers, and benefits of a multidisciplinary team approach in T2D therapy can help healthcare professionals adopt multidisciplinary care for T2D (Tabar et al., 2022; Scherger, 2025).

1.9 Future Directions and Research Frontiers

1.9.1 Artificial Intelligence and Predictive Analytics

There are several reasons why artificial intelligence (AI) has been used in the medical industry. "A field of science and engineering concerned with the computational understanding of what is commonly called intelligent behavior with creation of artifacts that exhibit such behavior" is the backbone of AI. Healthcare could be enhanced by AI algorithms, particularly when combined with modern technologies. AI abilities are required for these objectives since modern medicine has had difficulty collecting, analyzing, and applying vast amounts of data to the solution of intricate clinical problems (Tabar et al., 2022).

Both of these tasks—classification, where the outcome variable is a class, and prediction, where the outcome variable is a value—can be accomplished with machine learning techniques. In the treatment of diabetes mellitus, these activities can also be used for screening, diagnosis, treatment recommendations, complication management, and illness likelihood prediction. A variety of machine learning techniques, each with unique features, have been used to achieve these clinical goals. Machine learning is a subset of artificial intelligence. In particular, they encompass of wide range of methods.

1.9.2 Personalized Medicine in Diabetes Care

Personalized medicine, which involves identifying unique patient data and then suggesting a treatment tailored to that patient's needs, is a new concept in the treatment of disease (Raciti et al., 2014). Personalized medicine is a technique for determining diseases.

Not every diabetic patient with the same age, duration of the disease, body mass index, and When one treatment is used for a particular disease or therapy, the response rate is 100%; when another treatment is used, the response rate is 0%; and for other patients, the effectiveness rate is 100%. The problem is that doctors cannot predict which treatment will work best for any given patient, so the treatment that is most commonly selected for the greatest number of patients—even if it doesn't work for some patients—is usually selected first.

1.10 Conclusion

Diabetes is more than high blood glucose—it is a systemic condition that affects nearly every organ through OxS, inflammation, endothelial dysfunction, and glycation. These processes drive both microvascular and macrovascular complications, from retinopathy and neuropathy to heart disease, stroke, and PAD, as well as less recognized issues like reproductive problems and poor wound healing.

Looking "beyond glucose" highlights the need for early detection and multifactorial strategies that combine glycemic control with blood pressure and lipid management, lifestyle changes, and cardioprotective therapies. This broader approach not only improves clinical care but also empowers patients to protect their long-term health and quality of life.

References

Astrup, A., & Finer, N. (2000). Redefining type 2 diabetes: "Diabesity" or "obesity dependent diabetes mellitus"? *Obesity Reviews, 1*(2), 57–59.

Banjac, J., Vuković, V., Pustahija, T., Bohucki, N., Berić, D. K., Medić, S., Petrović, V., & Ristić, M. (2023). Epidemiological characteristics of COVID-19 during seven consecutive epidemiological waves (2020–2022) in the North Bačka District, Serbia. *Viruses, 15*(11), 2221.

Basmatzou, T., & Hatziveis, K. (2016). Diabetes mellitus and influences on human fertility. *International Journal of Caring Sciences, 9*(1), 371–379.

Best, J. T., Buttriss, G., & Hines, A. (2021). *Pathophysiology, physical assessment, and pharmacology: Advanced integrative clinical concepts*. FA Davis.

Blair, Y., Wessells, H., Pop-Busui, R., Ang, L., & Sarma, A. V. (2022). Urologic complications in diabetes. *Journal of Diabetes and Its Complications, 36*(10), Article 108288.

Bonaventura, A., Carbone, S., Dixon, D. L., Abbate, A., & Montecucco, F. (2019). Pharmacologic strategies to reduce cardiovascular disease in type 2 diabetes mellitus: Focus on SGLT-2 inhibitors and GLP-1 receptor agonists. *Journal of Internal Medicine, 286*(1), 16–31.

Brown, C. D., Higgins, M., Donato, K. A., Rohde, F. C., Garrison, R., Obarzanek, E., Ernst, N. D., & Horan, M. (2000). Body mass index and the prevalence of hypertension and dyslipidemia. *Obesity Research, 8*(9), 605–619.

Chowdhury, S., & Chakraborty, P. (2017). Universal health coverage—There is more to it than meets the eye. *Journal of Family Medicine and Primary Care, 6*(2), 169–170.

Ducat, L., Rubenstein, A., Philipson, L. H., & Anderson, B. J. (2015). A review of the mental health issues of diabetes conference. *Diabetes Care, 38*(2), 333–338.

Dwivedi, S., & Sikarwar, M. S. (2024). Diabetic nephropathy: Pathogenesis, mechanisms, and therapeutic strategies. *Hormone and Metabolic Research, 56*(11), 713–725.
Erener, S. (2020). Diabetes, infection risk and COVID-19. *Molecular Metabolism, 39*, Article 101044.
Galicia-Garcia, U., Benito-Vicente, A., Jebari, S., Larrea-Sebal, A., Siddiqi, H., Uribe, K. B., Ostolaza, H., & Martin, C. (2020). Pathophysiology of type 2 diabetes mellitus. *International Journal of Molecular Sciences, 21*(17), 6275.
Garg, K., Brackett, S., Hirsch, I. B., & Garg, S. K. (2020). NAFLD/NASH and diabetes. *Diabetes Technology and Therapeutics, 22*(S1),:S-174.
Herman, W. H., & Schillinger, D. (2023). Rethinking diabetes in the United States. *Frontiers in Endocrinology, 14*, 1–6.
Hoogeveen, E. K. (2022). The epidemiology of diabetic kidney disease. *Kidney Dialysis, 2*(3), 433–442.
Hordon, L., Consultant, L. H., & Rheumatologist, M. (2017). Limited joint mobility and other musculoskeletal problems in diabetes. *Journal of Diabetes Nursing, 20*, 166–170.
Hosseini, S., Zabihi, A., JafarianAmiri, S., & Bijani, A. (2018). Polypharmacy among the elderly. *Journal of Midlife Health, 9*(2), 97–103.
Janoutová, J., Machaczka, O., Zatloukalová, A., & Janout, V. (2022). Is Alzheimer's disease a type 3 diabetes? A review. *Central European Journal of Public Health, 30*(3), 139–143.
Jha, R., Lopez-Trevino, S., Kankanamalage, H. R., & Jha, J. C. (2024). Diabetes and renal complications: An overview on pathophysiology, biomarkers and therapeutic interventions. *Biomedicines, 12*(5), 1098.
Jomova, K., Raptova, R., Alomar, S. Y., Alwasel, S. H., Nepovimova, E., Kuca, K., & Valko, M. (2023). Reactive oxygen species, toxicity, oxidative stress, and antioxidants: Chronic diseases and aging. *Archives of Toxicology, 97*(10), 2499–2574.
Kahn, R., & Sievenpiper, J. L. (2014). Dietary sugar and body weight: Have we reached a crisis in the epidemic of obesity and diabetes? *Diabetes Care, 37*(4), 957–962.
Khanna, P., & Kumaresan, M. (2024). Comprehensive care for women with diabetes mellitus and gynecological complications. In *Management of diabetic complications: calling for a team approach* (pp. 193–204). Springer.
Koop, M. A., Sleijser-Koehorst, M. L., Hooijmans, C. R., Tdlohreg, P. Q., Lutke Schipholt, I. J., Scholten-Peeters, G. G., Coppieters, M. W. (2023). The potential protective effects of pre-injury exercise on neuroimmune responses following experimentally-induced traumatic neuropathy: A systematic review with meta-analysis. *Frontiers in Immunology, 14*, 1215566.
Lee, R., Wong, T. Y., & Sabanayagam, C. (2015). Epidemiology of diabetic retinopathy, diabetic macular edema and related vision loss. *Eye and Vision, 2*, 17.
Lee, W., Lloyd, J. T., Giuriceo, K., Day, T., Shrank, W., & Rajkumar, R. (2020). Systematic review and meta-analysis of patient race/ethnicity, socioeconomics, and quality for adult type 2 diabetes. *Health Services Research, 55*(5), 741–772.
Luk, A., Wild, S. H., Jones, S., Anjana, R. M., Hivert, M. F., McCaffrey, J., Gregg, E. W., & Misra, S. (2025). Early-onset type 2 diabetes: The next major diabetes transition. *Lancet, 405*(10325), 1234–1245.
Maisey, A. (2016). A practical approach to gastrointestinal complications of diabetes. *Diabetes Therapy, 7*(3), 379–386.
Mauricio, D., Gratacòs, M., & Franch-Nadal, J. (2023). Diabetic microvascular disease in non-classical beds: The hidden impact beyond the retina, the kidney, and the peripheral nerves. *Cardiovascular Diabetology, 22*(1), 21.
Mesarič, K. K, Pajek, J., Zakrajšek, B. L., Bogataj, Š, & Kodrič, J. (2023). Cognitive behavioral therapy for lifestyle changes in patients with obesity and type 2 diabetes: A systematic review and meta-analysis. *Science and Reports, 13*(1), 40141.
Mogensen, C. E., Christensen, C. K., & Vittinghus, E. (1983). The stages in diabetic renal disease: With emphasis on the stage of incipient diabetic nephropathy. *Diabetes, 32*(Suppl 2), 64–78.

Mosenzon, O., Cheng, A. Y., Rabinstein, A. A., & Sacco, S. (2023). Diabetes and stroke: What are the connections? *Journal of Stroke, 25*(1), 26–38.
Naik, P. P., & Farrukh, S. N. (2020). Clinical significance of diabetic dermatopathy. *Diabetes, Metabolic Syndrome and Obesity, 13*, 4823–4827.
Norris, S. L., Zhang, X., Avenell, A., Gregg, E., Bowman, B., Serdula, M., Brown, T. J., Schmid, C. H., & Lau, J. (2004). Long-term effectiveness of lifestyle and behavioral weight loss interventions in adults with type 2 diabetes: A meta-analysis. *American Journal of Medicine, 117*(10), 762–774.
Pal, D., Mitra, D., Hazra, S., & Ghosh, D. (2024). Protective effect of Aloe vera (L.) on diabetes-induced oxidative stress linked spermiological co-morbidity in human and rat: an in-vitro analysis. *Reproductive Sciences, 31*(9), 2685–2699.
Palmer, S. C., Tendal, B., Mustafa, R. A., Vandvik, P. O., Li, S., Hao, Q., et al. (2021). Sodium-glucose cotransporter protein-2 inhibitors and glucagon-like peptide-1 receptor agonists for type 2 diabetes: Systematic review and network meta-analysis of randomised controlled trials. *BMJ, 372*, Article n457.
Raciti, G. A., Nigro, C., Longo, M., Parrillo, L., Miele, C., Formisano, P., & Beguinot, F. (2014). Personalized medicine and type 2 diabetes: Lesson from epigenetics. *Epigenomics, 6*(2), 229–238.
Samsu, N. (2021). Diabetic nephropathy: Challenges in pathogenesis, diagnosis, and treatment. *BioMed Research International, 2021*, 1497449.
Scherger, J. E. (2025). Rethinking diabetes: What science reveals about diet, insulin, and successful treatments. *Family Medicine, 57*(2), 138–139.
Signorelli, S. S., Marino, E., Scuto, S., & Di Raimondo, D. (2020). Pathophysiology of peripheral arterial disease: A review on oxidative disorders. *International Journal of Molecular Sciences, 21*(12), 4393.
Stanimirovic, J., Radovanovic, J., Banjac, K., Obradovic, M., Essack, M., Zafirovic, S., Gluvic, Z., Gojobori, T., & Isenovic, E. R. (2022). Role of C-reactive protein in diabetic inflammation. *Mediators of Inflammation, 2022*, 3706508.
Stolar, M. (2010). Glycemic control and complications in type 2 diabetes mellitus. *American Journal of Medicine, 123*(3 Suppl), S3-11.
Sun, J. K., & Aiello, L. P. (2022). *Nonproliferative and proliferative diabetic retinopathy. In: Albert and Jakobiec's principles and practice of ophthalmology* (pp. 2955–2993). Springer.
Tabar, Z. F., Moghadamnia, A. R., Bijani, A., Hosseini, S. R., & Moghadamnia, A. A. (2022). Drug interactions in elderly (Amirkola Health and Ageing Project). *Caspian Journal of Internal Medicine, 13*(4), 786–794.
Tatulashvili, S., Fagherazzi, G., Dow, C., Cohen, R., Fosse, S., & Bihan, H. (2020). Socioeconomic inequalities and type 2 diabetes complications: A systematic review. *Diabetes & Metabolism, 46*(2), 89–99.
Twarda-Clapa, A., Olczak, A., Białkowska, A. M., & Koziołkiewicz, M. (2022). Advanced glycation end-products (AGEs): Formation, chemistry, classification, receptors, and diseases related to AGEs. *Cells, 11*(8), 1312.
Yan, L. J. (2014). Pathogenesis of chronic hyperglycemia: From reductive stress to oxidative stress. *Journal of Diabetes Research, 2014*, Article 137919.
Yang, Y., Zhao, B., Wang, Y., Lan, H., Liu, X., Hu, Y., & Cao, P. (2025). Diabetic neuropathy: Cutting-edge research and future directions. *Signal Transduction and Targeted Therapy, 10*(1), 132.
Yung, J. H., & Giacca, A. (2020). Role of c-Jun N-terminal kinase (JNK) in obesity and type 2 diabetes. *Cells, 9*(3), 706.
Zakir, M., Ahuja, N., Surksha, M. A., Sachdev, R., Kalariya, Y., Nasir, M., et al. (2023). Cardiovascular complications of diabetes: From microvascular to macrovascular pathways. *Cureus, 15*(9), Article e44028.
Zhang, W., Tong, L., Jin, B., & Sun, D. (2025). Diabetic testicular dysfunction and spermatogenesis impairment: Mechanisms and therapeutic prospects. *Frontiers in Endocrinology, 16*, 1653975.

Zhao, X., An, X., Yang, C., Sun, W., Ji, H., & Lian, F. (2023). The crucial role and mechanism of insulin resistance in metabolic disease. *Frontiers in Endocrinology, 14*, 1149239.
Zhu, J., & Jiang, Y. (2023). The role of diabetes in the pathophysiology and prognosis of ischemic stroke. *Frontiers in Endocrinology, 14*, 1207537.

Chapter 2
Silent Damage: Recognizing Early Signs of Diabetic Disabilities

Shahnaz Alom, Farak Ali, and Bibhuti Bhusan Kakoti

Abstract The metabolic disease known as diabetes mellitus often has long-term effects that gradually harm several organ systems. Neuropathy, retinopathy, nephropathy, and vascular dysfunction are diabetic impairments that may begin to develop before the onset of any clinical symptoms. Patients face a significant risk from this "silent damage" since early warning signs are often unrecognized, which may result in irreversible effects and a worse quality of life. The purpose of this chapter is to highlight the significance of detecting subtle deficiencies in sensory function, vision, ankle reflexes, microalbuminuria, and intermittent claudication as early warning symptoms of diabetes. To detect issues early and halt or postpone the progression of damage, routine testing such as nerve conduction studies, retinal exams, and renal function tests may be beneficial. Encouraging people to monitor their symptoms and report them early also requires training them how to do so and collaborating with other medical providers. Globally, and especially in middle- and low-income nations, the number of diabetics is on the rise. As a result, we need to shift our focus from reactive treatment to proactive detection and prevention of diabetes. To halt the gradual but constant development of diabetic complications, it is crucial to be aware of, consistently assess, and use integrated healthcare strategies. Lower impairment, better patient outcomes, and fewer long-term socioeconomic repercussions of diabetes-related disabilities may result from recognizing and addressing early signs.

Keywords Diabetic complications · Early detection · Microvascular damage · Neuropathy · Preventive care

---

Shahnaz Alom and Farak Ali—These authors are equally contributed.

S. Alom · F. Ali
Girijananda Chowdhury Institute of Pharmaceutical Science, Girijananda Chowdhury University-Tezpur Campus, Tezpur, India

S. Alom · F. Ali · B. B. Kakoti (✉)
Department of Pharmaceutical Sciences, Faculty of Science and Engineering, Dibrugarh University, Dibrugarh, India
e-mail: bibhutikakoti@dibru.ac.in

K. Adhikary et al. (eds.), *Healing Beyond Blood Sugar*,
https://doi.org/10.1007/978-981-95-8946-3_2

2.1 Introduction

Diabetes has become a global threat to humanity as it poses serious risks to people's health. A study released by the International Diabetes Federation estimates that the number of people with diabetes, defined as those between the ages of 20 and 79, would rise from 537 million in 2021 to 783 million in 2045. Diabetes has been steadily increasing in incidence due to urbanization, destructive lifestyles, and an ageing population (Luzi et al., 2024). Several complications arise from diabetes, including cardiopathy, nephropathy, stroke, neuropathy, heart attack, peripheral arterial disease, nerve damage, and blood vessel and heart problems, which may have a devastating impact on people's health, finances, and social lives (Aljuraiban et al., 2024; Janssen et al., 2020; Maniruzzaman et al., 2020). According to the World Health Organization (WHO), diabetes is among the leading causes of long-term disability and death. Half of all people with diabetes go undiagnosed until their symptoms are already severe, according to estimates. The long-term effects of diabetes make it easy for many individuals to ignore the disease's warning signs. People sometimes fail to recognize the seriousness of hyperglycaemia as a health condition, as its consequences take time to manifest, unlike other illnesses (Alom et al., 2025; Jaber & James, 2023; Ramachandran, 2014).

Severe hypoglycaemia and ketoacidosis are examples of the more extreme consequences of diabetes. In contrast, retinopathy, nephropathy, neuropathy, and cardiovascular disease are examples of the chronic, debilitating complications that impact many organ systems. The lack of universally accepted diagnostic criteria makes it difficult to provide reliable estimates of the frequency of diabetes complications. But one or more of these diabetic complications will affect most people with diabetes. Severe blindness, kidney failure, dialysis or a transplant, heart attacks, strokes, and amputations are some of the end-stage effects of diabetes. The silent damage is used to describe the slow but steady worsening of diabetes-related problems, which are not immediately apparent and often go undetected until the disease has progressed significantly (Yau et al., 2012). With the proper "life-long" diabetes treatment and a healthy lifestyle, many of these potentially fatal or crippling complications may be avoided. The risk of complications is associated with the length of time that diabetes has been present and with the level of glycaemic control that has been maintained. Glycated haemoglobin, or HbA1c, is a standard method for monitoring this control over a period of two to three months. Complication risk varies across people with diabetes; some people have difficulties while having lower HbA1c readings, which seem to indicate adequate glycaemic control (Nickerson & Dutta, 2012).

Neuropathy, retinopathy, and nephropathy are three microvascular consequences of diabetes (Nathan, 1993; Tommerdahl et al., 2022). Based on data from cohort studies, the estimated prevalence of diabetic neuropathy among adults and youths ranges from 2.4% to 75.1% (Jaiswal et al., 2017; Janghorbani et al., 2006). Following the exclusion of other possible causes, diabetic neuropathy is defined as a clinically diverse set of neurological illnesses characterized by impairment of the peripheral nervous system (Pop-Busui et al., 2017). Diffuse neuropathy, mononeuropathy, radiculopathy, and other neuropathies are the four forms of diabetic peripheral neuropathy, and their patterns of neurological impairments determine whether the condition is painful or not (Jensen et al., 2021; Ziegler et al., 2021). The most prevalent kind of diabetic peripheral neuropathy is diffuse neuropathy, which affects 75% to 90% of patients (Ziegler et al., 2021). Ulceration, infection, deformity, and amputation are lower-extremity problems that may develop in patients with diabetic peripheral neuropathy. Improving the diagnosis and treatment of diabetic peripheral neuropathy may be achieved through research that elucidates the complex pathogenetic pathways involved (Nkonge et al., 2023). The key to avoiding long-term disability is early detection of diabetes-related problems. Silently developing over the years, symptoms of diabetes often manifest only after the disease has progressed, causing microvascular and macrovascular damage. In addition to lowering the risk of consequences, early detection enables more targeted treatment approaches, such as improved blood pressure management, better cholesterol regulation, or tighter glycemic control. Lifestyle therapies, such as changing one's diet, increasing physical activity, and quitting smoking, have a far better chance of success if started before severe organ damage occurs (Yang et al., 2024).

2.2 Diabetes and Its Complications

The pathophysiology of diabetes complications is very complicated, and the disease itself is relatively standard. Hyperglycaemia causes oxidative stress and an overabundance of advanced glycation end products (AGEs) in the early phases of type 2 diabetes (T2DM) (Domingueti et al., 2016). Damage to respiratory chain components due to oxidative stress may be exacerbated as the illness progresses through protein glycation and mitochondrial DNA (mtDNA) damage (Bhatti et al., 2022). Once inflammation is promoted by metabolic imbalance, senescence, or cell death may occur as a result of glycation product binding to receptors (Phoenix et al., 2022; Takahashi et al., 2022). The structural alterations may cause a variety of vascular problems associated with diabetes (Teodoro et al., 2019). Numerous new hypoglycemic medications, including SGLT2i, DPP4i, and GLP-1RAs, have been used in clinical practice to enhance these processes. Nevertheless, several diabetes-related problems may still arise from early hyperglycaemia (El Mouhayyar et al., 2020). An underlying driver is necessary for the development of metabolic memory, also known as hyperglycemic memory. The persistence of cellular alterations and features shows the organism's ability to recover from a previous metabolic state. This process may be crucial in the development of diabetes and its long-term problems (Reddy et al., 2015).

Inflammation, immunology, oxidative stress, mitochondrial dysfunction, ageing, and other forms of cell death are the fundamental processes that underlie the consequences of diabetes (Galicia-Garcia et al., 2020). The formation of a heritable phenotype may be influenced by epigenetic processes such as noncoding RNAs (ncRNAs), DNA methylation, and histone modifications, all of which do not alter

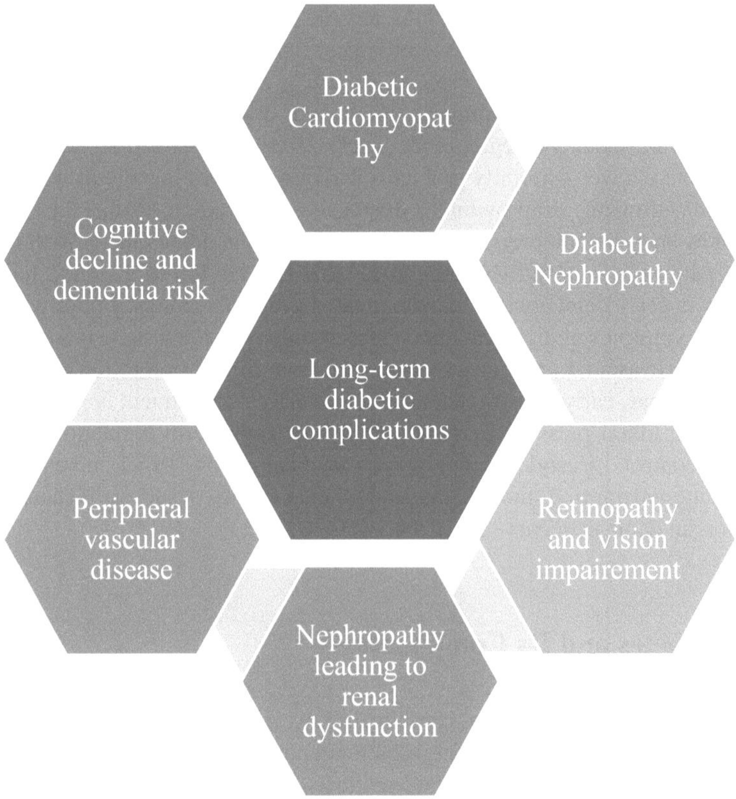

Fig. 2.1 Schematic representation of long-term diabetic complications

DNA sequences (Goldberg et al., 2007). Epigenetic alterations regulate physiological and pathological mechanisms linked to metabolic memory and diabetes consequences (Chen & Natarajan, 2022). As a result, the many changes that contribute to hyperglycaemic memory are the primary emphasis of this section. The various long-term diabetic complications are illustrated in Fig. 2.1 and are discussed.

2.2.1 Diabetic Cardiomyopathy

Diabetic cardiovascular diseases, such as arterial vasculopathy and diabetic cardiomyopathy (DCM), are the leading causes of mortality for diabetic individuals (Chib et al., 2025; Fang et al., 2004). Myocardial cells and vascular endothelial cells are targeted by inflammation, immune cell regulation, and the formation of cytotoxic free radicals, all of which are enhanced by elevated blood glucose (Johnson et al., 2022; Xie et al., 2022). These glucose-induced pathways cause injured cells to release more toxic irritants, which in turn encourage the transformation of non-cardiomyocyte cells into cardiomyocytes (Cheng et al., 2023). Then, adipokines and adhesion molecules, such as adiponectin, activate these fibroblasts to migrate and aggregate, which worsens the damage to the heart and blood vessels (El-Mesallamy et al., 2011). Clinical trial data, however, show that metabolic complications put diabetic cardiovascular disease patients at risk even with rigorous blood glucose management.

DM may lead to DCM, a cardiovascular condition that affects the heart's structure and function. This happens even when no other recognized cardiac risk factors, such as hypertension or coronary atherosclerotic heart disease, are present (Jia et al., 2018). Pathophysiology of DCM is characterized by cardiac autonomic neuropathy, aberrant calcium transients in cardiomyocytes, myocardial interstitial fibrosis, and metabolic dysfunction in cardiomyocytes, according to previous research (Marwick et al., 2018; Palomer et al., 2018). In rats that were diabetic after being induced with streptozotocin (STZ), fibronectin mRNA expression remained elevated even after blood glucose levels normalized (Roy et al., 1990). Metabolic memory may be involved in the onset and progression of DCM, given the disease's causes and symptoms (Zhan et al., 2023). Endothelial dysfunction, atherosclerosis, and other vascular problems may result from elevated blood glucose, which can affect the microvascular and macrovascular systems (Li et al., 2023a, 2023b). According to Jax, the perivascular fibrosis of microvessels and other structural changes may affect upstream arteries, causing endothelial dysfunction and, eventually, atherosclerosis (Jax, 2010). When it comes to controlling how blood vessels function, the endothelium, the largest organ in the body, plays a crucial role. Dysfunction of the endothelial cells is exacerbated by oxidative stress, inflammation, and aberrant mitochondrial metabolism brought on by chronic hyperglycaemia (Wang et al., 2022). An essential role in the development of diabetic coronary artery vasculopathy and DCM is related to inflammation, oxidative stress, and fibrosis. There are likely intricate regulatory mechanisms at work in these processes, as evidenced by the involvement of non-coding RNAs (ncRNAs) such as miR-320 and miR-27a. The functions of other microRNAs, including miR-423, miR-499, and miR-199a, in metabolic memory and the diabetic heart remain unclear, however, and need more research (Yang et al., 2024).

2.2.2 Diabetic Neuropathy

Diabetic neuropathy (DN) is the most common long-term effect of diabetes mellitus, which may manifest in a variety of ways, including problems with the eyes, feet, and cardiovascular system. Both central and peripheral nerves may be affected by the condition. One-third of individuals with peripheral neuropathy have distant peripheral neuropathy (DPN) (Hanewinckel et al., 2016). About 20% of people with diabetes may get neuropathic pain as a result of DPN; the most frequent symptom is numbness and loss of feeling in the distal symmetrical limbs. Acute pain, electrical pain, pruritus, hyperalgesia, and evoked pain are the most common forms of pain

(Sloan et al., 2018). Not only that, but when hyperglycaemia and metabolic problems work together, they weaken the immune system and its ability to fight off infections. This hidden wound has the potential to grow into a major amputation (Jeffcoate et al., 2018). Distal symmetric polyneuropathy, characterized by a stocking-glove distribution, is a hallmark of DN. Affected nerve conduction velocity and altered sensory function are symptoms of this condition, which may be caused by axonal atrophy, damage to unmyelinated neurons, myelin loss in myelinated nerves, and other reasons (Elafros et al., 2022; Li et al., 2023a, 2023b). Cell autophagy and cell metabolism, two of SCs' regulatory activities, are impaired or rendered dysfunctional due to hyperglycaemia, hyperlipidaemia, and the many signalling pathways involved (Liu et al., 2020; Sloan et al., 2021). Sensory neurons, particularly those in the dorsal root ganglia, are more susceptible to damage than motor neurons in the absence of glial cells such as Schwann cells (SCs) (Cernea & Raz, 2021). Sensory neurons are particularly vulnerable, both structurally and functionally. Unlike other types of neurons, sensory neurons rarely develop myelinated nerve fibres (Feldman et al., 2017). Neuronal demyelination and neuronal damage, the primary causes of peripheral neuropathy, are caused by oxidative stress, metabolic abnormalities, microangiopathy, and other variables caused by diabetes. This destruction of standard nerve cell structure and function occurs through specific signal transduction pathways (Modrak et al., 2020). DPN develops as a consequence of many metabolic processes, including oxidative stress and mitochondrial malfunction. In most cases, DPN develops as a result of one of four conditions: hyperglycaemia, dyslipidaemia, insulin resistance, or microvascular disease. The PKC, polyol, AGE, hexosamine, and PARP pathways are most often activated in response to hyperglycaemia and dyslipidaemia. Inflammation, metabolic disorders, oxidative stress, and mitochondrial dysfunction are among the detrimental neurological consequences resulting from the activation of insulin pathways, microvascular diseases, and other pathways (Zhu et al., 2024).

The exact function of microvascular alterations in DPN is still up for debate. The process of DPN involves microvascular alterations that result in an inadequate blood and oxygen supply. Endothelial cell failure has been observed in the sciatic nerve due to decreased neural blood flow and intra-neural oxygen tension (Cameron et al., 2001). Additionally, patients with DPN exhibited aberrant vascular alterations in their peroneal nerves, such as a reduction in proteins associated with vascular tight junctions, thickening of the nerve's microvascular basement membrane, proliferation and swelling of the vascular endothelium, and degeneration of the pericytes. Ischemia and hypoxia in peripheral nerve tissue are the consequences of these aberrant alterations, which lead to vascular constriction and affect blood flow (Takeshita et al., 2020). Damage to SCs, neurons, and nerves may result from oxidative stress and inflammation, which are worsened by hypoxia in the brain's microenvironment (Gonçalves et al., 2017).

2.2.3 Retinopathy and Vision Impairment

Diabetic retinopathy (DR) ranks high among the most common causes of blindness worldwide, which is a neurovascular consequence of DM that is unique to specific tissues (Teo et al., 2021). Unfortunately, most studies on DR have focused on microangiopathy, neovascularization, and neurodegeneration in inflammatory and hypoxic environments. Additionally, its exact pathophysiology is still a mystery. Patients with DR are first treated with panretinal photocoagulation to avoid vision loss. However, due to the laser's destructive nature, several ocular consequences may occur, including problems with visual acuity and damage to the visual field. Other therapies have varying degrees of restrictions and side effects; for instance, injecting anti-vascular endothelial growth factor (VEGF) medications into the eye does not entirely prevent the development of DR, and repeated injections increase the risk of endophthalmitis (Wykoff, 2017). As a neurovascular consequence of diabetes, DR is very tissue-specific (Oshitari, 2021). A well-functioning retina is the result of the coordinated efforts of several different types of cells that interact with one another. In the early stages of DR, the neurovascular unit (NVU), comprising blood vessels, glial cells, and neurons, undergoes fundamental pathogenic alterations (Hammes, 2018). There are two groups of six phases that comprise DR, based on international clinical grading standards. Microangiomas and tiny blebs comprise stage 1 of non-proliferative diabetic retinopathy (NPDR), which is followed by stage 2, characterized by hard exudates, and stage 3, marked by cotton-like soft exudates. Stage 4 involves neovascularization and vitreous bleeding; stage 5 involves proliferation of fibrovascular and vitreous tissue; and stage 6 involves retinal detachment and stretching leading to blindness (Wang et al., 2024). This second type is known as proliferative diabetic retinopathy (PDR). The majority of DR cases begin with NPDR, the first stage. Raised blood sugar levels lead to the death of pericytes and increased blood vessel permeability (Beltramo & Porta, 2013). Deterioration of endothelium-pericyte communication and weakening of the basement membrane may follow pericyte loss (Bianchi et al., 2016). Retinal ischemia and hypoxia may occur as a consequence of microaneurysms and capillary blockage caused by the loss of pericytes and endothelial cells (Liu et al., 2019). Afterwards, PDR develops as a result of abnormal neovascularization caused by increased amounts of VEGF and intravitreal angiopoietin (Gupta et al., 2013).

Before the development of microangiopathy, there is evidence of decreased retinal thickness and loss of retinal ganglion cells (RGCs), suggesting that DR is a neurodegenerative form of microangiopathy (Sloan et al., 2021). Patients with diabetes are at increased risk for permanent eyesight loss due to anomalies in axonal degeneration and neuronal cell death. Elevated levels of various inflammatory cytokines and chemokines may be detected in patients' blood, vitreous, and aqueous humour throughout the early and chronic phases of DR (Enders et al., 2023). The role of increased DNA methylation in the development of DR is increasingly recognized (Hoke et al., 2021). In the retina, elevated levels of reactive oxygen species (ROS) cause oxidative stress due to the overproduction of intracellular AGEs. Activation of the protein kinase C (PKC), polyol, and hexosamine pathways, as well as disruption of antioxidant defences, can all be caused by chronic hyperglycaemia (Wang et al., 2024).

2.2.4 Nephropathy Leading to Renal Dysfunction

Diabetic neuropathy (DN) is one of the most common forms of chronic kidney disease (CKD) and end-stage renal disease (ESRD) globally, especially in those with T2DM (Arroyave et al., 2020; Gross et al., 2005; Shaw et al., 2010). Along with the current GFR and prior Glomerular filtration rate (GFR) trajectory, proteinuria has traditionally been considered the gold standard for evaluating and monitoring renal function. On the other hand, proteinuria isn't enough to track DN development, as around a third of patients have a decline in renal function before reaching albuminuria (Lee & Choi, 2015; Perkins et al., 2010).

Nephromegaly and a modified Doppler are early morphological indicators of renal injury; however, proteinuria and GFR are the most reliable methods for determining the extent of damage (Zhang et al., 2018). Between 10 and 20 years after the start of diabetes, the average annual incidence of DN is 3% (Magee et al., 2017). Evidence of proteinuria $\geq$300 mg/day in a diabetic patient was previously used to identify DN (American Diabetes Association, 2004b). Albumin in the urine is an indication of DN, but by the time it appears in the urine, the glomeruli have already sustained significant damage. To determine whether individuals are at risk of kidney impairment, new urine biomarkers are needed. Various potential early indicators, including α-1 microglobulin, β-1 microglobulin, nephrin, cystatin C, and others, were identified in a proteomic investigation of non-albumin proteinuria (NAP) (Ballantyne et al., 1993). Unfortunately, neither these markers nor their calibration is now accessible worldwide, even though they may be used as sensitive early indicators of tubule damage (Kim et al., 2014). Another potential urinary biomarker, kininogen-1, was also discovered by precipitating proteins from morning pee and then resolving them using 2D electrophoresis. Additionally, confirmation in bigger cohorts is needed for this kallikrein-kinin system protein (Vitova et al., 2017). Table 2.1 summarizes the different stages of DN.

The main risk factors of diabetic nephropathy, according to several epidemiological studies, are ethnicity, family history, obesity, hypertension, dyslipidaemia, gestational diabetes, and insulin resistance (Raile et al., 2007). Proteinuria, smoking, high systolic blood pressure, and an increased glycosylated haemoglobin level (HbA1c) are other potential risk factors (Sulaiman, 2019). Although nephropathy is the best indicator of death in diabetic patients, there are substantial individual differences in how it develops. Research using high-throughput technology and genome-wide transcriptome investigations has shown that genetic variables activate inflammatory signalling pathways and cause oxidative stress (Hameed et al., 2018; Kato & Natarajan, 2014). Epigenetic processes, including DNA methylation, non-coding RNAs, and histone modifications, may play a significant role in the development of

Table 2.1 Diabetic nephropathy staging (Gheith et al., 2016; Tervaert et al., 2010)

Stages	Staging of DN by Tervaert et al	Staging of DN by Gheith et al
Stage 1	The thickening of the glomerular basement membrane	Starting from the beginning and continuing for five years. No albuminuria, borderline GFR, and hypertension. However, renal plasma flow increased, and kidney size grew by 20%
Stage 2	Mild to severe enlargement of the mesangium	Two years after the start, with thickening of the basement membrane and proliferation of the mesangial vessels, a normal glomerular filtration rate, and no outward signs
Stage 3	Nodular sclerosis	Microalbuminuria (30–300 mg/day) and glomerular damage 5–10 years after initiation, with or without hypertension
Stage 4	A more advanced form of diabetic glomerulosclerosis characterized by vascular lesions and tubulointerstitial lesions	Proteinuria that cannot be reversed, persistent high blood pressure, and a glomerular filtration rate (GFR) $\leq$60 ml/min/1.73 m^2
Stage 5	–	A GFR below 15 ml/min/1.73 m^2 indicates end-stage renal disease

diabetic nephropathy, according to the available evidence. Consequently, variations in the promoter regions of the genes encoding the cytokines TNF-α, IL-6, and IL-1β, as well as changes in their expression, have been associated with DN vulnerability. Inflammation and the resulting remodelling of tissues may cause a local metabolic environment dysregulation, which in turn can cause damage to the kidneys. Instances of oxidative stress, the polyol pathway, the diacylglycerol-protein kinase C (DAG) route, the hexosamine pathway, and other cellular signalling pathways are activated by excess intracellular glucose (Ni et al., 2015; Sulaiman, 2019).

2.2.5 *Peripheral Vascular Disease*

Peripheral arterial disease (PAD) occurs when the arteries in the lower and upper extremities become partially or fully blocked. Even though neuropathy has gotten a lot of attention, PAD is a significant risk factor for leg ulcers and amputations (Peters et al., 2007; Zhang et al., 2020). This means that PAD is likely being untreated since it is not being correctly identified. When the noncardiac, non-intracranial peripheral arteries of the lower and upper limbs become totally or partially blocked, it may cause tissue loss or restricted blood flow; this condition is known as peripheral artery disease (PAD) (Kullo & Rooke, 2016). While atherosclerosis is the most common cause, other conditions, such as embolism, thrombosis, fibromuscular dysplasia, or vasculitis, may also lead to this condition. Possible indicators of systemic atherosclerosis in intracranial and coronary arteries that are not located at the periphery include atherosclerotic PAD. Most DM cases affect the distal arteries, particularly the dorsalis pedis artery, which supplies blood to the lower extremities (Marso & Hiatt, 2006).

Coronary heart disease (CHD) and cerebrovascular disease (CVD) are both influenced by the main risk factors for PAD, which include DM, hypertension, smoking, and hyperlipidaemia. On the other hand, such risks have varying effects on vascular disorders (Forrest et al., 2000). A recent systematic review found that DM was a significant risk factor for PAD, right up there with smoking and hypertension/ hypercholesterolemia, according to community-based studies assessing the worldwide incidence and risk factors of PAD (Song et al., 2019). Along with more conventional risk factors (such as advanced age, smoking, high blood pressure, high cholesterol, and poor kidney function), diabetes was shown to be an essential predictor of PAD incidence and development in many community-based studies (Ramos et al., 2009; Weragoda et al., 2016). It increased the likelihood of lower limb amputation, length of hospital stays, and death. Although the basic risk factors for PAD in those without DM are still prominent in those with DM, other relationships have also been found. These factors include a longer duration of diabetes, an elevated glycated haemoglobin (HbA1c) level, abdominal obesity, being male, and neuropathy (Akalu & Birhan, 2020; Soyoye et al., 2016). Atherosclerosis is the central pathophysiological theme of PAD in DM. Atherosclerosis is the first step; occlusion and reduced blood flow are the outcomes. Predating the diagnosis of impaired fasting glucose and DM, pathogenic alterations may be seen in subclinical atherosclerosis (Drexel et al., 2005). As with other vascular beds, these alterations are observed in individuals with diabetes. Endothelial dysfunction, inflammation, platelet aggregation, and vascular smooth muscle cell (VSMC) dysfunction are among the pathogenetic pathways identified in the onset of atherosclerosis (Soyoye et al., 2021).

2.2.6 Cognitive Decline and Dementia Risk

Dementia is a devastating neurological disease which drastically affects routine tasks. Over 60% of the world's 5,50,000 dementia diagnoses and approximately 100,000 new cases occur in poor and middle-income nations (Chowdhary et al., 2022). Dementia often begins in old age, but diabetes greatly increases the chance of developing the disease by worsening damage to neurons and blood vessels. Patients with diabetes are 73% more likely to develop dementia than those without the disease, with a 56% greater chance of developing alzheimer's disease (AD) (Gudala et al., 2013). Consistent with previous research, people with diabetes had up to a twofold increased chance of getting dementia, with particular increases in the risks of AD and vascular dementia (Biessels et al., 2006).

Scientists have investigated the relationship between diabetes and cognitive decline. Among 1455 adult diabetes patients followed for 15 years, 101 got dementia and 77 had AD, suggesting a 66% higher risk, according to a meta-analysis by Leibson et al. (1997). Dementia risk was double in Mexican patients with T2DM compared to non-diabetics (Salinas et al., 2016). Diabetes almost quadruples the risk of AD and dementia, according to considerable prospective cohort research in Rotterdam, Netherlands (Ott et al., 1999). According to a meta-analysis of 243 prospective studies and 153 randomized control trials, diabetes significantly increases the risk of AD by 69% (Yu et al., 2020). Furthermore, another research found that cognitive impairment and dementia are 1.25 to 1.91 times more common in diabetic patients, and that these risks are present even in the early stages of the disease (Xue et al., 2019). Diabetes and its consequences, including insulin resistance, rapid variations in blood glucose, altered blood flow rate, and chronic inflammation, may raise the risk of dementia, according to biological research. Animal studies on diabetes have shown that reduced granule cell proliferation in the CA1 and CA3 hippocampus regions leads to neuronal death and, ultimately, dementia. Brain shrinkage, changed brain vasculature, decreased synaptic plasticity, and malfunctioning of neuroglial cells are all symptoms of diabetic brain injury that reduce brain function (Chen et al., 2018; Mohammed Faheem & El Askary, 2017). The brains of diabetes patients may experience alterations similar to those shown in early-stage AD, according to imaging and neuropathological investigations (Mayeda et al., 2015). Neuronal injury and cognitive deficits may result from hypoglycaemia, which can cause significant vascular damage to the brain (Hendrie et al., 2017; Song et al., 2022). Dementia is more likely to develop in diabetes individuals with diabetes who have severe hypoglycaemia. In particular, among AD patients, the incidence of dementia is directly proportional to the frequency with which they have severe hypoglycaemia episodes. Regardless of whether or not dementia is present, the risk of death may be increased by as little as one severe episode (Cao et al., 2024; Han et al., 2022).

2.3 The Silent Progression of Damage

2.3.1 Understanding the Physiology of Micro vs. Macro Vascular Complications

Individuals who have diabetes mellitus and related microvascular problems seem to be more vulnerable to accelerated atherosclerosis, which may lead to cardiovascular and cerebrovascular events as well as early mortality (Kalofoutis et al., 2007). Arterioles, capillaries, and venules comprise microvessels, the fundamental functional unit of the cardiovascular system. Their structure and cellular makeup are distinct from those of macrovessels. While macrovessels are responsible for delivering blood to organs, microvessels ensure that nutrients are delivered correctly and maintain blood pressure stability (Orasanu & Plutzky, 2009). The microcirculation can adjust blood flow in response to specific metabolic demands because of regulatory mechanisms that govern vascular permeability and myogenic responses. Before obvious hyperglycaemia and vascular pathological alterations appear, abnormalities in microvascular function may already be present (Orasanu & Plutzky, 2009). A condition known asdiabetic microangiopathy develops when the microvasculature under goes pathognomonic alterations. These changes impact the capillary basement membrane, which includes arterioles in the retina, heart, skin, and muscle, by thickening them. Multiple clinical issues, including hypertension, delayed wound healing, and tissue hypoxia, are induced by this thickening, which in turn leads to irregularity in vascular function. Neovascularization originating from the vasa vasorum may also predict platelet rupture, encourage atherosclerosis, and link macro- and microangiopathy. The mechanism by which microvascular disease contributes to macrovascular atherosclerosis and other systemic consequences of diabetes remains unclear (Chawla et al., 2016).

2.3.2 Common Pathways for the Development of Micro and Macrovascular Complications

2.3.2.1 Oxidative Stress

The development of micro- and macrovascular complications in diabetes is triggered by oxidative stress, which is caused by an excess of reactive oxygen species (ROS). This stress activates additional harmful pathways, including elevated polyol pathway activity, nonenzymatic glycation, and increased PKC levels (Jakus & Rietbrock, 2004). Additionally, it renders inactive two vital enzymes that prevent atherosclerosis: prostacyclin synthase and endothelial nitric oxide synthase (Jakus & Rietbrock, 2004). The Damage to cells, particularly mitochondrial DNA, may occur as a result of ROS interacting with DNA and proteins, a process accelerated by hyperglycaemia. Early mitochondrial DNA damage, accompanied by hyperglycaemia-induced ROS overproduction, was observed in research on human retinal endothelial cells (ECs). The microvasculature may retain pathogenic "memory" in the form of ROS-mediated cellular damage, which persists even when glucose levels are normalized (Giacco & Brownlee, 2010). Several experimental findings suggest that the excessive generation of superoxide by mitochondria is the primary cause of metabolic problems in diabetes (Xie et al., 2008). In individuals with T2DM, atherosclerosis and cardiomyopathy are caused by the inhibition of anti-atherosclerotic enzymes and the formation of ROS through mitochondrial processes involving free fatty acids. Subjects without diabetes or impaired glucose tolerance who were in the highest quintile of insulin resistance had a 2.0-fold higher risk of cardiovascular disease compared to those in the lowest quintile, even after accounting for various known risk factors, such as smoking, systolic blood pressure, high-density lipoprotein, triglycerides, and LDL cholesterol (Duncan, 2011). Numerous processes associated with oxidative stress promote macrovascular problems in diabetes, including AGE formation, PKC activation, increased polyol flow, and hexosamine production. Several pro-inflammatory and pro-atherosclerotic target genes in vascular smooth muscle cells

(VSMCs), ECs, and macrophages may be activated by elevated glucose concentrations through the NF-κB pathway (Giacco & Brownlee, 2010). The process of accelerated atherosclerosis is fuelled by hyperglycaemia, which in turn triggers oxidative stress.

2.3.2.2 Advanced Glycation End Products (AGE)

AGEs are a diverse collection of compounds generated when plasma proteins undergo non-enzymatic glycation. This process alters the molecular structure of proteins, disrupting enzyme activity and interfering with receptor functionality, which causes a disturbance in their normal functioning. By cross-linking with proteins, lipids, and nucleic acids, AGEs alter the structure and function of both extracellular and intracellular components, resulting in various complications associated with diabetes. The process begins when AGEs bind to receptors for AGEs (RAGE) that are located in the plasma membrane (Chawla et al., 2016). This leads to an increase in the expression of transcription factors, such as NF-κB, and the genes it targets, as well as the production of chemicals that promote inflammation and generate free radicals. Soluble AGEs activate monocytes, while their migration is inhibited by AGEs in the basement membrane. AGE-bound RAGE enhances endothelial permeability to macromolecules. To create ROS, AGEs inhibit endothelial nitric oxide function (Schmidt et al., 1994). AGEs also alter LDL particles, which speed up atherosclerosis when combined with vascular injury. According to Kalousová et al., there is a notable increase in AGE in T2DM patients when compared to both healthy individuals and those with T1DM ($4.14\% \pm 0.86 \times 10^1$ AU/g vs. $4.08 \pm 0.71 \times 10^2$ AU/g, $P < 0.001$) (Kalousová et al., 2002). According to Kilhovd et al., there was a notable rise in AGE levels in T2DM patients as compared to non-diabetic control participants (7.4 [4.4–10.9] vs. 4.2 [1.6–6.4] U/ml, $P < 0.0001$). Also, those with T2DM had higher AGE levels in their blood compared to those without coronary heart disease (8.1 [6.4–10.9] vs. 7.1 [3.5–9.8] U/ml, $P = 0.03$) (Kilhovd et al., 1999).

2.3.2.3 Vasa Vasorum Neovascularization

Plaque load increases due to vasa vasorum proliferation, which in turn promotes atherosclerosis (Tian et al., 2013). During the formation of atherosclerotic plaques, many biological processes, including inflammation, plaque perfusion, and concurrent intra-plaque bleeding, are associated with the growth of vasa vasorum. The adventitial layer and the artery lumen both expand toward the intima as neovascularization progresses (Hayden & Tyagi, 2004). Increased angiogenesis and neovasculature microangiopathy both contribute to the acceleration of diabetic atherosclerosis in T2DM (Chawla et al., 2016). An essential part of homeostatic systems, the early angiogenic response in the adventitial vasa vasorum appears to be triggered by hypoxia, as indicated by the finding of enhanced hypoxia-inducible factor and vascular endothelial growth factor (VEGF) activity (Xu et al., 2015). VEFG is a multi-role cytokine that increases vascular permeability to macromolecules, promotes monocyte chemotaxis, and stimulates the generation of tissue factors; all of these contribute to microvascular problems. Experimental models of diabetic kidney illness have also shown an upregulation of VEGF (Bonnefond et al., 2013). On the other hand, a VEGF gene transfer experiment in rats has revealed that VEGF therapy may reduce diabetic neuropathy and restore vasa nervorum microcirculation (Orasanu & Plutzky, 2009). Due to its potent angiogenic inhibition, a neurotropic factor called pigment epithelium-derived factor (PEDF) in the eye may counteract the effects of VEGF (Schratzberger et al., 2001). In proliferative diabetic retinopathy, VEGF levels are higher while PEDF levels are lower. One possible cause of diabetic nephropathy is low PEDF levels. Proliferative retinopathy may be increased by other growth factors, such as insulin-like growth factor 1, basic fibroblast growth factor, and hepatocyte growth factor (Gao et al., 2001).

2.3.2.4 Inflammation at Low Grades

It is well known that inflammation is a significant risk factor for both atherosclerosis and T2DM. One of the first steps in atherogenesis is the loss of vascular cells' nonadhesive ability and the adherence of monocytes to ECs, both of which occur in response to hyperglycemia. There is evidence that monocyte adherence to arterial ECsis triggered by hyperglycemia (Syed Ikmal et al., 2013). The fact that both hyperglycemia and AGEs may enhance EC generation of superoxide, as shown in Fig. 2.2, suggests that they are associated with oxidative stress. Additionally, glucose triggers the matrix-degrading enzyme metalloproteinase, leading to vascular smooth muscle cell proliferation, migration, and altered activity, as well as arterial remodelling and plaque rupture. The development of IR is known to be influenced by an elevated level of tumour necrosis factor alpha. As mentioned before, IR itself has an inflammatory effect. Diabetes is associated with an increase in the levels of several inflammatory markers, including C-reactive protein, fibrinogen, plasminogen activator inhibitor-1, and interleukin-6. Research has shown that monocytes get activated when glucose levels are high, leading to the production of inflammatory mediators, including protein kinase-C (PKC) and NF-κB, which in turn promote oxidative stress (Otsuka et al., 2005).

2.3.3 Interlink Between Microvascular and Macrovascular Complications

Diabetes can lead to heart involvement due to both macrovascular and microvascular factors, including fatty acid and glucose derangements, hypertrophy, and loss of function resulting from glycation. Cardiomyopathy and atherosclerosis in large arteries may be linked to a microvascular component in diabetes (Laakso, 2011). Small

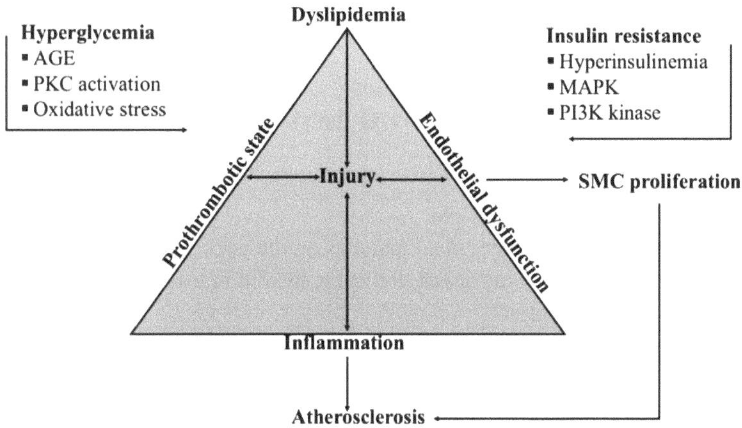

Figure2 The atherosclerotic process is driven by insulin resistance and hyperglycaemia

artery and capillary alterations may cause long-term issues in diabetic individuals, including retinopathy, nephropathy, and neuropathy, as well as other heart disease symptoms. Implementing and maintaining optimal blood glucose management at an early stage can help prevent microvascular disease. Controlling blood pressure and dyslipidemia is crucial for avoiding macrovascular diseases, as well as managing blood sugar levels. Patients with microvascular problems are at risk for accelerated atherosclerosis and early mortality. Neovascularization from the vasa vasorum may link macroangiopathy and microangiopathy. A better understanding of variable responses to treatment therapies may improve outcomes in T2DM, including both microvascular and macrovascular consequences. A more rigorous study on the interlinking theory will clarify whether microvascular difficulties precede macrovascular issues or are two endpoints of the same illness continuum (Chawla et al., 2016).

2.4 Early Warning Signs to Watch For

Since the effects of hyperglycaemia do not appear quickly, many people ignore the symptoms of diabetes even though the condition progresses slowly over time. Damage may begin years before symptoms appear, yet this fact is often overlooked. Unfortunately, vascular problems may be prevented and the illness can be quickly controlled if early signs are recognized. Because early-stage T2DM often has no symptoms, individuals must be aware of what to look out for (Ramachandran, 2014). Some common warning signs and symptoms of diabetes are given below:

i. Weight loss for no apparent reason
ii. Frequent irritation and anger issues
iii. Frequent urination
iv. Constant exhaustion

v. Dry mouth
vi. Skin rash
vii. Foot numbness and burning sensation
viii. Recurrent infections, particularly in the skin, urinary tract, oral cavity, and genitourinary regions
ix. Slow wound healing
x. Reduced or impaired eyesight
xi. The occurrence of velvety black patches on the neck, armpits, or groin region, known as Acanthosis nigricans, indicates insulin resistance
xii. Reactive hypoglycemia
xiii. Impotence or erectile dysfunction

The T2DM, characterized by very high blood sugar levels, and T1DM, characterized by a fast onset of severe hyperglycemia, both often cause the characteristic diabetic symptoms, including polyuria, polydipsia, and polyphagia. T1DM and long-term undiagnosed T2DM are the only two conditions known to cause severe weight loss. Undiagnosed diabetes may manifest itself in a variety of ways, including unexplained weight loss, extreme tiredness, irritability, and persistent discomfort. Mild or slowly progressing symptoms may sometimes go unrecognized (Ramachandran, 2014).

2.4.1 Importance of Recognizing Prediabetes

The risk of vascular consequences, including cardiovascular illnesses, is substantial even in prediabetic phases like Impaired fasting glycemia (IFG) and Impaired glucose tolerance (IGT). More than 316 million individuals (6.9% of the world population) have IGT, according to the latest estimates by the International Diabetes Federation (IDF). Over 70 per cent of them reside in LMICs (Magliano et al., 2021). Also, keep in mind that one-third of people with IGT are in the working-age range of 20–39 years, which means they are very likely to spend a lot of time at high risk of getting diabetes and/or its complications (Magliano et al., 2021). Two to three hours after a meal, some prediabetic individuals may have reactive hypoglycemia. This indicates that insulin metabolism is compromised, which might lead to diabetes in the near future. The risks associated with undetected diabetes might be mitigated if those exhibiting these symptoms or who have risk factors for diabetes had regular medical examinations. Many individuals who would otherwise be silent victims of the metabolic abnormalities associated with diabetes may benefit from an improvement in their health (Ramachandran, 2014).

2.5 Screening and Diagnostic Approaches

People who are initially asymptomatic may still benefit from screening for T2DM due to the availability of accurate testing and the fact that the illness can be slowed and its negative consequences mitigated by lifestyle modifications and medication [7, 8]. Although no evidence screening for T2DM reduces mortality after 10 years of follow-up, studies have shown that patients with impaired glucose tolerance and impaired fasting glucose can delay the development of T2DM through lifestyle and pharmacological interventions. Some studies even suggest that lifestyle changes are more effective than pharmacologic interventions [12, 13].

2.5.1 Screening

2.5.1.1 Non-pregnant Adult

Although there are some minor variations, many professional organizations have released guidelines for screening for T2DM (Table 2.2). Screening people who are overweight or obese between the ages of 40 and 70 is recommended by the U.S. Preventive Services Task Force (USPSTF), which recently revised its guidelines. Individuals whose findings are out of the ordinary should be referred to behavioural counselling programs that emphasize the importance of exercise and a balanced diet. It is recommended that clinicians check patients who are at a greater risk (Selph et al., 2015). The guidelines for screening for prediabetes are part of the American Diabetes Association's (ADA) recommendations to test a larger population based on risk, which includes all individuals 45 years and above, regardless of risk (American Diabetes Association, 2003; Engelgau et al., 2000). Although the majority of prediction models overestimate the likelihood of diabetes, several risk prediction calculators are available to provide more accurate estimates. One of two validated risk assessments should be used to assist in deciding who should be examined, according to the Canadian Task Force on Preventive Health Care (Buijsse et al., 2011; Mann et al., 2010).

2.5.1.2 Pregnant Women

Pregnancy complications, including congenital disabilities and foetal mortality, are more likely in women with hyperglycaemia. There is a three- to fourfold greater risk of baby abnormalities in women with gestational diabetes mellitus (GDM) who have fasting hyperglycaemia (Ashique et al., 2025; Sheffield, 2002). In preeclampsia, caesarean section, congenital abnormalities, macrosomia (and later childhood/adolescent obesity), shoulder dystocia, nerve palsy, bone fracture, jaundice, and infant mortality are some of the maternal and foetal issues that screening

Table 2.2 A review of the guidelines for the screening of T2DM (Pippitt et al., 2016)

Parameters	As per the American Association of clinical endocrinologists	As per the American Diabetes Association
Skin condition	Acanthosis nigricans	Acanthosis nigricans
Medications	Antipsychotic medications for schizophrenia or severe bipolar disorder Hypertensive patient with blood pressure >140/90 mmHg and on antihypertensive medications Chronic glucocorticoid exposure	Hypertensive patient with blood pressure >140/90 mmHg and on antihypertensive medications
Family history	Heart disease, stroke, or a history of T2DM in the family	T2DM in a first-degree relative
HDL level	HDL cholesterol level <35 mg/dl (0.91 mmol/L) Triglyceride level >250 mg/dl (2.8 mmol/L)	HDL cholesterol level <35 mg/dl Triglyceride level >250 mg/dl
Ethnicity	Asian, black, Hispanic, Native American (Alaska Native or American Indian), or Pacific Islander	Black, Hispanic/Latino, Asian American, Native American/Alaska, and Native Hawaiian/Pacific Islander
Weight; lifestyle	Overweight or obese; sedentary lifestyle	Obesity, physical inactivity
Metabolism of glucose	Problems with glucose tolerance, fasting glucose, and metabolic syndrome	Previous tests have shown an A1C > 5.7%, poor glucose tolerance, or impaired fasting glucose
Ovarian condition	Polycystic ovary syndrome	Polycystic ovary syndrome
Sleeping	Obstructive sleep apnea, chronic sleep deprivation, and night-shift work are all examples of sleep disorders that should be evaluated every three years for patients with glucose intolerance (A1C > 5.7%, impaired glucose tolerance, or impaired fasting glucose on prior tests)	-
Liver condition	Non-alcoholic fatty liver disease	-

aims to decrease (Crowther et al., 2005; Mann et al., 2010). The risk factors for pregnant women to develop T2DM are listed in Table 2.2. Gestational diabetes mellitus (GDM), such as obesity, advanced maternal age (older than 35 years), a history of GDM, a family history of diabetes, or belonging to a high-risk ethnic group, the American Diabetes Association recommends screening during the first trimester (American Diabetes Association, 2015a). A 50 g non-fasting oral glucose challenge test and a 100 g fasting oral glucose tolerance test are both recommended for screening for GDM. If the first test comes back positive, the second test is used for diagnosis (Garrison, 2015).

2.5.1.3 Children

Adolescents and children under the age of 18 with a body mass index (BMI) above the 85th percentile for their age and gender, a weight-to-height ratio above the 85th percentile, or a weight over 120% of the ideal [50th percentile] for their height should be screened by the American Diabetes Association. Causes of T2DM in the family, acanthosis nigricans, high blood pressure, high cholesterol, polycystic ovarian syndrome, or being a member of a high-risk ethnic group are all factors to consider. Moreover, 35 Patients at risk should undergo screening every two years beginning at age 10, or when puberty starts if the child is less than 10 years old, according to the American Academy of Paediatrics and the American Diabetes Association (2015c), Copeland et al., (2013).

2.5.1.4 Older Adult

The value of screening for T2DM and prediabetes depends on whether or not therapy will increase the patient's life expectancy or quality of life, even though over half of the elderly population has prediabetes, and the risk of both conditions is greater in the elderly population as a whole (Kirkman et al., 2012). Although the American Diabetes Association endorses screening as a potential measure to prevent problems that can cause functional impairment in the elderly, no organizations have yet proposed regular screening in this population. While the objectives of therapy may vary in older people, the criteria for diagnosis remain the same (American Diabetes Association, 2015b). There is no set age at which screening should end; rather, it is a matter for the doctor and patient to decide together, taking into account factors including life expectancy and any co-morbidities (Kirkman et al., 2012).

2.5.2 Diagnostic Approaches

Diabetic diagnosis is possible when one random plasma glucose test is 200 mg/dL (11.1 mmol/L) or above, and characteristic hyperglycaemia symptoms are present. Oral glucose tolerance testing with a 75-g glucose load or a fasting plasma glucose level of 126 mg/dL (7.0 mmol/L) or higher, or an A1C level of 6.5% or higher, can also be used to make the diagnosis (American Diabetes Association, 2014). However, it is recommended to repeat the tests the following day to confirm the diagnosis. Repeat testing or testing using a different modality could be helpful if the findings do not align with the clinical picture or are inconsistent (American Diabetes Association, 2004a).

2.5.2.1 A1C Level

The A1C is a measure of the glycosylation percentage of the haemoglobin A1C chain; it provides a rough idea of the typical blood glucose levels over the last 2–3 months, estimated from the body's sluggish red blood cell turnover (Cohen et al., 2010). In 2010, A1C was first included in the ADA standards as a method for diagnosing diabetes. Attempts to standardize laboratory tests have not eliminated the limitations of A1C testing; in some individuals, there is only a partial correlation between the A1C level and the actual glucose level. There are several reasons for showing falsely low A1C values, including haemolytic anaemias, chronic liver disease, pregnancy, sudden blood loss and patients receiving antiretroviral medications for HIV. In contrast, causes of erroneously high A1C levels include aplastic anaemias, hyperbilirubinemia, hypertriglyceridemia, and previous splenectomy. Some racial and ethnic groups may have a higher prevalence of hemoglobinopathies and haemoglobin variations, which may cause A1C levels to fluctuate (Lapolla et al., 2011; Malkani & Mordes, 2011).

2.5.2.2 Fasting Plasma Glucose

According to the National Health and Nutrition Examination Survey data, fasting plasma glucose levels may detect up to one-third more instances of undiagnosed diabetes than A1C readings (Picón et al., 2012). The only reliable way to assess fasting plasma glucose is with a venous blood sample; readings from an elevated glucometer or a continuous glucose monitor are not diagnostic (American Diabetes Association, 2015a).

2.5.2.3 Special Tests

It is now widely acknowledged that diabetes may be categorized into a spectrum of illnesses. This spectrum includes T1DM, T2DM and GDM, prediabetes, neonatal diabetes, juvenile maturity-onset diabetes, and latent autoimmune diabetes in adults (American Diabetes Association, 2014; Palmer & Hirsch, 2003). The causes of these illnesses overlap to some extent. T1DM often have autoimmune indicators such as autoantibodies against at least one of the following: zinc transporter, insulin, islet cells, and insulinoma-associated antigen-2 (Handelsman et al., 2015; Hosszúfalusi et al., 2003). Autoantibodies are not present in people with idiopathic T1DM, and these tests may not be as specific for patients with T2DM or latent autoimmune diabetes in adults (Patel & Macerollo, 2010). Notwithstanding these reservations, autoantibody testing for T2DM should be performed routinely, according to the American Association of Clinical Endocrinologists.16 The effectiveness of additional testing in improving patient outcomes related to diabetes etiology classification needs more investigation. Some of the special tests are summarised in Table3.

Table 2.3 Special tests for diabetes classification (Pippitt et al., 2016)

Test	Description	Clinical
Zinc transporter 8 autoantibody C peptide	Linked to autoimmune-mediated diabetes, even in individuals who do not have autoantibodies Indicates the body's natural insulin production; conditions such as T1DM or low or undetectable insulin levels	Patients with negative autoimmune antibodies who are clinically suspected of having T1DM or latent autoimmune diabetes in the adult (LADA) should be considered
Genetic testing	Necessary for the identification of monogenic diabetes syndromes, such as newborn diabetes and young people with mature-onset diabetes Very costly	Consider this in children only if they've been diagnosed before six months, if they have no autoantibodies, or if there's a family history of the disease but none of the typical risk factors for T2DM, such as being overweight, being from a low-risk ethnic group, or having insulin resistance
Insulinoma-associated antigen-2 Insulin autoantibody Islet cell autoantibody glutamic acid decarboxylase 65	T2DM-related autoimmune antibodies Islet cell autoantibodies or a single positive test for glutamic acid decarboxylase 65 may be more prevalent in LADA	Differentiate between T2DM, T1DM, and LADA

2.6 Importance of Early Detection

Hyperglycaemia is the hallmark of T2DM, a metabolic disorder that progresses over time. Several problems, including cardiovascular disease, renal disease, retinopathy, and others, may develop as a result of chronically high blood glucose levels (Ali et al., 2022). Many health concerns may be exacerbated by delaying the diagnosis of diabetes. Complications with the cardiovascular system, kidneys, nervous system, and eyes might develop when blood glucose levels stay high for a long time (Zheng et al., 2018). Because there may be no outward signs of diabetes in its early stages, it can be easily missed. Complications may arise from untreated high blood sugar, which can damage blood vessels and the neurological system. Consequently, these risks may be successfully reduced with early detection and treatment of diabetes. Individuals at risk for T2DM may be identified using alternative approaches in addition to recognized risk factors. Three other methods for prediabetes diagnosis are as follows.

Glycated albumin (GA) is a newly developed biomarker that may help individuals with diabetes track their blood sugar levels over shorter periods (Koga & Kasayama,

2010). Similar to HbA1c, GA indicates the average glucose level over 2–3 weeks and may be used for diabetes management (Yazdanpanah et al., 2017). The improved early detection and treatment of diabetes is a result of its increased sensitivity and specificity (Sumner et al., 2016). Nearly 80% of African prediabetics were detected when HbA1c with GA was used, compared to only HbA1c (78% vs. 50%, $P < 0.001$). When testing fasting glucose, a GA of ≥17.1% may detect the majority of undiagnosed diabetes. GA decreased the incidence of false-positive screenings by 33.75%, as measured by fasting glucose. In high-risk populations, particularly those with normal fasting glucose, abnormal GA is a crucial marker for OGTT screening (He et al., 2017).

Continuous glucose monitoring (CGM) is another novel method that tracks patients' glucose changes, including postprandial excursions in real time (Vigersky et al., 2012). There are several benefits to using CGM (Continuous Glucose Monitoring) instead of more conventional glucose monitoring techniques, such as frequent blood tests or fingerstick measures. To begin, continuous glucose monitoring (CGM) records a patient's ever-changing glucose profile throughout the day. Thus, glycemic variability may be better understood, and trends or patterns can be more precisely identified than with intermittent testing (Carlson et al., 2017). Additionally, continuous glucose monitors can detect when blood sugar levels rise or fall in response to various factors, including food, physical activity, emotional stress, and prescription medications. For healthcare professionals and patients to create tailored treatment plans and make informed decisions about nutrition, exercise, and medication adjustments, this data is crucial. Clinical glucose monitors (CGMs) show promise as a diagnostic and treatment tool for those with prediabetes and other high-risk populations for developing diabetes. Those who were monitored continuously for at least 24 h showed impaired glucose tolerance if their fasting blood glucose level was less than 100 mg/dL (Nomura et al., 2011). By delivering continuous blood glucose data, the integration of CGM into standard clinical practice improves prediabetes care. Enhanced sensors and smaller devices are just two examples of the recent technological advancements in continuous glucose monitoring (CGM) that have led to more reliable and user-friendly solutions. Central glucose monitoring (CGM) has gained popularity due to patients' growing desire for improved blood glucose management and overall well-being. Nevertheless, there are issues, such as the fact that it is expensive, which restrict its application to specific areas and patient groups (Ribet et al., 2017).

Glycated serum protein (GSP) is a novel biomarker that indicates the effectiveness of blood sugar management in individuals with diabetes (Raghav & Ahmad, 2014). A few other metabolic parameters may affect GSP detection, making it a quick, easy, and repeatable method. In cases of renal impairment and anaemia, GSP provides more accurate diabetes monitoring than HbA1c because of its greater sensitivity and specificity. Researchers found a strong positive correlation between fructosamine levels and HbA1c. This suggests that both fructosamine and HbA1c could be helpful glycemic markers for cancer patients with diabetes, chemotherapy patients taking

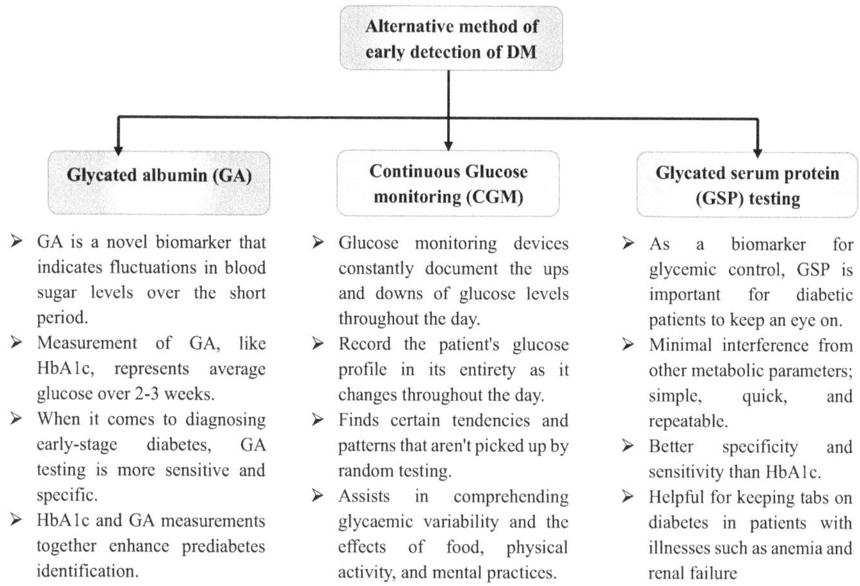

Fig. 2.3 Three alternative methods of early detection of T2DM

glucocorticoids, and those with anaemia, hypoalbuminemia, or impaired renal function (Toyoshima et al., 2023). GSP testing may help detect diabetes and its consequences at an earlier stage. Research conducted in 2016 indicated that GSP was effective in predicting diabetes in overweight and obese youths (aged 10–18) using 2 h glucose and HbA1c readings. Diabetic complication screening and prediction may potentially benefit from GSP detection, according to certain studies (Chan et al., 2016). To ensure the precision and dependability of biomarkers, such as GA, CGM, and GSP tests, it is essential to validate diagnostic models for prediabetes. These biomarkers may be validated to demonstrate that they accurately represent glycemic management, continually monitor glucose levels, and capture short-term fluctuations in glycemic levels. Verifying the accuracy and reliability of these diagnostic methods is crucial for detecting prediabetes early, which in turn allows for better treatment choices and improved health outcomes for patients (Zhang et al., 2023). A summary of the above discussion is given in Fig. 2.3.

2.7 Conclusion

It is crucial to detect and prevent T2DM early, as its incidence and effects are on the rise. Different fasting glucose and HbA1c cutoffs make prediabetes diagnosis challenging. That is why we need new ways to pinpoint populations most at risk. The lack of clarity around prediabetes makes its diagnosis difficult (17). Estimating prevalence across populations is made more difficult by the lack of unanimity on prediabetes diagnosis. We need biomarkers that are more specific and sensitive for future studies. To get an accurate diagnosis of prediabetes, it is necessary to optimize glucose and HbA1c thresholds and implement dynamic monitoring. Determining the best ways to avoid or manage prediabetes is crucial in the fight against the development of T2DM. It is critical to thoroughly describe the decision-making process that is based on the model's output when using the new diagnostic model. By following this procedure, we can determine whether a person is at high risk or requires further evaluation and care. Specific patient features, supplementary clinical considerations, and the adoption of applicable regulations or standards are among the factors that influence this decision-making process. To better comprehend the possible diagnostic signs and how they might be used in clinical practice, it is helpful to build a thorough framework for the decision-making process. By incorporating several criteria into their decision-making process, healthcare providers are better equipped to meet the specific needs of their patients through the use of individualized treatments and management plans made possible by this framework. In conclusion, the increasing prevalence of T2DM necessitates a global agreement on the diagnosis of prediabetes, methods for preventing and treating the disease, and the need for more targeted and individualised approaches. Hyperglycemia is not defined solely by glucose or haemoglobin A1c levels, but rather as a spectrum.

2.8 Availability of Data

None.

Acknowledgements The images were created using a PowerPoint presentation and www.Grammarly.com to correct the grammar of this manuscript.

Author Contributions Shahnaz Alom and Farak Ali were involved in the conceptualization, writing of the original draft, mechanistic insight, input on critical points, editing; Bibhuti Bhusan Kakoti was involved in the conceptualization, manuscript writing, reviewing, and conceptualization of figures and approved the version to be published.

Funding None.

Conflict of Interest None.

References

Akalu, Y., & Birhan, A. (2020). Peripheral arterial disease and its associated factors among type 2 diabetes mellitus patients at Debre Tabor General Hospital, Northwest Ethiopia. *Journal of Diabetes Research, 2020*, 1–9. https://doi.org/10.1155/2020/9419413

Ali, M. K., Pearson-Stuttard, J., Selvin, E., & Gregg, E. W. (2022). Interpreting global trends in type 2 diabetes complications and mortality. *Diabetologia, 65*(1), 3–13. https://doi.org/10.1007/s00125-021-05585-2

Aljuraiban, G. S., Alharbi, F. J., Aljohi, A. O., Almeshari, A. Z., Alotaibi, M. N., AlShammari, S. S., Al-Musharaf, S., Aldhwayan, M. M., & Abudawood, M. (2024). Systemic immune-inflammation index in relation to diabetes markers in Saudi adults: A retrospective study. *Medicina, 60*(3), 442. https://doi.org/10.3390/medicina60030442

Alom, S., Ali, F., Bezbaruah, R., & Kakoti, B. B. (2025). In-vitro and in-silico analysis of phyto-constituents of Enhydra fluctuans as an antidiabetic agent. *Advances in Traditional Medicine.* https://doi.org/10.1007/s13596-025-00821-1

American Diabetes Association. (2003). Screening for type 2 diabetes. *Diabetes Care, 26*(suppl_1), s21–s24. https://doi.org/10.2337/diacare.26.2007.S21

American Diabetes Association. (2004a). Diagnosis and classification of diabetes mellitus. *Diabetes Care, 27*(suppl_1), s5–s10. https://doi.org/10.2337/diacare.27.2007.S5

American Diabetes Association. (2004b). Nephropathy in diabetes. *Diabetes Care, 27*(suppl_1), s79–s83. https://doi.org/10.2337/diacare.27.2007.S79

American Diabetes Association. (2014). Diagnosis and classification of diabetes mellitus. *Diabetes Care, 37*(Supplement_1), S81–S90. https://doi.org/10.2337/dc14-S081

American Diabetes Association. (2015a). 2. Classification and diagnosis of diabetes. *Diabetes Care, 38*(Supplement_1), S8–S16. https://doi.org/10.2337/dc15-S005

American Diabetes Association. (2015b). 10. Older adults. *Diabetes Care, 38*(Supplement_1), S67–S69. https://doi.org/10.2337/dc15-S013

American Diabetes Association. (2015c). 11. Children and adolescents. *Diabetes Care, 38*(Supplement_1), S70–S76. https://doi.org/10.2337/dc15-S014

Arroyave, F., Montaño, D., & Lizcano, F. (2020). Diabetes mellitus is a chronic disease that can benefit from therapy with induced pluripotent stem cells. *International Journal of Molecular Sciences, 21*(22), 8685. https://doi.org/10.3390/ijms21228685

Ashique, S., Ghazanfar, S., Mojgani, N., & Tonelli, F. M. P. (2025). *Postbiotics in metabolic disorders* (1st ed.). CRC Press. https://doi.org/10.1201/9781003607779

Ballantyne, F. C., Gibbons, J., & O'Reilly, D. S. (1993). Urine Albumin should replace total protein for the assessment of glomerular proteinuria. *Annals of Clinical Biochemistry: International Journal of Laboratory Medicine, 30*(1), 101–103. https://doi.org/10.1177/000456329303000119

Beltramo, E., & Porta, M. (2013). Pericyte loss in diabetic retinopathy: Mechanisms and consequences. *Current Medicinal Chemistry, 20*(26), 3218–3225. https://doi.org/10.2174/09298673113209990022

Bhatti, J. S., Sehrawat, A., Mishra, J., Sidhu, I. S., Navik, U., Khullar, N., Kumar, S., Bhatti, G. K., & Reddy, P. H. (2022). Oxidative stress in the pathophysiology of type 2 diabetes and related complications: Current therapeutics strategies and future perspectives. *Free Radical Biology and Medicine, 184*, 114–134. https://doi.org/10.1016/j.freeradbiomed.2022.03.019

Bianchi, E., Ripandelli, G., Taurone, S., Feher, J., Plateroti, R., Kovacs, I., Magliulo, G., Orlando, M. P., Micera, A., Battaglione, E., & Artico, M. (2016). Age and diabetes related changes of the retinal capillaries: An ultrastructural and immunohistochemical study. *International Journal of Immunopathology and Pharmacology, 29*(1), 40–53. https://doi.org/10.1177/0394632015615592

Biessels, G. J., Staekenborg, S., Brunner, E., Brayne, C., & Scheltens, P. (2006). Risk of dementia in diabetes mellitus: A systematic review. *The Lancet Neurology, 5*(1), 64–74. https://doi.org/10.1016/S1474-4422(05)70284-2

Bonnefond, A., Saulnier, P.-J., Stathopoulou, M. G., Grarup, N., Ndiaye, N. C., Roussel, R., Nezhad, M. A., Dechaume, A., Lantieri, O., Hercberg, S., Lauritzen, T., Balkau, B., El-Sayed Moustafa, J. S., Hansen, T., Pedersen, O., Froguel, P., Charpentier, G., Marre, M., Hadjadj, S., & Visvikis-Siest, S. (2013). What is the contribution of two genetic variants regulating VEGF levels to type

2 diabetes risk and to microvascular complications? *PLoS ONE, 8*(2), Article e55921. https://doi.org/10.1371/journal.pone.0055921
Buijsse, B., Simmons, R. K., Griffin, S. J., & Schulze, M. B. (2011). Risk assessment tools for identifying individuals at risk of developing type 2 diabetes. *Epidemiologic Reviews, 33*(1), 46–62. https://doi.org/10.1093/epirev/mxq019
Cameron, N. E., Eaton, S. E. M., Cotter, M. A., & Tesfaye, S. (2001). Vascular factors and metabolic interactions in the pathogenesis of diabetic neuropathy. *Diabetologia, 44*(11), 1973–1988. https://doi.org/10.1007/s001250100001
Cao, F., Yang, F., Li, J., Guo, W., Zhang, C., Gao, F., Sun, X., Zhou, Y., & Zhang, W. (2024). The relationship between diabetes and the dementia risk: A meta-analysis. *Diabetology & Metabolic Syndrome, 16*(1), 101. https://doi.org/10.1186/s13098-024-01346-4
Carlson, A. L., Mullen, D. M., & Bergenstal, R. M. (2017). Clinical use of continuous glucose monitoring in adults with type 2 diabetes. *Diabetes Technology & Therapeutics, 19*(S2), S-4–S-11. https://doi.org/10.1089/dia.2017.0024
Cernea, S., & Raz, I. (2021). Management of diabetic neuropathy. *Metabolism, 123*, Article 154867. https://doi.org/10.1016/j.metabol.2021.154867
Chan, C. L., Pyle, L., Kelsey, M., Newnes, L., Zeitler, P. S., & Nadeau, K. J. (2016). Screening for type 2 diabetes and prediabetes in obese youth: Evaluating alternate markers of glycemia—1,5-anhydroglucitol, fructosamine, and glycated albumin: Alternative glycemic markers in obese youth. *Pediatric Diabetes, 17*(3), 206–211. https://doi.org/10.1111/pedi.12258
Chawla, A., Chawla, R., & Jaggi, S. (2016). Microvasular and macrovascular complications in diabetes mellitus: Distinct or continuum? *Indian Journal of Endocrinology and Metabolism, 20*(4), 546. https://doi.org/10.4103/2230-8210.183480
Chen, R., Shi, J., Yin, Q., Li, X., Sheng, Y., Han, J., Zhuang, P., & Zhang, Y. (2018). Morphological and pathological characteristics of brain in diabetic encephalopathy. *Journal of Alzheimer's Disease, 65*(1), 15–28. https://doi.org/10.3233/JAD-180314
Chen, Z., & Natarajan, R. (2022). Epigenetic modifications in metabolic memory: What are the memories, and can we erase them? *American Journal of Physiology-Cell Physiology, 323*(2), C570–C582. https://doi.org/10.1152/ajpcell.00201.2022
Cheng, Y., Wang, Y., Yin, R., Xu, Y., Zhang, L., Zhang, Y., Yang, L., & Zhao, D. (2023). Central role of cardiac fibroblasts in myocardial fibrosis of diabetic cardiomyopathy. *Frontiers in Endocrinology, 14*, 1162754. https://doi.org/10.3389/fendo.2023.1162754
Chib, S., Dutta, B. J., Chalotra, R., Abubakar, M., Kumar, P., Singh, T. G., & Singh, R. (2025). Role of flavonoids in mitigating the pathological complexities and treatment hurdles in Alzheimer's disease. *Phytotherapy Research, 39*(2), 747–775. https://doi.org/10.1002/ptr.8406
Chowdhary, N., Barbui, C., Anstey, K. J., Kivipelto, M., Barbera, M., Peters, R., Zheng, L., Kulmala, J., Stephen, R., Ferri, C. P., Joanette, Y., Wang, H., Comas-Herrera, A., Alessi, C., Suharya (Dy), K., Mwangi, K. J., Petersen, R. C., Motala, A. A., Mendis, S., & Dua, T. (2022). Reducing the risk of cognitive decline and dementia: WHO recommendations. *Frontiers in Neurology, 12*, 765584. https://doi.org/10.3389/fneur.2021.765584
Cohen, R. M., Haggerty, S., & Herman, W. H. (2010). HbA1c for the diagnosis of diabetes and prediabetes: Is it time for a mid-course correction? *The Journal of Clinical Endocrinology & Metabolism, 95*(12), 5203–5206. https://doi.org/10.1210/jc.2010-2352
Copeland, K. C., Silverstein, J., Moore, K. R., Prazar, G. E., Raymer, T., Shiffman, R. N., Springer, S. C., Thaker, V. V., Anderson, M., Spann, S. J., & Flinn, S. K. (2013). Management of Newly Diagnosed Type 2 Diabetes Mellitus (T2DM) in children and adolescents. *Pediatrics, 131*(2), 364–382. https://doi.org/10.1542/peds.2012-3494
Crowther, C. A., Hiller, J. E., Moss, J. R., McPhee, A. J., Jeffries, W. S., & Robinson, J. S. (2005). Effect of treatment of gestational diabetes mellitus on pregnancy outcomes. *New England Journal of Medicine, 352*(24), 2477–2486. https://doi.org/10.1056/NEJMoa042973

Domingueti, C. P., Dusse, L. M. S., Carvalho, M. D. G., De Sousa, L. P., Gomes, K. B., & Fernandes, A. P. (2016). Diabetes mellitus: The linkage between oxidative stress, inflammation, hypercoagulability and vascular complications. *Journal of Diabetes and Its Complications, 30*(4), 738–745. https://doi.org/10.1016/j.jdiacomp.2015.12.018

Drexel, H., Aczel, S., Marte, T., Benzer, W., Langer, P., Moll, W., & Saely, C. H. (2005). Is atherosclerosis in diabetes and impaired fasting glucose driven by elevated LDL cholesterol or by decreased HDL cholesterol? *Diabetes Care, 28*(1), 101–107. https://doi.org/10.2337/diacare.28.1.101

Duncan, J. G. (2011). Mitochondrial dysfunction in diabetic cardiomyopathy. *Biochimica et Biophysica Acta (BBA)—Molecular Cell Research, 1813*(7), 1351–1359. https://doi.org/10.1016/j.bbamcr.2011.01.014

El Mouhayyar, C., Riachy, R., Khalil, A. B., Eid, A., & Azar, S. (2020). SGLT2 inhibitors, GLP-1 agonists, and DPP-4 inhibitors in diabetes and microvascular complications: A review. *International Journal of Endocrinology, 2020*, 1–11. https://doi.org/10.1155/2020/1762164

Elafros, M. A., Andersen, H., Bennett, D. L., Savelieff, M. G., Viswanathan, V., Callaghan, B. C., & Feldman, E. L. (2022). Towards prevention of diabetic peripheral neuropathy: Clinical presentation, pathogenesis, and new treatments. *The Lancet Neurology, 21*(10), 922–936. https://doi.org/10.1016/S1474-4422(22)00188-0

El-Mesallamy, H. O., Hamdy, N. M., Salman, T. M., & Mahmoud, S. (2011). Adiponectin and E-selectin concentrations in relation to inflammation in obese type 2 diabetic patients with coronary heart disease(s). *Minerva Endocrinologica, 36*(3), 163–170.

Enders, J., Elliott, D., & Wright, D. E. (2023). Emerging nonpharmacologic interventions to treat diabetic peripheral neuropathy. *Antioxidants & Redox Signaling, 38*(13–15), 989–1000. https://doi.org/10.1089/ars.2022.0158

Engelgau, M. M., Narayan, K. M., & Herman, W. H. (2000). Screening for type 2 diabetes. *Diabetes Care, 23*(10), 1563–1580. https://doi.org/10.2337/diacare.23.10.1563

Fang, Z. Y., Prins, J. B., & Marwick, T. H. (2004). Diabetic cardiomyopathy: Evidence, mechanisms, and therapeutic implications. *Endocrine Reviews, 25*(4), 543–567. https://doi.org/10.1210/er.2003-0012

Feldman, E. L., Nave, K.-A., Jensen, T. S., & Bennett, D. L. H. (2017). New horizons in diabetic neuropathy: Mechanisms, bioenergetics, and pain. *Neuron, 93*(6), 1296–1313. https://doi.org/10.1016/j.neuron.2017.02.005

Forrest, K.Y.-Z., Becker, D. J., Kuller, L. H., Wolfson, S. K., & Orchard, T. J. (2000). Are predictors of coronary heart disease and lower-extremity arterial disease in type 1 diabetes the same? *Atherosclerosis, 148*(1), 159–169. https://doi.org/10.1016/S0021-9150(99)00217-8

Galicia-Garcia, U., Benito-Vicente, A., Jebari, S., Larrea-Sebal, A., Siddiqi, H., Uribe, K. B., Ostolaza, H., & Martín, C. (2020). Pathophysiology of type 2 diabetes mellitus. *International Journal of Molecular Sciences, 21*(17), 6275. https://doi.org/10.3390/ijms21176275

Gao, G., Li, Y., Zhang, D., Gee, S., Crosson, C., & Ma, J. (2001). Unbalanced expression of VEGF and PEDF in ischemia-induced retinal neovascularization. *FEBS Letters, 489*(2–3), 270–276. https://doi.org/10.1016/S0014-5793(01)02110-X

Garrison, A. (2015). Screening, diagnosis, and management of gestational diabetes mellitus. *American Family Physician, 91*(7), 460–467.

Gheith, O., Farouk, N., Nampoory, N., Halim, M. A., & Al-Otaibi, T. (2016). Diabetic kidney disease: World wide difference of prevalence and risk factors. *Journal of Nephropharmacology, 5*(1), 49–56.

Giacco, F., & Brownlee, M. (2010). Oxidative stress and diabetic complications. *Circulation Research, 107*(9), 1058–1070. https://doi.org/10.1161/CIRCRESAHA.110.223545

Goldberg, A. D., Allis, C. D., & Bernstein, E. (2007). Epigenetics: A landscape takes shape. *Cell, 128*(4), 635–638. https://doi.org/10.1016/j.cell.2007.02.006

Gonçalves, N. P., Vægter, C. B., Andersen, H., Østergaard, L., Calcutt, N. A., & Jensen, T. S. (2017). Schwann cell interactions with axons and microvessels in diabetic neuropathy. *Nature Reviews Neurology, 13*(3), 135–147. https://doi.org/10.1038/nrneurol.2016.201

Gross, J. L., De Azevedo, M. J., Silveiro, S. P., Canani, L. H., Caramori, M. L., & Zelmanovitz, T. (2005). Diabetic nephropathy: Diagnosis, prevention, and treatment. *Diabetes Care, 28*(1), 164–176. https://doi.org/10.2337/diacare.28.1.164

Gudala, K., Bansal, D., Schifano, F., & Bhansali, A. (2013). Diabetes mellitus and risk of dementia: A meta-analysis of prospective observational studies. *Journal of Diabetes Investigation, 4*(6), 640–650. https://doi.org/10.1111/jdi.12087

Gupta, N., Mansoor, S., Sharma, A., Sapkal, A., Sheth, J., Falatoonzadeh, P., Kuppermann, B., & Kenney, M. (2013). Diabetic retinopathy and VEGF. *The Open Ophthalmology Journal, 7*(1), 4–10. https://doi.org/10.2174/1874364101307010004

Hameed, I., Masoodi, S. R., Malik, P. A., Mir, S. A., Ghazanfar, K., & Ganai, B. A. (2018). Genetic variations in key inflammatory cytokines exacerbates the risk of diabetic nephropathy by influencing the gene expression. *Gene, 661*, 51–59. https://doi.org/10.1016/j.gene.2018.03.095

Hammes, H.-P. (2018). Diabetic retinopathy: Hyperglycaemia, oxidative stress and beyond. *Diabetologia, 61*(1), 29–38. https://doi.org/10.1007/s00125-017-4435-8

Han, E., Han, K., Lee, B.-W., Kang, E. S., Cha, B.-S., Ko, S.-H., & Lee, Y. (2022). Severe hypoglycemia increases dementia risk and related mortality: A nationwide, population-based cohort study. *The Journal of Clinical Endocrinology & Metabolism, 107*(5), e1976–e1986. https://doi.org/10.1210/clinem/dgab860

Handelsman, Y., Bloomgarden, Z. T., Grunberger, G., Umpierrez, G., Zimmerman, R. S., Bailey, T. S., Blonde, L., Bray, G. A., Cohen, A. J., Dagogo-Jack, S., Davidson, J. A., Einhorn, D., Ganda, O. P., Garber, A. J., Garvey, W. T., Henry, R. R., Hirsch, I. B., Horton, E. S., Hurley, D. L., & Zangeneh, F. (2015). American Association of Clinical Endocrinologists and American College of Endocrinology—Clinical practice guidelines for developing a diabetes mellitus comprehensive care plan—2015—Executive summary. *Endocrine Practice, 21*(4), 413–437. https://doi.org/10.4158/EP15672.GL

Hanewinckel, R., Van Oijen, M., Ikram, M. A., & Van Doorn, P. A. (2016). The epidemiology and risk factors of chronic polyneuropathy. *European Journal of Epidemiology, 31*(1), 5–20. https://doi.org/10.1007/s10654-015-0094-6

Hayden, M. R., & Tyagi, S. C. (2004). Vasa vasorum in plaque angiogenesis, metabolic syndrome, type 2 diabetes mellitus, and atheroscleropathy: A malignant transformation. *Cardiovascular Diabetology, 3*(1), 1. https://doi.org/10.1186/1475-2840-3-1

He, X., Ying, L., Ma, X., Shen, Y., Su, H., Peng, J., Wang, Y., Bao, Y., Zhou, J., & Jia, W. (2017). An additional measurement of glycated albumin can help prevent missed diagnosis of diabetes in Chinese population. *Clinica Chimica Acta, 475*, 188–192. https://doi.org/10.1016/j.cca.2017.10.018

Hendrie, H. C., Zheng, M., Li, W., Lane, K., Ambuehl, R., Purnell, C., Unverzagt, F. W., Torke, A., Balasubramanyam, A., Callahan, C. M., & Gao, S. (2017). Glucose level decline precedes dementia in elderly African Americans with diabetes. *Alzheimer's & Dementia, 13*(2), 111–118. https://doi.org/10.1016/j.jalz.2016.08.017

Hoke, A., Cerri, F., Fisgin, A., Riva, N., & Quattrini, A. (2021). Normal structure and pathological features in peripheral neuropathies. *Journal of the Peripheral Nervous System, 26*(S2). https://doi.org/10.1111/jns.12462

Hosszúfalusi, N., Vatay, Á., Rajczy, K., Prohászka, Z., Pozsonyi, É., Horváth, L., Grosz, A., Gerõ, L., Madácsy, L., Romics, L., Karádi, I., Füst, G., & Pánczél, P. (2003). Similar genetic features and different islet cell autoantibody pattern of Latent Autoimmune Diabetes in Adults (LADA) compared with adult-onset type 1 diabetes with rapid progression. *Diabetes Care, 26*(2), 452–457. https://doi.org/10.2337/diacare.26.2.452

Jaber, F. A., & James, J. W. (2023). Early prediction of diabetic using data mining. *SN Computer Science, 4*(2), 169. https://doi.org/10.1007/s42979-022-01594-z

Jaiswal, M., Divers, J., Dabelea, D., Isom, S., Bell, R. A., Martin, C. L., Pettitt, D. J., Saydah, S., Pihoker, C., Standiford, D. A., Dolan, L. M., Marcovina, S., Linder, B., Liese, A. D., Pop-Busui, R., & Feldman, E. L. (2017). Prevalence of and risk factors for diabetic peripheral neuropathy in youth with type 1 and type 2 diabetes: SEARCH for diabetes in youth study. *Diabetes Care, 40*(9), 1226–1232. https://doi.org/10.2337/dc17-0179

Jakus, V., & Rietbrock, N. (2004). Advanced glycation end-products and the progress of diabetic vascular complications. *Physiological Research, 53*(2), 131–142.

Janghorbani, M., Rezvanian, H., Kachooei, A., Ghorbani, A., Chitsaz, A., Izadi, F., & Amini, M. (2006). Peripheral neuropathy in type 2 diabetes mellitus in Isfahan, Iran: Prevalence and risk factors. *Acta Neurologica Scandinavica, 114*(6), 384–391. https://doi.org/10.1111/j.1600-0404.2006.00716.x

Janssen, L. M. M., Hiligsmann, M., Elissen, A. M. J., Joore, M. A., Schaper, N. C., Bosma, J. H. A., Stehouwer, C. D. A., Sep, S. J. S., Koster, A., Schram, M. T., & Evers, S. M. A. A. (2020). Burden of disease of type 2 diabetes mellitus: Cost of illness and quality of life estimated using the Maastricht Study. *Diabetic Medicine, 37*(10), 1759–1765. https://doi.org/10.1111/dme.14285

Jax, T. W. (2010). Metabolic memory: A vascular perspective. *Cardiovascular Diabetology, 9*(1), 51. https://doi.org/10.1186/1475-2840-9-51

Jeffcoate, W. J., Vileikyte, L., Boyko, E. J., Armstrong, D. G., & Boulton, A. J. M. (2018). Current challenges and opportunities in the prevention and management of diabetic foot ulcers. *Diabetes Care, 41*(4), 645–652. https://doi.org/10.2337/dc17-1836

Jensen, T. S., Karlsson, P., Gylfadottir, S. S., Andersen, S. T., Bennett, D. L., Tankisi, H., Finnerup, N. B., Terkelsen, A. J., Khan, K., Themistocleous, A. C., Kristensen, A. G., Itani, M., Sindrup, S. H., Andersen, H., Charles, M., Feldman, E. L., & Callaghan, B. C. (2021). Painful and non-painful diabetic neuropathy, diagnostic challenges and implications for future management. *Brain, 144*(6), 1632–1645. https://doi.org/10.1093/brain/awab079

Jia, G., Hill, M. A., & Sowers, J. R. (2018). Diabetic cardiomyopathy: An update of mechanisms contributing to this clinical entity. *Circulation Research, 122*(4), 624–638. https://doi.org/10.1161/CIRCRESAHA.117.311586

Johnson, J., Jaggers, R. M., Gopalkrishna, S., Dahdah, A., Murphy, A. J., Hanssen, N. M. J., & Nagareddy, P. R. (2022). Oxidative stress in neutrophils: Implications for diabetic cardiovascular complications. *Antioxidants & Redox Signaling, 36*(10–12), 652–666. https://doi.org/10.1089/ars.2021.0116

Kalofoutis, C., Piperi, C., Kalofoutis, A., Harris, F., Phoenix, D., & Singh, J. (2007). Type II diabetes mellitus and cardiovascular risk factors: Current therapeutic approaches. *Experimental and Clinical Cardiology, 12*(1), 17–28.

Kalousová, M., Skrha, J., & Zima, T. (2002). Advanced glycation end-products and advanced oxidation protein products in patients with diabetes mellitus. *Physiological Research, 51*(6), 597–604.

Kato, M., & Natarajan, R. (2014). Diabetic nephropathy—Emerging epigenetic mechanisms. *Nature Reviews Nephrology, 10*(9), 517–530. https://doi.org/10.1038/nrneph.2014.116

Kilhovd, B. K., Berg, T. J., Birkeland, K. I., Thorsby, P., & Hanssen, K. F. (1999). Serum levels of advanced glycation end products are increased in patients with type 2 diabetes and coronary heart disease. *Diabetes Care, 22*(9), 1543–1548. https://doi.org/10.2337/diacare.22.9.1543

Kim, S. S., Song, S. H., Kim, I. J., Kim, W. J., Jeon, Y. K., Kim, B. H., Kwak, I. S., Lee, E. K., & Kim, Y. K. (2014). Nonalbuminuric proteinuria as a biomarker for tubular damage in early development of nephropathy with type 2 diabetic patients. *Diabetes/metabolism Research and Reviews, 30*(8), 736–741. https://doi.org/10.1002/dmrr.2546

Kirkman, M. S., Briscoe, V. J., Clark, N., Florez, H., Haas, L. B., Halter, J. B., Huang, E. S., Korytkowski, M. T., Munshi, M. N., Odegard, P. S., Pratley, R. E., & Swift, C. S. (2012). Diabetes in older adults. *Diabetes Care, 35*(12), 2650–2664. https://doi.org/10.2337/dc12-1801

Koga, M., & Kasayama, S. (2010). Clinical impact of glycated albumin as another glycemic control marker. *Endocrine Journal, 57*(9), 751–762. https://doi.org/10.1507/endocrj.K10E-138

Kullo, I. J., & Rooke, T. W. (2016). Peripheral artery disease. *New England Journal of Medicine, 374*(9), 861–871. https://doi.org/10.1056/NEJMcp1507631

Laakso, M. (2011). Heart in diabetes: A microvascular disease. *Diabetes Care, 34*(Supplement_2), S145–S149. https://doi.org/10.2337/dc11-s209

Lapolla, A., Mosca, A., & Fedele, D. (2011). The general use of glycated haemoglobin for the diagnosis of diabetes and other categories of glucose intolerance: Still a long way to go. *Nutrition, Metabolism and Cardiovascular Diseases, 21*(7), 467–475. https://doi.org/10.1016/j.numecd.2011.02.006

Lee, S.-Y., & Choi, M. E. (2015). Urinary biomarkers for early diabetic nephropathy: Beyond albuminuria. *Pediatric Nephrology, 30*(7), 1063–1075. https://doi.org/10.1007/s00467-014-2888-2

Leibson, C. L., Rocca, W. A., Hanson, V. A., Cha, R., Kokmen, E., O'Brien, P. C., & Palumbo, P. J. (1997). Risk of dementia among persons with diabetes mellitus: A population-based cohort study. *American Journal of Epidemiology, 145*(4), 301–308. https://doi.org/10.1093/oxfordjournals.aje.a009106

Li, J., Guan, R., & Pan, L. (2023a). Mechanism of Schwann cells in diabetic peripheral neuropathy: A review. *Medicine, 102*(1), Article e32653. https://doi.org/10.1097/MD.0000000000032653

Li, Y., Liu, Y., Liu, S., Gao, M., Wang, W., Chen, K., Huang, L., & Liu, Y. (2023b). Diabetic vascular diseases: Molecular mechanisms and therapeutic strategies. *Signal Transduction and Targeted Therapy, 8*(1), 152. https://doi.org/10.1038/s41392-023-01400-z

Liu, C., Ge, H.-M., Liu, B.-H., Dong, R., Shan, K., Chen, X., Yao, M.-D., Li, X.-M., Yao, J., Zhou, R.-M., Zhang, S.-J., Jiang, Q., Zhao, C., & Yan, B. (2019). Targeting pericyte–Endothelial cell crosstalk by circular RNA-cPWWP2A inhibition aggravates diabetes-induced microvascular dysfunction. *Proceedings of the National Academy of Sciences, 116*(15), 7455–7464. https://doi.org/10.1073/pnas.1814874116

Liu, Y., Shao, S., & Guo, H. (2020). Schwann cells apoptosis is induced by high glucose in diabetic peripheral neuropathy. *Life Sciences, 248*, Article 117459. https://doi.org/10.1016/j.lfs.2020.117459

Luzi, L., Massarini, S., Ferrulli, A., Senesi, P., Carruba, M., Romano, C., Di Lembo, S., Bianchi, M., Bulgheroni, P., Villa, M., Serra, F., & Lenzi, A. (2024). Urban diabetes: Analysis of diabetes prevalence in cities of the Lombardy region participating in the cities changing diabetes project. *Acta Diabetologica, 61*(12), 1569–1576. https://doi.org/10.1007/s00592-024-02324-y

Magee, C., Grieve, D. J., Watson, C. J., & Brazil, D. P. (2017). Diabetic nephropathy: A tangled web to unweave. *Cardiovascular Drugs and Therapy, 31*(5–6), 579–592. https://doi.org/10.1007/s10557-017-6755-9

Magliano, D. J., Boyko, E. J., & IDF Diabetes Atlas 10th Edition Scientific Committee. (2021). *IDF diabetes atlas* (10th ed.). International Diabetes Federation. http://www.ncbi.nlm.nih.gov/books/NBK581934/

Malkani, S., & Mordes, J. P. (2011). Implications of using hemoglobin A1C for diagnosing diabetes mellitus. *The American Journal of Medicine, 124*(5), 395–401. https://doi.org/10.1016/j.amjmed.2010.11.025

Maniruzzaman, M., Rahman, Md. J., Ahammed, B., & Abedin, Md. M. (2020). Classification and prediction of diabetes disease using machine learning paradigm. *Health Information Science and Systems, 8*(1), 7. https://doi.org/10.1007/s13755-019-0095-z

Mann, D. M., Bertoni, A. G., Shimbo, D., Carnethon, M. R., Chen, H., Jenny, N. S., & Muntner, P. (2010). Comparative validity of 3 diabetes mellitus risk prediction scoring models in a multiethnic US cohort: The multi-ethnic study of atherosclerosis. *American Journal of Epidemiology, 171*(9), 980–988. https://doi.org/10.1093/aje/kwq030

Marso, S. P., & Hiatt, W. R. (2006). Peripheral arterial disease in patients with diabetes. *Journal of the American College of Cardiology, 47*(5), 921–929. https://doi.org/10.1016/j.jacc.2005.09.065

Marwick, T. H., Ritchie, R., Shaw, J. E., & Kaye, D. (2018). Implications of underlying mechanisms for the recognition and management of diabetic cardiomyopathy. *Journal of the American College of Cardiology, 71*(3), 339–351. https://doi.org/10.1016/j.jacc.2017.11.019

Mayeda, E. R., Whitmer, R. A., & Yaffe, K. (2015). Diabetes and cognition. *Clinics in Geriatric Medicine, 31*(1), 101–115. https://doi.org/10.1016/j.cger.2014.08.021

Modrak, M., Talukder, M. A. H., Gurgenashvili, K., Noble, M., & Elfar, J. C. (2020). Peripheral nerve injury and myelination: Potential therapeutic strategies. *Journal of Neuroscience Research, 98*(5), 780–795. https://doi.org/10.1002/jnr.24538

Mohammed Faheem, N., & El Askary, A. (2017). Neuroprotective role of curcumin on the hippocampus against the structural and serological alterations of streptozotocin-induced diabetes in sprague dawely rats. *Iranian Journal of Basic Medical Sciences, 20*(6). https://doi.org/10.22038/ijbms.2017.8839

Nathan, D. M. (1993). Long-term complications of diabetes mellitus. *New England Journal of Medicine, 328*(23), 1676–1685. https://doi.org/10.1056/NEJM199306103282306

Ni, W., Tang, L., & Wei, W. (2015). Research progress in signalling pathway in diabetic nephropathy. *Diabetes/metabolism Research and Reviews, 31*(3), 221–233. https://doi.org/10.1002/dmrr.2568

Nickerson, H. D., & Dutta, S. (2012). Diabetic complications: Current challenges and opportunities. *Journal of Cardiovascular Translational Research, 5*(4), 375–379. https://doi.org/10.1007/s12265-012-9388-1

Nkonge, K. M., Nkonge, D. K., & Nkonge, T. N. (2023). Screening for diabetic peripheral neuropathy in resource-limited settings. *Diabetology & Metabolic Syndrome, 15*(1), 55. https://doi.org/10.1186/s13098-023-01032-x

Nomura, K., Saitoh, T., Kim, G. U., & Yamanouchi, T. (2011). Glycemic profiles of healthy individuals with low fasting plasma glucose and HbA1c. *ISRN Endocrinology, 2011*, 1–6. https://doi.org/10.5402/2011/435047

Orasanu, G., & Plutzky, J. (2009). The pathologic continuum of diabetic vascular disease. *Journal of the American College of Cardiology, 53*(5), S35–S42. https://doi.org/10.1016/j.jacc.2008.09.055

Oshitari, T. (2021). The pathogenesis and therapeutic approaches of diabetic neuropathy in the retina. *International Journal of Molecular Sciences, 22*(16), 9050. https://doi.org/10.3390/ijms22169050

Otsuka, A., Azuma, K., Iesaki, T., Sato, F., Hirose, T., Shimizu, T., Tanaka, Y., Daida, H., Kawamori, R., & Watada, H. (2005). Temporary hyperglycaemia provokes monocyte adhesion to endothelial cells in rat thoracic aorta. *Diabetologia, 48*(12), 2667–2674. https://doi.org/10.1007/s00125-005-0005-6

Ott, A., Stolk, R. P., Van Harskamp, F., Pols, H. A. P., Hofman, A., & Breteler, M. M. B. (1999). Diabetes mellitus and the risk of dementia: The Rotterdam study. *Neurology, 53*(9), 1937–1937. https://doi.org/10.1212/WNL.53.9.1937

Palmer, J. P., & Hirsch, I. B. (2003). What's in a name: Latent autoimmune diabetes of adults, type 1.5, adult-onset, and type 1 diabetes. *Diabetes Care, 26*(2), 536–538. https://doi.org/10.2337/diacare.26.2.536

Palomer, X., Pizarro-Delgado, J., & Vázquez-Carrera, M. (2018). Emerging actors in diabetic cardiomyopathy: Heartbreaker biomarkers or therapeutic targets? *Trends in Pharmacological Sciences, 39*(5), 452–467. https://doi.org/10.1016/j.tips.2018.02.010

Patel, P., & Macerollo, A. (2010). Diabetes mellitus: Diagnosis and screening. *American Family Physician, 81*(7), 863–870.

Perkins, B. A., Ficociello, L. H., Roshan, B., Warram, J. H., & Krolewski, A. S. (2010). In patients with type 1 diabetes and new-onset microalbuminuria the development of advanced chronic kidney disease may not require progression to proteinuria. *Kidney International, 77*(1), 57–64. https://doi.org/10.1038/ki.2009.399

Peters, E. J. G., Armstrong, D. G., & Lavery, L. A. (2007). Risk factors for recurrent diabetic foot ulcers. *Diabetes Care, 30*(8), 2077–2079. https://doi.org/10.2337/dc07-0445

Phoenix, A., Chandran, R., & Ergul, A. (2022). Cerebral microvascular senescence and inflammation in diabetes. *Frontiers in Physiology, 13*, Article 864758. https://doi.org/10.3389/fphys.2022.864758

Picón, M. J., Murri, M., Muñoz, A., Fernández-García, J. C., Gomez-Huelgas, R., & Tinahones, F. J. (2012). Hemoglobin A1c versus oral glucose tolerance test in postpartum diabetes screening. *Diabetes Care, 35*(8), 1648–1653. https://doi.org/10.2337/dc11-2111

Pippitt, K., Li, M., & Gurgle, H. E. (2016). Diabetes mellitus: Screening and diagnosis. *American Family Physician, 93*(2), 103–109.

Pop-Busui, R., Boulton, A. J. M., Feldman, E. L., Bril, V., Freeman, R., Malik, R. A., Sosenko, J. M., & Ziegler, D. (2017). Diabetic neuropathy: A position statement by the American Diabetes Association. *Diabetes Care, 40*(1), 136–154. https://doi.org/10.2337/dc16-2042

Raghav, A., & Ahmad, J. (2014). Glycated serum albumin: A potential disease marker and an intermediate index of diabetes control. *Diabetes & Metabolic Syndrome: Clinical Research & Reviews, 8*(4), 245–251. https://doi.org/10.1016/j.dsx.2014.09.017

Raile, K., Galler, A., Hofer, S., Herbst, A., Dunstheimer, D., Busch, P., & Holl, R. W. (2007). Diabetic nephropathy in 27,805 children, adolescents, and adults with type 1 diabetes. *Diabetes Care, 30*(10), 2523–2528. https://doi.org/10.2337/dc07-0282

Ramachandran, A. (2014). Know the signs and symptoms of diabetes. *The Indian Journal of Medical Research, 140*(5), 579–581.

Ramos, R., Quesada, M., Solanas, P., Subirana, I., Sala, J., Vila, J., Masiá, R., Cerezo, C., Elosua, R., Grau, M., Cordón, F., Juvinyà, D., Fitó, M., Isabel Covas, M., Clarà, A., Ángel Muñoz, M., & Marrugat, J. (2009). Prevalence of symptomatic and asymptomatic peripheral arterial disease and the value of the ankle-brachial index to stratify cardiovascular risk. *European Journal of Vascular and Endovascular Surgery, 38*(3), 305–311. https://doi.org/10.1016/j.ejvs.2009.04.013

Reddy, M. A., Zhang, E., & Natarajan, R. (2015). Epigenetic mechanisms in diabetic complications and metabolic memory. *Diabetologia, 58*(3), 443–455. https://doi.org/10.1007/s00125-014-3462-y

Ribet, F., Stemme, G., & Roxhed, N. (2017). Ultra-miniaturization of a planar amperometric sensor targeting continuous intradermal glucose monitoring. *Biosensors and Bioelectronics, 90*, 577–583. https://doi.org/10.1016/j.bios.2016.10.007

Roy, S., Sala, R., Cagliero, E., & Lorenzi, M. (1990). Overexpression of fibronectin induced by diabetes or high glucose: Phenomenon with a memory. *Proceedings of the National Academy of Sciences, 87*(1), 404–408. https://doi.org/10.1073/pnas.87.1.404

Salinas, R. M., Hiriart, M., Acosta, I., Sosa, A. L., & Prince, M. J. (2016). Type 2 diabetes mellitus as a risk factor for dementia in a Mexican population. *Journal of Diabetes and Its Complications, 30*(7), 1234–1239. https://doi.org/10.1016/j.jdiacomp.2016.06.005

Schmidt, A. M., Hori, O., Brett, J., Yan, S. D., Wautier, J. L., & Stern, D. (1994). Cellular receptors for advanced glycation end products. Implications for induction of oxidant stress and cellular dysfunction in the pathogenesis of vascular lesions. *Arteriosclerosis and Thrombosis: A Journal of Vascular Biology, 14*(10), 1521–1528. https://doi.org/10.1161/01.ATV.14.10.1521

Schratzberger, P., Walter, D. H., Rittig, K., Bahlmann, F. H., Pola, R., Curry, C., Silver, M., Krainin, J. G., Weinberg, D. H., Ropper, A. H., & Isner, J. M. (2001). Reversal of experimental diabetic neuropathy by VEGF gene transfer. *Journal of Clinical Investigation, 107*(9), 1083–1092. https://doi.org/10.1172/JCI12188

Selph, S., Dana, T., Blazina, I., Bougatsos, C., Patel, H., & Chou, R. (2015). Screening for type 2 diabetes mellitus: A systematic review for the U.S. preventive services task force. *Annals of Internal Medicine, 162*(11), 765–776. https://doi.org/10.7326/M14-2221

Shaw, J. E., Sicree, R. A., & Zimmet, P. Z. (2010). Global estimates of the prevalence of diabetes for 2010 and 2030. *Diabetes Research and Clinical Practice, 87*(1), 4–14. https://doi.org/10.1016/j.diabres.2009.10.007

Sheffield, J. (2002). Maternal diabetes mellitus and infant malformations. *Obstetrics & Gynecology, 100*(5), 925–930. https://doi.org/10.1016/S0029-7844(02)02242-1

Sloan, G., Selvarajah, D., & Tesfaye, S. (2021). Pathogenesis, diagnosis and clinical management of diabetic sensorimotor peripheral neuropathy. *Nature Reviews Endocrinology, 17*(7), 400–420. https://doi.org/10.1038/s41574-021-00496-z

Sloan, G., Shillo, P., Selvarajah, D., Wu, J., Wilkinson, I. D., Tracey, I., Anand, P., & Tesfaye, S. (2018). A new look at painful diabetic neuropathy. *Diabetes Research and Clinical Practice, 144*, 177–191. https://doi.org/10.1016/j.diabres.2018.08.020

Song, J., Bai, H., Xu, H., Xing, Y., & Chen, S. (2022). HbA1c variability and the risk of dementia in patients with diabetes: A meta-analysis. *International Journal of Clinical Practice, 2022*(1), 7706330. https://doi.org/10.1155/2022/7706330

Song, P., Rudan, D., Zhu, Y., Fowkes, F. J. I., Rahimi, K., Fowkes, F. G. R., & Rudan, I. (2019). Global, regional, and national prevalence and risk factors for peripheral artery disease in 2015: An updated systematic review and analysis. *The Lancet. Global Health, 7*(8), e1020–e1030. https://doi.org/10.1016/S2214-109X(19)30255-4

Soyoye, D. O., Abiodun, O. O., Ikem, R. T., Kolawole, B. A., & Akintomide, A. O. (2021). Diabetes and peripheral artery disease: A review. *World Journal of Diabetes, 12*(6), 827–838. https://doi.org/10.4239/wjd.v12.i6.827

Soyoye, D. O., Ikem, R. T., Kolawole, B. A., Oluwadiya, K. S., Bolarinwa, R. A., & Adebayo, O. J. (2016). Prevalence and correlates of peripheral arterial disease in Nigerians with type 2 diabetes. *Advances in Medicine, 2016*, 1–6. https://doi.org/10.1155/2016/3529419

Sulaiman, M. K. (2019). Diabetic nephropathy: Recent advances in pathophysiology and challenges in dietary management. *Diabetology & Metabolic Syndrome, 11*(1), 7. https://doi.org/10.1186/s13098-019-0403-4

Sumner, A. E., Duong, M. T., Aldana, P. C., Ricks, M., Tulloch-Reid, M. K., Lozier, J. N., Chung, S. T., & Sacks, D. B. (2016). A1C combined with glycated albumin improves detection of prediabetes in Africans: The Africans in America study. *Diabetes Care, 39*(2), 271–277. https://doi.org/10.2337/dc15-1699

Syed Ikmal, S. I. Q., Zaman Huri, H., Vethakkan, S. R., & Wan Ahmad, W. A. (2013). Potential biomarkers of insulin resistance and atherosclerosis in type 2 diabetes mellitus patients with coronary artery disease. *International Journal of Endocrinology, 2013*, 1–11. https://doi.org/10.1155/2013/698567

Takahashi, P., Xavier, D. J., Lima, J. E. B. F., Evangelista, A. F., Collares, C. V. A., Foss-Freitas, M. C., Rassi, D. M., Donadi, E. A., Passos, G. A., & Sakamoto-Hojo, E. T. (2022). Transcript expression profiles and MicroRNA regulation indicate an upregulation of processes linked to oxidative stress, DNA repair, cell death, and inflammation in type 1 diabetes mellitus patients. *Journal of Diabetes Research, 2022*, 1–15. https://doi.org/10.1155/2022/3511329

Takeshita, Y., Sato, R., & Kanda, T. (2020). Blood-Nerve Barrier (BNB) pathology in diabetic peripheral neuropathy and in vitro human BNB model. *International Journal of Molecular Sciences, 22*(1), 62. https://doi.org/10.3390/ijms22010062

Teo, Z. L., Tham, Y.-C., Yu, M., Chee, M. L., Rim, T. H., Cheung, N., Bikbov, M. M., Wang, Y. X., Tang, Y., Lu, Y., Wong, I. Y., Ting, D. S. W., Tan, G. S. W., Jonas, J. B., Sabanayagam, C., Wong, T. Y., & Cheng, C.-Y. (2021). Global prevalence of diabetic retinopathy and projection of burden through 2045. *Ophthalmology, 128*(11), 1580–1591. https://doi.org/10.1016/j.ophtha.2021.04.027

Teodoro, J. S., Nunes, S., Rolo, A. P., Reis, F., & Palmeira, C. M. (2019). Therapeutic options targeting oxidative stress, mitochondrial dysfunction and inflammation to hinder the progression of vascular complications of diabetes. *Frontiers in Physiology, 9*, 1857. https://doi.org/10.3389/fphys.2018.01857

Tervaert, T. W. C., Mooyaart, A. L., Amann, K., Cohen, A. H., Cook, H. T., Drachenberg, C. B., Ferrario, F., Fogo, A. B., Haas, M., De Heer, E., Joh, K., Noël, L. H., Radhakrishnan, J., Seshan, S. V., Bajema, I. M., & Bruijn, J. A. (2010). Pathologic classification of diabetic nephropathy. *Journal of the American Society of Nephrology, 21*(4), 556–563. https://doi.org/10.1681/ASN.2010010010

Tian, J., Hu, S., Sun, Y., Yu, H., Han, X., Cheng, W., Ban, X., Zhang, S., Yu, B., & Jang, I.-K. (2013). Vasa vasorum and plaque progression, and responses to atorvastatin in a rabbit model of atherosclerosis: Contrast-enhanced ultrasound imaging and intravascular ultrasound study. *Heart, 99*(1), 48–54. https://doi.org/10.1136/heartjnl-2012-302775

Tommerdahl, K. L., Shapiro, A. L. B., Nehus, E. J., & Bjornstad, P. (2022). Early microvascular complications in type 1 and type 2 diabetes: Recent developments and updates. *Pediatric Nephrology, 37*(1), 79–93. https://doi.org/10.1007/s00467-021-05050-7

Toyoshima, M. T. K., Cukier, P., Damascena, A. S., Batista, R. L., De Azevedo Correa, F., Zanatta Kawahara, E., Minanni, C. A., Hoff, A. O., & Nery, M. (2023). Fructosamine and glycated hemoglobin as biomarkers of glycemic control in people with type 2 diabetes mellitus and cancer (GlicoOnco study). *Clinics, 78*, Article 100240. https://doi.org/10.1016/j.clinsp.2023.100240

Vigersky, R. A., Fonda, S. J., Chellappa, M., Walker, M. S., & Ehrhardt, N. M. (2012). Short- and long-term effects of real-time continuous glucose monitoring in patients with type 2 diabetes. *Diabetes Care, 35*(1), 32–38. https://doi.org/10.2337/dc11-1438

Vitova, L., Tuma, Z., Moravec, J., Kvapil, M., Matejovic, M., & Mares, J. (2017). Early urinary biomarkers of diabetic nephropathy in type 1 diabetes mellitus show involvement of kallikrein-kinin system. *BMC Nephrology, 18*(1), 112. https://doi.org/10.1186/s12882-017-0519-4

Wang, M., Li, Y., Li, S., & Lv, J. (2022). Endothelial dysfunction and diabetic cardiomyopathy. *Frontiers in Endocrinology, 13*, Article 851941. https://doi.org/10.3389/fendo.2022.851941

Wang, Z., Zhang, N., Lin, P., Xing, Y., & Yang, N. (2024). Recent advances in the treatment and delivery system of diabetic retinopathy. *Frontiers in Endocrinology, 15*, 1347864. https://doi.org/10.3389/fendo.2024.1347864

Weragoda, J., Seneviratne, R., Weerasinghe, M. C., & Wijeyaratne, S. (2016). Risk factors of peripheral arterial disease: A case control study in Sri Lanka. *BMC Research Notes, 9*(1), 508. https://doi.org/10.1186/s13104-016-2314-x

Wykoff, C. C. (2017). Impact of intravitreal pharmacotherapies including antivascular endothelial growth factor and corticosteroid agents on diabetic retinopathy. *Current Opinion in Ophthalmology, 28*(3), 213–218. https://doi.org/10.1097/ICU.0000000000000364

Xie, L., Xiao, Y., Tai, S., Yang, H., Zhou, S., & Zhou, Z. (2022). Emerging roles of Sodium Glucose Cotransporter 2 (SGLT-2) inhibitors in diabetic cardiovascular diseases: Focusing on immunity, inflammation and metabolism. *Frontiers in Pharmacology, 13*, Article 836849. https://doi.org/10.3389/fphar.2022.836849

Xie, L., Zhu, X., Hu, Y., Li, T., Gao, Y., Shi, Y., & Tang, S. (2008). Mitochondrial DNA oxidative damage triggering mitochondrial dysfunction and apoptosis in high glucose-induced HRECs. *Investigative Opthalmology & Visual Science, 49*(9), 4203. https://doi.org/10.1167/iovs.07-1364

Xu, J., Lu, X., & Shi, G.-P. (2015). Vasa vasorum in atherosclerosis and clinical significance. *International Journal of Molecular Sciences, 16*(5), 11574–11608. https://doi.org/10.3390/ijms160511574

Xue, M., Xu, W., Ou, Y.-N., Cao, X.-P., Tan, M.-S., Tan, L., & Yu, J.-T. (2019). Diabetes mellitus and risks of cognitive impairment and dementia: A systematic review and meta-analysis of 144 prospective studies. *Ageing Research Reviews, 55*, Article 100944. https://doi.org/10.1016/j.arr.2019.100944

Yang, T., Qi, F., Guo, F., Shao, M., Song, Y., Ren, G., Linlin, Z., Qin, G., & Zhao, Y. (2024). An update on chronic complications of diabetes mellitus: From molecular mechanisms to therapeutic strategies with a focus on metabolic memory. *Molecular Medicine, 30*(1), 71. https://doi.org/10.1186/s10020-024-00824-9

Yazdanpanah, S., Rabiee, M., Tahriri, M., Abdolrahim, M., Rajab, A., Jazayeri, H. E., & Tayebi, L. (2017). Evaluation of glycated albumin (GA) and GA/HbA1c ratio for diagnosis of diabetes and glycemic control: A comprehensive review. *Critical Reviews in Clinical Laboratory Sciences, 54*(4), 219–232. https://doi.org/10.1080/10408363.2017.1299684

Yu, J.-T., Xu, W., Tan, C.-C., Andrieu, S., Suckling, J., Evangelou, E., Pan, A., Zhang, C., Jia, J., Feng, L., Kua, E.-H., Wang, Y.-J., Wang, H.-F., Tan, M.-S., Li, J.-Q., Hou, X.-H., Wan, Y., Tan, L., Mok, V., & Vellas, B. (2020). Evidence-based prevention of Alzheimer's disease: Systematic review and meta-analysis of 243 observational prospective studies and 153 randomised controlled trials. *Journal of Neurology, Neurosurgery & Psychiatry, 91*(11), 1201–1209. https://doi.org/10.1136/jnnp-2019-321913

Zhan, J., Jin, K., Ding, N., Zhou, Y., Hu, G., Yuan, S., Xie, R., Wen, Z., Chen, C., Li, H., & Wang, D. W. (2023). Positive feedback loop of miR-320 and CD36 regulates the hyperglycemic memory-induced diabetic diastolic cardiac dysfunction. *Molecular Therapy—Nucleic Acids, 31*, 122–138. https://doi.org/10.1016/j.omtn.2022.12.009

Zhang, J., Liu, J., & Qin, X. (2018). Advances in early biomarkers of diabetic nephropathy. *Revista Da Associação Médica Brasileira, 64*(1), 85–92. https://doi.org/10.1590/1806-9282.64.01.85

Zhang, J., Zhang, Z., Zhang, K., Ge, X., Sun, R., & Zhai, X. (2023). Early detection of type 2 diabetes risk: Limitations of current diagnostic criteria. *Frontiers in Endocrinology, 14*, 1260623. https://doi.org/10.3389/fendo.2023.1260623

Zhang, Y., Lazzarini, P. A., McPhail, S. M., Van Netten, J. J., Armstrong, D. G., & Pacella, R. E. (2020). Global disability burdens of diabetes-related lower-extremity complications in 1990 and 2016. *Diabetes Care, 43*(5), 964–974. https://doi.org/10.2337/dc19-1614

Zheng, Y., Ley, S. H., & Hu, F. B. (2018). Global aetiology and epidemiology of type 2 diabetes mellitus and its complications. *Nature Reviews Endocrinology, 14*(2), 88–98. https://doi.org/10.1038/nrendo.2017.151

Zhu, J., Hu, Z., Luo, Y., Liu, Y., Luo, W., Du, X., Luo, Z., Hu, J., & Peng, S. (2024). Diabetic peripheral neuropathy: Pathogenetic mechanisms and treatment. *Frontiers in Endocrinology, 14*, 1265372. https://doi.org/10.3389/fendo.2023.1265372

Ziegler, D., Papanas, N., Schnell, O., Nguyen, B. D. T., Nguyen, K. T., Kulkantrakorn, K., & Deerochanawong, C. (2021). Current concepts in the management of diabetic polyneuropathy. *Journal of Diabetes Investigation, 12*(4), 464–475. https://doi.org/10.1111/jdi.13401

Chapter 3
Nerve Under Siege: Managing Diabetic Neuropathy and Pain

Shahnaz Alom, Farak Ali, Md. Abubakar, Samiksha Yogi, and Hans Raj Bhat

Abstract Diabetic neuropathy is a painful consequence of diabetes mellitus that affects millions of people. It is characterized by nerve injury resulting from elevated blood glucose levels. Numerous symptoms, including pain, numbness, muscular weakness, autonomic dysfunction, and foot ulcers, may be brought on by diabetic neuropathy, which can seriously impact a person's quality of life. According to estimates, the incidence of neuropathy is above 50% in patients with chronic illness and around 8% in people with a recent diagnosis. Sensorimotor and autonomic neuropathies are the two most common forms of diabetic neuropathy. Pain, paraesthesia, and a lack of sensation are symptoms of sensorimotor neuropathy, while myocardial infarction, arrhythmia, and unexpected death are symptoms of autonomic neuropathy. In addition to glycaemic management, there is no other treatment for preventing sensorimotor and autonomic neuropathies. Patients with cardiovascular autonomic neuropathy should undergo extensive diabetic treatment, multifactorial cardiovascular risk reduction, and lifestyle modification. Tricyclic antidepressants, serotonin and norepinephrine reuptake inhibitors, gabapentin, pregabalin, and opioids are used to alleviate sensory neuropathy. The goal of this chapter is to provide a comprehensive analysis of the pathophysiology of diabetic neuropathy, along with a discussion of the underlying molecular mechanisms and pathways. This includes

Shahnaz Alom, Farak Ali, Md. Abubakar—These authors are equally contributed.

S. Alom · F. Ali
Girijananda Chowdhury Institute of Pharmaceutical Science, Girijananda Chowdhury University-Tezpur Campus, Tezpur 784501, India

S. Alom · F. Ali · H. R. Bhat (✉)
Department of Pharmaceutical Sciences, Faculty of Science and Engineering, Dibrugarh University, Dibrugarh 786004, India
e-mail: pharmahans@gmail.com

Md. Abubakar · S. Yogi
Department of Pharmacology and Toxicology, National Institute of Pharmaceutical Education and Research, Hajipur 844102, India

S. Yogi
Department of Surgery, School of Medicine, Washington University in St. Louis, St. Louis, MO, USA

K. Adhikary et al. (eds.), *Healing Beyond Blood Sugar*,
https://doi.org/10.1007/978-981-95-8946-3_3

the influence of hyperglycemiaon nerve function, aberrant glucose metabolism, the involvement of advanced glycation end products (AGEs), and inflammatory and immune-mediated processes.

Keywords Diabetes · Neuropathy · Autonomic neuropathies · Neuropathic pain · Hyperglycemia · Sensorimotor neuropathy

3.1 Introduction

A consequence of diabetes mellitus, diabetic neuropathy is brought on by the vascular and metabolic abnormalities linked to the disease. Research has shown that diabetic neuropathy develops in 50–66% of diabetes individuals with diabetes during the course of their condition (Strand et al., 2024). Autonomic dysfunction, muscle weakness, paresthesia, discomfort, and nerve injury are the hallmark symptoms of the disorder (Sloan et al., 2018). Peripheral sensory neuropathy, autonomic neuropathy, polyradiculopathy, polyneuropathy and mononeuropathy/focal neuropathy are some types of diabetic neuropathy (Deli et al., 2013; Pop-Busui et al., 2017; Sloan et al., 2018). When a person has diabetes, they are most likely to get peripheral sensorimotor neuropathy. Symptoms such as tingling, numbness, and discomfort are common and typically affect the lower extremities first (Pop-Busui et al., 2017). Several bodily systems, including those related to the heart and the gastrointestinal system, become dysregulated in individuals with autonomic neuropathy, characterized by a disruption of autonomic nerve activity (Moţăţăianu et al., 2018; Pop-Busui et al., 2017). Muscle weakness and soreness are symptoms of proximal neuropathy, which most often impacts the hip, thigh, and buttocks. Extreme pain and weak muscles may be symptoms of focal neuropathy, a condition characterized by the sudden onset of neurological impairments in specific nerves. To understand the pathogenesis of diabetic neuropathy and develop treatment planstailored to each patient's particular needs, accurate categorization of the condition is crucial (Strand et al., 2024). The effects of diabetic neuropathy go far beyond the symptoms themselves, and neuropathic pain may be experienced by 25–50% of those with the condition. As a result of crippling pain, limited mobility, and diminished emotional well-being, patients with diabetic neuropathy often encounter a significant decline in their quality of life. Patients' health-related quality of life is already reduced when neuropathic pain, which is usually characterized as a burning or stabbing sensation, becomes persistent and resistant to traditional therapies (Pop-Busui et al., 2017). Autonomic neuropathy makes things worse for those who already have it since it may lead to a lot of consequences, such as sexual dysfunction, gastroparesis, and orthostatic hypotension (Moţăţăianu et al., 2018). There is evidence that the incidence of orthostatic hypotension due to cardiovascular autonomic neuropathy might approach 50% after 15 years of having type 2 diabetes (Ang et al., 2014). It is crucial to comprehend the pathogenesis of diabetic neuropathy and develop effective treatments, as the disease significantly impacts a patient's physical, emotional, and social well-being (Strand et al., 2024). This article summarizes the current knowledge on the pathophysiology of diabetic neuropathy, a condition characterized by damage and dysfunction of the nervous system brought on by diabetes mellitus. This evidence review will cover factors at the molecular, cellular, and systemic levels that contribute to the onset and progression of diabetic neuropathy. Novel therapeutic strategies for diabetic neuropathy, based on its pathophysiological mechanisms, are also explored in this chapter. Additionally, this chapter aimed to guide the future of DN management by highlighting the existing problems and difficulties, particularly from the standpoint of the molecular pathways that contribute to its advancement.

3.2 Epidemiology

The prevalence of DN appears to be higher in individuals with type 2 diabetes (T2DM) compared to those with type 1 diabetes (T1DM), according to a previous study (Hicks & Selvin, 2019). For instance, adolescents with T2DM were much more likely to have DN than those with T1DM (26% vs. 8%, respectively) (Jaiswal et al., 2013). DN was found in 42% of individuals with T2DM at baseline in the ACCORD study, a seminal randomized trial evaluating the impact of glycemic therapies on microvascular complications (Ismail-Beigi et al., 2010). In contrast, the Diabetes Control and Complications Trial (DCCT) found that DN was present in only 6% of individuals with T1DM at baseline (Martin et al., 2014; The Diabetes Control & Complications Trial Research Group, 1993). There should be considerable care when comparing studies, given the significant variation in reported prevalence rates resulting from methodological and demographic variables (Smith et al., 2022a). For example, the average duration of diabetes at baseline in the ACCORD trial was 10 years, whereas in the DCCT it was six years. The Michigan Neuropathy Screening Instrument was employed to identify DN, whereas the DCCT relied on clinical evidence and nerve conduction investigations (Ismail-Beigi et al., 2010; Martin et al., 2014). Risk factors for DN were also found in these groundbreaking investigations. A total of 1,441 individuals with T1DM were followed for 14 years as part of the DCCT and its Epidemiology of Diabetes Interventions and Complications (EDIC) studies. Risk variables for DN, including age, duration of diabetes, and chronic hyperglycemia, increased the condition's incidence from 6% at baseline to 30% at final follow-up (Martin et al., 2014; The Diabetes Control & Complications Trial Research Group, 1993). Along with height, macroalbuminuria, pulse rate, beta-blocker usage, and persistent albuminuria, these risk variables were recently confirmed in a DCCT/EDIC data review (Braffett et al., 2020). Some of these results are supported by the Pittsburgh Epidemiology of Diabetes Complications research, which included 400 individuals with T1DM; 16% of those aged 18–29 had DN, compared to 58% of those aged 30 and higher (Maser et al., 1989). Previous longitudinal studies in Africa and Europe have also shown similar patterns (Barbosa et al., 2019; Jarso et al., 2011).

The increased frequency of DN in T2DM may be due to additional cardiometabolic risk factors such as central obesity, dyslipidemia, and hypertension (Callaghan et al., 2016, 2018). Due to their variability from standard T1DM and T2DM phenotypes, the World Health Organization has labelled additional diabetes subtypes as "hybrid" and "unclassified" (Smith et al., 2022b). Future research may look at stratifying these subtypes.

3.3 Forms of Diabetic Neuropathy

Diabetic neuropathy has been classified into many clinical conditions. The most prevalent type is a distal, symmetrical, predominantly sensory polyneuropathy that gradually worsens over time, primarily affecting the lower extremities, particularly the legs and feet. The other forms are listed below: Acute ophthalmoplegia affecting the third (and less frequently the sixth) cranial nerve on one side; acute mononeuropathy of the limbs or trunk, including a painful thoracolumbar radiculopathy; an acute or subacute painful, asymmetrical, primarily motor multiple neuropathy affecting the upper lumbar roots and the proximal leg muscles (diabetic amyotrophy); a more symmetrical, proximal motor weakness and wasting, typically without pain and with variable sensory loss, usually without pain and with variable sensory loss, following a subacute or chronic course; and an autonomic neuropathy involving bowel, bladder, sweating, and circulatory reflexes. Tables 3.1 and 3.2 show that several kinds of neuropathy, including subacute proximal neuropathies, autonomic and distal symmetrical neuropathies, and others, often coexist or overlap (Deli et al., 2013).

3.3.1 Sensorimotor Neuropathy

3.3.1.1 Diabetic Polyneuropathy in the Distal Sensory Nervous System

Up to 50% of diabetic patients may experience symptoms of the most common type of neuropathy, which can include burning pain, electrical or stabbing sensations, paresthesia, hyperesthesia, and intense deep pain (Boulton et al., 2005). In most cases, these symptoms worsen and disrupt sleep throughout the night. This, together with daytime unpleasant sensations, often reduces the individual's capacity to carry out everyday tasks (Tesfaye & Selvarajah, 2012). A lack of ankle reflexes, together with diminished or missing sensations of vibration, pressure, pain, and warmth (mediated by both large and tiny fibres), is a common finding when examining the lower limbs (Boulton et al., 2005; Deli et al., 2013). Although proximal weakness and atrophy may occur in some individuals, distal sensory neuropathy and moderate muscle weakness are more common in most patients. Interestingly, a diagnosis may only be determined by examination or, in rare instances, when a patient presents with

Table 3.1 Symptoms, diagnosis, and treatments of autonomic diabetic neuropathies (Boulton et al., 2005; Deli et al., 2013)

	Gastrointestinal complications	Cardiac complications	Sudomotor (skin) complications	Sexual complications	Pupillomotor complications	Bladder complications
Sign and symptoms	Dysregulation of glucose and gastroparesis, nausea, vomiting, early fullness, bloating, burp, or pain in the abdomen, constipation	Intolerance to exercise, early weariness, and weaknesses during exercise, vertigo, light-headedness, weakness, postural hypotension, exhaustion, and syncope	Hyperhidrosis, dry skin, anhidrosis, heat intolerance	Vaginal dryness, erectile dysfunction	Blurred vision, trouble adjusting to different lighting conditions, and a decrease in the ability to perceive subtle bodily sensations	Urinary retention, incontinence, frequency, urgency, and nocturia

(continued)

Table 3.1 (continued)

	Gastrointestinal complications	Cardiac complications	Sudomotor (skin) complications	Sexual complications	Pupillomotor complications	Bladder complications
Diagnosis	Endoscopy, manometry, gastric emptying study, barium study, and electrophysiology	123I-metaiodobenzylguanidine (MIBG) scan, heart rate variability (HRV), thallium scan, blood pressure measurements (both standing and supine), and catecholamine levels	Measurements of quantitative submotor axon reflex, perspiration, and cutaneous blood flow	Pap smear, nocturnal penile tumescence, penile-brachial pressure index, heart rate variability, and history and physical examination	Heart rate variability, pupillometry	Post-void sonography, cystometrogram
Treatment	Medications such as antibiotics, antiemetics (Phenergan, Compazine, Tangan, and scopolamine), prokinetic drugs (metoclopramide, domperidone, erythromycin), gastric pacing, pancreatic extracts, tricyclic antidepressants, and enteral feeds	A combination of angiotensin-converting enzyme inhibitors, beta-blockers, and graded supervised exercise, octreotide, clonidine, midodrine, and mechanical measures	Vasodilators, emollients, skin lubricants, botulinum toxin, glycopyrrolate, and scopolamine	Injection of prostaglandin E1, sex therapy, prosthesis or sexual device, psychiatric counselling, vardenafil, tadalafil, and sildenafil, vaginal lubricants	Driving at night with caution and identifying any odd myocardial infarction symptoms	Intermittent catheterization, Bethanechol

Table 3.2 Characteristics of various types of neuropathies that are disabling in diabetic patients (Attal et al., 2010; Deli et al., 2013)

Types	Pain	Distal symmetrical sensory loss	Sensory ataxia	Autonomic dysfunction	Weakness	Electrophysiological test	Progression	Nerve biopsy	CSF protein
CIPD	Occasional	The variable primarily focuses on proprioception	Common	Uncommon	Frequent, often severe proximal and distal	Demyelinated, mixed axonal	Weeks/ months	Demyelination and variable axon loss	Increased
LDP	Common in distal limbs	Length-dependent; primarily based on temperature and pain perceptions	Rare	Common	Distal symmetrical, minor weakness	Distal symmetrical, axonal pattern	Years	Severe damage to the axons	Variable
Focal/ MFDN	Common in most situations	Variable	Uncommon	Uncommon	Common, asymmetrical- in the root or nerve region	Multifocal, axonal pattern	Weeks/ months	Variable	Increased

* CIPD—Chronic inflammatory demyelinating polyneuropathy, LDP—Length-dependent polyneuropathy, MFDN—Multifocal diabetic neuropathy, CSF—cerebrospinal fluid

a painless foot ulcer (Boulton et al., 2005). This is because it is possible for up to half of the patients not to exhibit any symptoms. Painful neuropathy symptoms may affect as many as one-third of community-based diabetes patients (10–35%). Antiglycemic medication treatment, which includes insulin and hypoglycemic medications, may cause insulin neuritis, a type of small-fibre neuropathy that can cause pain and paresthesia in specific individuals early in their diabetes course (Bansal et al., 2006). Multiple sclerosis in diabetic patients with radiculopathies. These disorders are similar to mononeuropathies. Painful unilateral or asymmetrical multiple neuropathy syndrome is more common in elderly adults with mild or undiagnosed diabetes. The haphazard involvement of several nerves characterizes Mononeuritis multiplex. Like mononeuropathy, many nerves are involved in a sequential or atypical fashion, with the first nerve experiencing a sudden beginning. It is essential to distinguish between systemic vasculitis and nerve infarctions caused by blockage of the vasa nervosum (Bansal et al., 2006). Radiculoplexus neuropathies are a kind of diabetic illness that mainly affects people with moderate diabetes; they manifest subacutely with pain and weakness (Table 3.2). The three primary forms of diabetic radiculoplexus neuropathy involve the cervical plexus, the thoracic plexus, and the lumbar region of the spine (Tracy & Dyck, 2008). About one percent of people with diabetes may develop diabetic lumbosacral radiculoplexus neuropathy, which is likely the most dangerous kind of diabetic neuropathy (Pop-Busui, 2010; Tracy & Dyck, 2008). Diabetes polyradiculopathy, diabetic amyotrophy, diabetic mononeuritis multiplex, diabetic proximal neuropathy, Bruns-Garland syndrome, and others have been used to describe it (Tracy & Dyck, 2008). The pain, which may be very intense, typically begins in the hips or lower back and radiates down one side of the body to the thigh and knee. It's deep and agonizing, with sharp, stabbing pains that tend to be worst at night. Despite pain being the most severe symptom initially, the central issue is the weakening and atrophy of the muscles, most noticeably in the pelvic girdle and thighs, although it may also affect the distal leg muscles (Bansal et al., 2006; Tracy & Dyck, 2008). An essential but uncommon consequence of diabetes mellitus is diabetic thoracic radiculopathies. Extensive workups for underlying abdominal or chest pathology are generally prompted by the intense pain and dysaesthesia that commonly accompany these conditions, which manifest along the trunk, chest, or abdominal wall (Deli et al., 2013). They may include several dermatomes and exhibit symmetrical patterns (Abbott et al., 2011). The most well-known form of radiculoplexus neuropathy is diabetic lumbosacral neuropathy, but very rarely, the cervical segment may also be affected (Tracy & Dyck, 2008).

3.3.1.2 Diabetic Acute Mononeuropathy/Focal Neuropathy

The oculomotor, trochlear, and facial nerves are the most often affected areas of the skull in diabetic individuals with neuropathy. Diabetic oculomotor palsy is characterized by third-nerve palsy with pupillary sparing, which is caused by nerve infarction (Bansal et al., 2006). The femoral, sciatic, and peroneal nerves are the most commonly affected, in that order (Bansal et al., 2006; Tracy & Dyck, 2008).

However, diabetes has been associated with isolated involvement of nearly all major peripheral nerves; for instance, carpal tunnel syndrome is three times more common in diabetic patients than in the normal population, and it is the second most common neuropathic disease in diabetic patients. Affected nerves in the upper limb are relatively uncommon (Bansal et al., 2006). It seems nerve entrapment, rather than nerve infarction, is more likely in these instances. Periods of transition in the diabetes condition, such as after an episode of hyper- or hypoglycaemia, the initiation or adjustment of insulin therapy, or fast weight loss, are common occurrences of mononeuropathies (Deli et al., 2013).

3.3.1.3 Diabetic Radiculopathies and Multiple Mononeuropathies

Radiculoplexus neuropathies are a kind of diabetic condition that primarily affects people with moderate diabetes; they manifest subacutely with pain and weakness (Table 3.2). Diabetic radiculoplexus neuropathy may manifest in three primary ways: asymmetrical (in the cervical spine), symmetrical (in the thoracic spine), and lumbosacral (in the sacral region) (Tracy & Dyck, 2008). About one percent of people with diabetes may develop diabetic lumbosacral radiculoplexus neuropathy, which is likely the mostdangerous kind of diabetic neuropathy (Pop-Busui, 2010; Tracy & Dyck, 2008). Diabeticpolyradiculopathy, diabetic amyotrophy, Bruns-Garland syndrome, diabetic mononeuritis multiplex, proximal diabetic neuropathy, and a host of other terms have been used to describe it (Tracy & Dyck, 2008). Excruciating pain often worsens at night and starts in the lower back or hip and travels down one leg to the knee; the pain is deep and throbbing with sharp, stabbing jags on top of it. Muscle weakness and atrophy, most noticeably in the pelvic girdle and thighs, but also in the distal leg, becoming the most problematic symptom once pain has subsided (Bansal et al., 2006; Tracy & Dyck, 2008). An essential but uncommon consequence of diabetes mellitus is diabetic thoracic radiculopathies. Extensive workups for underlying abdominal or chest pathology are generally prompted by the intense pain and dysaesthesia that commonly accompany these conditions, which manifest along the trunk, chest, or abdominal wall (Tracy & Dyck, 2008). They may include several dermatomes and exhibit symmetrical patterns (Abbott et al., 2011). The most well-known form of radiculoplexus neuropathy is diabetic lumbosacral neuropathy, but very rarely, the cervical segment may also be affected (Tracy & Dyck, 2008). Multiple Mononeuropathies are similar to mononeuropathies. Older people with modest or undiagnosed diabetes are more likely to develop a painful condition of asymmetrical or unilateral neuropathies. A condition known as mononeuritis multiplex occurs when multiple nerves are damaged in a random distribution. Like mononeuropathy, mononeuritis multiplex involves a sudden onset and affects the nerves sequentially or irregularly, rather than affecting one nerve at a time. To avoid confusion with systemic vasculitis, it is essential to understand that nerve infarctions occur when the vasa nervorum become occluded (Bansal et al., 2006).

3.3.2 *Autonomic Neuropathy*

A common condition affecting the cholinergic, adrenergic, and peptidergic autonomic fibres in a condition of diabetes without additional reasons is diabetic autonomic neuropathy. There are two forms of this condition: one that is only identifiable via testing, and another that is defined by the existence of symptoms and indications (Spallone et al., 2011) (Table 3.1).

3.3.2.1 Gastrointestinal Autonomic Neuropathy

Autonomic (sympathetic and parasympathetic) and enteric neural systems interact with the underlying rhythmicity created by the interstitial cells of Cajal, situated within the smooth muscle, to influence the motor, sensory, and secretory activities of the gastrointestinal tract. Diagnosing gastrointestinal autonomic neuropathy is often an exclusionary process due to the difficulty of evaluating gastrointestinal autonomic function in people (Boulton et al., 2005; Chandrasekharan & Srinivasan, 2007; Spallone et al., 2011; Tesfaye & Selvarajah, 2012). In addition to impaired oral medication absorption, poor glycaemic control, malnutrition, abnormal postprandial regulation of blood pressure, poor quality of life, and a high rate of hospitalization, diabetes is linked to gastrointestinal symptoms like nausea, bloating, abdominal pain, diarrhoea, constipation, and delayed gastric emptying (Boulton et al., 2005; Chandrasekharan & Srinivasan, 2007; Pop-Busui, 2010; Spallone et al., 2011; Tesfaye & Selvarajah, 2012). These sensations are experienced by up to 75% of individuals with diabetes (Chandrasekharan & Srinivasan, 2007).

3.3.2.2 Cardiovascular Autonomic Neuropathy (CAN)

The inability of the circulatory system to regulate itself automatically is known as CAN. In diabetes, CAN is caused by a combination of factors, including how well the blood sugar is controlled, how long the disease has been going on, the rate of neuronal death due to ageing, and the difference between the two blood pressure readings (Spallone et al., 2011). One of the main ways that diabetes affects the nervous system is through the activation of metabolic and redox pathways within cells, which, along with impaired nerve perfusion, lead to the development and worsening of diabetic neuropathies (Pop-Busui, 2010). The initial signs of autonomic neuropathy in diabetics are often linked to parasympathetic denervation and early enhancement of sympathetic tone because neuropathy manifests first in the longest fibres. Autonomic dysfunction symptoms could not manifest until a considerable amount of time has passed once diabetes begins. However, in T2DM, subclinical CAN may be found within a year of diagnosis, and in T1DM, it can be found within two years of diagnosis (Pop-Busui, 2010). Orthostatic hypotension, irregular blood pressure control, exercise intolerance, resting tachycardia, poor heart rate variability, and other symptoms are present in this condition (Chandrasekharan & Srinivasan, 2007; Price & Hackett, 2008; Tesfaye & Selvarajah, 2012) (Table 3.1). Silent myocardial ischaemia, coronary artery disease, stroke, diabetic nephropathy development, perioperative morbidity, and overall mortality are all strongly related to CAN. Still, not all research has shown this to be the case. Patient categorization based on cardiovascular risk factors is possible using CAN evaluation, including those with and without preexisting cardiovascular disease (Tesfaye & Selvarajah, 2012).

3.3.2.3 Complications of Diabetic Autonomic Neuropathy

3.3.2.3.1 Sudomotor (Skin) dysfunction in Diabetes

The 'glove and stocking' distribution of thermoregulatory sweating loss, which first occurs in diabetic autonomic neuropathy, may spread to the upper limbs and anterior abdomen, following the well-known length dependence of diabetic neuropathy. Global anhidrosis, often seen with severe autonomic neuropathy, is the result of this process (Freeman, 2005). Hyperhidrosis may also be caused by diabetic autonomic neuropathy. A compensatory mechanism involving proximal areas, such as the head and trunk, which are spared in dying-back neuropathy, might lead to excessive sweating. There are rare instances of gustatory sweating, which is defined as an abnormal production of perspiration that spreads over the whole body (facial, neck, shoulders, and chest) after the ingestion of any meal, including those without a spicy flavour (Freeman, 2005).

3.3.2.3.2 Urinary Bladder Dysfunction in Diabetes

Between 43 and 87% of people with T1DM and 25% of those with T2DM have bladder dysfunction, according to estimates (Boulton et al., 2005; Davies et al., 2006; Tesfaye et al., 2010). Diabetic neuropathy, particularly peripheral and autonomic neuropathy, is the leading cause of bladder dysfunction in T2DM. Research on both animals and humans has shown that polyneuropathy, a condition that primarily affects sensory and autonomic nerve fibres, is the root cause of diabetic cystopathy (Burakgazi et al., 2012). Even when there is clear evidence of a bladder problem, patients may not have any symptoms in the early stages. The most common first sign of lower urinary tract involvement is impaired bladder sensation. Decreased bladder sensation, increased bladder capacity, and asymptomatic urine retention all contribute to delayed micturition reflexes (Burakgazi et al., 2012; Tesfaye et al., 2010). Until a patient develops a UTI due to an increase in residual urine volume, they may not realize that their bladder is dysfunctional (Boulton et al., 2005; Burakgazi et al., 2012; Tesfaye et al., 2010). Stream weakening, hesitancy, and straining are frequent signs (Burakgazi et al., 2012; Tesfaye et al., 2010). Overstretched bladder, decreased bladder contractility, increased residual urine, and impaired uroflow are symptoms of diabetic cystopathy (Burakgazi et al., 2012). Impairment of the feeling of bladder fullness is a hallmark of this condition.

3.3.2.3.3 Erectile Dysfunction (ED) in Diabetes

The inability to maintain an erection due to endothelial dysfunction and autonomic neuropathy impacts 30–40% of men with diabetes. An early indicator of cardiovascular risk, ED is closely associated with endothelial dysfunction. Although there are effective therapies for erectile dysfunction, managing this illness may be quite challenging at times. The possible link between late-onset hypogonadism and diabetes has garnered a lot of attention recently, although neither condition is causally related, and there is no evidence to support treating borderline hypogonadism in diabetics (Price & Hackett, 2008). Recognizing erectile dysfunction and its comorbidities, such as endothelial dysfunction, is essential for effective therapy of ED (Palumbo, 2007).

3.4 Etiology of Diabetic Neuropathy

The effects of diabetes on the neurological system are complicated and multidimensional, and the disease is both debilitating and progressive. Although diabetes may affect any part of the nervous system, patients with type 2 diabetes mellitus (T2DM) are more likely to have cardiovascular autonomic neuropathy and distal symmetric polyneuropathy, the two most frequent types of diabetic neuropathy (Feldman et al., 2019; Hansen et al., 2023; Pop-Busui et al., 2017). When discussing distal symmetric polyneuropathy, the term "diagnostic neuropathy" is usually used. Impairments in sensory axons tend to be more severe and length-dependent. In contrast, autonomic axons are also affected, and motor neurons are affected to a lesser degree, although this is usually the case in more advanced stages of the illness (Feldman et al., 2019). In addition to the more common generalized forms, chronic inflammatory demyelinating polyneuropathy, proximal motor neuropathy (such as diabetic amyotrophy), cranial, truncal, or focal limb neuropathy may also manifest with focal or multifocal presentations (Boulton et al., 2005). The etiologic impact of hyperglycemia and metabolic syndrome is associated with many of the risk factors that contribute to the advancement of diabetic neuropathy. The rate of painful diabetic neuropathy is correlated with the severity and duration of hyperglycemia. This is particularly true in T2DM, which is associated with a higher prevalence of chronic, painful sensorineural involvement in the lower limbs compared to T1DM (Strand et al., 2024). Additionally, compared to T2DM, T1DM appears to benefit more from tighter glucose control in the early stages of the disease, particularly in reducing the risk of neuropathy (Callaghan et al., 2012; Pop-Busui et al., 2017). Higher body mass, dyslipidemia, hypertension, comorbid hypertension, and renal impairment are additional connections, particularly those linked to other characteristics of the metabolic syndrome (Strand et al., 2024; Van Acker et al., 2009). Due to the challenges in preserving neuronal health in proportionately longer tissues and the consistent underlying neurotrophic factors, individuals who are taller than average are more prone to experiencing neuropathic symptoms to a greater extent than those who are shorter (Feldman et al., 2017). Finally, there is strong evidence that hereditary factors play a role in the associations between ACE and MTHFR gene variants (Lyssenko & Vaag, 2023). Nerve fibre alterations are an early indicator of diabetic neuropathy's multi-system presentation, which might occur before the disease's obvious symptoms appear (Kirthi et al., 2021). The primary pathophysiologic mechanisms are believed to include the polyol pathway, microvascular damage, and glycosylation end-products (Stevens & Shakher, 2011; Zochodne, 2019). However, there is likely a complex network of related variables. Sorbitol is produced by the polyol pathway when there is an increase in glucose concentration inside nerve terminals. A reduction in sodium–potassium adenosine triphosphatase and nicotinamide adenine phosphate (NADPH) synthesis follows an increase in sorbitol and fructose levels. This molecular change enhances the protective barrier against oxidative damage and vasodilation, resulting in persistent ischemia and inadequate responses to metabolic pressures. A thickening of the capillary basement membrane and hyperplastic endothelial tissue develops in neuronal and proximal vascular tissue. Diabetic problems such as cutaneous wounds, retinopathy, ischemic stroke, and hearing loss are caused by microvascular damage, which is impacted by these alterations (Hall et al., 2022). Due to hyperglycemia, increased amounts of reactive oxygen species in the damaged neural tissue cause further oxidative and inflammatory damage. Further vascular complications in diabetes are caused by these naturally occurring species, which can be neutralized. As a result, proteins, lipids, nucleic acids, and altered intracellular signalling pathways undergo direct structural and functional modifications (Sies, 1999; Volpe et al., 2018).

3.5 Molecular Mechanism and Pathways

The damage to nerve structure and function by hyperglycemia is substantial. Several hypotheses have been advanced to account for the detrimental effects of hyperglycemia on the nerves of diabetic patients. It is thought that hyperglycemia, by causing the production of reactive nitrogen species (RNS) and reactive oxygen species (ROS), contributes to nerve injury and dysfunction (Bhatti et al., 2022; Dewanjee et al., 2018). Tissues experience increased oxidative stress when the levels of ROS and RNS are high. Lipids in the myelin sheath that encases neurons are vulnerable to oxidative stress caused by these reactive species. Neuropathy pain results from an increase in the generation of spontaneous impulses inside neurons and dorsal nerve ganglia, which is caused by hyperexcitability in afferent nociceptors and central neurons, due to the destruction of peripheral myelin (Dewanjee et al., 2018). Hyperglycemia may alter the structure and function of nerves in more ways than simply destroying their myelin sheath. Research on the consequences of hyperglycemia in rats has indicated that, under hyperglycemic conditions, nerve conduction velocity, the number of large myelinated fibres, and nerve fibre diameter are all reduced (Malone et al., 1996). Although further study in human models is required, the earlier onset of hyperglycemia may influence subsequent alterations in nerve morphology and conduction velocity, as these changes were more severe in hyperglycemic rats at a younger age (Strand et al., 2024). Other pathways have been linked to nerve injury caused by hyperglycemia, including the polyol pathway, the promotion of mitochondrial dysfunction, and the production of advanced glycation end-products (AGEs) (Bhatti et al., 2022; Dewanjee et al., 2018). Hyperglycemia, like oxidative stress-induced degradation of myelin sheath lipids, may lead to mitochondrial damage by increasing oxidative stress. Axonal injury and diabetic neuropathy are outcomes of mitochondrial damage, leading to inadequate ATP generation (Bhatti et al., 2022). An additional complication of hyperglycemia is an increase in glycation, the mechanism by which glucose and other substances contribute to the AGE production. Researchers have found that patients with diabetic neuropathy have higher levels of the AGE receptor (RAGE) in their peripheral nerve endothelium and Schwann cells. This leads them to suspect that AGEs may play a role in the development of diabetic neuropathy by damaging the endothelial cells' ability to maintain blood flow (Dewanjee et al., 2018). Additionally, hyperglycemia causes extra glucose to be processed through the polyol pathway. Excessive consumption and eventual depletion of nicotinamide adenine dinucleotide phosphate (NADPH) result from amplifying this process (Luna et al., 2021). The production of reduced glutathione (GSH)- an antioxidant that helps protect cells from reactive oxygen species (ROS) and other chemicals requires NADPH. The depletion of glutathione (GSH) reserves increases damage to nerve vasculature and endothelial cells, potentially leading to diabetic neuropathy (Luna et al., 2021). Several hypothesised processes contribute to the development of diabetic neuropathy, including metabolic pathways, inflammatory pathways, and immune-mediated pathways (Christensen et al., 2020; Dewanjee et al., 2018; Eid et al., 2019; Luna et al., 2021). Two substances known to mediate immunological and inflammatory responses, nuclear factor-κB (NF-κB) and tumour necrosis factor-α (TNF-α), have been linked to diabetic neuropathy. Inflammatory stimuli stimulate the transcriptional factor NF-κB, which is present in the perineurium, epineurial arteries, and endoneurium of individuals with diabetes, as well as in Schwann cells cultivated in a high-glucose medium (Dewanjee et al., 2018). Furthermore, demyelinating polyneuropathies have been shown to involve the overexpression of the p65 component of NF-κB, suggesting that NF-κB may play a role in the onset of inflammatory demyelination, as seen in diabetic neuropathy (Dewanjee et al., 2018). The inflammatory protein TNF-α controls the activity of immune cells. Research has shown that high blood sugar levels may raise TNF-α levels, and this in turn increases the risk of developing diabetic neuropathy (Luna et al., 2021). All things considered, there are several ways in which hyperglycemia may worsen nerve damage and dysfunction, which in turn can lead to diabetic neuropathy. Once these pathways are understood, future research may focus on finding strategies to disrupt them to stop diabetic neuropathy from becoming worse.

3.6 Role of Hyperglycaemia and Hyperlipidaemia in the Pathogenesis of Diabetic Neuropathy

The pathophysiology of diabetic neuropathy can only be understood by examining the mechanisms by which the peripheral nervous system utilizes substrates for energy, particularly in the context of diabetes. Through glycolysis and the tricarboxylic acid cycle (for glucose) and β-oxidation (for fatty acids), NADH and FADH2 are produced in Schwann cells, DRG neurons, and axons (Feldman et al., 2019). Each β-oxidation cycle that occurs when long-chain fatty acids are delivered into Schwann cells produces one molecule of acetyl-CoA, which is then sent to the tricarboxylic acid cycle for the synthesis of NADH and FADH2. Substrate overload, as seen in diabetes, causes the transport system to become saturated, leading to the conversion of acetyl-CoA molecules to acylcarnitines. Toxic buildup of acylcarnitines in diabetic neuropathy worsens the condition by killing off Schwann cells and dorsal root ganglia neurons. One theory suggests that mitochondrial malfunction and an abnormal integrated stress response in Schwann cells are involved in the axonal degeneration that might be induced by the accumulation of acylcarnitines produced by these cells (Viader et al., 2013). To generate ATP via oxidative phosphorylation, NADH and FADH2 are transported throughout the mitochondria by Complexes I-IV. Innate cellular antioxidants, including catalase, glutathione, and superoxide dismutase, can neutralize modest quantities of reactive oxygen species (ROS) produced as a result of oxidative phosphorylation (Russell et al., 2008; Vincent, 2013; Vincent et al. 2004, 2008, 2011, 2009b). However, when there is an excessive substrate load, as seen in diabetes, oxidative phosphorylation fails, leading to a decrease in ATP synthesis and an increase in ROS levels. This, in turn, causes mitochondrial failure as well as metabolic and oxidative damage to Schwann cells and DRG neurons (Chowdhury et al., 2013; Fernyhough, 2015; Fernyhough & McGavock, 2014). Axonal disruption and damage are exacerbated when mitochondria that aren't working properly don't generate enough energy and can't usually transport molecules along axons. Inflammation and elevated reactive oxygen species (ROS) are the outcomes of glucose metabolism via the hexosamine and polyol pathways, respectively. Mitochondrial injury is a significant contributor to inflammation, which in turn leads to ongoing dysfunction of the neurological system (Feldman et al., 2017). Glycation of several structural and functional proteins leads to the formation of advanced glycation end-products (AGEs) when glucose levels are elevated. By interacting with the AGE-specific receptor (RAGE), AGEs influence gene expression and intracellular signalling, leading to the production of pro-inflammatory chemicals and free radicals, and cause proteins to lose or change their function. Figure 3.1 illustrates that hyperlipidemia leads to an increase in free fatty acids, which can damage the peripheral nervous system, particularly Schwann cells, through the generation of reactive oxygen species (ROS) and systemic and local inflammation triggered by the activation of macrophages, which in turn produce cytokines and chemokines.

Other lipids in diabetic neuropathy negatively impact the peripheral nerve system. In neurons, the conversion of cholesterol to oxysterols causes tissue destruction (Jang & Lee, 2011; Vincent et al., 2011). On the other hand, reactive oxygen species (ROS) oxidize plasma lipoproteins, especially low-density lipoproteins (LDLs), which bind to oxidized LDL receptor 1 (LOX1) (Vincent et al., 2009a), Toll-like receptor 4 (TLR4) (Vincent et al., 2004), and RAGE (Vincent et al., 2007). Oxidized low-density lipoprotein (LDL) binding to these receptors initiates a cascade of signalling events, including caspase 3 activation and nuclear DNA degradation (Vincent et al., 2007), which in turn induce further inflammation and ROS buildup, leading to persistent and worsening nerve injury (Cotter & Cameron, 2003; Keller et al., 1999; Vincent et al., 2009a) (Fig. 3.1).

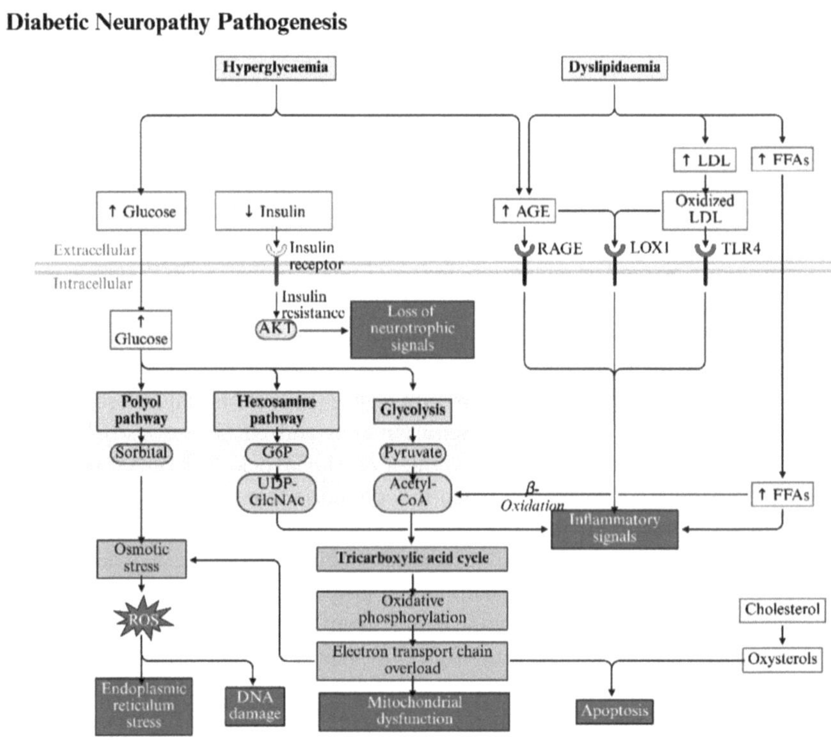

Fig. 3.1 Pathogenesis of diabetic neuropathy. The pathological changes in neurons, glia, and vascular cells caused by hyperglycaemia, dyslipidaemia, and altered insulin signalling include DNA damage, endoplasmic reticulum stress, mitochondrial dysfunction, neurodegeneration, loss of neurotrophic signalling, and macrophage activation, all of which can lead to nerve dysfunction and, eventually, neuropathy. Due to metabolic deficiencies making different cell types more or less vulnerable to damage, the role of these pathways in neuropathy development changes over time, with the illness profile and cell type. The figure was prepared using www.Biorender.com and adapted from (Feldman et al., 2019)

FFAs, free fatty acids; Glucosamine-6-P, AGE, advanced glycation end-product; LDL, low-density lipoprotein; glucosamine 6-phosphate; RAGE, AGE-specific receptor; LOX1, oxidized LDL receptor 1; UDP-GlcNAc, uridine diphosphate N-acetylglucosamine; ROS, reactive oxygen species; TLR4, Toll-like receptor 4.

3.7 Nerve Fibre Pathology and Clinical Manifestations

Large sensory fibres are often affected by distal sensory neuropathy, while it may also impact tiny fibres. Unmyelinated somatic and autonomic fibres are the most common targets of distal small-fibre neuropathy. Degeneration of sympathetic pre- and post-ganglionic fibres is one of the several autonomic fibres involved in diabetic autonomic neuropathy (Tesfaye et al., 2010). Along with somatic large and small nerve fibres, they are simultaneously engaged. In diabetic autonomic neuropathy, the distal sudomotor fibres are involved first, followed by the cardiovagal function, and finally, the autonomic pathways are widely involved. Acute small fibre neuropathy, rather than large fibre neuropathy, might develop due to a fast decrease in hyperglycemia, a complication of diabetes treatment (Sasaki et al., 2020). After 10 years of diabetes, the majority of people will begin to have distal sensory neuropathy, the most prevalent form of diabetic neuropathy. Chronic symmetrical length-dependent sensorimotor polyneuropathy is the most frequent kind of diabetic peripheral neuropathy. Initially, most people with neuropathy will not have any symptoms at all, and others may even have mild or non-existent neuropathy. Pathologic changes to the nerves appear to be linked to alterations in microvessels, as observed in diabetic retinopathy and nephropathy. One of the most significant risk factors is probably total exposure to hyperglycemia. Strict glycemic management may stabilize and even improve this risk factor. Statistical analysis has shown a correlation between this polyneuropathy and nephropathy and retinopathy (Tesfaye et al., 2010). A verified diagnosis of diabetic sensorimotor polyneuropathy requires both a neuropathy symptom and an impairment in nerve conduction. Diabetic sensorimotor polyneuropathy may be associated with the following symptoms: loss of sensation, positive sensory neuropathic symptoms (such as numbness, tingling, burning, or sharp pain) primarily in the legs, feet, or toes; or a symmetrical reduction of distal sensation or clearly diminished or nonexistent ankle reflexes. Neuropathic pain and autonomic dysfunction can progress with time (Tesfaye et al., 2010). Orthostatic hypotension affects 25–50% of individuals with diabetic autonomic neuropathy. The vagal and adrenergic limbs of the baroreflex are both impaired in diabetic orthostatic hypotension. Diabetic neuropathic pain care mainly includes ruling out alternative sources of painful peripheral neuropathy, enhancing glycemic control as a preventative measure, and using pain medicines (Schreiber, 2015). Symptoms include hypesthesia, positive paresthesia symptoms, or a lack of vibratory sensitivity, which are signs of sensory impairments. Pain may develop, although it is uncommon (Sasaki et al., 2020). Diabetic distal sensory neuropathy may cause a burning feeling when the patient is farther away from blood vessels. Some individuals experience distal burning pain; however, nerve conduction investigations of large myelinated fibres show normal or near-normal results. Some patients report experiencing a sensation of rickling, stabbing, or burning in the ball or pads of their feet (Tesfaye et al., 2010).

3.8 Diagnosis Evaluation

3.8.1 Diabetes Mellitus and Pre-Diabetes Diagnosis

Neuropathy is another symptom that has been linked to pre-diabetes. According to the latest ADA recommendations, HgbA1c, fasting plasma glucose, or 2-h postprandial glucose levels may be used to diagnose diabetes. This statement suggested using the A1c test with a cutoff of $\geq$ 6.5% to diagnose diabetes. Diabetes may still be diagnosed using the previously defined glucose criteria: a fasting plasma glucose level of 7 mmol/L or a 2-h postprandial glucose level of 11.1 mmol/L (Basevi et al., 2011). Fasting plasma glucose levels between 5.6 and 6.9 mmol/l or 2-h postprandial glucose values between 7.8 and 11.0 mmol/l on the oral glucose tolerance test are the diagnostic criteria for pre-diabetes. Notably, 110 mg/dL (6.1 mmol/L) is the cutoff for impaired fasting glucose, according to the World Health Organization and many other diabetes organizations (Basevi et al., 2011). Accordingly, it is acceptable to consider an A1c range of 5.7% to 6.4% as identifying those at high risk for developing diabetes in the future, a condition also known as pre-diabetes (Deli et al., 2013). When A1c levels are high, the likelihood of developing diabetes increases at an accelerated rate, just as they do with glucose readings. Those with an A1c level of more than 6.0% should be considered at very high risk and should undergo the most rigorous therapies with the most careful follow-up. This guideline includes medical care and lifestyle standards (Basevi et al., 2011).

3.8.2 Sensorimotor Neuropathy Diagnosis

The sensory impairments, rather than motor nerve failure, are the hallmark of diabetic peripheral neuropathy (DPN). These symptoms often manifest at the extremities' far ends and move closer together in a "stocking glove" pattern as the disease worsens or the patient's diabetes progresses (Edwards et al., 2008). Damage to larger nerve fibres occurs later than to smaller ones in the standard form (Hartemann et al., 2011). Different types of DPN cause different symptoms; for example, problems with proprioception and light touch might be caused by significant fibre illness. Paraesthesia, dysaesthesia, and neuropathic pain are symptoms of small-fibre illness, which affects pain and temperature perception (Edwards et al., 2008) (Table 3.3). Only the most severe cases result in distal impairment. Mild, asymptomatic DPN is commonly indicated by diminished or nonexistent deep-tendon reflexes, mainly the Achilles tendon reflex. Ulceration and neurorthropathy (Charcot's joints) in the foot are two late consequences that may manifest in more advanced cases of asymptomatic neuropathy (Edwards et al., 2008). When diagnosing DPN, taking the patient's temperature, joint position, pinprick sensation, and muscular power at the bedside is essential. A 128 Hz tuning fork is recommended for vibration testing. A 10-g monofilament is suggested for assessing touch sensitivity (Bansal et al., 2006; Baron et al., 2010). The diagnosis of neuropathic pain has been facilitated with the development of numerous questionnaires (Bansal et al., 2006; Baron et al., 2010; Hartemann et al., 2011). The DN4 questionnaire stands out due to its ease of use, quick completion time, and excellent diagnostic performance. It can diagnose neuropathic pain with an accuracy of 90% and a sensitivity of 83% for scores of 4/10 or above (Hartemann et al., 2011). One significant benefit of screening techniques is that they may help non-specialists detect possible patients with neuropathy. But these techniques can't substitute human clinicians' discretion since they miss 10–20% of individuals with neuropathy that doctors diagnose (Cruccu et al., 2010). Although electrophysiological testing is not typically recommended for diagnosing chronic sensorimotor diabetic neuropathy, as it may be normal in cases of damage to small-diameter fibres, it is a dependable procedure for ruling out other possible causes in cases of mononeuropathies or radiculopathies, such as demyelinating polyneuropathies. When the clinical presentation is unusual and the cause of the diabetes is unclear (symmetrical symptoms or involvement of the upper limbs), these methods are beneficial (Bansal et al., 2006; Hartemann et al., 2011; Tesfaye et al., 2010). In terms of laboratory testing, skin biopsies may be used to evaluate neuropathies characterized by distal loss of unmyelinated nerve fibres. Laser-evoked potentials are the gold standard for assessingAδ pathway dysfunction, also known as small fibre neuropathy (Cruccu et al., 2010).

3.8.3 Autonomic Neuropathy Diagnosis

While questionnaires exist to assess the severity of orthostatic symptoms in dysautonomic disorders, none have undergone validation for cardiovascular autonomic neuropathy (CAN), and there is a dearth of validated translations into other languages (Spallone et al., 2011). It is essential to assess diabetic patients for the existence of CAN if they exhibit signs of autonomic dysfunction, such as unexplained tachycardia, orthostatic hypotension, and poor exercise tolerance, among others. Patients at higher risk of CAN, owing to a history of poor glycaemic control, cardiovascular risk factors, DPN, and macro- and microangiopathic diabetic complications, should undergo screening for CAN at the diagnosis of T2DM and 5 years after the diagnosis of T1DM (Tesfaye et al., 2010). Tests for cardiovascular autonomic reflexes, such as the heart rate response to standing, deep breathing, and the Valsalva manoeuvre, as well as the blood pressure reaction to standing, are the foundation of CAN diagnosis (Spallone et al., 2011; Tesfaye et al., 2010) (Table 3.1). One of the tools that may measure GI symptoms is the Diabetes Bowel Symptom Questionnaire. The diagnosis of gastroparesis is best accomplished with objective measurements of stomach

Table 3.3 Characterization and evaluation of both positive and negative sensory indicators and symptoms in neuropathic pain patients (Baron et al., 2010)

	Symptoms	Sign	Diagnosis
Negative sign and symptoms	Thermohypoaesthesia, hypoalgesia, hypoaesthesia, and pallhypoaesthesia	Decreased sensitivity to: vibration, painful stimuli, cold or warm stimuli, nonpainful stimuli	Apply a painter's brush, cotton swab, tuning fork, or pinprick objects heated to 10 or 45 °C to the skin
Spontaneous pain or sensations	Superficial discomfort, paroxysmal pain, and paraesthesia	Persistent non-painful feeling, severe, extremely rapid electrical shocks that last only seconds, persistently painful feeling	Number each episode: Intensity grade (0–10), Evoking threshold, Area in cm^2
Evoked pain	Both mechanical static and mechanical dynamic allodynia, pinprick or mechanical puncture hyperalgesia, temporal summation, heat allodynia, cold allodynia, and deep somatic mechanical allodynia	When applied to skin, commonly painless stimuli cause pain Pressure stimulation on skin that is typically painless may cause pain Stimuli that are often perceived as stingy but not unpleasant may actually cause pain Repeated exposure to identical, single-noxious stimuli is perceived as an increase inthe intensity of pain Cold stimuli that are often painless cause pain Thermal stimuli that are non-painful induce pain Non-painful pressure on deep somatic tissues induces pain	Caressing the skin using a paintbrush, etc. Physically applying light, moderate pressure on the skin Using a little touch to gently puncture the skin gently Pricking the skin with a safety pin every < 3 s for 30 s Rub 20 °C objects against skin Rub 40 °C objects against the skin Pressure is applied gently to muscles or joints

emptying. Unfortunately, diabetic gastroparesis cannot be detected by a specialized test; it can only be diagnosed by exclusion after thorough gastrointestinal investigations (Deli et al., 2013). Complete patient histories (including sexual, medical, drug, alcohol, cigarette, and psychological aspects) are essential diagnostic processes in emergency departments. The gold standard for characterizing erectile dysfunction (ED) symptom frequency and severity is the use of validated questionnaires (Tesfaye et al., 2010). All patients with ED and cardiovascular illness should have their cardiac risk factors examined and maintained because of the possibility of harmful or unexpected medication interactions. Patients who do not show improvement when using phosphodiesterase-5 inhibitors may benefit from specialised testing to determine the cause of their condition. Complete urodynamic testing is the gold standard for identifying the specific kind of dysfunctional bladder. Autonomic dysfunction in DPN may be better identified by evaluating sudomotor dysfunction. Table 3.1 shows that the quantitative sudomotor axon reflex test has a sensitivity of 75% for diagnosing distal small-fibre polyneuropathy (Tesfaye et al., 2010).

3.9 Management Strategies to Delay Disease Progression

The DN care focuses on preventing neuropathy development, symptom reduction, and complication alleviation from insensate or painless DN (Fonseca, 2007; Khadilkar et al., 2012). An individual's pathologic processes dictate the efficacy of DN treatment (Fonseca, 2007). Several clinical recommendations have been developed based on existing research to help prevent and manage DN. The recommendations encompass a wide range of approaches to prevent, slow the progression of, and treat DN symptoms. Treatments for DN might therefore be either symptomatic or preventative (Khadilkar et al., 2012). However, a few alternatives for treating DN target the underlying nerve damage. So far, most DN management approaches have focused on preventing the disease's progression. To identify the first symptoms of neuropathy and begin treatment promptly, screening for DN is essential in clinical practice (Pop-Busui et al., 2017). Based on the research, Table 3.4 highlights the current management strategies for preventing the progression of DN.

3.9.1 Monitoring of Blood Glucose Level

The most crucial step in preventing DN is to monitor blood glucose levels and make lifestyle changes (Pop-Busui et al., 2017; Smith et al., 2022b). Patients with T1DM and T2DM may slow the development of cardiovascular autonomic neuropathy and distal symmetrical polyneuropathy by reducing their sugar intake (Pop-Busui et al., 2017; Zilliox & Russell, 2019). According to the Diabetes Control and Clinical Trials, this approach seems to work better with T1DM; after 6.5 years of intense

Table 3.4 Management strategies to delay disease progression

Strategies	Treatment	Mode of action	References
Monitoring of blood glucose level	Diabetes management options include insulin, anti-diabetic medications, electrical stimulation, and percutaneous nerve stimulation. Non-management options include making dietary changes to maintain stable glucose levels, engaging in regular physical activity, and undergoing physiotherapy. Surgical procedures, such as pancreatic transplant and bariatric surgery, are also available	Slows the progression of distal symmetric polyneuropathy in individuals with type 2 diabetes mellitus (T2DM) and prevents the development of cardiovascular autonomic neuropathy and distal symmetric polyneuropathy in people with type 1 diabetes mellitus (T1DM)	Gæde et al. (1999), Pop-Busui et al. (2017), and Smith et al. (2022b)
Lifestyle changes	Treatment plans that include physiotherapy and rehabilitation, glucose-controlled diets, counselling, and supervised training	Minimize the potential for DN and cardiometabolic complications	Smith et al. (2022b)
Foot care for diabetic patients	Five steps to prevent foot ulcers: (1) identifying high-risk feet; (2) regularly checking and examining those feet; (3) educating patients, their families, and healthcare professionals; (4) wearing appropriate footwear regularly; and (5) managing symptoms that may indicate a future ulcer	Reduces or eliminates the need for amputations	Schaper et al. (2016)

(continued)

Table 3.4 (continued)

Strategies	Treatment	Mode of action	References
Pharmacological and non-pharmacological interventions	Here are three steps that might be helpful: First, there is first-line therapy with tricyclic antidepressants (TCAs), selective serotonin reuptake inhibitors (SNRIs), pregabalin, and gabapentin; second-line therapy with tramadol and other weak opioids and SNRIs; and third-line therapy with potentopioids, cannabinoids, and anticonvulsants Supplements containing antioxidants as alternatives: vitamin B_{12}, α-lipoic acid, and acetyl-L-carnitine	Treat and manage symptoms of diabetic neuropathy and its associated pain	American Diabetes Association (2021), Ansari et al. (2021), and Rutkove (2009, 89, 90, 133)

treatment, patients' DN is decreased by 60% (Nathan, 1993). After receiving extensive therapy to reduce blood glucose levels, T2DM patients with neuropathy had an improvement in vibration perception, according to a 1998 United Kingdom Prospective Diabetes Study report (Lancet, 1998). On the other hand, from 1998 to 2015, rigorous glycaemic management did not significantly affect neuropathy in T2DM patients. While strict glycaemic control may help DM patients avoid or postpone the development of DN, Rodríguez-Gutiérrez et al. felt that this approach is insufficient for T2DM patients because they are more likely to have other untreated risk factors, such as cardiometabolic factors (Rodríguez-Gutiérrez & Montori, 2016). There appears to be a growing consensus that glycaemic monitoring alone cannot slow the progression of DN in T2DM patients. Several clinical studies across different nations have revealed that these individuals often have metabolic syndrome, which includes obesity, hyperglycaemia, and dyslipidaemia. These conditions are major risk factors for neuropathy (Pop-Busui et al., 2022). To encourage individualized therapy based on glycaemic objectives, the American Diabetes Association (ADA) has developed specific recommendations for children, adolescents, adults, pregnant women, and the elderly (Ismail, 2023).

3.9.2 Lifestyle Changes

In addition to monitoring blood sugar levels, people with T2DM should modify their lifestyle to reduce cardiometabolic risk factors, decrease their likelihood of developing DN, and slow its progression. Some examples of lifestyle changes include eating healthily and exercising regularly (Pop-Busui et al., 2022). Based on research conducted on animals, it has been discovered that sustained exercise has several benefits. Firstly, it lowers blood sugar levels and produces oxidative and nitrosative stress. Secondly, it improves the bioenergetics of the mitochondria in both the nerve cell body and the distal axon. Lastly, it increases axonal transport and counteracts the inflammatory effects of dyslipidaemia, lipotoxicity, and obesity. Lastly, it improves nerve regeneration after metabolic injury. However, different results were observed in clinical research. Patients with DPN showed considerable improvements in peroneal and sural motor nerve function in a 2006 clinical study that examined the effects of long-term exercise training on the patients (Balducci et al., 2006). There was a slowing of motor and sensory neuropathy development across the four-year trial period, indicating that exercise may alter the normal progression of DN. However, new research on the impact of exercise on DN has shown conflicting results. Regardless of the type of 12-week physical exercise training-sedentary controls, aerobic, isokinetic strength, or a combination of the two neither improved nor worsened the sensory or motor nerve electrodiagnostic findings (i.e., sural, median, and ulnar sensory nerve responses) in older T2DM patients with length-dependent distal symmetric polyneuropathy, according to a RCT by Stubbs et al. (2019). Nevertheless, it has been demonstrated that a subgroup of individuals can specifically enhance their sensory nerve function through an organized, short-term aerobic exercise program. Recent meta-analysis of 13 RCTs with 592 patients who underwent peripheral nerve conduction testing from 2014 to 2022 lends credence to this conclusion. Patients with DN showed the most significant improvements in peripheral nerve conduction, glycaemic management, and balance when exercising in conjunction with an endurance and sensorimotor training program (Streckmann et al., 2022). In healthcare settings outside of research, implementing supervised exercise programs may be difficult owing to patient compliance issues and a lack of resources (such as money, facilities, and qualified personnel) to oversee the programs (Smith et al., 2022b). Dietary monitoring has been proposed in the literature as a potential strategy for delaying disease progression and prevention. Most studies included nutrition as one of several multifactorial lifestyle measures for DN prevention, although there is little data on the efficacy of diet alone. In particular, the Diabetes Prevention Program found that reducing the prevalence of type 2 diabetes mellitus (T2DM) and reversing symptoms of metabolic syndrome may be achieved through dietary counselling and exercise (Knowler, 2002; Orchard et al., 2005). Additionally, to lower DN risk factors, the ADA recommends limiting consumption of processed foods and those high in calories. The best way for patients to avoid developing DN is to eat foods high in polyunsaturated fats and antioxidants (Pop-Busui et al., 2022). The functions of mitochondria in distal axons are further diminished by oxidative stress and pro-inflammatory cellular damage responses inducible by lipid metabolites and persistent cellular hyperglycemia (Zilliox & Russell, 2019). Several dietary supplements, such as the antioxidant α-lipoic acid (ALA), are recommended for use in combating oxidative damage. Additionally, it is recommended to take supplements that contain nicotine riboside, as this helps generate nicotinamide adenine dinucleotide (NAD+), which in turn protects neurons from oxidative damage and delays the onset of DN (Cantó et al., 2012); these supplements can also activate molecular pathways that protect against dyslipidaemia and obesity (Chandarasekaran, 2016). Consequently, DN may be effectively alleviated with dietary control. Axonal regeneration, improved glucose and lipid metabolism, and a longer duration of effect in BM patients can only be achieved when exercise-based intervention is also implemented (Zilliox & Russell, 2019).

3.9.3 *Foot Care for Diabetic Patients*

The amputations of the lower limbs are more common in DN patients. The significance of yearly foot examinations and regular foot care in preventing lower limb amputations was highlighted in a recent systematic review that examined the 5-year mortality rate of patients with above-the-knee amputation (40–90%) and below-the-knee amputation (40–82%) (Thorud et al., 2016). Diabetic patients should get education on how to properly care for their feet, including how to recognize the foot that is at risk, how to examine and check their feet daily, what footwear is appropriate, and how to treat pre-ulcerative lesions accurately and promptly (Schaper et al., 2016). Healthcare professionals and family members should also get the education. The best methods for preventing diabetic foot issues are not well-established, despite the existence of foot care recommendations. Correct diabetic foot care was associated with a decrease in the severity of amputations, shorter hospital stays, and lower mortality rates, according to a meta-analysis of 19 trials. The research, however, lacked quality (Buggy & Moore, 2017). Another meta-analysis of 12 RCTs found insufficient high-quality data to conclude that educational measures alone may reduce the occurrence of diabetic foot ulcers (DFUs) and amputations. To effectively prevent DFUs, the authors agreed that educational interventions should be supplemented with additional strategies (Dorresteijn et al., 2014).

3.9.4 *Pharmacological Interventions*

To decrease the risk of diabetic peripheral neuropathy (DPN) and autonomic neuropathy in diabetic patients, it is recommended that they improve their blood glucose control, lipid and blood pressure levels, and abstain from smoking and excessive alcohol consumption (American Diabetes Association, 2011; Hartemann et al., 2011).

3.9.4.1 Preventive Measures

Several medicines have been attempted to stop the course of diabetic neuropathy, which is based on its aetiology. Currently, only palliative therapies are available after subjective symptoms begin, although this might improve clinical results (Obrosova,

2009). According to a review of research on experimental peripheral diabetic neuropathy, no pharmaceutical drug has been shown to alleviate nerve conduction velocity deficit (Obrosova, 2009). This is even though all of these drugs have been demonstrated to relieve painful or insensitive neuropathy symptoms. Painful and insensitive neuropathy is caused by oxidative-nitrosative stress, imbalances in growth factors, increased aldose reductase, protein kinase C, and poly(ADP-ribose) polymerase activities, as well as a deficiency of C-peptide, according to animal studies that employed genetic and pharmacological methods (Obrosova, 2009). According to recent research, some subjective symptoms and reduced conduction velocity may have improved with therapy with aldose reductase inhibitors (Deli et al., 2013). The results of this study lend support to the notion that the polyol pathway plays a crucial role in the development and progression of diabetic neuropathy in humans. However, one subgroup analysis (4 studies employing tolrestat) favoured treatment (Chalk et al., 2007), and there was no overall significant difference between the treated and control groups in a Cochrane meta-analysis involving 32 trials (standardized mean difference: $-0.25, 95\%$ CI: -0.56 to 0.05). Neither foot ulceration nor nerve conduction metrics generally improved (27 trials vs. 1 research study). None of the studies looked at people's quality of life. At the same time, the majority of side effects were mild or uncommon; three drugs- sorbinil (a chemical with severe hypersensitivity responses), zenarestat (which caused an increase in creatinine), and tolrestat (which altered liver function) had dose-limiting adverse events that caused their removal from human usage (Chalk et al., 2007). To control blood pressure, avoid or treat cardiovascular disease and nephropathy, angiotensin-converting enzyme inhibitors and angiotensin receptor blockers are often prescribed to diabetic patients. Despite some promising results in prospective evaluations and small-scale investigations, there has been a lack of large-scale research on the effects of angiotensin-converting enzyme inhibitors and angiotensin receptor blockers on neuropathy (Edwards et al., 2008).

3.9.4.2 Symptomatic Treatment

Guidelines for painful DN are now the main emphasis due to the lack of information on insensate or painless DN treatment. These include pharmacotherapies such as opioids, topical analgesics, tricyclic antidepressants (TCAs), anticonvulsants, serotonin and norepinephrine reuptake inhibitors (SNRIs), and intravenous (IV) drugs. The primary advantages and disadvantages of these strategies are summarized in Table 3.5.

3.9.4.2.1 Anticonvulsants

For painful DN, pregabalin and gabapentin are suggested as first- or second-line therapy (Smith et al., 2022b). The Food and Drug Administration (FDA) in the United States has approved pregabalin for this purpose, but gabapentin is only authorized

Table 3.5 Advantages and disadvantages of pharmacotherapies

Pharmacotherapies	Advantages	Disadvantages	Evidence level
Anticonvulsants-pregabalin and gabapentin	i. Anticonvulsants are a great pain reliever for DN patients (Derry et al., 2019; Wiffen et al., 2017) ii. Pregabalin has been approved for treating painful DN in the UK and the USA (Smith et al., 2022b)	i. Gabapentin is not authorized for treating painful DN in the USA (Smith et al., 2022b) ii. Recent instances of abuse have been reported in the UK (Smith et al., 2022b) iii. Some of the adverse effects of anticonvulsants include sleepiness, dizziness, headache, diarrhoea, and nausea, and they are also linked to tachyphylaxis (Smith et al., 2022b) iv. In rare cases, pregabalin has been associated with severe respiratory depression (Smith et al., 2022b)	Moderate level (Derry et al., 2019; Wiffen et al., 2017)
Serotonin and norepinephrine reuptake inhibitors (SNRIs)-duloxetine and venlafaxine	i. Pain in DN is greatly alleviated by duloxetine (Smith et al., 2022b) ii. For painful DN, duloxetine has received approval in the US and UK (Smith et al., 2022b)	i. The adverse effects of SNRIs are comparable to those of anticonvulsants (Smith et al., 2022b) ii. Sleep issues and sexual dysfunction could be more obvious (Pop-Busui et al., 2017) iii. For painful DN, venlafaxine is not authorized (Smith et al., 2022b)	Duloxetine-moderate level, venlafaxine- low level (Gallagher et al., 2015; Smith et al., 2022b)

(continued)

Table 3.5 (continued)

Pharmacotherapies	Advantages	Disadvantages	Evidence level
Tricyclic antidepressants-amitriptyline	i. There have been thousands of patients who have benefited from amitriptyline for painful DN (Moore et al. 2015b) ii. For neuropathic pain, the UK approved amitriptyline (Smith et al., 2022b)	i. Many unwanted effects may be experienced when using amitriptyline, including trouble sleeping, constipation, erectile dysfunction, arrhythmias, and postural hypotension (Smith et al., 2022b) ii. In the USA, amitriptyline is not authorized (Smith et al., 2022b)	Low level (Moore et al. 2015b)
Opioids- tapentadol and tramadol	i. According to the FDA, tapentadol may be used to treat neuropathic pain (Smith et al., 2022b) ii. Tramadol is an effective analgesic for DN (Freeman et al., 2007; Harati et al., 1998) iii. The UK and the USA have authorized tramadol for moderate to severe pain (Smith et al., 2022b) iv. There may be less potential for misuse of tramadol (Dunn et al., 2019)	i. There is no UK approval for the use of tapentadol for neuropathic pain (Smith et al., 2022b) ii. Substance addiction and misuse are associated with opioids (Staudt et al., 2022) iii. Constipation, headache, dizziness, lethargy, nausea, and sleepiness are some of the many adverse effects of opioids (Smith et al., 2022b) iv. Combining tramadol with SNRIs or SSRIs is not recommended (Attal et al., 2010)	Low level (Duehmke et al., 2017; Freo et al., 2019)

(continued)

Table 3.5 (continued)

Pharmacotherapies	Advantages	Disadvantages	Evidence level
Topical analgesics- topical capsaicin	i. DN patients report much less pain when treated with 0.075% capsaicin (Mason et al., 2004) ii. In cases of DN, an 8% capsaicin solution considerably reduces pain (Freynhagen et al., 2021; Van Nooten et al., 2017) iii. 8% capsaicin may be as effective as duloxetine and even more helpful than anticonvulsants (Van Nooten et al., 2017)	i. To get an adequate response, some individuals may need to apply 8% capsaicin two or three times (Freynhagen et al., 2021) ii. Capsaicin used topically has the potential to disrupt opioid signalling (Polydefkis et al., 2004) iii. Topically analgesics can only alleviate localized discomfort (Smith et al., 2022b)	0.075% capsaicin- low level (Kulkantrakorn et al., 2019; Mason et al., 2004) 8% capsaicin - moderate level (Freynhagen et al., 2021; Van Nooten et al., 2017)
Intravenous (IV) medication- lidocaine and ketamine	Intravenous medicines often alleviate pain in DN (Aiyer et al., 2018; Zhu et al., 2019)	i. Currently, clinical guidelines for DN do not recommend IV medicines (Smith et al., 2022b) ii. It's possible that IV lidocaine won't work in the long run (Zhu et al., 2019) iii. IV drugs are only available for use in hospitals and may cause a variety of unwanted side effects, such as nausea, vertigo, and sleep problems (Moulin et al., 2019; Staudt et al., 2022)	Low level (Aiyer et al., 2018; Zhu et al., 2019)

to treat postherpetic neuralgia. Both have wider UK licencing for the treatment of peripheral neuropathic pain. Still, after several instances of abuse, the government has begun to control both drugs more strictly (Smith et al., 2022b). As a therapy for painful DN, these medications have moderate evidence. There was a 30% reduction in pain intensity (risk ratio 1.1, 8 RCTs, 2320 participants) and a 50% reduction (risk ratio 1.3, 11 RCTs, 2931 participants) in comparison to placebo, according to a recent Cochrane systematic review (Derry et al., 2019). Similarly, with gabapentin 1200 mg or more, there was a moderate effect compared to placebo (7 RCTs, 1439 participants) and a significant benefit compared to placebo (6 RCTs, 1331 participants) (Wiffen et al., 2017). Carbamazepine, valproic acid, lamotrigine, and phenytoin are among the other anticonvulsants that have been studied; however, the evidence for their effectiveness is limited (Birse et al., 2012; Gill et al., 2011; Wiffen et al., 2013, 2014). It's unclear exactly how pregabalin and gabapentin work. Although they are linked to tachyphylaxis, their binding to the 2 ~ subunit of calcium channels gives the impression of producing analgesic effects. A list of common adverse effects for both drugs includes lethargy, vertigo, headache, diarrhoea, and nausea. Dosage adjustments should be considered for individuals at higher risk, such as those over 65 years of age, those with respiratory or neurological diseases, or those with renal impairment. This recommendation followed a review of worldwide safety data published in 2021 by the UK's Medicines and Healthcare products Regulatory Agency (MHRA) regarding pregabalin. The agency stated that the drug is associated with rare cases of severe respiratory depression (Smith et al., 2022b).

3.9.4.2.2 Serotonin and Norepinephrine Reuptake Inhibitors (SNRIs)

When dealing with painful DN, duloxetine is suggested as either a first- or second-line therapy (Smith et al., 2022b). In the US and UK, it is only recommended for DN and not for other types of neuropathic pain. Duloxetine, an SNRI, somewhat blocks dopamine reuptake and blocks descending pain pathways. The usual adverse effects are comparable to anticonvulsants, with the potential for more obvious erectile dysfunction and sleep disturbances (Pop-Busui et al., 2017). A prior Cochrane systematic review (8 studies, 2728 participants) indicated that 60 to 120 mg is effective in treating painful DN, whereas lower dosages are not; hence, the evidence level for duloxetine is also moderate (Lunn et al., 2014). A large-scale, multi-centre, double-blind RCT showed that 60 mg of duloxetine daily for 12 weeks substantially decreased DN pain compared to placebo (Gao et al., 2015). Some comparative studies have shown that duloxetine is equally effective as gabapentin, pregabalin, and amitriptyline (a tricyclic antidepressant) (Smith et al., 2022b), while others have shown conflicting findings (Alam et al., 2020). In contrast, duloxetine outperformed pregabalin in other studies (Alam et al., 2020; Tanenberg et al., 2014; Tesfaye et al., 2013). The American Academy of Neurology and the European Federation of Neurological Societies Task Force both suggest venlafaxine, an SSRI and selective serotonin reuptake inhibitor (SNRI), as a first- or second-line therapy for painful DN (Attal et al., 2010; Bril et al., 2011); however, its usage does not need a prescription. While NICE discourages the use of this medicine in settings where specialists are absent, other clinical guidelines acknowledge its effectiveness without offering specific guidance (Pop-Busui et al., 2017; Tesfaye et al., 2011). Venlafaxine is not included in the most current American Diabetes Association compendium on managing painful DN (Pop-Busui et al., 2022). For venlafaxine, the evidence is weak. There is minimal evidence to support the use of venlafaxine in treating painful DN, according to a recent Cochrane systematic review (6 RCTs, 460 participants). A substantial placebo effect tainted these trials, even if dosages between 150 and 225 mg were beneficial (Gallagher et al., 2015). Although no study has compared venlafaxine with duloxetine for DN, the latter was more effective in treatingchemotherapy-induced peripheral neuropathy (Farshchian et al., 2018).

3.9.4.2.3 Tricyclic Antidepressants

Amitriptyline, on the other hand, is suggested for painful DN as a first- or second-line therapy (Pop-Busui et al., 2017; Smith et al., 2022b). Although it lacks a license for usage in the United States, it is the only TCA approved for treating neuropathic pain in the United Kingdom. The treatment of major depressive illness is its primary usage. There is minimal evidence for amitriptyline. Although amitriptyline has been shown to alleviate DN pain in many RCTs (Boyle et al., 2012; Smith et al., 2022b), a prior Cochrane systematic review found that the findings given are probably skewed because of the small sample sizes (5 studies, 654 participants). However, the authors emphasized that it should be compared against the fact that amitriptyline has benefited thousands of patients (Moore et al. 2015a). Althoughamitriptyline's antidepressant and analgesic effects are well-established, the precise mechanism by which it exerts these effects remains a mystery. It inhibits noradrenaline and serotonin reuptake at nerve terminals andthe CNS's sodium, potassium, and N-methyl-D-aspartate (NMDA) channels. These channels are involved in the development of neuropathic pain. Postural hypotension, which may be particularly troublesome in older patients and requires strict monitoring, is one of the common adverse effects along with sleep difficulties, dry mouth, constipation, sexual dysfunction, arrhythmias, migraines, and others (Smith et al., 2022b). The effectiveness of desipramine and nortriptyline in alleviating painful DN has also been studied. There is evidence that desipramine, like amitriptyline, may help painful DN symptoms, according to severalRCTs (Max et al., 1991, 1992; Sindrup et al., 1990). In addition, a small-scale, double-blind RCT indicated that nortriptyline considerably decreased pain levels in DN patients (Gómez-Pérez et al., 1996). Despite this, prior Cochrane systematic reviews have found no evidence to support their use in neuropathic pain management (Derry et al., 2019; Hearn et al., 2014). This is because the studies that did evaluate them had significant methodological flaws and biases. The American Diabetes Association asserts that these medications are superior to amitriptyline for specific age groups and comorbidities, a view also shared by the American Academy of Neurology (Bril et al., 2011; Pop-Busui et al., 2017). Although a new study in cryptogenic sensory polyneuropathy showed that nortriptyline was effective in lowering neuropathic pain, no current studies have evaluated desipramine and nortriptyline in DN (Barohn et al., 2021).

3.9.4.2.4 Opioids

Opioids may be considered as a therapeutic option for painful DN according to some clinical recommendations (Bril et al., 2011; Cruccu et al., 2010), or as a component of combination therapy in cases when pain cannot be managed alone (Tesfaye et al., 2011). On the other hand, opioids pose a serious problem when it comes to addiction and misuse (Staudt et al., 2022). Because of these and other dangers, opioids are not recommended by the American Diabetes Association for painful DN (Pop-Busui et al., 2022). NICE states that only tramadol should be used as an acute salvage therapy [98]. In the United States and the United Kingdom, Tramadol is authorized for treating moderate to severe pain, not specifically neuropathic pain (Smith et al., 2022b). It binds most strongly to the μ, κ, and δ receptors in the middle of the cell. Furthermore, it should not be used in combination with SNRIs/SSRIs, as it inhibits the reuptake of noradrenaline and serotonin (Cruccu et al., 2010). There may be less potential for tramadol abuse when compared to other opioids (Dunn et al., 2019). There is limited evidence to support the effectiveness of tramadol. Two large RCTs (Freeman et al., 2007; Harati et al., 1998) showed that tramadol considerably reduced pain in DN patients compared to a placebo. A later RCT provided further evidence of tramadol's analgesic effectiveness in patients with polyneuropathy, which included people with diabetes (Sindrup et al., 2012). But there isn't much data on tramadol for neuropathic pain, and the studies that have been conducted have been tiny and probably biased, according to a recent Cochrane systematic review (Duehmke et al., 2017). Tapentadol is licensed for the treatment of neuropathic pain in the US but not in the UK. While tapentadol and tramadol have analgesic effects, tapentadol binds to the receptor more strongly (Alam et al., 2020). Tapentadol and tramadol often cause the following adverse effects: lightheadedness, somnolence, headache, nausea, and constipation (Smith et al., 2022b). There is currently insufficient data to recommend tapentadol. While it has shown promise in alleviating painful DN in several studies, further high-quality RCTs are required (Freo et al., 2019; Smith et al., 2022b). There is a lack of evidence to support the use of methadone and oxycodone as treatments for neuropathic pain (Gaskell et al., 2016; McNicol et al., 2017). Efficacy, safety, and effect on quality of life can only be determined by conducting more RCTs (McNicol et al., 2013).

3.9.4.2.5 Topical Analgesics

In cases when oral drugs are not tolerated, such as in cases of localized pain, topical analgesics may be considered as an option for uncomfortable DN, according to some clinical recommendations (Bril et al., 2011; Cruccu et al., 2010). Topical capsaicin has just received approval from the FDA to treat painful DN; however, the drug does not yet possess the appropriate licensing to be used for this purpose in the UK. It is believed to alleviate pain by influencing nerve fibre neurotrophic signalling and membrane potential (Anand & Bley, 2011). The evidence level varies from moderate to low depending on the strength of the topical capsaicin. In an RCT examining 0.025% capsaicin gel versus placebo, individuals with severe DN reported no statistically significant difference in pain reduction (Kulkantrakorn et al., 2013). The use of 0.075% capsaicin, as opposed to a placebo, considerably alleviates neuropathic pain, according to a prior meta-analysis that included 6 RCTs and 656 patients (Mason et al., 2004). There has been no significant difference between 0.075% capsaicin and placebo in a double-masked RCT that is adequately powered, since the meta-analysis (Kulkantrakorn et al., 2019). A recent meta-analysis of 25 RCTs showed that an 8% capsaicin patch effectively reduced pain by $\geq$ 30% compared to a placebo. In addition, it shares a profile of effectiveness with duloxetine and may be more advantageous than anticonvulsants (Van Nooten et al., 2017). Even while it may only take one application to reduce pain, a post hoc analysis of the PACE multi-centre open-label trial found that some patients might need two or even three applications before they saw any benefit (Freynhagen et al., 2021). The potential for topical capsaicin to injure tiny nerve fibres and disrupt nociceptive signals is a source of concern (Polydefkis et al., 2004). $\alpha 2$ adrenergic receptor agonist, topical clonidine, is more effective in individuals whose nociceptors have been altered by capsaicin (Campbell et al., 2012). Notwithstanding these reservations, capsaicin used topically has the potential to be less unpleasant than other oral pain relievers (Van Nooten et al., 2017). Since no high-quality RCTs have demonstrated the effectiveness of topical lidocaine or ketamine for DN, the level of evidence for these medications is relatively poor (Smith et al., 2022b).

3.9.4.2.6 Intravenous (IV) Medication

Although there is some weak evidence that intravenous medication may alleviate painful DN, current medical guidelines do not support this treatment. A new meta-analysis of 26 studies found that intravenous lidocaine reduces neuropathic pain in the short term (Zhu et al., 2019). Following the comprehensive review, an RCT including 34 patients with refractory neuropathic pain indicated that intravenous lidocaine had no more analgesic impact than the control infusion. Sleepiness, vertigo, nausea, and stomach aches were the most frequently reported adverse effects after infusion in this trial (Moulin et al., 2019). Administering intravenous ketamine at subanaesthetic doses has the dual effect of reducing pain and preventing hyperalgesia (Staudt et al., 2022). All 13 trials that looked at intravenous ketamine for neuropathic pain showed that it was effective in reducing pain, according to a recent meta-analysis (Wiffen et al., 2014). Ketamine sometimes causes several unpleasant side effects, such as light-headedness, lethargy, nausea, vomiting, and dizziness (Moulin et al., 2019).

3.9.4.3 Combination Therapy

Regrettably, there is a dearth of evidence-based research on combination treatment for neuropathic pain, which is a significant problem (Chou et al., 2009). Because of the substantial risk of serotonin syndrome, it is not possible to mix SNRIs with TCAs based on their pharmacological and pharmacokinetic profiles. Combinations of TCAs with gabapentin, pregabalin, or SNRI are also viable options. It is possible to mix opioids with any of these medications. Most recently, the AAN recommended adding venlafaxine to gabapentin for improved response, while the EFNS recommendations favoured a combination of gabapentin, opioids and TCA gabapentin (Basevi et al., 2011; Ziegler et al., 2011). The COMBO-DN multicentre, double-blind, parallel-group study in diabetic peripheral neuropathic pain, which was recently published, investigated whether the combination of both medications is more effective than increasing the dose of each drug to its maximum recommended dose in patients who are not responding to standard doses of duloxetine or pregabalin (Tesfaye et al., 2013). The initial 8 weeks of treatment consisted of 300 mg of pregabalin (groups 3, 4) or 60 mg of duloxetine (groups 1 and 2). Groups 2 and 3 got a combination of 60 mg of duloxetine and 300 mg of pregabalin daily, while group 4 received 600 mg of pregabalin daily. After that, only non-responders were given 120 mg of duloxetine per day for the 8 weeks of combination/high-dose treatment. A total of 804 individuals underwent evaluation for first treatment, with 339 undergoing evaluations for combination/high-dose therapy. With a p-value of 0.068, the 50% response rates for combination and high-dose monotherapy were 52.1% and 39.3%, respectively. According to exploratory analyses of the first 8 weeks of treatment without multiple comparison correction, 60 mg/day of duloxetine was shown to be better than 300 mg/day of pregabalin ($p < 0.001$) (Tesfaye et al., 2013). The combination treatment was deemed adequate, safe, and well-tolerated; however, it did not show a noticeable improvement over high-dose monotherapy.

3.10 Novel Therapies

Numerous innovative treatments are being studied, including neuromodulation devices like spinal cord stimulation (SCS), frequency-modulated electromagnetic neural stimulation (FREMS), transcutaneous electrical nerve stimulation (TENS), and neuromuscular electrical stimulation (NMES). The American Academy of Neurology has recommended that nutraceuticals, including acetyl-L-carnitine (ALC), α-lipoic acid (ALA), and vitamin $B_{12,}$ should be investigated further for their potential safety and effectiveness in DN (Bril et al., 2011). Although the American Diabetes Association previously said that there was insufficient evidence for the use of nutraceuticals in diabetes, they have now acknowledged this and included them in their monograph for the treatment of painful DN (Pop-Busui et al., 2022). Although nutraceuticals have great promise as a therapy for DN owing to their accessibility, low cost, and generally positive perception of safety, questions persist about their regulation, particularly about the absence of quality and manufacturing standards (Le et al., 2022; Yilmaz et al., 2017). Furthermore, there is a lack of high-quality research, so the existing evidence for their safety is poor to extremely low (Han et al., 2012; Rolim et al., 2019).

3.10.1 Devices for Neuromodulation

3.10.1.1 SCS (Spinal Cord Stimulation)

When dealing with very painful DN, several professional recommendations advise SCS (Pop-Busui et al., 2022; Tesfaye et al., 2011). The three distinct SCS treatments that use various electrical impulses are conventional (tonic pulse, 40–80 Hz), high-frequency (tonic pulse, 1–10 kHz), and burst stimulation (intermittent stimulation, variable parameters). There is no known precise mechanism by which SCS reduces pain (O'Connell et al., 2021). The 10 kHz SCS system was authorized by the FDA in 2021 for refractory painful DN in the USA, and SCS is approved in the UK for refractory neuropathic pain (Smith et al., 2022b). For SCS, the evidence is insufficient. A recent systematic review found two randomized controlled trials (RCTs) examining SCS for painful DN (Henson et al., 2021). Although both randomised controlled trials demonstrated a substantial reduction in pain, their design was of poor quality and likely prone to high risks of bias (Henson et al., 2021). The effectiveness of SCS in treating chronic pain, which is not solely due to DN, was the subject of a recent Cochrane systematic review (15 RCTs, 908 participants), which reported low-quality data and indicated that any therapeutic benefit disappeared once trials were sham-controlled. In addition, it brought attention to the fact that this treatment is associated with several very significant side effects, including infection, lead failure/displacement, and the need for further surgical operations (O'Connell et al., 2021). Although dorsal root ganglion stimulation has been suggested as a non-pharmacological option to pharmaceutical therapy for painful DN, no randomized controlled trials (RCTs) evaluating its effectiveness have been found.

3.10.1.2 Fragmentation Reconstruction by Electromagnetic Stimulation (FREMS)

The evidence for FREMS as a therapy for DN is so weak that clinical recommendations do not recommend it. While the placebo device showed no effects, the FREMS device lowered vibration thresholds and discomfort levels, enhanced sensory touch perception, and increased motor nerve conductivity in a preliminary randomized controlled trial ($n = 31$) (Bosi et al., 2005). There was no statistically significant difference between the control and intervention groups in a later multicentre, double-masked RCT ($n = 110$) that primarily assessed whether FREMS enhanced peripheral nerve conductivity. Furthermore, whereas FREMS alleviated some pain during administration, the effects did not last after stimulation (Bosi et al., 2013). Also, there were no statistically significant changes in pain levels between baseline and 12 weeks after 10 FREMS sessions, according to the newly published FREMSTOP trial ($n = 25$) (Crasto et al., 2022).

3.10.1.3 TENS (Transcutaneous Electrical Nerve Stimulation)

Nonpharmacological therapy options for chronic pain include transcutaneous electrical nerve stimulation (TENS), yet no professional recommendations suggest using it for painful DN. A meta-analysis indicated that TENS substantially lowers pain scores by 0.44 (95% CI 0.79 to 0.09), but the included studies had poor methodological quality, so the level of evidence for TENS is low (Stein et al., 2013). Some preliminary research in DN patients suggests that TENS may enhance vibration perception thresholds, balance, and gait metrics when compared to sham devices (Najafi et al., 2013, 2017). Electrical stimulation with percutaneous needles, sometimes referred to as PENS (percutaneous electrical nerve stimulation), is a method that is somewhat similar to TENS. Although PENS has been recommended as a therapy for painful DN by the American Academy of Neurology (Bril et al., 2011). Compared to sham needles, PENS considerably reduced pain, physical activity, and sleep ratings in a single randomized controlled trial ($n = 50$) of individuals with T2DM and DN (Hamza et al., 2000). Further studies with well-constructed RCTs are necessary to understand the effects of TENS and PENS further.

3.10.1.4 Neuromuscular Electrical Stimulation (NMES)

NMES may be used as a nonpharmacological adjuvant therapy for DN. In contrast to TENS and other forms of peripheral nerve stimulation, this method simulates exercise by depolarizing neurons and evoking muscular contractions. Currently, a double-masked RCT (clinicaltrials.gov identifier NCT03767478) is being conducted to examine NMES in DN (Smith et al., 2022b).

3.10.2 Nutraceuticals

3.10.2.1 α-Lipoic Acid (ALA)

Although ALA's promise has only been acknowledged in a few clinical recommendations (Pop-Busui et al., 2022; Tesfaye et al., 2011). It remains the most promising nutraceutical for the treatment of DN. A naturally occurring antioxidant called ALA may alleviate DN symptoms by lowering oxidative stress levels. This stress has various metabolic effects on microvessels and neurons. There are certain countries in which it is authorized to treat DN; however, the United States and the United

Kingdom are not among them (Pop-Busui et al., 2022). There is insufficient evidence to support the use of ALA. Intervention groups receiving 300–600 mg of IV ALA daily had significantly faster motor and sensory nerve conduction velocities than the control groups, according to a prior meta-analysis of 15 RCTs. Nevertheless, a large number of the studies that were considered had questionable quality and were very susceptible to bias (Han et al., 2012). Oral ALA has also been studied; a Russian-Israeli double-blind randomized controlled trial (SYDNEY II) with 181 participants found that 600 mg of ALA daily for 5 weeks alleviated neuropathy symptoms more than a placebo, and was better than 1200 mg and 1800 mg (Ziegler et al., 2006). In contrast, the NATHAN 1 trial determined that the composite primary endpoints of NIS-LL score and a battery of neurophysiology tests were not significantly impacted by 600 mg per day ALA over four years (Ziegler et al., 2011). Even if the NIS-LL scores are much higher than they were at baseline, the FDA will not approve the drug if the main objective is not met (Feldman et al., 2019; Ziegler et al., 2011).

3.10.2.2 Riboflavin (Vitamin B_{12})

Vitamin B_{12} insufficiency, peripheral neuropathy, and diabetes management often occur together. To begin, a diagnosis of DN cannot be made without first ruling out vitamin B_{12} deficiency, which is a separate cause of peripheral neuropathy (Pop-Busui et al., 2017). Additionally, a lack of vitamin B_{12} may be a side effect of the diabetes medication metformin. Individuals taking metformin were found to have lower vitamin B_{12} levels and a substantially increased risk of vitamin B_{12} insufficiency compared to those taking alternative diabetic therapies, according to a recent meta-analysis of 31 studies (Yang et al., 2019). Therefore, individuals on metformin, especially those with anaemia or peripheral neuropathy, should have their vitamin B_{12} levels checked regularly, according to the American Diabetes Association (American Diabetes Association, 2021). A 2022 MHRA investigation found a significantly higher-than-expected rate of vitamin B_{12} insufficiency in patients using metformin, indicating that these guidelines are not consistently followed in the UK. There is limited evidence for vitamin B_{12}, although it is believed to alleviate DN by reducing neuropathic pain and promoting myelin formation and repair (Jayabalan & Low, 2016; Okada et al., 2010; Zhang et al., 2013). Although most research has focused on the oral administration of vitamin B_{12}, injection is also an option. After one year, the effects of oral vitamin B_{12} (1000 g/day) vs placebo were examined in a significant double-blind RCT that included individuals with DN and autonomic neuropathy who had been using metformin for at least four years. While there was no statistically significant improvement in cardiovascular autonomic reflex assessments and neuropathy clinical examination scores, there were notable improvements in neuropathy symptoms, pain outcomes, QoL, sural nerve conduction velocity, action potential amplitude, and skin conductance in the feet of the 44 participants in the intervention group compared to baseline. Furthermore, no reported side effects were observed among participants (Didangelos et al., 2021). Although this study has promising results, further high-quality studies are needed to establish its effectiveness and safety in DN. Vitamin B_{12} is not suitable for all patients with DN at this time, as it is only prescribed for those who are deficient in it (Pop-Busui et al., 2022). Research on its effectiveness in T1DM is limited, as moststudies have focused on T2DM and metformin. In a recent study, Li et al. compared the effects of vitamin B_{12} (0.5 mg three times daily) and ALC (500 mg three times daily) in a multi-centre double-blind RCT that included individuals with T1DM and T2DM (Li et al., 2016). Although the vitamin B_{12} group did not improve the sural and typical peroneal nerve action potential amplitudes, both groups exhibited increased nerve conductivity. They experienced a dramatic decrease in neuropathy symptoms and impairment at 24 weeks. The agents were generally well-tolerated, and the adverse effects, including nausea, hiccups, stomach pain, and gastrointestinal problems, were comparable in the two groups. The authors failed to include any variations across diabetes subtypes, which may have provided valuable information and should be considered in future studies (Li et al., 2016). The rare but documented adverse effects of vitamin B_{12} in the general population include sensitivity and acne (Smith et al., 2022b).

3.10.2.3 Acetyl L-carnitine (ALC)

ALC's function in neuronal glucose and lipid metabolism has led to its suggestion as a potential therapy for DN. In hyperglycemic and hyperlipidemic states, maintaining optimal mitochondrial function is crucial, and this is achieved by promoting the transport of long-chain fatty acids (Rolim et al., 2019). Very little evidence has been found. According to a recent Cochrane systematic review, four trials involving 907 people examined ALC's effects in DN at doses of 2000 mg/day, 15,000 mg/day, and 3000 mg/day. Reviewers found very little evidence that ALC is more effective than placebo in reducing pain in DN at 6 and 12 months. There was a lack of high-quality data to establish safety, and little evidence was available for other endpoints, including sensations and symptoms. To understand outcomes like nerve conductivity, further high-quality research is required (Smith et al., 2022b).

3.11 Problems and Challenges in Diabetic Neuropathy Management

The introduction of various therapies, innovative therapeutic techniques, patient access to healthcare facilities, and knowledge-sharing initiatives about DN have been undertaken in response to the rapidly increasing incidence of the illness to slow its development. Disappointingly, several DN management issues require attention. This section goes into detail on the problems and challenges associated with enhancing DN management from the perspectives of knowledge, therapy, patient adherence, and facility accessibility (Ismail, 2023).

3.11.1 Problems in Treating Diabetic Neuropathy (DN)

Research has shown that 50% of people with DM would have DN symptoms at some point (Pop-Busui et al., 2010, 2013, 2017; Rolim et al., 2019; Ziegler et al., 2015). Roughly 20%–30% of people newly diagnosed with or in the early stages of T2DM have DN (Andersen et al., 2018). Also, the severe and agonizing pain might make it challenging to treat DN patients with symptomatic (painful) variations. A common complaint is persistent pain in the lower limbs, which worsens at night and is noticeable even at rest (Khadilkar et al., 2012). The precise mechanism by which this disease develops remains a mystery, regrettably. Despite encouraging results in pre-clinical investigations, several clinical trials were unsuccessful. As a result, uncertainties surrounding pharmacological targets hinder the development of innovative drugs that target diseases. Additionally, aldose reductase has been the subject of much investigation owing to its potential benefits in reversing DN, since Dvornik et al. uncovered its function in the DN pathogenesis (Dvornik et al., 1973). A possible next step in the fight against DN might be to inhibit this enzyme (Zhu, 2013). One strategy to prevent the polyol pathway from becoming overactive is to usealdose reductase inhibitors (ARIs). Nonetheless, no randomised controlled trial (RCT) demonstrating an advantage of ARIs over placebo in patients with DN was identified in a prior comprehensive review (Chalk et al., 2007). Although ARIs have been around for 30 years, their high side effect incidence has prevented them from being the standard therapy for DN (Veves, 2007). Other possible treatments involving the antagonistic effects of diacylglycerol buildup on PKC activation have also been the subject of similar concerns. The PKC inhibitor ruboxistaurin (RBX) has been shown to have therapeutic benefits in DN through a comprehensive evaluation of RCTs. Nevertheless, those trials could not provide enough data to prove that it effectively treated DN (Bansal et al., 2013). Patients with less severe DN have also shown that RBX is more successful in alleviating symptoms (Bansal et al., 2013; Vinik et al., 2005). In conclusion, several novel medicines that target RAGE activation have also been thoroughly investigated in animal models (Saleh et al., 2019), with some exhibiting promising therapeutic results for humans (El-Mesallamy et al., 2011). However, the high toxicity levels of these medications pose a significant challenge in clinical trials (Kobayashi & Zochodne, 2020; Pop-Busui et al., 2022). The industry is unwilling to invest more money in these medications due to uncertainties and the fact that they do not work very well in enhancing nerve function in T2DM-induced DN (Kobayashi & Zochodne, 2020). As a result, patients are left with fewer pharmaceutical options. Their only hope for slowing the disease's advancement is a mix of anti-diabetic drugs and various forms of therapy.

3.11.2 Problems with DN Medication Adherence

Despite the global establishment of diabetes care standards, several reasons exist why not all patients can follow them. A significant issue in many countries is that patients with type 2 diabetes mellitus (T2DM) often fail to adhere to their treatment regimens (Masaba & Mmusi-Phetoe, 2021; Whittemore et al., 2019). It is associated with a lack of understanding of the causes and course of diabetes, insecurity in one's financial situation, a lack of support from family and friends, difficulties in interacting between patients and healthcare providers, complicated treatment plans, and insufficient health insurance (Ismail, 2023). Concerned about the potential adverse effects of the drugs, several patients willingly discontinued therapy and began using traditional remedies instead. In addition, inadequate healthcare is a factor in people not following their diabetes treatment plans for self-care (Masaba & Mmusi-Phetoe, 2021). Ineffective communication between patients and healthcare professionals may undermine patient adherence, even when free drugs are provided by the government (Masaba & Mmusi-Phetoe, 2021). Especially when patients do not understand how their illness develops, cultural beliefs and myths are likely to impact their trust in their physicians' advice and prescriptions (Rezaei et al., 2019; Whittemore et al., 2019). As a result, improving the patient's adherence rate requires providing them with suitable health education and counselling. After receiving health education and counselling, patients' clinical results considerably enhanced (i.e., 86.8% adherence rate), as shown by Awodele and Osuolale (Awodele & Osuolale, 2015). Additionally, a complex treatment plan can increase the likelihood of non-adherence. Polypharmacy, the use of various pharmaceuticals by a single patient, is more common among patients with multiple comorbidities. Patients with diabetes and no other health problems were more likely to take their prescriptions as prescribed in a cross-sectional study than those with multiple medical conditions, who were more likely to require numerous medications (Alqarni et al., 2018; Hatah et al., 2020; Paraidathathu et al., 2013). Particularly in rural areas of low-income countries, there is a lack of understanding about the importance of diabetes treatment, which further complicates matters (Whittemore et al., 2019). However, community and healthcare professionals can collaborate to enhance people's knowledge, thereby addressing the problem. Patients' understanding and compliance with dietary guidelines grow when they get positive reinforcement from loved ones (Masaba & Mmusi-Phetoe, 2021). In addition, when given additional information about the advantages, older individuals with various comorbidities showed higher drug adherence (Huber & Reich, 2016; Rwegerera, 2014).

3.11.3 Poor Management in DN Due to Poverty

Even though there is a worldwide standard for managing diabetes, not all countries can afford it, particularly those in poorer nations where poverty is prevalent. Patients often fail to adhere due to financial constraints. Medications for diabetes were out of reach for 51% of Nigerian diabetic patients, the majority of whom were female and without jobs. The high expense of medicine meant that 69% of people had to buy smaller quantities (Awodele & Osuolale, 2015). Assistance from high-income nations is crucial in mitigating the impact of these challenges. Through international collaborative relationships, national programs may be implemented in healthcare facilities, medical schools, and hospitals (Karachaliou et al., 2020). The results show that the 12-month Kerala Diabetes Prevention Programme, which consisted of a peer support education group, reduced cardiovascular risk variables and enhanced lifestyle improvements. Improvements in diabetes symptoms, however, did not reach statistical significance (Thankappan et al., 2018).

3.11.4 The Coronavirus (COVID-2019) Pandemic Restricts Facility and Patient Education

Diabetes mellitus (DM) treatment and management have been profoundly affected by the 2019 coronavirus disease (COVID-19). People were put on lockdown for an extended period because of the pandemic. Appropriate guidelines for DM patients to attend hospital follow-ups were lacking in many low-income nations. Additionally, individuals in low-income countries were less likely to take precautions, including social distancing, wearing protective clothing, and seeking medical attention, due to inadequate sick pay and social security coverage (Ismail, 2023). Also, many patients had trouble getting their hands on the medications they needed for diabetes control since it involves going to healthcare centres to get prescriptions. During the COVID-19 pandemic, insulin was severely limited. While emergency services prioritized treating COVID-19 patients, several private hospitals' outpatient clinics and endocrinologists were temporarily closed. The treatment of diabetic patients, particularly those who required hospital admission, was affected by these challenges (Nouhjah & Jahanfar, 2020). In summary, patients experienced stress as a result of the disruption of their regular diabetic treatment, and their obesity increased as a result of their lack of physical exercise, both of which exacerbated their hyperglycemic states and problems associated with diabetes (Ghosal et al., 2020). In the wake of the COVID-19 pandemic, innovative approaches to diabetes care have emerged, such as telehealth, remote patient monitoring, online glucose monitoring through internet- and smartphone-enabled wearable tech, and free educational videos and ebooks on self-management of diabetes through mobile applications (Hartmann-Boyce et al., 2020; Wang et al., 2020). But since these standards are based on wealthier nations, they won't help patients in low-income countries that struggle with things like inadequate healthcare planning, low levels of education, and extreme poverty. Some proposals were made to enhance the treatment of DM patients, such as shifting from active to passive follow-up, creating community centres outside of hospitals (such as mosques, churches, and community centres) where patients can go for visits and training, and increasing the number of primary healthcare centres and outpatient clinics to treat non-communicable diseases. These centres took innovative steps, such as allowing patients to self-monitor their blood glucose levels without paying extra, providing doctors with guidelines for clinical management cases during disease outbreaks, having trained investigators conduct needs assessments, contacting patients via landlines for consultations with endocrinologists and physicians, and using patients' cell phones to spread educational and intervention information through text messages (Nouhjah & Jahanfar, 2020).

3.12 Emerging Research and Future Directions

Understanding the pathogenesis of diabetic neuropathy has made significant progress in recent years. Inflammatory pathways, oxidative stress, mitochondrial dysfunction, and immune-mediated pathways have been investigated in recent years (Feldman et al., 2019; Strand et al., 2024), but earlier research has focused on microvascular damage and chronic hyperglycemia. Recent advances in our understanding of these intricate processes and their connection to neuropathic pain have paved the way for novel targeted treatment approaches. For neuropathic pain caused by diabetic neuropathy, the FDA has authorized many possible treatments, including pregabalin, duloxetine, capsaicin, and spinal cord stimulation (Qureshi et al., 2022). In recent years, there has been a rise in interest in spinal cord stimulation (SCS) as a potential new therapeutic target. When oral medicines, vitamins, and other conservative approaches fail to alleviate neuropathic pain, SCS is often explored (Basem et al., 2023). A more recent alternative, high-frequency SCS (10 kHz), has outperformed more traditional therapies by more than 80% at the 24-month follow-up. Additionally, research has shown changes in neurological evaluations, specifically improvements in sensory abilities. Patients do not have many choices regarding treatments that may change their sickness. Novel disease-modifying treatment alternatives are required since rigorous glucose management has a limited impact on avoiding diabetic neuropathy. The beneficial effects of neuropathy may be enhanced by incorporating physical activity and dietary changes. From a disease-modifying perspective, however, further study is required to determine the impact of exercise in preventing and curing diabetic neuropathy. Oral drugs that may slow or stop the worsening of diabetic neuropathy do not exist at this time (Callaghan et al., 2020).

3.13 Conclusions

Understanding the pathogenesis of diabetic neuropathy is crucial for effective treatment. Sensory, motor, and autonomic neuropathy are part of diabetic peripheral neuropathy. Diabetic peripheral neuropathy develops in the peripheral nervous system and can affect both large and small nerve fibres. To fully comprehend the condition and its effects on patients, one must have an in-depth understanding of its complex impact on multiple organs. A disruption of the hexosamine, protein kinase C, or polymerase pathways, an increase in sorbitol levels, or damage caused by oxidative stress are all potential contributors to peripheral nerve injury. Endothelial dysfunction, impaired repair mechanisms, and neurovascular damage have all been linked (Bodman et al., 2025). Prevention is crucial for diabetic neuropathy since it affects so many organ systems, and there is currently no treatment. Educating patients about the dangers and signs of early peripheral neuropathy is essential. Patients diagnosed with diabetes or prediabetes should also get education about healthy eating habits. Diabetic neuropathy may grow silently, but if symptoms appear, they can be quite restricting; therefore, patient awareness is crucial. In addition to reducing lipids, blood pressure, and blood sugar, losing weight simplifies blood sugar regulation; thus, exercise and weight reduction should be addressed. In addition, patients should be aware of the need for foot protection and should refrain from invasive foot operations (Strand et al., 2024).

Treatment options for insensate or painless DN are limited. First- and second-linepharmacotherapies for individuals with painful DN include anticonvulsants, SNRIs, and TCAs. Many adverse effects are associated with these pharmacotherapies, and the evidence for their efficacy is of moderate to low quality. The use of opioids as a third-line pharmacotherapy is sometimes advised. However, new guidelines caution against its use altogether due to the hazards. Recent trials of 8% topical capsaicin demonstrate effectiveness for painful DN, while the evidence for topical analgesics is moderate to poor. Medications administered intravenously are not yet advised; their use is restricted to instances where there is no improvement and more research is needed. Novel nonpharmacological treatments for DN, such as neuromodulation devices, may enhance nerve conductivity and pain relief. Despite the related procedural risks and low-quality data, SCS has just been authorized for severe, painful DN. The effectiveness of other non-invasive neuromodulation devices, such as TENS and NMES, remains unknown due to a lack of sufficient evidence. Novel disease-modifying nutraceuticals, including ALA, vitamin B_{12}, and ALC, have been investigated. Still, neither the US nor the UK has found enough evidence to approve them, and there are growing safety concerns about them due to the absence of restrictions (Smith et al., 2022b). The psychological and social effects of DN, as well as its morbidity, have recently attracted a lot of attention. Managing DN symptoms and stopping the disease from progressing are the main goals of current clinical recommendations. Unfortunately, the efficacy of current therapy is compromised since most of these recommendations do not address the underlying causes that contribute to DN. To address the challenges that prevent the current treatment of DN from being effective, it is essential to determine the mechanisms and risk factors of DN (Ismail, 2023).

3.14 Availability of Data

None.

Acknowledgements The images were created using www.biorander.com and www.Grammarly.com to correct the grammar of this manuscript.

Author Contributions Shahnaz Alom, Farak Ali, and Md. Abubakar were involved in the conceptualization, writing of the original draft, and providing mechanistic insights; they also provided input on critical points and edited the manuscript, Samiksha Yogi contributed to the manuscript writing and editing, Hans Raj Bhatwere involved in the conceptualization, manuscript writing, reviewing, and conceptualization of figures, and approved the version to be published.

Funding None.

Conflict of Interest None.

References

Abbott, C. A., Malik, R. A., Van Ross, E. R. E., Kulkarni, J., & Boulton, A. J. M. (2011). Prevalence and characteristics of painful diabetic neuropathy in a large community-based diabetic population in the U.K. *Diabetes Care, 34*(10), 2220–2224. https://doi.org/10.2337/dc11-1108

Aiyer, R., Mehta, N., Gungor, S., & Gulati, A. (2018). A systematic review of NMDA receptor antagonists for treatment of neuropathic pain in clinical practice. *The Clinical Journal of Pain, 34*(5), 450–467. https://doi.org/10.1097/AJP.0000000000000547

Alam, U., Sloan, G., & Tesfaye, S. (2020). Treating pain in diabetic neuropathy: Current and developmental drugs. *Drugs, 80*(4), 363–384. https://doi.org/10.1007/s40265-020-01259-2

Alqarni, A. M., Alrahbeni, T., Al Qarni, A., & Al Qarni, H. M. (2018). Adherence to diabetes medication among diabetic patients in the Bisha governorate of Saudi Arabia & A cross-sectional survey. *Patient Preference and Adherence, 13*, 63–71. https://doi.org/10.2147/PPA.S176355

American Diabetes Association. (2011). Standards of medical care in diabetes—2011. *Diabetes Care, 34*(Supplement_1), S11–S61. https://doi.org/10.2337/dc11-S011

American Diabetes Association. (2021). 3. prevention or delay of type 2 diabetes: Standards of medical care in diabetes—2021. *Diabetes Care, 44*(Supplement_1), S34–S39. https://doi.org/10.2337/dc21-S003

Anand, P., & Bley, K. (2011). Topical capsaicin for pain management: Therapeutic potential and mechanisms of action of the new high-concentration capsaicin 8% patch. *British Journal of Anaesthesia, 107*(4), 490–502. https://doi.org/10.1093/bja/aer260

Andersen, S. T., Witte, D. R., Dalsgaard, E.-M., Andersen, H., Nawroth, P., Fleming, T., Jensen, T. M., Finnerup, N. B., Jensen, T. S., Lauritzen, T., Feldman, E. L., Callaghan, B. C., & Charles, M. (2018). Risk factors for incident diabetic polyneuropathy in a cohort with screen-detected type 2 diabetes followed for 13 years: ADDITION-Denmark. *Diabetes Care, 41*(5), 1068–1075. https://doi.org/10.2337/dc17-2062

Ang, L., Jaiswal, M., Martin, C., & Pop-Busui, R. (2014). Glucose control and diabetic neuropathy: Lessons from recent large clinical trials. *Current Diabetes Reports, 14*(9), 528. https://doi.org/10.1007/s11892-014-0528-7

Ansari, P., Hannan, J. M. A., Azam, S., & Jakaria, M. (2021). Challenges in diabetic micro-complication management: Focus on diabetic neuropathy. *International Journal of Translational Medicine, 1*(3), 175–186. https://doi.org/10.3390/ijtm1030013

Attal, N., Cruccu, G., Baron, R., Haanpää, M., Hansson, P., Jensen, T. S., & Nurmikko, T. (2010). EFNS guidelines on the pharmacological treatment of neuropathic pain: 2010 revision. *European Journal of Neurology, 17*(9), 1113. https://doi.org/10.1111/j.1468-1331.2010.02999.x

Awodele, O., & Osuolale, J. (2015). Medication adherence in type 2 diabetes patients: Study of patients in Alimosho General Hospital, Igando, Lagos, Nigeria. *African Health Sciences, 15*(2), 513. https://doi.org/10.4314/ahs.v15i2.26

Balducci, S., Iacobellis, G., Parisi, L., Di Biase, N., Calandriello, E., Leonetti, F., & Fallucca, F. (2006). Exercise training can modify the natural history of diabetic peripheral neuropathy. *Journal of Diabetes and Its Complications, 20*(4), 216–223. https://doi.org/10.1016/j.jdiacomp.2005.07.005

Bansal, D., Badhan, Y., Gudala, K., & Schifano, F. (2013). Ruboxistaurin for the treatment of diabetic peripheral neuropathy: A systematic review of randomized clinical trials. *Diabetes & Metabolism Journal, 37*(5), 375. https://doi.org/10.4093/dmj.2013.37.5.375

Bansal, V., Kalita, J., & Misra, U. K. (2006). Diabetic neuropathy. *Postgraduate Medical Journal, 82*(964), 95–100. https://doi.org/10.1136/pgmj.2005.036137

Barbosa, M., Saavedra, A., Oliveira, S., Reis, L., Rodrigues, F., Severo, M., Sittl, R., Maier, C., & Carvalho, D. M. (2019). Prevalence and determinants of painful and painless neuropathy in type 1 diabetes mellitus. *Frontiers in Endocrinology, 10*, 402. https://doi.org/10.3389/fendo.2019.00402

Barohn, R. J., Gajewski, B., Pasnoor, M., Brown, A., Herbelin, L. L., Kimminau, K. S., Mudaranthakam, D. P., Jawdat, O., Dimachkie, M. M., Patient Assisted Intervention for Neuropathy: Comparison of Treatment in Real Life Situations (PAIN-CONTRoLS) Study Team, Iyadurai, S., Stino, A., Kissel, J., Pascuzzi, R., Brannagan, T., Wicklund, M., Ahmed, A., Walk, D., Smith, G., … Cash, T. (2021). Patient assisted intervention for neuropathy: Comparison of treatment in real life situations (PAIN-CONTRoLS): Bayesian adaptive comparative effectiveness randomized trial. *JAMA Neurology, 78*(1), 68. https://doi.org/10.1001/jamaneurol.2020.2590

Baron, R., Binder, A., & Wasner, G. (2010). Neuropathic pain: Diagnosis, pathophysiological mechanisms, and treatment. *The Lancet Neurology, 9*(8), 807–819. https://doi.org/10.1016/S1474-4422(10)70143-5

Basem, J. I., Bah, F. N., & Mehta, N. D. (2023). A brief review on the novel therapies for painful diabetic neuropathy. *Current Pain and Headache Reports, 27*(9), 299–305. https://doi.org/10.1007/s11916-023-01126-1

Basevi, V., Di Mario, S., Morciano, C., Nonino, F., & Magrini, N. (2011). Comment on: American diabetes association. Standards of medical care in diabetes—2011. *Diabetes Care, 34*(Suppl. 1), S11–S61, e53–e53. https://doi.org/10.2337/dc11-0174

Bhatti, J. S., Sehrawat, A., Mishra, J., Sidhu, I. S., Navik, U., Khullar, N., Kumar, S., Bhatti, G. K., & Reddy, P. H. (2022). Oxidative stress in the pathophysiology of type 2 diabetes and related complications: Current therapeutics strategies and future perspectives. *Free Radical Biology and Medicine, 184*, 114–134. https://doi.org/10.1016/j.freeradbiomed.2022.03.019

Birse, F., Derry, S., & Moore, R. A. (2012). Phenytoin for neuropathic pain and fibromyalgia in adults. *Cochrane Database of Systematic Reviews, 5*. https://doi.org/10.1002/14651858.CD009485.pub2

Bodman, M. A., Dreyer, M. A., & Varacallo, M. A. (2025). Diabetic peripheral neuropathy. In *StatPearls*. StatPearls Publishing. http://www.ncbi.nlm.nih.gov/books/NBK442009/

Bosi, E., Bax, G., Scionti, L., Spallone, V., Tesfaye, S., Valensi, P., & Ziegler, D. (2013). Frequency-modulated electromagnetic neural stimulation (FREMS) as a treatment for symptomatic diabetic neuropathy: Results from a double-blind, randomised, multicentre, long-term, placebo-controlled clinical trial. *Diabetologia, 56*(3), 467–475. https://doi.org/10.1007/s00125-012-2795-7

Bosi, E., Conti, M., Vermigli, C., Cazzetta, G., Peretti, E., Cordoni, M. C., Galimberti, G., & Scionti, L. (2005). Effectiveness of frequency-modulated electromagnetic neural stimulation in the treatment of painful diabetic neuropathy. *Diabetologia, 48*(5), 817–823. https://doi.org/10.1007/s00125-005-1734-2

Boulton, A. J. M., Vinik, A. I., Arezzo, J. C., Bril, V., Feldman, E. L., Freeman, R., Malik, R. A., Maser, R. E., Sosenko, J. M., & Ziegler, D. (2005). Diabetic neuropathies. *Diabetes Care, 28*(4), 956–962. https://doi.org/10.2337/diacare.28.4.956

Boyle, J., Eriksson, M. E. V., Gribble, L., Gouni, R., Johnsen, S., Coppini, D. V., & Kerr, D. (2012). Randomized, placebo-controlled comparison of amitriptyline, duloxetine, and pregabalin in patients with chronic diabetic peripheral neuropathic pain. *Diabetes Care, 35*(12), 2451–2458. https://doi.org/10.2337/dc12-0656

Braffett, B. H., Gubitosi-Klug, R. A., Albers, J. W., Feldman, E. L., Martin, C. L., White, N. H., Orchard, T. J., Lopes-Virella, M., Lachin, J. M., Pop-Busui, R., & The DCCT/EDIC Research Group. (2020). Risk factors for diabetic peripheral neuropathy and cardiovascular autonomic neuropathy in the diabetes control and complications trial/epidemiology of diabetes interventions and complications (DCCT/EDIC) study. *Diabetes, 69*(5), 1000–1010. https://doi.org/10.2337/db19-1046

Bril, V., England, J., Franklin, G. M., Backonja, M., Cohen, J., Del Toro, D., Feldman, E., Iverson, D. J., Perkins, B., Russell, J. W., & Zochodne, D. (2011). Evidence-based guideline: Treatment of painful diabetic neuropathy [RETIRED]: Report of the American Academy of Neurology, the American Association of Neuromuscular and Electrodiagnostic Medicine, and the American Academy of Physical Medicine and Rehabilitation. *Neurology, 76*(20), 1758–1765. https://doi.org/10.1212/WNL.0b013e3182166ebe

Buggy, A., & Moore, Z. (2017). The impact of the multidisciplinary team in the management of individuals with diabetic foot ulcers: A systematic review. *Journal of Wound Care, 26*(6), 324–339. https://doi.org/10.12968/jowc.2017.26.6.324

Burakgazi, A. Z., Alsowaity, B., Burakgazi, Z. A., Unal, D., & Kelly, J. J. (2012). Bladder dysfunction in peripheral neuropathies. *Muscle & Nerve, 45*(1), 2–8. https://doi.org/10.1002/mus.22178

Callaghan, B. C., Gallagher, G., Fridman, V., & Feldman, E. L. (2020). Diabetic neuropathy: What does the future hold? *Diabetologia, 63*(5), 891–897. https://doi.org/10.1007/s00125-020-05085-9

Callaghan, B. C., Gao, L., Li, Y., Zhou, X., Reynolds, E., Banerjee, M., Pop-Busui, R., Feldman, E. L., & Ji, L. (2018). Diabetes and obesity are the main metabolic drivers of peripheral neuropathy. *Annals of Clinical and Translational Neurology, 5*(4), 397–405. https://doi.org/10.1002/acn3.531

Callaghan, B. C., Little, A. A., Feldman, E. L., & Hughes, R. A. (2012). Enhanced glucose control for preventing and treating diabetic neuropathy. *Cochrane Database of Systematic Reviews, 6*. https://doi.org/10.1002/14651858.CD007543.pub2

Callaghan, B. C., Xia, R., Banerjee, M., De Rekeneire, N., Harris, T. B., Newman, A. B., Satterfield, S., Schwartz, A. V., Vinik, A. I., Feldman, E. L., & Strotmeyer, E. S. (2016). Metabolic syndrome components are associated with symptomatic polyneuropathy independent of glycemic status. *Diabetes Care, 39*(5), 801–807. https://doi.org/10.2337/dc16-0081

Campbell, C. M., Kipnes, M. S., Stouch, B. C., Brady, K. L., Kelly, M., Schmidt, W. K., Petersen, K. L., Rowbotham, M. C., & Campbell, J. N. (2012). Randomized control trial of topical clonidine for treatment of painful diabetic neuropathy. *Pain, 153*(9), 1815–1823. https://doi.org/10.1016/j.pain.2012.04.014

Cantó, C., Houtkooper, R. H., Pirinen, E., Youn, D. Y., Oosterveer, M. H., Cen, Y., Fernandez-Marcos, P. J., Yamamoto, H., Andreux, P. A., Cettour-Rose, P., Gademann, K., Rinsch, C., Schoonjans, K., Sauve, A. A., & Auwerx, J. (2012). The NAD+ precursor nicotinamide riboside enhances oxidative metabolism and protects against high-fat diet-induced obesity. *Cell Metabolism, 15*(6), 838–847. https://doi.org/10.1016/j.cmet.2012.04.022

Chalk, C., Benstead, T. J., & Moore, F. (2007). Aldose reductase inhibitors for the treatment of diabetic polyneuropathy. *Cochrane Database of Systematic Reviews, 1*. https://doi.org/10.1002/14651858.CD004572.pub2

Chandarasekaran, K. (2016). *Nicotinamide adenine dinucleotide (NAD)*. https://doi.org/10.1036/1097-8542.452150

Chandrasekharan, B., & Srinivasan, S. (2007). Diabetes and the enteric nervous system. *Neurogastroenterology & Motility, 19*(12), 951–960. https://doi.org/10.1111/j.1365-2982.2007.01023.x

Chou, R., Carson, S., & Chan, B. K. S. (2009). Gabapentin versus tricyclic antidepressants for diabetic neuropathy and post-herpetic neuralgia: Discrepancies between direct and indirect meta-analyses of randomized controlled trials. *Journal of General Internal Medicine, 24*(2), 178–188. https://doi.org/10.1007/s11606-008-0877-5

Chowdhury, S. K. R., Smith, D. R., & Fernyhough, P. (2013). The role of aberrant mitochondrial bioenergetics in diabetic neuropathy. *Neurobiology of Disease, 51*, 56–65. https://doi.org/10.1016/j.nbd.2012.03.016

Christensen, D. H., Knudsen, S. T., Gylfadottir, S. S., Christensen, L. B., Nielsen, J. S., Beck-Nielsen, H., Sørensen, H. T., Andersen, H., Callaghan, B. C., Feldman, E. L., Finnerup, N. B., Jensen, T. S., & Thomsen, R. W. (2020). Metabolic factors, lifestyle habits, and possible polyneuropathy in early type 2 diabetes: A nationwide study of 5,249 patients in the Danish Centre for Strategic Research in type 2 diabetes (DD2) cohort. *Diabetes Care, 43*(6), 1266–1275. https://doi.org/10.2337/dc19-2277

Cotter, M. A., & Cameron, N. E. (2003). Effect of the NAD(P)H oxidase inhibitor, apocynin, on peripheral nerve perfusion and function in diabetic rats. *Life Sciences, 73*(14), 1813–1824. https://doi.org/10.1016/S0024-3205(03)00508-3

Crasto, W., Altaf, Q., Selvaraj, D. R., Jack, B., Patel, V., Nawaz, S., Murthy, N., Sukumar, N., Saravanan, P., & Tahrani, A. A. (2022). Frequency rhythmic electrical modulation system (FREMS) to alleviate painful diabetic peripheral neuropathy: A pilot, randomised controlled trial (The FREMSTOP study). *Diabetic Medicine, 39*(3), Article e14710. https://doi.org/10.1111/dme.14710

Cruccu, G., Sommer, C., Anand, P., Attal, N., Baron, R., Garcia-Larrea, L., Haanpaa, M., Jensen, T. S., Serra, J., & Treede, R.-D. (2010). EFNS guidelines on neuropathic pain assessment: Revised 2009. *European Journal of Neurology, 17*(8), 1010–1018. https://doi.org/10.1111/j.1468-1331.2010.02969.x

Davies, M., Brophy, S., Williams, R., & Taylor, A. (2006). The prevalence, severity, and impact of painful diabetic peripheral neuropathy in type 2 diabetes. *Diabetes Care, 29*(7), 1518–1522. https://doi.org/10.2337/dc05-2228

Deli, G., Bosnyak, E., Pusch, G., Komoly, S., & Feher, G. (2013). Diabetic neuropathies: Diagnosis and management. *Neuroendocrinology, 98*(4), 267–280. https://doi.org/10.1159/000358728

Derry, S., Bell, R. F., Straube, S., Wiffen, P. J., Aldington, D., & Moore, R. A. (2019). Pregabalin for neuropathic pain in adults. *Cochrane Database of Systematic Reviews, 5*. https://doi.org/10.1002/14651858.CD007076.pub3

Dewanjee, S., Das, S., Das, A. K., Bhattacharjee, N., Dihingia, A., Dua, T. K., Kalita, J., & Manna, P. (2018). Molecular mechanism of diabetic neuropathy and its pharmacotherapeutic targets. *European Journal of Pharmacology, 833*, 472–523. https://doi.org/10.1016/j.ejphar.2018.06.034

Didangelos, T., Karlafti, E., Kotzakioulafi, E., Margariti, E., Giannoulaki, P., Batanis, G., Tesfaye, S., & Kantartzis, K. (2021). Vitamin B12 supplementation in diabetic neuropathy: A 1-year, randomized, double-blind. *Placebo-Controlled Trial. Nutrients, 13*(2), 395. https://doi.org/10.3390/nu13020395

Dorresteijn, J. A., Kriegsman, D. M., Assendelft, W. J., & Valk, G. D. (2014). Patient education for preventing diabetic foot ulceration. *Cochrane Database of Systematic Reviews, 12*. https://doi.org/10.1002/14651858.CD001488.pub5

Duehmke, R. M., Derry, S., Wiffen, P. J., Bell, R. F., Aldington, D., & Moore, R. A. (2017). Tramadol for neuropathic pain in adults. *Cochrane Database of Systematic Reviews, 6*. https://doi.org/10.1002/14651858.CD003726.pub4

Dunn, K. E., Bergeria, C. L., Huhn, A. S., & Strain, E. C. (2019). A systematic review of laboratory evidence for the abuse potential of tramadol in humans. *Frontiers in Psychiatry, 10*, 704. https://doi.org/10.3389/fpsyt.2019.00704

Dvornik, D., Simard-Duquesne, N., Krami, M., Sestanj, K., Gabbay, K. H., Kinoshita, J. H., Varma, S. D., & Merola, L. O. (1973). Polyol Accumulation in galactosemic and diabetic rats: Control by an aldose reductase inhibitor. *Science, 182*(4117), 1146–1148. https://doi.org/10.1126/science.182.4117.1146

Edwards, J. L., Vincent, A. M., Cheng, H. T., & Feldman, E. L. (2008). Diabetic neuropathy: Mechanisms to management. *Pharmacology & Therapeutics, 120*(1), 1–34. https://doi.org/10.1016/j.pharmthera.2008.05.005

Eid, S., Sas, K. M., Abcouwer, S. F., Feldman, E. L., Gardner, T. W., Pennathur, S., & Fort, P. E. (2019). New insights into the mechanisms of diabetic complications: Role of lipids and lipid metabolism. *Diabetologia, 62*(9), 1539–1549. https://doi.org/10.1007/s00125-019-4959-1

El-Mesallamy, H. O., Hamdy, N. M., Ezzat, O. A., & Reda, A. M. (2011). Levels of soluble advanced glycation end product-receptors and other soluble serum markers as indicators of diabetic neuropathy in the foot. *Journal of Investigative Medicine: The Official Publication of the American Federation for Clinical Research, 59*(8), 1233–1238. https://doi.org/10.2130/JIM.0b013e318231db64

Farshchian, N., Alavi, A., Heydarheydari, S., & Moradian, N. (2018). Comparative study of the effects of venlafaxine and duloxetine on chemotherapy-induced peripheral neuropathy. *Cancer Chemotherapy and Pharmacology, 82*(5), 787–793. https://doi.org/10.1007/s00280-018-3664-y

Feldman, E. L., Callaghan, B. C., Pop-Busui, R., Zochodne, D. W., Wright, D. E., Bennett, D. L., Bril, V., Russell, J. W., & Viswanathan, V. (2019). Diabetic neuropathy. *Nature Reviews Disease Primers, 5*(1), 41. https://doi.org/10.1038/s41572-019-0092-1

Feldman, E. L., Nave, K.-A., Jensen, T. S., & Bennett, D. L. H. (2017). New horizons in diabetic neuropathy: Mechanisms, bioenergetics, and pain. *Neuron, 93*(6), 1296–1313. https://doi.org/10.1016/j.neuron.2017.02.005

Fernyhough, P. (2015). Mitochondrial dysfunction in diabetic neuropathy: A series of unfortunate metabolic events. *Current Diabetes Reports, 15*(11), 89. https://doi.org/10.1007/s11892-015-0671-9

Fernyhough, P., & McGavock, J. (2014). Mechanisms of disease: Mitochondrial dysfunction in sensory neuropathy and other complications in diabetes. *Handbook of Clinical Neurology, 126*, 353–377. https://doi.org/10.1016/B978-0-444-53480-4.00027-8

Fonseca, V. A. (2007). Clinical diabetes: Translating research into practice. *Annals of Internal Medicine, 146*(2), 152. https://doi.org/10.7326/0003-4819-146-2-200701160-00020

Freeman, R. (2005). Autonomic peripheral neuropathy. *The Lancet, 365*(9466), 1259–1270. https://doi.org/10.1016/S0140-6736(05)74815-7

Freeman, R., Raskin, P., Hewitt, D. J., Vorsanger, G. J., Jordan, D. M., Xiang, J., Rosenthal, N. R., & for the CAPSS-237 Study Group. (2007). Randomized study of tramadol/acetaminophen versus placebo in painful diabetic peripheral neuropathy. *Current Medical Research and Opinion, 23*(1), 147–161. https://doi.org/10.1185/030079906X162674

Freo, U., Romualdi, P., & Kress, H. G. (2019). Tapentadol for neuropathic pain: A review of clinical studies. *Journal of Pain Research, 12*, 1537–1551. https://doi.org/10.2147/JPR.S190162

Freynhagen, R., Argoff, C., Eerdekens, M., Engelen, S., & Perrot, S. (2021). Progressive response to repeat application of capsaicin 179 mg (8% w/w) cutaneous patch in peripheral neuropathic pain: Comprehensive new analysis and clinical implications. *Pain Medicine, 22*(10), 2324–2336. https://doi.org/10.1093/pm/pnab113

Gæde, P., Vedel, P., Parving, H.-H., & Pedersen, O. (1999). Intensified multifactorial intervention in patients with type 2 diabetes mellitus and microalbuminuria: The Steno type 2 randomised study. *The Lancet, 353*(9153), 617–622. https://doi.org/10.1016/S0140-6736(98)07368-1

Gallagher, H. C., Gallagher, R. M., Butler, M., Buggy, D. J., & Henman, M. C. (2015). Venlafaxine for neuropathic pain in adults. *Cochrane Database of Systematic Reviews, 6*. https://doi.org/10.1002/14651858.CD011091.pub2

Gao, Y., Guo, X., Han, P., Li, Q., Yang, G., Qu, S., Yue, L., Wang, C. -N., Skljarevski, V., Dueñas, H., Raskin, J., & Gu, L. (2015). Treatment of patients with diabetic peripheral neuropathic pain in China: A double-blind randomised trial of duloxetine vs. placebo. *International Journal of Clinical Practice, 69*(9), 957–966. https://doi.org/10.1111/ijcp.12641

Gaskell, H., Derry, S., Stannard, C., & Moore, R. A. (2016). Oxycodone for neuropathic pain in adults. *Cochrane Database of Systematic Reviews,* 7. https://doi.org/10.1002/14651858.CD010692.pub3

Ghosal, S., Sinha, B., Majumder, M., & Misra, A. (2020). Estimation of effects of nationwide lockdown for containing coronavirus infection on worsening of glycosylated haemoglobin and increase in diabetes-related complications: A simulation model using multivariate regression analysis. *Diabetes & Metabolic Syndrome: Clinical Research & Reviews, 14*(4), 319–323. https://doi.org/10.1016/j.dsx.2020.03.014

Gill, D., Derry, S., Wiffen, P. J., & Moore, R. A. (2011). Valproic acid and sodium valproate for neuropathic pain and fibromyalgia in adults. *Cochrane Database of Systematic Reviews.* https://doi.org/10.1002/14651858.CD009183.pub2

Gómez-Pérez, F. J., Choza, R., Ríos, J. M., Reza, A., Huerta, E., Aguilar, C. A., & Rull, J. A. (1996). Nortriptyline-fluphenazine vs. Carbamazepine in the symptomatic treatment of diabetic neuropathy. *Archives of Medical Research, 27*(4), 525–529.

Hall, B. E., Macdonald, E., Cassidy, M., Yun, S., Sapio, M. R., Ray, P., Doty, M., Nara, P., Burton, M. D., Shiers, S., Ray-Chaudhury, A., Mannes, A. J., Price, T. J., Iadarola, M. J., & Kulkarni, A. B. (2022). Transcriptomic analysis of human sensory neurons in painful diabetic neuropathy reveals inflammation and neuronal loss. *Scientific Reports, 12*(1), 4729. https://doi.org/10.1038/s41598-022-08100-8

Hamza, M. A., White, P. F., Craig, W. F., Ghoname, E. S., Ahmed, H. E., Proctor, T. J., Noe, C. E., Vakharia, A. S., & Gajraj, N. (2000). Percutaneous electrical nerve stimulation: A novel analgesic therapy for diabetic neuropathic pain. *Diabetes Care, 23*(3), 365–370. https://doi.org/10.2337/diacare.23.3.365

Han, T., Bai, J., Liu, W., & Hu, Y. (2012). Therapy of endocrine disease: A systematic review and meta-analysis of α-lipoic acid in the treatment of diabetic peripheral neuropathy. *European Journal of Endocrinology, 167*(4), 465–471. https://doi.org/10.1530/EJE-12-0555

Hansen, C. S., Määttä, L. L., Andersen, S. T., & Charles, M. H. (2023). The epidemiology of diabetic neuropathy. In S. Tesfaye, C. H. Gibbons, R. A. Malik, & A. Veves (Eds.), *Diabetic neuropathy* (pp. 5–36). Springer International Publishing. https://doi.org/10.1007/978-3-031-15613-7_2

Harati, Y., Gooch, C., Swenson, M., Edelman, S., Greene, D., Raskin, P., Donofrio, P., Cornblath, D., Sachdeo, R., Siu, C. O., & Kamin, M. (1998). Double-blind randomized trial of tramadol for the treatment of the pain of diabetic neuropathy. *Neurology, 50*(6), 1842–1846. https://doi.org/10.1212/WNL.50.6.1842

Hartemann, A., Attal, N., Bouhassira, D., Dumont, I., Gin, H., Jeanne, S., Said, G., & Richard, J.-L. (2011). Painful diabetic neuropathy: Diagnosis and management. *Diabetes & Metabolism, 37*(5), 377–388. https://doi.org/10.1016/j.diabet.2011.06.003

Hartmann-Boyce, J., Morris, E., Goyder, C., Kinton, J., Perring, J., Nunan, D., Mahtani, K., Buse, J. B., Del Prato, S., Ji, L., Roussel, R., & Khunti, K. (2020). Diabetes and COVID-19: Risks, management, and learnings from other national disasters. *Diabetes Care, 43*(8), 1695–1703. https://doi.org/10.2337/dc20-1192

Hatah, E., Rahim, N., Makmor-Bakry, M., Mohamed Shah, N., Mohamad, N., Ahmad, M., Haron, N. H., Sze Hwe, C., Tan Meng Wah, A., Hassan, F., Shaik Rahmat, S., Robert, S. A., & Abdullah, N. (2020). Development and validation of Malaysia medication adherence assessment tool (MyMAAT) for diabetic patients. *PLOS ONE, 15*(11), e0241909. https://doi.org/10.1371/journal.pone.0241909

Hearn, L., Moore, R. A., Derry, S., Wiffen, P. J., & Phillips, T. (2014). Desipramine for neuropathic pain in adults. In The Cochrane Collaboration (Ed.), *Cochrane Database of Systematic Reviews* (p. CD011003.pub2). John Wiley & Sons, Ltd. https://doi.org/10.1002/14651858.CD011003.pub2

Henson, J. V., Varhabhatla, N. C., Bebic, Z., Kaye, A. D., Yong, R. J., Urman, R. D., & Merkow, J. S. (2021). Spinal cord stimulation for painful diabetic peripheral neuropathy: A systematic review. *Pain and Therapy, 10*(2), 895–908. https://doi.org/10.1007/s40122-021-00282-9

Hicks, C. W., & Selvin, E. (2019). Epidemiology of peripheral neuropathy and lower extremity disease in diabetes. *Current Diabetes Reports, 19*(10), 86. https://doi.org/10.1007/s11892-019-1212-8

Huber, C. A., & Reich, O. (2016). Medication adherence in patients with diabetes mellitus: Does physician drug dispensing enhance quality of care? Evidence from a large health claims database in Switzerland. *Patient Preference and Adherence, 10*, 1803–1809. https://doi.org/10.2147/PPA.S115425

Ismail, C. A. N. (2023). Issues and challenges in diabetic neuropathy management: A narrative review. *World Journal of Diabetes, 14*(6), 741–757. https://doi.org/10.4239/wjd.v14.i6.741

Ismail-Beigi, F., Craven, T., Banerji, M. A., Basile, J., Calles, J., Cohen, R. M., Cuddihy, R., Cushman, W. C., Genuth, S., Grimm, R. H., Hamilton, B. P., Hoogwerf, B., Karl, D., Katz, L., Krikorian, A., O'Connor, P., Pop-Busui, R., Schubart, U., Simmons, D., … Hramiak, I. (2010). Effect of intensive treatment of hyperglycaemia on microvascular outcomes in type 2 diabetes: An analysis of the ACCORD randomised trial. *The Lancet, 376*(9739), 419–430. https://doi.org/10.1016/S0140-6736(10)60576-4

Jaiswal, M., Lauer, A., Martin, C. L., Bell, R. A., Divers, J., Dabelea, D., Pettitt, D. J., Saydah, S., Pihoker, C., Standiford, D. A., Rodriguez, B. L., Pop-Busui, R., Feldman, E. L., & for the SEARCH for Diabetes in Youth Study Group. (2013). Peripheral neuropathy in adolescents and young adults with type 1 and type 2 diabetes from the SEARCH for diabetes in youth follow-up cohort. *Diabetes Care, 36*(12), 3903–3908. https://doi.org/10.2337/dc13-1213

Jang, E.-R., & Lee, C. S. (2011). 7-Ketocholesterol induces apoptosis in differentiated PC12 cells via reactive oxygen species-dependent activation of NF-κB and Akt pathways. *Neurochemistry International, 58*(1), 52–59. https://doi.org/10.1016/j.neuint.2010.10.012

Jarso, G., Ahmed, A., & Feleke, Y. (2011). The prevalence, clinical features and management of periphral neuropathy among diabetic patients in Tikur Anbessa and St. Paul's Specialized University Hospitals, Addis Ababa, Ethiopia. *Ethiopian Medical Journal, 49*(4), 299–311.

Jayabalan, B., & Low, L. (2016). Vitamin B supplementation for diabetic peripheral neuropathy. *Singapore Medical Journal, 57*(02), 55–59. https://doi.org/10.11622/smedj.2016027

Karachaliou, F., Simatos, G., & Simatou, A. (2020). The challenges in the development of diabetes prevention and care models in low-income settings. *Frontiers in Endocrinology, 11*, 518. https://doi.org/10.3389/fendo.2020.00518

Keller, J. N., Hanni, K. B., & Markesbery, W. R. (1999). Oxidized low-density lipoprotein induces neuronal death: Implications for calcium, reactive oxygen species, and caspases. *Journal of Neurochemistry, 72*(6), 2601–2609. https://doi.org/10.1046/j.1471-4159.1999.0722601.x

Khadilkar, S., Mukadana, A., & Deshmukh, S. (2012). Diabetic neuropathy: Pain and its management. In *Symptom oriented pain management* (pp. 316–316). Jaypee Brothers Medical Publishers (P) Ltd. https://doi.org/10.5005/jp/books/11597_31

Kirthi, V., Perumbalath, A., Brown, E., Nevitt, S., Petropoulos, I. N., Burgess, J., Roylance, R., Cuthbertson, D. J., Jackson, T. L., Malik, R. A., & Alam, U. (2021). Prevalence of peripheral neuropathy in pre-diabetes: A systematic review. *BMJ Open Diabetes Research & Care, 9*(1), Article e002040. https://doi.org/10.1136/bmjdrc-2020-002040

Knowler, W. C. (2002). Reduction in the incidence of type 2 diabetes with lifestyle intervention or metformin. *New England Journal of Medicine, 346*(6), 393–403. https://doi.org/10.1056/NEJMoa012512

Kobayashi, M., & Zochodne, D. W. (2020). Diabetic polyneuropathy: Bridging the translational gap. *Journal of the Peripheral Nervous System, 25*(2), 66–75. https://doi.org/10.1111/jns.12392

Kulkantrakorn, K., Chomjit, A., Sithinamsuwan, P., Tharavanij, T., Suwankanoknark, J., & Napunnaphat, P. (2019). 0.075% capsaicin lotion for the treatment of painful diabetic neuropathy: A randomized, double-blind, crossover, placebo-controlled trial. *Journal of Clinical Neuroscience, 62*, 174–179. https://doi.org/10.1016/j.jocn.2018.11.036

Kulkantrakorn, K., Lorsuwansiri, C., & Meesawatsom, P. (2013). 0.025% capsaicin gel for the treatment of painful diabetic neuropathy: A randomized, double-blind, crossover, Placebo-controlled trial. *Pain Practice, 13*(6), 497–503. https://doi.org/10.1111/papr.12013

Lancet. (1998). Intensive blood-glucose control with sulphonylureas or insulin compared with conventional treatment and risk of complications in patients with type 2 diabetes (UKPDS 33). *The Lancet, 352*(9131), 837–853. https://doi.org/10.1016/S0140-6736(98)07019-6

Le, Y., Wang, B., & Xue, M. (2022). Nutraceuticals use and type 2 diabetes mellitus. *Current Opinion in Pharmacology, 62*, 168–176. https://doi.org/10.1016/j.coph.2021.12.004

Li, S., Chen, X., Li, Q., Du, J., Liu, Z., Peng, Y., Xu, M., Li, Q., Lei, M., Wang, C., Zheng, S., Zhang, X., Yu, H., Shi, J., Tao, S., Feng, P., & Tian, H. (2016). Effects of acetyl-L-carnitine and methylcobalamin for diabetic peripheral neuropathy: A multicenter, randomized, double-blind, controlled trial. *Journal of Diabetes Investigation, 7*(5), 777–785. https://doi.org/10.1111/jdi.12493

Luna, R., Talanki Manjunatha, R., Bollu, B., Jhaveri, S., Avanthika, C., Reddy, N., Saha, T., & Gandhi, F. (2021). A comprehensive review of neuronal changes in diabetics. *Cureus*. https://doi.org/10.7759/cureus.19142

Lunn, M. P., Hughes, R. A., & Wiffen, P. J. (2014). Duloxetine for treating painful neuropathy, chronic pain or fibromyalgia. *Cochrane Database of Systematic Reviews, 10*. https://doi.org/10.1002/14651858.CD007115.pub3

Lyssenko, V., & Vaag, A. (2023). Genetics of diabetes-associated microvascular complications. *Diabetologia, 66*(9), 1601–1613. https://doi.org/10.1007/s00125-023-05964-x

Malone, J. I., Lowitt, S., Korthals, J. K., Salem, A., & Miranda, C. (1996). The effect of hyperglycemia on nerve conduction and structure is age dependent. *Diabetes, 45*(2), 209–215. https://doi.org/10.2337/diab.45.2.209

Martin, C. L., Albers, J. W., Pop-Busui, R., & for the DCCT/EDIC Research Group. (2014). Neuropathy and related findings in the diabetes control and complications trial/epidemiology of diabetes interventions and complications study. *Diabetes Care, 37*(1), 31–38. https://doi.org/10.2337/dc13-2114

Masaba, B. B., & Mmusi-Phetoe, R. M. (2021). Determinants of non-adherence to treatment among patients with type 2 diabetes in Kenya: A systematic review. *Journal of Multidisciplinary Healthcare, 13*, 2069–2076. https://doi.org/10.2147/JMDH.S270137

Maser, R. E., Steenkiste, A. R., Dorman, J. S., Nielsen, V. K., Bass, E. B., Manjoo, Q., Drash, A. L., Becker, D. J., Kuller, L. H., Greene, D. A., & Orchard, T. J. (1989). Epidemiological correlates of diabetic neuropathy: Report From Pittsburgh epidemiology of diabetes complications study. *Diabetes, 38*(11), 1456–1461. https://doi.org/10.2337/diab.38.11.1456

Mason, L., Moore, R. A., Derry, S., Edwards, J. E., & McQuay, H. J. (2004). Systematic review of topical capsaicin for the treatment of chronic pain. *BMJ, 328*(7446), 991. https://doi.org/10.1136/bmj.38042.506748.EE

Max, M. B., Kishore-Kumar, R., Schafer, S. C., Meister, B., Gracely, R. H., Smoller, B., & Dubner, R. (1991). Efficacy of desipramine in painful diabetic neuropathy: A placebo-controlled trial. *Pain, 45*(1), 3–9. https://doi.org/10.1016/0304-3959(91)90157-S

Max, M. B., Lynch, S. A., Muir, J., Shoaf, S. E., Smoller, B., & Dubner, R. (1992). Effects of desipramine, amitriptyline, and fluoxetine on pain in diabetic neuropathy. *New England Journal of Medicine, 326*(19), 1250–1256. https://doi.org/10.1056/NEJM199205073261904

McNicol, E. D., Ferguson, M. C., & Schumann, R. (2017). Methadone for neuropathic pain in adults. *Cochrane Database of Systematic Reviews, 1*. https://doi.org/10.1002/14651858.CD012499.pub2

McNicol, E. D., Midbari, A., & Eisenberg, E. (2013). Opioids for neuropathic pain. *Cochrane Database of Systematic Reviews, 1*. https://doi.org/10.1002/14651858.CD006146.pub2

Moore, R., Spinhirne, A., Lai, M. J., Preisser, S., Li, Y., Kang, T., & Bleris, L. (2015a). CRISPR-based self-cleaving mechanism for controllable gene delivery in human cells. *Nucleic Acids Research, 43*(2), 1297–1303. https://doi.org/10.1093/nar/gku1326

Moore, R. A., Derry, S., Aldington, D., Cole, P., & Wiffen, P. J. (2015b). Amitriptyline for neuropathic pain in adults. *Cochrane Database of Systematic Reviews, 5*. https://doi.org/10.1002/14651858.CD008242.pub3

Moţăţăianu, A., Maier, S., Bajko, Z., Voidazan, S., Bălaşa, R., & Stoian, A. (2018). Cardiac autonomic neuropathy in type 1 and type 2 diabetes patients. *BMC Neurology, 18*(1), 126. https://doi.org/10.1186/s12883-018-1125-1

Moulin, D. E., Morley-Forster, P. K., Pirani, Z., Rohfritsch, C., & Stitt, L. (2019). Intravenous lidocaine in the management of chronic peripheral neuropathic pain: A randomized-controlled trial. *Canadian Journal of Anesthesia/journal Canadien D'anesthésie, 66*(7), 820–827. https://doi.org/10.1007/s12630-019-01395-8

Najafi, B., Crews, R. T., & Wrobel, J. S. (2013). A novel plantar stimulation technology for improving protective sensation and postural control in patients with diabetic peripheral neuropathy: A double-blinded. *Randomized Study. Gerontology, 59*(5), 473–480. https://doi.org/10.1159/000352072

Najafi, B., Talal, T. K., Grewal, G. S., Menzies, R., Armstrong, D. G., & Lavery, L. A. (2017). Using plantar electrical stimulation to improve postural balance and plantar sensation among patients with diabetic peripheral neuropathy: A randomized double blinded study. *Journal of Diabetes Science and Technology, 11*(4), 693–701. https://doi.org/10.1177/1932296817695338

Nathan, D. M. (1993). The effect of intensive treatment of diabetes on the development and progression of long-term complications in insulin-dependent diabetes mellitus. *New England Journal of Medicine, 329*(14), 977–986. https://doi.org/10.1056/NEJM199309303291401

Nouhjah, S., & Jahanfar, S. (2020). Challenges of diabetes care management in developing countries with a high incidence of COVID-19: A brief report. *Diabetes & Metabolic Syndrome: Clinical Research & Reviews, 14*(5), 731–732. https://doi.org/10.1016/j.dsx.2020.05.012

Obrosova, I. G. (2009). Diabetic painful and insensate neuropathy: Pathogenesis and potential treatments. *Neurotherapeutics, 6*(4), 638–647. https://doi.org/10.1016/j.nurt.2009.07.004

O'Connell, N. E., Ferraro, M. C., Gibson, W., Rice, A. S., Vase, L., Coyle, D., & Eccleston, C. (2021). Implanted spinal neuromodulation interventions for chronic pain in adults. *Cochrane Database of Systematic Reviews, 4*. https://doi.org/10.1002/14651858.CD013756.pub2

Okada, K., Tanaka, H., Temporin, K., Okamoto, M., Kuroda, Y., Moritomo, H., Murase, T., & Yoshikawa, H. (2010). Methylcobalamin increases Erk1/2 and Akt activities through the methylation cycle and promotes nerve regeneration in a rat sciatic nerve injury model. *Experimental Neurology, 222*(2), 191–203. https://doi.org/10.1016/j.expneurol.2009.12.017

Orchard, T. J., Temprosa, M., Goldberg, R., Haffner, S., Ratner, R., Marcovina, S., Fowler, S., & for the Diabetes Prevention Program Research Group. (2005). The effect of metformin and intensive lifestyle intervention on the metabolic syndrome: The diabetes prevention program randomized trial. *Annals of Internal Medicine, 142*(8), 611–619. https://doi.org/10.7326/0003-4819-142-8-200504190-00009

Palumbo, P. J. (2007). Metabolic risk factors, endothelial dysfunction, and erectile dysfunction in men with diabetes. *The American Journal of the Medical Sciences, 334*(6), 466–480. https://doi.org/10.1097/MAJ.0b013e318126c198

Paraidathathu, T., Azuana, Islahudin, F., & Ahmad. (2013). Medication adherence in patients with type 2 diabetes mellitus treated at primary health clinics in Malaysia. *Patient Preference and Adherence, 525*. https://doi.org/10.2147/PPA.S44698

Polydefkis, M., Hauer, P., Sheth, S., Sirdofsky, M., Griffin, J. W., & McArthur, J. C. (2004). The time course of epidermal nerve fibre regeneration: Studies in normal controls and in people with diabetes, with and without neuropathy. *Brain, 127*(7), 1606–1615. https://doi.org/10.1093/brain/awh175

Pop-Busui, R. (2010). Cardiac autonomic neuropathy in diabetes. *Diabetes Care, 33*(2), 434–441. https://doi.org/10.2337/dc09-1294

Pop-Busui, R., Ang, L., Boulton, A., Feldman, E., Marcus, R., Mizokami-Stout, K., Singleton, J. R., & Ziegler, D. (2022). Diagnosis and treatment of painful diabetic peripheral neuropathy. *ADA Clinical Compendia, 2022*(1), 1–32. https://doi.org/10.2337/db2022-01

Pop-Busui, R., Boulton, A. J. M., Feldman, E. L., Bril, V., Freeman, R., Malik, R. A., Sosenko, J. M., & Ziegler, D. (2017). Diabetic neuropathy: A position statement by the American Diabetes Association. *Diabetes Care, 40*(1), 136–154. https://doi.org/10.2337/dc16-2042

Pop-Busui, R., Evans, G. W., Gerstein, H. C., Fonseca, V., Fleg, J. L., Hoogwerf, B. J., Genuth, S., Grimm, R. H., Corson, M. A., Prineas, R., & the ACCORD Study Group. (2010). Effects of cardiac autonomic dysfunction on mortality risk in the action to control cardiovascular risk in diabetes (ACCORD) trial. *Diabetes Care, 33*(7), 1578–1584. https://doi.org/10.2337/dc10-0125

Pop-Busui, R., Lu, J., Brooks, M. M., Albert, S., Althouse, A. D., Escobedo, J., Green, J., Palumbo, P., Perkins, B. A., Whitehouse, F., Jones, T. L. Z., & for the BARI 2D Study Group. (2013). Impact of glycemic control strategies on the progression of diabetic peripheral neuropathy in the bypass angioplasty revascularization investigation 2 diabetes (BARI 2D) cohort. *Diabetes Care, 36*(10), 3208–3215. https://doi.org/10.2337/dc13-0012

Price, D., & Hackett, G. (2008). Management of erectile dysfunction in diabetes: An update for 2008. *Current Diabetes Reports, 8*(6), 437–443. https://doi.org/10.1007/s11892-008-0076-0

Qureshi, Z., Ali, M. N., & Khalid, M. (2022). An insight into potential pharmacotherapeutic agents for painful diabetic neuropathy. *Journal of Diabetes Research, 2022*, 1–19. https://doi.org/10.1155/2022/9989272

Rezaei, M., Valiee, S., Tahan, M., Ebtekar, F., & Ghanei Gheshlagh, R. (2019). Barriers of medication adherence in patients with type-2 diabetes: A pilot qualitative study. *Diabetes, Metabolic Syndrome and Obesity: Targets and Therapy, 12*, 589–599. https://doi.org/10.2147/DMSO.S197159

Rodríguez-Gutiérrez, R., & Montori, V. M. (2016). Glycemic control for patients with type 2 diabetes mellitus: Our evolving faith in the face of evidence. *Circulation: Cardiovascular Quality and Outcomes, 9*(5), 504–512. https://doi.org/10.1161/CIRCOUTCOMES.116.002901

Rolim, L. C., Da Silva, E. M., Flumignan, R. L., Abreu, M. M., & Dib, S. A. (2019). Acetyl-L-carnitine for the treatment of diabetic peripheral neuropathy. *Cochrane Database of Systematic Reviews, 6*. https://doi.org/10.1002/14651858.CD011265.pub2

Russell, J. W., Berent-Spillson, A., Vincent, A. M., Freimann, C. L., Sullivan, K. A., & Feldman, E. L. (2008). Oxidative injury and neuropathy in diabetes and impaired glucose tolerance. *Neurobiology of Disease, 30*(3), 420–429. https://doi.org/10.1016/j.nbd.2008.02.013

Rutkove, S. B. (2009). A 52-year-old woman with disabling peripheral neuropathy: Review of diabetic polyneuropathy. *JAMA, 302*(13), 1451. https://doi.org/10.1001/jama.2009.1377

Rwegerera, G. M. (2014). Adherence to anti-diabetic drugs among patients with Type 2 diabetes mellitus at Muhimbili National Hospital, Dar es Salaam, Tanzania- A cross-sectional study. *Pan African Medical Journal, 17*. https://doi.org/10.11604/pamj.2014.17.252.2972

Saleh, I., Maritska, Z., Parisa, N., & Hidayat, R. (2019). Inhibition of receptor for advanced glycation end products as new promising strategy treatment in diabetic retinopathy. *Open Access Macedonian Journal of Medical Sciences, 7*(23), 3921–3924. https://doi.org/10.3889/oamjms.2019.759

Sasaki, H., Kawamura, N., Dyck, P. J., Dyck, P. J. B., Kihara, M., & Low, P. A. (2020). Spectrum of diabetic neuropathies. *Diabetology International, 11*(2), 87–96. https://doi.org/10.1007/s13340-019-00424-7

Schaper, N. C., Van Netten, J. J., Apelqvist, J., Lipsky, B. A., Bakker, K., & on behalf of the International Working Group on the Diabetic Foot (IWGDF). (2016). Prevention and management of foot problems in diabetes: A Summary Guidance for Daily Practice 2015, based on the IWGDF Guidance Documents. *Diabetes/metabolism Research and Reviews, 32*(S1), 7–15. https://doi.org/10.1002/dmrr.2695

Schreiber, A. K. (2015). Diabetic neuropathic pain: Physiopathology and treatment. *World Journal of Diabetes, 6*(3), 432. https://doi.org/10.4239/wjd.v6.i3.432

Sies, H. (1999). Glutathione and its role in cellular functions. *Free Radical Biology & Medicine, 27*(9–10), 916–921. https://doi.org/10.1016/s0891-5849(99)00177-x

Sindrup, S., Gram, L., Skjold, T., Grodum, E., Brosen, K., & Beck-Nielsen, H. (1990). Clomipramine vs desipramine vs placebo in the treatment of diabetic neuropathy symptoms. A double-blind cross-over study. *British Journal of Clinical Pharmacology, 30*(5), 683–691. https://doi.org/10.1111/j.1365-2125.1990.tb03836.x

Sindrup, S. H., Konder, R., Lehmann, R., Meier, T., Winkel, M., Ashworth, J., Baron, R., & Jensen, T. S. (2012). Randomized controlled trial of the combined monoaminergic and opioid investigational compound GRT9906 in painful polyneuropathy. *European Journal of Pain, 16*(6), 849–859. https://doi.org/10.1002/j.1532-2149.2011.00069.x

Sloan, G., Shillo, P., Selvarajah, D., Wu, J., Wilkinson, I. D., Tracey, I., Anand, P., & Tesfaye, S. (2018). A new look at painful diabetic neuropathy. *Diabetes Research and Clinical Practice, 144*, 177–191. https://doi.org/10.1016/j.diabres.2018.08.020

Smith, S., Normahani, P., Lane, T., Hohenschurz-Schmidt, D., Oliver, N., & Davies, A. H. (2022a). Pathogenesis of distal symmetrical polyneuropathy in diabetes. *Life, 12*(7), 1074. https://doi.org/10.3390/life12071074

Smith, S., Normahani, P., Lane, T., Hohenschurz-Schmidt, D., Oliver, N., & Davies, A. H. (2022b). Prevention and management strategies for diabetic neuropathy. *Life, 12*(8), 1185. https://doi.org/10.3390/life12081185

Spallone, V., Bellavere, F., Scionti, L., Maule, S., Quadri, R., Bax, G., Melga, P., Viviani, G. L., Esposito, K., & Morganti, R. (2011). Recommendations for the use of cardiovascular tests in diagnosing diabetic autonomic neuropathy☆. *Nutrition, Metabolism and Cardiovascular Diseases, 21*(1), 69–78. https://doi.org/10.1016/j.numecd.2010.07.005

Staudt, M. D., Prabhala, T., Sheldon, B. L., Quaranta, N., Zakher, M., Bhullar, R., Pilitsis, J. G., & Argoff, C. E. (2022). Current strategies for the management of painful diabetic neuropathy. *Journal of Diabetes Science and Technology, 16*(2), 341–352. https://doi.org/10.1177/1932296820951829

Stein, C., Eibel, B., Sbruzzi, G., Lago, P. D., & Plentz, R. D. M. (2013). Electrical stimulation and electromagnetic field use in patients with diabetic neuropathy: Systematic review and meta-analysis. *Brazilian Journal of Physical Therapy, 17*(2), 93–104. https://doi.org/10.1590/S1413-35552012005000083

Stevens, M., & Shakher, J. (2011). Update on the management of diabetic polyneuropathies. *Diabetes, Metabolic Syndrome and Obesity: Targets and Therapy, 289*. https://doi.org/10.2147/DMSO.S11324

Strand, N., Anderson, M. A., Attanti, S., Gill, B., Wie, C., Dawodu, A., Pagan-Rosado, R., Harbell, M. W., & Maloney, J. A. (2024). Diabetic neuropathy: Pathophysiology review. *Current Pain and Headache Reports, 28*(6), 481–487. https://doi.org/10.1007/s11916-024-01243-5

Streckmann, F., Balke, M., Cavaletti, G., Toscanelli, A., Bloch, W., Décard, B. F., Lehmann, H. C., & Faude, O. (2022). Exercise and neuropathy: Systematic review with meta-analysis. *Sports Medicine, 52*(5), 1043–1065. https://doi.org/10.1007/s40279-021-01596-6

Stubbs, E. B., Fisher, M. A., Miller, C. M., Jelinek, C., Butler, J., McBurney, C., & Collins, E. G. (2019). Randomized controlled trial of physical exercise in diabetic veterans with length-dependent distal symmetric polyneuropathy. *Frontiers in Neuroscience, 13*, 51. https://doi.org/10.3389/fnins.2019.00051

Tanenberg, R. J., Clemow, D. B., Giaconia, J. M., & Risser, R. C. (2014). Duloxetine compared with pregabalin for diabetic peripheral neuropathic pain management in patients with suboptimal pain response to gabapentin and treated with or without antidepressants: A post hoc analysis. *Pain Practice, 14*(7), 640–648. https://doi.org/10.1111/papr.12121

Tesfaye, S., Boulton, A. J. M., Dyck, P. J., Freeman, R., Horowitz, M., Kempler, P., Lauria, G., Malik, R. A., Spallone, V., Vinik, A., Bernardi, L., Valensi, P., & on behalf of the Toronto Diabetic Neuropathy Expert Group. (2010). Diabetic neuropathies: Update on definitions, diagnostic criteria, estimation of severity, and treatments. *Diabetes Care, 33*(10), 2285–2293. https://doi.org/10.2337/dc10-1303

Tesfaye, S., & Selvarajah, D. (2012). Advances in the epidemiology, pathogenesis and management of diabetic peripheral neuropathy. *Diabetes/metabolism Research and Reviews, 28*(S1), 8–14. https://doi.org/10.1002/dmrr.2239

Tesfaye, S., Vileikyte, L., Rayman, G., Sindrup, S. H., Perkins, B. A., Baconja, M., Vinik, A. I., Boulton, A. J. M., & on behalf of The Toronto Expert Panel on Diabetic Neuropathy. (2011). Painful diabetic peripheral neuropathy: Consensus recommendations on diagnosis, assessment and management. *Diabetes/metabolism Research and Reviews, 27*(7), 629–638. https://doi.org/10.1002/dmrr.1225

Tesfaye, S., Wilhelm, S., Lledo, A., Schacht, A., Tölle, T., Bouhassira, D., Cruccu, G., Skljarevski, V., & Freynhagen, R. (2013). Duloxetine and pregabalin: High-dose monotherapy or their combination? The "COMBO-DN study"—A multinational, randomized, double-blind, parallel-group study in patients with diabetic peripheral neuropathic pain. *Pain, 154*(12), 2616–2625. https://doi.org/10.1016/j.pain.2013.05.043

Thankappan, K. R., Sathish, T., Tapp, R. J., Shaw, J. E., Lotfaliany, M., Wolfe, R., Absetz, P., Mathews, E., Aziz, Z., Williams, E. D., Fisher, E. B., Zimmet, P. Z., Mahal, A., Balachandran, S., D'Esposito, F., Sajeev, P., Thomas, E., & Oldenburg, B. (2018). A peer-support lifestyle intervention for preventing type 2 diabetes in India: A cluster-randomized controlled trial of the Kerala Diabetes Prevention Program. *PLOS Medicine, 15*(6), Article e1002575. https://doi.org/10.1371/journal.pmed.1002575

The Diabetes Control and Complications Trial Research Group. (1993). The effect of intensive treatment of diabetes on the development and progression of long-term complications in insulin-dependent diabetes mellitus. *New England Journal of Medicine, 329*(14), 977–986. https://doi.org/10.1056/NEJM199309303291401

Thorud, J. C., Plemmons, B., Buckley, C. J., Shibuya, N., & Jupiter, D. C. (2016). Mortality after nontraumatic major amputation among patients with diabetes and peripheral vascular disease: A systematic review. *The Journal of Foot and Ankle Surgery, 55*(3), 591–599. https://doi.org/10.1053/j.jfas.2016.01.012

Tracy, J. A., & Dyck, P. J. B. (2008). The spectrum of diabetic neuropathies. *Physical Medicine and Rehabilitation Clinics of North America, 19*(1), 1–26. https://doi.org/10.1016/j.pmr.2007.10.010

Van Acker, K., Bouhassira, D., De Bacquer, D., Weiss, S., Matthys, K., Raemen, H., Mathieu, C., & Colin, I. M. (2009). Prevalence and impact on quality of life of peripheral neuropathy with or without neuropathic pain in type 1 and type 2 diabetic patients attending hospital outpatients clinics. *Diabetes & Metabolism, 35*(3), 206–213. https://doi.org/10.1016/j.diabet.2008.11.004

Van Nooten, F., Treur, M., Pantiri, K., Stoker, M., & Charokopou, M. (2017). Capsaicin 8% patch versus oral neuropathic pain medications for the treatment of painful diabetic peripheral neuropathy: A systematic literature review and network meta-analysis. *Clinical Therapeutics, 39*(4), 787-803.e18. https://doi.org/10.1016/j.clinthera.2017.02.010

Veves, A. (2007). Aldose reductase inhibitors for the treatment of diabetic neuropathy. In A. Veves & R. A. Malik (Eds.), *Diabetic neuropathy* (pp. 309–320). Humana Press. https://doi.org/10.1007/978-1-59745-311-0_18

Viader, A., Sasaki, Y., Kim, S., Strickland, A., Workman, C. S., Yang, K., Gross, R. W., & Milbrandt, J. (2013). Aberrant Schwann cell lipid metabolism linked to mitochondrial deficits leads to axon degeneration and neuropathy. *Neuron, 77*(5), 886–898. https://doi.org/10.1016/j.neuron.2013.01.012

Vincent. (2013). Biology of diabetic neuropathy. In *Handbook of clinical neurology* (Vol. 115, pp. 591–606). Elsevier. https://doi.org/10.1016/B978-0-444-52902-2.00034-5

Vincent, A., Edwards, J., Sadidi, M., & Feldman, E. (2008). The antioxidant response as a drug target in diabetic neuropathy. *Current Drug Targets, 9*(1), 94–100. https://doi.org/10.2174/138945008783431754

Vincent, A. M., Callaghan, B. C., Smith, A. L., & Feldman, E. L. (2011). Diabetic neuropathy: Cellular mechanisms as therapeutic targets. *Nature Reviews Neurology, 7*(10), 573–583. https://doi.org/10.1038/nrneurol.2011.137

Vincent, A. M., Hayes, J. M., McLean, L. L., Vivekanandan-Giri, A., Pennathur, S., & Feldman, E. L. (2009a). Dyslipidemia-induced neuropathy in mice. *Diabetes, 58*(10), 2376–2385. https://doi.org/10.2337/db09-0047

Vincent, A. M., Kato, K., McLean, L. L., Soules, M. E., & Feldman, E. L. (2009b). Sensory neurons and Schwann cells respond to oxidative stress by increasing antioxidant defense mechanisms. *Antioxidants & Redox Signaling, 11*(3), 425–438. https://doi.org/10.1089/ars.2008.2235

Vincent, A. M., Perrone, L., Sullivan, K. A., Backus, C., Sastry, A. M., Lastoskie, C., & Feldman, E. L. (2007). Receptor for advanced glycation end products activation injures primary sensory neurons via oxidative stress. *Endocrinology, 148*(2), 548–558. https://doi.org/10.1210/en.2006-0073

Vincent, A. M., Russell, J. W., Low, P., & Feldman, E. L. (2004). Oxidative stress in the pathogenesis of diabetic neuropathy. *Endocrine Reviews, 25*(4), 612–628. https://doi.org/10.1210/er.2003-0019

Vinik, A. I., Bril, V., Kempler, P., Litchy, W. J., Tesfaye, S., Price, K. L., & Bastyr, E. J. (2005). Treatment of symptomatic diabetic peripheral neuropathy with the protein kinase C β-inhibitor ruboxistaurin mesylate during a 1-year, randomized, placebo-controlled, double-blind clinical trial. *Clinical Therapeutics, 27*(8), 1164–1180. https://doi.org/10.1016/j.clinthera.2005.08.001

Volpe, C. M. O., Villar-Delfino, P. H., Dos Anjos, P. M. F., & Nogueira-Machado, J. A. (2018). Cellular death, reactive oxygen species (ROS) and diabetic complications. *Cell Death & Disease, 9*(2), 119. https://doi.org/10.1038/s41419-017-0135-z

Wang, A., Zhao, W., Xu, Z., & Gu, J. (2020). Timely blood glucose management for the outbreak of 2019 novel coronavirus disease (COVID-19) is urgently needed. *Diabetes Research and Clinical Practice, 162*, Article 108118. https://doi.org/10.1016/j.diabres.2020.108118

Whittemore, R., Vilar-Compte, M., De La Cerda, S., Marron, D., Conover, R., Delvy, R., Lozano-Marrufo, A., & Pérez-Escamilla, R. (2019). Challenges to diabetes self-management for adults with type 2 diabetes in low-resource settings in Mexico City: A qualitative descriptive study. *International Journal for Equity in Health, 18*(1), 133. https://doi.org/10.1186/s12939-019-1035-x

Wiffen, P. J., Derry, S., Bell, R. F., Rice, A. S., Tölle, T. R., Phillips, T., & Moore, R. A. (2017). Gabapentin for chronic neuropathic pain in adults. *Cochrane Database of Systematic Reviews, 2*. https://doi.org/10.1002/14651858.CD007938.pub4

Wiffen, P. J., Derry, S., & Moore, R. A. (2013). Lamotrigine for chronic neuropathic pain and fibromyalgia in adults. *Cochrane Database of Systematic Reviews, 5*. https://doi.org/10.1002/14651858.CD006044.pub4

Wiffen, P. J., Derry, S., Moore, R. A., & Kalso, E. A. (2014). Carbamazepine for chronic neuropathic pain and fibromyalgia in adults. *Cochrane Database of Systematic Reviews, 5*. https://doi.org/10.1002/14651858.CD005451.pub3

Yang, W., Cai, X., Wu, H., & Ji, L. (2019). Associations between metformin use and vitamin B_{12} levels, anemia, and neuropathy in patients with diabetes: A meta-analysis. *Journal of Diabetes, 11*(9), 729–743. https://doi.org/10.1111/1753-0407.12900

Yilmaz, Z., Piracha, F., Anderson, L., & Mazzola, N. (2017). Supplements for diabetes mellitus: A review of the literature. *Journal of Pharmacy Practice, 30*(6), 631–638. https://doi.org/10.1177/0897190016663070

Zhang, M., Han, W., Hu, S., & Xu, H. (2013). Methylcobalamin: A potential vitamin of pain killer. *Neural Plasticity, 2013*, 1–6. https://doi.org/10.1155/2013/424651

Zhu, B., Zhou, X., Zhou, Q., Wang, H., Wang, S., & Luo, K. (2019). Intra-venous lidocaine to relieve neuropathic pain: A systematic review and meta-analysis. *Frontiers in Neurology, 10*, 954. https://doi.org/10.3389/fneur.2019.00954

Zhu, C. (2013). Aldose reductase inhibitors as potential therapeutic drugs of diabetic complications. In O. Oguntibeju (Ed.), *Diabetes mellitus—Insights and perspectives*. InTech. https://doi.org/10.5772/54642

Ziegler, D., Ametov, A., Barinov, A., Dyck, P. J., Gurieva, I., Low, P. A., Munzel, U., Yakhno, N., Raz, I., Novosadova, M., Maus, J., & Samigullin, R. (2006). Oral treatment with α-lipoic acid improves symptomatic diabetic polyneuropathy. *Diabetes Care, 29*(11), 2365–2370. https://doi.org/10.2337/dc06-1216

Ziegler, D., Low, P. A., Litchy, W. J., Boulton, A. J. M., Vinik, A. I., Freeman, R., Samigullin, R., Tritschler, H., Munzel, U., Maus, J., Schütte, K., & Dyck, P. J. (2011). Efficacy and safety of antioxidant treatment with α-lipoic acid over 4 years in diabetic polyneuropathy. *Diabetes Care, 34*(9), 2054–2060. https://doi.org/10.2337/dc11-0503

Ziegler, D., Strom, A., Lobmann, R., Reiners, K., Rett, K., & Schnell, O. (2015). High prevalence of diagnosed and undiagnosed polyneuropathy in subjects with and without diabetes participating in a nationwide educational initiative (PROTECT study). *Journal of Diabetes and Its Complications, 29*(8), 998–1002. https://doi.org/10.1016/j.jdiacomp.2015.09.008

Zilliox, L. A., & Russell, J. W. (2019). Physical activity and dietary interventions in diabetic neuropathy: A systematic review. *Clinical Autonomic Research, 29*(4), 443–455. https://doi.org/10.1007/s10286-019-00607-x

Zochodne, D. W. (2019). The challenges of diabetic polyneuropathy: A brief update. *Current Opinion in Neurology, 32*(5), 666–675. https://doi.org/10.1097/WCO.0000000000000723

Chapter 4
Non-healing Foot Ulcers in Diabetes: Challenges in Wound Healing and Strategies For Limb Preservation

Krishnendu Adhikary, Sumana Roy Chowdhury, Krishnendu Ganguly, and Sabina Yasmin

Abstract Chronic foot ulcers, especially those that fail to heal, represent a major and escalating global health burden, primarily impacting individuals with diabetes mellitus, peripheral arterial disease (PAD), and other systemic conditions. These non-healing ulcers contribute significantly to morbidity, diminished quality of life, frequent hospitalizations, and, in severe cases, limb loss. The pathogenesis of diabetic foot ulcers is multifactorial, involving ischemia, infection, neuropathy, and impaired wound healing mechanisms. Effective management demands a comprehensive, multidisciplinary approach targeting both local wound conditions and systemic metabolic derangements. Limb preservation, a critical goal in the management of chronic diabetic foot ulcersaims to prevent amputation while promoting wound healing and functional recovery. Therapeutic strategies include offloading pressure from the ulcer site, aggressive infection control, vascular interventions for revascularization, and advanced wound care modalities such as bioengineered skin substitutes, negative pressure wound therapy (NPWT), and topical growth factors. Moreover, stem cell therapy and regenerative medicine approaches are emerging as promising options for enhancing tissue repair and regeneration. This review highlights the complexity of diabetic foot ulcers, emphasizing the systemic and local interplay that hampers healing. It also outlines both established and emerging interventions designed to improve limb salvage and long-term outcomes. A deeper understanding of the molecular and cellular mechanisms underlying chronic wound healing may lead to innovative therapies, ultimately reducing the global burden of diabetic foot ulcers and lowering amputation rates.

K. Adhikary · S. R. Chowdhury · K. Ganguly
Department of Medical Laboratory Technology, Paramedical College Durgapur, Durgapur, India

K. Adhikary
Research and Development Cell, Lovely Professional University, Jalandhar, Phagwara, Punjab, India

S. Yasmin (✉)
Department of Pharmaceutical Chemistry, College of Pharmacy, King Khalid University, Abha, Saudi Arabia
e-mail: sahussain@kku.edu.sa

K. Adhikary et al. (eds.), *Healing Beyond Blood Sugar*,
https://doi.org/10.1007/978-981-95-8946-3_4

Keywords Chronic foot ulcers · Non-healing wounds · Limb preservation · Diabetes mellitus · Peripheral arterial disease · Advanced wound care · Revascularization · Stem cell therapy · Regenerative medicine

4.1 Introduction

Diabetic foot ulcers (DFUs) are a serious complication of diabetes, affecting 15–25% of patients globally and contributing to 4–10% prevalence, particularly higher in developing countries due to limited healthcare access (Chang & Nguyen, 2021; Sorber & Abularrage, 2021). DFUs account for over 80% of non-traumatic lower-limb amputations in diabetics, with more than one million amputations annually (Zhang et al., 2022). They lead to significant physical, emotional, and financial burdens, including reduced quality of life, high treatment costs, and increased mortality—over 50% within five years post-amputation. Recurrence rates are high, with 40% of ulcers reappearing within a year. Key risk factors include poor glycemic control, neuropathy, vascular insufficiency, infection, and delayed care (Pourkazemi et al., 2020). The impact is especially severe in low- and middle-income countries due to lack of awareness, infrastructure, and financial resources, making DFUs a persistent global health challenge (Li et al., 2023).

This chapter provides an overview of non-healing diabetic foot ulcers (DFUs), exploring biological and clinical factors such as neuropathy, ischemia, oxidative stress, inflammation, and infection that hinder healing (Luo et al., 2022). It examines global patterns, risk factors, and disparities in healthcare access that influence DFU outcomes (Deng et al., 2023). Therapeutic approaches range from standard infection control to advanced options like stem cell therapy, growth factors, negative-pressure wound therapy, and bioengineered skin substitutes (Couturier et al., 2023). The chapter also highlights clinical gaps and research limitations that delay effective wound healing (Guo et al., 2023). Emphasizing a multidisciplinary approach involving endocrinologists, vascular surgeons, podiatrists, microbiologists, and rehabilitation specialists, it aims to inform better prevention and treatment strategies to reduce amputations and improve quality of life in diabetic patients (Bardill et al., 2022).

4.2 Pathophysiology of Diabetic Foot Ulcers

Diabetic foot ulcers arise from a complex interplay of neuropathy, ischemia, infection, and impaired tissue healing (Huang et al., 2023). Chronic hyperglycemia causes vascular and neural damage, weakening immune defense and skin integrity. Minor trauma or pressure, especially with reduced sensation or blood flow, can initiate ulcer formation. Progression to chronic ulcers reflects systemic, cellular, and molecular dysfunctions. Understanding these mechanisms is key to developing effective prevention, early intervention, and treatment strategies (Jeon et al., 2017).

4.2.1 Role of Peripheral Neuropathy

Neuropathy, particularly peripheral neuropathy, is a primary contributor to diabetic foot ulcer development. Chronic hyperglycemia damages nerves through oxidative stress, sorbitol accumulation, and microvascular injury, leading to sensory, motor, and autonomic dysfunction (Gallagher et al., 2024a, 2024b). Sensory loss reduces pain perception, allowing unnoticed trauma and callus formation. Motor neuropathy causes foot deformities like claw toes, altering pressure distribution (Lin et al., 2020b). Autonomic neuropathy leads to dry, cracked skin, increasing infection risk. Combined, these neuropathic changes make the foot highly vulnerable to chronic ulceration (Oni et al., 2020).

4.2.2 Ischemia and Peripheral Arterial Disease

Peripheral arterial disease (PAD) is a major contributor to delayed healing and tissue necrosis in diabetic foot ulcers. Diabetes accelerates atherosclerosis, leading to arterial narrowing and reduced oxygenation in the lower limbs, which impairs wound healing. Ischemic ulcers typically appear on distal areas such as the toes and heel as deep, painful, slow-to-granulate wounds (Bolton, 2019). Beyond macrovascular disease, diabetes also causes microvascular dysfunction, reducing capillary density and compromising immune cell function and antibiotic delivery (Gallagher et al., 2024a, 2024b). The combination of neuropathy and ischemia significantly increases ulcer and amputation risk. Early vascular assessments, including ankle-brachial index and Doppler studies, are essential for identifying patients needing revascularization or limb-preserving interventions (Lin et al., 2020b).

4.2.3 Infection and Formation of Biofilm

Infection is a major factor in the progression of superficial diabetic ulcers into deep, non-healing wounds. Diabetic patients are more susceptible due to impaired immunity, poor circulation, and elevated glucose levels that promote bacterial growth (Lin et al., 2020b). Biofilm formation further complicates infection control by shielding microbes from antibiotics and immune responses, leading to chronic inflammation and treatment resistance. Common pathogens include *Staphylococcus aureus*, *Pseudomonas aeruginosa*, and polymicrobial communities. Effective treatment involves debridement, targeted antibiotics, and strategies to disrupt biofilm and restore healing (Gallagher et al., 2024a, 2024b).

4.2.4 *Impaired Cellular and Molecular Repair Processes*

Diabetic foot ulcers persist due to disrupted molecular and cellular healing processes. Hyperglycemia impairs normal wound healing phases—hemostasis, inflammation, proliferation, and remodeling—leading to delayed tissue regeneration (Song et al., 2022). Fibroblast and keratinocyte activity is reduced, macrophages remain pro-inflammatory, and angiogenesis is hindered by low VEGF levels. Excess reactive oxygen species and AGEs damage cells and the extracellular matrix, while poor collagen deposition, mitochondrial dysfunction, and impaired signaling (e.g., nitric oxide) further stall healing. Emerging therapies targeting growth factors, antioxidants, stem cells, and biomaterials aim to restore proper healing dynamics (Tang et al., 2024) (Fig. 4.1).

4.3 Classification and Risk Factors

Diabetic foot ulcers result from systemic and local factors that compromise tissue integrity, blood flow, and infection defense. Identifying risk factors is crucial for early intervention and preventing complications like infection, gangrene, and amputation (Song et al., 2022). Ulcer recurrence reflects not only metabolic issues but also neuropathy, biomechanical stress, and impaired healing. Clinical grading systems help standardize assessment by evaluating depth, infection, and ischemia, guiding prognosis and treatment decisions (Tang et al., 2024).

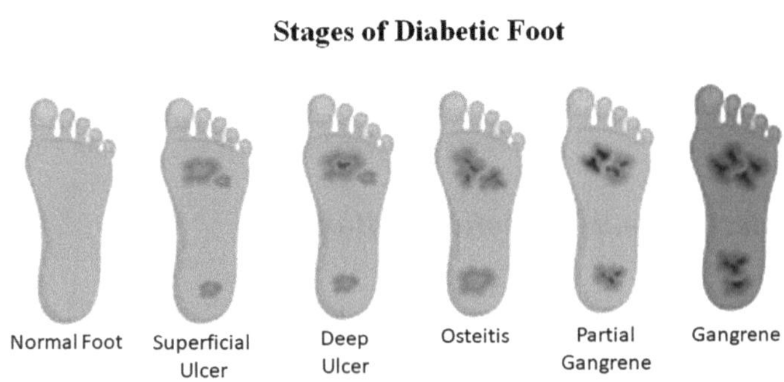

Fig. 4.1 Stages of diabetic foot ulcer. Comparison of normal foot with superficial ulcer, deep ulcer, osteitis, partial gangrene and gangrene

4.3.1 Clinical Risk Factors for Non-healing Ulcers

Diabetic foot ulcers are linked to multiple clinical risk factors, with poor glycemic control being a major contributor due to its role in neuropathy, vascular damage, and immune suppression (Adhikary et al., 2024a). Peripheral neuropathy reduces protective sensation, allowing unnoticed trauma to progress into ulcers. Peripheral arterial disease (PAD) further impairs tissue perfusion and healing. Infection is a common complication, particularly when neuropathy and ischemia coexist (Mitra et al., 2025).

Foot deformities like claw toes, hammer toes, and Charcot arthropathy alter pressure distribution, increasing ulcer risk. Ill-fitting footwear adds mechanical stress, while systemic conditions—such as chronic kidney disease, obesity, dyslipidemia, hypertension, and smoking—further impair circulation and healing (Adhikary et al., 2024b). Advanced age, long-standing diabetes, prior ulcers or amputations, and poor foot hygiene also increase vulnerability. Identifying and addressing these risk factors through regular foot exams, patient education, and screening can reduce ulcer incidence and recurrence (Adhikary et al., 2025).

4.3.2 Ulcer Grading Systems (Wagner, University of Texas, SINBAD)

Several classification systems are used to assess diabetic foot ulcer severity and guide treatment. The Wagner system grades ulcers by depth and tissue involvement, from Grade 0 (intact skin) to Grade 5 (extensive gangrene), but it overlooks key factors like infection and ischemia (Song et al., 2022). The University of Texas (UT) system offers a more comprehensive approach by incorporating depth, infection, and ischemia in a matrix format, making it more effective for predicting healing outcomes and amputation risk.

The SINBAD system (Site, Ischemia, Neuropathy, Bacterial infection, Area, Depth) offers a simplified, standardized method for assessing diabetic foot ulcers, particularly useful for population studies and audits due to its ease of use and reproducibility (Tang et al., 2024). Unlike Wagner and UT systems, SINBAD focuses on broad applicability. Together, these systems aid in evaluating ulcer severity, guiding treatment, and improving clinical communication and decision-making.

4.4 Diagnostic Approaches

4.4.1 Clinical Assessment and Wound Evaluation

Thorough clinical assessment is essential for managing non-healing diabetic foot ulcers and preventing complications such as infection and amputation. Evaluation begins with a detailed history, including diabetes duration, glycemic control, comorbidities, smoking, and mobility status to understand the patient's risk profile (Boulton et al., 2005; Singh et al., 2005). Physical examination includes identifying deformities (e.g., claw toes, Charcot foot), pressure points, calluses, and infection signs (Bakker et al., 2015). Wound depth and duration are assessed by palpation and edge characteristics, with plantar ulcers often linked to neuropathy and dorsal ulcers to trauma. Inflammation signs like erythema and maceration suggest infection (Snyder & Cardinal, 2010). Classification systems like Wagner and UT help guide prognosis and treatment by staging ulcers by depth, infection, and ischemia (Wagner, 1981; Lavery et al., 1996). Neuropathy is evaluated with tools such as monofilaments and tuning forks (Tesfaye et al., 2010), while vascular status is assessed using ABI, TBI, SPP, and $TcPO_2$ to predict healing (Faglia et al., 2006). Due to atypical infection presentations in diabetic patients, microbial cultures and imaging are often needed for diagnosis and management (Lipsky et al., 2012). An integrated approach combining history, physical exam, vascular and neurological assessment, and infection screening is essential for effective treatment and improved outcomes (Armstrong et al., 2017).

4.4.2 Imaging Modalities and Vascular Studies

In diabetic patients, untreated foot ulcers can lead to serious morbidity and limb loss. Imaging and vascular assessments are essential for diagnosing underlying pathology, determining tissue involvement, and guiding treatment (Conte et al., 2019). Vascular studies evaluate blood supply crucial for healing, while imaging reveals soft tissue and bone complications. Plain X-rays are typically the first step, useful for detecting foreign bodies, gas, or bone changes like osteomyelitis or Charcot arthropathy, though limited for soft tissue evaluation. MRI is the gold standard for assessing suspected deep infections, offering high sensitivity for osteomyelitis, abscesses, and sinus tracts (Lipsky et al., 2020a, 2020b). CT scans are used when MRI is unavailable, particularly for chronic bone changes. Ultrasound, though operator-dependent, is valuable for guiding drainage and assessing superficial abscesses, cellulitis, or edema.

Peripheral arterial disease (PAD) commonly impairs wound healing, making vascular evaluation crucial in non-healing diabetic foot ulcers. Ankle-brachial index (ABI) is a simple, noninvasive test but may yield falsely high results in diabetic patients due to arterial calcification. Thus, further studies like duplex ultrasonography, which combines Doppler flow and real-time imaging, are useful for detecting obstructions. Magnetic resonance angiography (MRA) and computed tomographic angiography (CTA) offer detailed vascular mapping essential for surgical planning. Digital subtraction angiography (DSA) remains the gold standard, especially when noninvasive results are inconclusive or during revascularization procedures, and can facilitate interventions such as angioplasty or stenting (Conte et al., 2016). Comprehensive vascular and imaging assessments guide treatment, reduce complications like amputations, and support a multimodal care approach.

4.4.3 Microbiological and Biochemical Diagnostics

Microbial and biochemical diagnostics are essential for detecting infections, guiding antimicrobial therapy, and identifying metabolic issues that hinder healing. Accurate pathogen identification is critical, as diabetic foot ulcers may be colonized by various bacteria. Superficial swabs often reflect colonizing flora rather than true pathogens; therefore, tissue samples from debrided or surgically removed areas are preferred for accurate cultures (Lipsky et al., 2020a, 2020b). Diabetic foot infections are often polymicrobial, typically involving Gram-negative bacilli, Gram-positive cocci (including MRSA), and, in severe or necrotic cases, anaerobes. Advances in microbiological techniques like PCR and 16S rRNA gene sequencing have improved detection of elusive or mixed pathogens, especially in patients with prior antibiotic use. These methods offer faster, more accurate results than traditional cultures but may detect non-pathogenic organisms, so findings must be interpreted cautiously (Lipsky et al., 2020a, 2020b).

Antibiotic susceptibility testing is essential for identifying pathogens and guiding therapy, particularly given the rise of multidrug-resistant organisms in diabetic foot infections. Empirical antibiotics are initiated based on disease severity and later adjusted per culture results to reduce adverse effects, resistance, and treatment failure (Edmonds et al., 2020; Lipsky et al., 2020a, 2020b). Molecular diagnostics, while highly sensitive, may detect non-viable or colonizing microbes and must be interpreted with caution (Lipsky et al., 2020a, 2020b). Biochemical markers like ESR, albumin, pre-albumin, lactate, and organ function tests offer insight into infection severity, nutritional status, tissue perfusion, and systemic involvement. For example, hypoalbuminemia correlates with poor healing, and abnormal renal or liver function may necessitate antibiotic dose adjustments. A comprehensive approach integrating microbiology and biochemistry enables precise, multidisciplinary management and improved outcomes in diabetic foot complications (Game et al., 2020a, 2020b).

4.5 Conventional Wound Management

4.5.1 Debridement Techniques

In diabetic patients with non-healing foot ulcers, debridement is a critical wound care intervention to remove necrotic tissue, reduce biofilm, and promote granulation. Sharp debridement is the preferred method, especially in infected or heavily exudative wounds, as it enables rapid removal of devitalized tissue and facilitates microbial sampling (Lipsky et al., 2020a, 2020b). Autolytic debridement, using moisture-retentive dressings like hydrogels or alginates, is less invasive and suitable for mild wounds or patients intolerant to sharp methods, though it is slower and ineffective in heavily infected or ischemic wounds (Armstrong et al., 2017).

Mechanical debridement, such as wet-to-dry dressings or irrigation, removes devitalized tissue through physical force but is non-selective, often damaging healthy tissue, and is less favored due to pain and availability of better methods. Enzymatic debridement uses topical agents like collagenase for selective tissue removal, especially in non-surgical candidates. However, it requires daily monitoring, acts slowly, and is unsuitable for infected or heavily exudative wounds (Lipsky et al., 2020a, 2020b).

Biological debridement, using germ-free larvae (maggot therapy), selectively digests dead tissue while preserving healthy tissue and is effective for chronic or failing lesions like diabetic foot ulcers, though it is typically reserved for cases where other therapies have failed or are unsuitable (Lipsky et al., 2020a, 2020b). Factors such as ulcer size, site, depth, bacterial contamination risk, ischemia potential, patient tolerance, and resources influence debridement choice. Multiple methods may be used throughout healing stages, with individualized and repeated adjustments necessary. Successful debridement removes healing barriers and prepares tissue for advanced treatments like growth factors or negative pressure therapy. Debridement is a fundamental part of wound care within a multidisciplinary approach, including vascular assessment, infection and metabolic control, and offloading (Armstrong et al., 2017).

4.5.2 Infection Control and Antibiotic Stewardship

Antibiotic stewardship is essential in managing diabetic foot ulcers, which are prone to infection due to poor immunity, reduced blood flow, and neuropathy that can delay symptom recognition. Delayed or improper infection control is a major contributor to poor healing and risk of amputation. Effective infection management involves appropriate antibiotic use and preventative measures to support healing and limit resistance. Diabetic foot ulcers may range from mild infections like cellulitis to severe conditions such as osteomyelitis or abscesses. While common signs include redness, swelling, and discharge, infections may be subtle due to impaired inflammatory responses in diabetics, necessitating regular monitoring by skilled clinicians. Debridement remains central to infection control, as removing devitalized tissue lowers microbial load and biofilm, both key contributors to persistent infections and antibiotic resistance (Lipsky et al., 2020a, 2020b).

Infection control in diabetic foot ulcers involves sterile wound cleansing, disinfected dressings, and appropriate offloading to promote healing and reduce bacterial colonization. Topical antimicrobials like PHMB, silver, or iodine may be used in heavily colonized wounds without systemic infection but should be limited to avoid toxicity and resistance. Antibiotic management is critical, as empiric broad-spectrum use can lead to multidrug-resistant organisms. Systemic antibiotics should only be used for clear infections and guided by culture and sensitivity testing. Accurate diagnosis and targeted therapy are best achieved through proper specimen collection, ideally from deep tissue post-debridement (Lipsky et al., 2020a, 2020b).

The duration of antibiotic therapy should match the severity of infection—longer courses may be needed for deep tissue or bone infections, often alongside surgery, while mild infections may respond to short courses. Regular reassessment is essential to evaluate effectiveness and adjust treatment if needed. Complex cases often require multidisciplinary input, including infectious disease specialists. In diabetic foot ulcers, infection prevention and antibiotic use must be ongoing, adaptive processes aimed at both treatment and resistance prevention. Education on foot hygiene, early reporting of wound changes, and adherence to treatment support infection control and healing (Lipsky et al., 2020a, 2020b).

4.5.3 Offloading and Pressure Redistribution

Recurrent mechanical stress is a key factor in the development and persistence of diabetic foot ulcers, especially in patients with peripheral neuropathy who lack pain sensation (Bus et al., 2016a, 2016b). Offloading, or relieving pressure on the affected area, is crucial to promote healing and prevent further injury. Without effective offloading, even advanced wound care fails. Total contact casting (TCC) is the gold standard for treating plantar ulcers, as it evenly redistributes pressure and significantly improves healing due to its non-removable nature (Lavery et al., 2014; Armstrong et al., 2017). However, TCC requires clinical expertise due to risks like skin breakdown and infection. Removable cast walkers (RCWs) offer comfort and convenience but are often removed by patients, reducing their effectiveness (Frykberg et al., 2020; Lazzarini et al., 2019). To improve adherence, "instant TCC" uses adhesives or wraps to make RCWs non-removable, combining the benefits of both approaches (Lipsky et al., 2020a, 2020b).

Custom orthotics and therapeutic shoes play a key role in pressure redistribution, particularly for patients with foot deformities or a history of ulcers. These devices address structural abnormalities, reduce shear stress, and offload high-pressure areas, especially after wound closure to help prevent recurrence (Tamir et al.,

2020). Insoles made from pressure-distributing materials like gels or layered foams can further reduce localized pressure. When conservative methods fail, surgical offloading—such as exostectomy, tendon lengthening, or reconstructive surgery—may be necessary for select patients with persistent structural defects or recurrent ulcers.

Patient education on activity modification—such as reducing walking and avoiding going barefoot—is vital for ulcer management. Pressure-mapping technology can help identify high-risk areas and guide optimal, adaptive offloading strategies as healing progresses (van Netten et al., 2020). When applied effectively, these interventions lower the risk of infection and amputation, improve healing, and support long-term limb preservation as part of comprehensive diabetic wound care (Armstrong et al., 2017; Lipsky et al., 2020a, 2020b).

4.5.4 System Optimization and Glycemic Control

Maintaining good glycemic control is critical for effective management of non-healing diabetic foot ulcers. Poor glucose regulation impairs wound healing by disrupting immune response, collagen formation, and angiogenesis (Jeffcoate et al., 2018). Strong evidence links controlled blood glucose—especially at ulcer onset—with faster healing and reduced complications. Keeping HbA1c within target levels lowers the risk of ulcer development, infection, and potential amputation. In poorly controlled type 2 diabetes, insulin is often necessary to achieve rapid stabilization when ulcers are present (Armstrong et al., 2017; Lipsky et al., 2020a, 2020b).

Systemic optimization is essential in managing diabetic foot ulcers and involves addressing comorbidities such as peripheral arterial disease, renal impairment, malnutrition, and glucose control, all of which affect healing outcomes (Martínez-Gómez et al., 2021). Multidisciplinary care tailors interventions to individual needs, including medication adjustments, cardiovascular risk reduction, and rehabilitation. Ongoing research supports the link between glycemic control and ulcer resolution. Effective management includes regular monitoring of metabolic parameters and overall health. As part of standard care, systemic optimization—alongside local wound management and infection control—can significantly improve outcomes in high-risk patients (Armstrong et al., 2017; Lipsky et al., 2020a, 2020b) (Fig. 4.2).

Over time, myelin loss can be exacerbated by diabetes-related low-grade inflammation that persists and sustained hyperglycemia, leading to peripheral neuropathy. The sensitive, voluntary, and autonomous nerves are harmed as a result of oxidative stress. Peripheral artery disease (PAD) weakens the lower- extremity zones and increases their susceptibility to secondary infections by causing hypercoagulability, severe limb ischemia, and inadequate blood flow, which results in hypoxia. Furthermore, those with diabetes also have decreased angiogenesis. Thus, foot ulcers are to be expected.

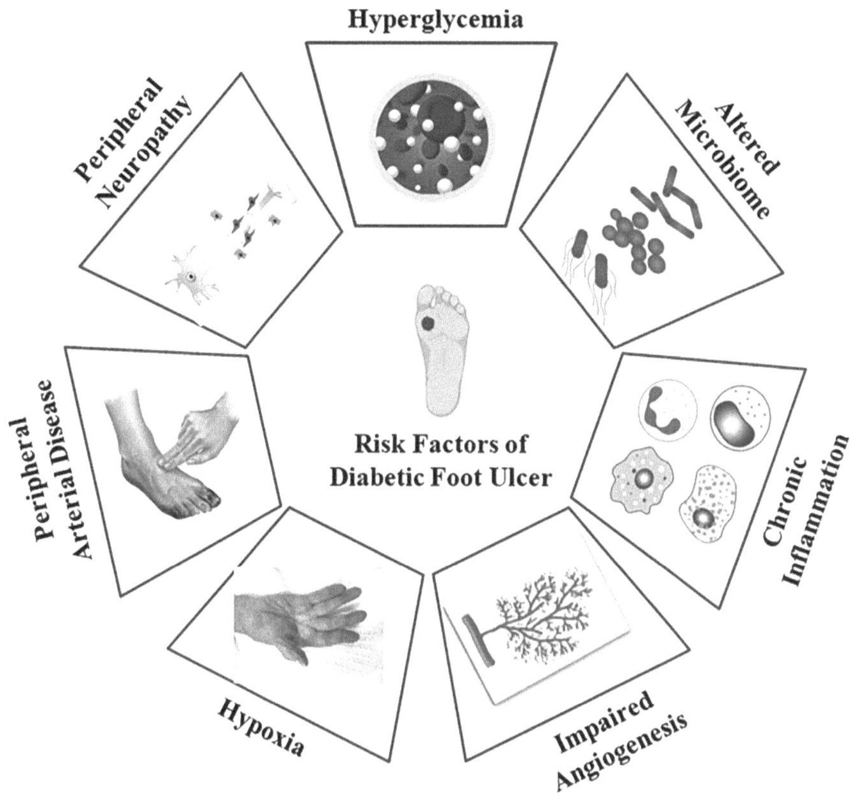

Fig. 4.2 The occurrence of ulcers in diabetes-related feet (DFUs) is linked to risk factors

4.6 Advanced Wound Care Strategies

4.6.1 Negative Pressure Wound Therapy (NPWT)

Negative Pressure Wound Therapy (NPWT) is an effective adjunct in managing chronic diabetic foot ulcers, supporting limb salvage by addressing impaired healing caused by vascular, immunological, and neuropathic complications of hyperglycemia (Lázaro-Martínez et al., 2014). Delivered via a vacuum-sealed dressing, NPWT improves blood flow, reduces edema, removes exudate, and promotes granulation tissue formation (Armstrong & Lavery, 2005; Blume et al., 2008). It helps resolve chronic inflammation and poor tissue regeneration common in diabetic ulcers (Game et al., 2016). Studies show NPWT accelerates healing, reduces amputation risk, and supports surgical closure preparation (Lavery et al., 2007; Liu et al., 2017). However, it requires careful wound evaluation to avoid risks like bleeding or infection and should be combined with debridement and antimicrobial therapy (Hingorani et al.,

2016). While cost and expertise limit use in low-resource settings, NPWT is most effective within multidisciplinary care teams (Armstrong et al., 2011).

When properly applied, Negative Pressure Wound Therapy (NPWT) supports limb salvage and functional recovery in chronic diabetic ulcers, both pre- and post-reconstructive surgery. It is a key component of advanced wound care, supported by clinical guidelines, systematic reviews, and randomized trials (Game et al., 2016). While further research is needed to refine treatment protocols based on ulcer characteristics and comorbidities, NPWT effectively enhances mechanical and biological healing processes. Despite cost and clinical challenges, it offers significant benefits in improving outcomes and preventing amputation within a comprehensive care model.

4.6.2 Bioengineered Tissue and Skin Substitutes

Genetically modified allografts and tissue-engineered skin substitutes are emerging as key treatments for diabetic foot ulcers (DFUs), addressing barriers such as neuropathy, poor perfusion, and infection (Hingorani et al., 2016). Standard care often fails in chronic cases, which are associated with delayed healing and increased risk of amputation (Armstrong et al., 2017). Bioengineered products provide structural support and biochemical signaling that promote tissue regeneration (Lipsky et al., 2020a, 2020b). Examples include Apligraf—a bilayered living skin equivalent shown to enhance healing by releasing growth factors (Veves et al., 2001)—and acellular matrices like GraftJacket and DermACELL, which facilitate angiogenesis and epithelialization (Driver et al., 2015; Winters et al., 2016). Despite demonstrated efficacy, challenges remain due to variability in ulcer characteristics, patient adherence, high costs, and limited accessibility (Game et al., 2016; Lavery et al., 2020). Even with advanced care, 30–50% of DFUs may not fully heal (Armstrong et al., 2017). However, when used within limb salvage programs and combined with other therapies like negative pressure wound therapy, skin substitutes improve closure rates and reduce infection risks (Han et al., 2012; Kirsner et al., 2012). These solutions offer significant clinical value but must be integrated into comprehensive care models for optimal outcomes.

4.6.3 Topical Growth Factors and Peptides

Topical growth factors and peptides offer a targeted approach for treating diabetic foot ulcers (DFUs), particularly when systemic complications hinder healing. Chronic diabetic wounds involve impaired cell function, persistent inflammation, poor neovascularization, and disrupted extracellular matrix regulation, increasing infection and amputation risk (Lipsky et al., 2020a, 2020b). Agents like epidermal growth factor (EGF), fibroblast growth factor (FGF), and platelet-derived growth factor

(PDGF) promote cellular proliferation, angiogenesis, and tissue repair at the wound site (Game et al., 2016).

Various fibroblast growth factors (FGFs), recombinant human EGF (rhEGF), and umbilical cord-derived factors have demonstrated clinical effectiveness in accelerating wound closure and healing in DFUs compared to standard care (Martínez-Sánchez et al., 2019). These bioactive agents enhance granulation, re-epithelialization, and reduce chronic inflammation. Platelet-rich plasma (PRP), rich in cytokines and growth factors, also supports healing and reduces infection-related complications. Randomized trials show that topical EGF can reduce wound size in over 70% of patients without notable side effects (Fernández-Montequín et al., 2009).

The effectiveness of growth factor therapies for DFUs is limited by patient adherence, wound characteristics (e.g., size, depth, infection, ischemia), and variability in individual responses (Game et al., 2016). Chronic wounds differ enzymatically from acute wounds, often degrading exogenous growth factors and reducing their efficacy (Barrientos et al., 2014). Current research focuses on advanced delivery systems—such as hydrogels, nanoparticles, and slow-release formulations—to improve bioavailability at the wound site (Anitua et al., 2015). Additionally, high costs and limited access in resource-constrained settings remain major barriers, even when local efficacy is observed (Hingorani et al., 2016).

Topical growth factors and peptides play an increasing role in multifactorial DFU care by promoting healing even in the presence of infection or ischemia, thus reducing morbidity and risk of limb loss (Lavery et al., 2020). Emerging formulations and combination strategies—such as pairing growth factors with cellular therapies or negative pressure wound therapy (NPWT)—offer promise for more individualized, effective treatment. As adjuncts to standard care, including infection control, offloading, glycemic management, and vascular optimization, these agents help overcome biological barriers to healing and support limb salvage.

4.6.4 Hyperbaric Oxygen Therapy (HBOT)

Hyperbaric oxygen therapy (HBOT) is a promising adjunct for diabetic foot ulcers (DFUs) complicated by hypoxia, a common barrier to healing in diabetes. Reduced oxygen delivery—often due to peripheral arterial disease, neuropathy, or chronic inflammation—impairs tissue repair and increases infection and amputation risk (Lipsky et al., 2020a, 2020b). HBOT enhances oxygen availability to ischemic tissues, promoting healing by improving oxygen diffusion and blood flow (Thackham et al., 2008).

HBOT supports wound healing by promoting oxygen-dependent processes such as angiogenesis, fibroblast activation, collagen synthesis, and reduction of inflammation and edema (Heyboer et al., 2017). It also enhances leukocyte function, improving infection control in diabetic ulcers (Kranke et al., 2015). Clinical evidence from randomized controlled trials and meta-analyses shows that HBOT improves wound healing and reduces ulcer size, though its impact on minor amputations and side effects remains unclear (Löndahl et al., 2010; Zhao et al., 2020).

Despite its benefits, HBOT has medical and logistical limitations. It requires specialized facilities and trained personnel, making it less accessible in resource-limited settings (Santema et al., 2018). Not all patients are ideal candidates—those with infections, poor vascular supply, or comorbidities may face increased risks such as oxygen toxicity, barotrauma, or hypoglycemia (Heyboer et al., 2017). Additionally, treatment demands high patient compliance, as optimal outcomes are linked to extended protocols of 20–40 sessions (Löndahl et al., 2011).

HBOT should be integrated into a comprehensive wound care plan that includes infection control, debridement, metabolic management, and vascular assessment. Its effectiveness varies by dose and patient response, as shown in clinical trials. When appropriately applied in complex DFU cases, HBOT can enhance healing and reduce the risk of major amputations (Kranke et al., 2015).

Hyperbaric oxygen therapy (HBOT) is a clinically supported adjunct for diabetic foot ulcers, working by countering hypoxia and activating key wound healing pathways. While resource-intensive, HBOT remains a valuable tool in managing complex diabetic complications, promoting healing, and aiding in limb preservation (Kranke et al., 2015).

4.7 Limb Preservation and Revascularization

4.7.1 Surgical and Endovascular Revascularization

Surgical debridement and revascularization are key interventions for non-healing diabetic foot ulcers (DFUs), addressing underlying limb ischemia commonly caused by peripheral arterial disease (PAD), which impairs blood flow and oxygenation, increasing the risk of limb loss (Hingorani et al., 2016). Both open surgical bypass and minimally invasive endovascular approaches can restore perfusion, enhance the wound environment, support healing, and aid in limb salvage (Conte et al., 2019).

Surgical revascularization, including bypass grafting with prosthetic or autologous veins, is often used for severe DFU cases, particularly when small distal vessels (e.g., crural or pedal arteries) are involved and endovascular options are unsuitable (Farber & Eberhardt, 2016). Complex cases may also require free flap transfer or limb-salvage reconstruction, though frail or elderly patients may not tolerate surgery well due to higher perioperative risk (Faglia et al., 2012). Endovascular approaches—such as PTA, subintimal angioplasty, and stenting—are favored for their minimally invasive nature and quicker recovery. Angiosome-directed revascularization has improved healing and limb salvage by targeting ulcer-specific arterial supply (Iida et al., 2013). Hybrid techniques combining open and endovascular methods offer flexibility for complex or multilevel disease (Setacci et al., 2014).

Effective revascularization requires detailed planning, including perfusion assessment (e.g., ABI, toe pressure, $TcPO_2$) and imaging (e.g., CT angiography, DSA) (Mills et al., 2014). Long-term success depends on multidisciplinary care addressing infection prevention, metabolic control, offloading, and post-procedure surveillance to reduce complications like restenosis or graft failure (Abularrage et al., 2018). Ultimately, both surgical and endovascular approaches improve perfusion and reduce major amputation risk, with therapy choice guided by patient health, anatomy, and resource availability—both offering comparable one-year limb salvage rates (Conte et al., 2019).

4.7.2 Multidisciplinary Limb Salvage Protocols

Diabetic foot ulcers (DFUs), often complicated by comorbidities such as peripheral neuropathy, PAD, poor glycemic control, and inflammation, require individualized, multidisciplinary limb salvage strategies (Armstrong et al., 2017). Comprehensive care includes wound assessment, infection control—particularly for biofilm-related infections (Lipsky et al., 2020a, 2020b)—and vascular evaluation to guide revascularization (Hingorani et al., 2016). Systemic factors like renal function and nutrition must also be managed to support healing (Brownrigg et al., 2015).

Biomechanical offloading using total contact casting, orthotics, or specialized footwear is critical to reduce pressure and prevent further injury, especially in patients with sensory deficits (Bus et al., 2016a, 2016b). In advanced cases, surgical interventions like grafts or flaps may support limb salvage (Atter et al., 2012). Multidisciplinary models have shown superior outcomes, including higher healing rates, fewer amputations, and improved survival compared to standard care (Wu et al., 2018).

Specialty foot clinics focused on prevention, education, and risk reduction improve long-term outcomes, though implementation challenges include care coordination, provider availability, patient compliance, and access (Game et al., 2020a, 2020b). Global guidelines strongly support early multidisciplinary intervention and continuous patient follow-up to reduce limb loss and enhance care quality (Schaper et al., 2020).

4.8 Emerging Therapies

Emerging treatments for diabetic patients with non-healing ulcers—such as growth factor injections, stem cells, genetically engineered skin substitutes, oxygen-based therapies, and negative pressure wound therapy (NPWT)—aim to enhance wound closure and preserve limbs. Chronic hyperglycemia impairs healing by affecting vascular growth, collagen synthesis, and immune function, increasing the risk of infection and amputation (Armstrong et al., 2017). Platelet-derived growth factors have shown promise in promoting granulation tissue and healing (Game & Jeffcoate, 2016), while NPWT and oxygen therapies improve perfusion and cellular regeneration (Lázaro-Martínez et al., 2021a, 2021b). Despite their potential, these interventions face challenges such as cost, accessibility, and limited high-quality evidence (Hingorani et al., 2016).

4.8.1 Stem Cell Therapy and Regenerative Medicine

Regenerative medicine and stem cell therapy are emerging options for treating diabetic foot ulcers (DFUs), especially when conventional treatments fail. DFUs often involve impaired angiogenesis, chronic inflammation, and poor cell proliferation, hindering healing (Falanga, 2005). Mesenchymal stem cells (MSCs) from sources like bone marrow, adipose tissue, and umbilical cord blood promote tissue repair via neovascularization, immunomodulation, and paracrine signaling (Dash et al., 2021). MSCs can be delivered locally or via injection, showing potential for limb salvage in chronic DFUs (Han et al., 2021). Advances in tissue engineering, including 3D bioprinting combined with stem cells, offer customized treatment but face challenges such as cell viability, immune rejection, and high costs (Briquez et al., 2015). Further research is needed to establish standardized protocols and assess long-term safety.

4.8.2 Gene Therapy and Exosome-Based Treatments

Gene therapy and exosome-based therapies offer promising advancements for treating non-healing diabetic foot ulcers (DFUs) by addressing biological barriers to healing. Gene therapy, using vectors to deliver genes encoding proteins like VEGF or PDGF, has shown to enhance angiogenesis and tissue regeneration in chronic wounds (Blome et al., 2020; Luo et al., 2021). Exosome-based therapy, a cell-free alternative, delivers bioactive molecules such as microRNAs and peptides that modulate inflammation, stimulate angiogenesis, and support fibroblast function (Li et al., 2019). Despite challenges in large-scale production and patient-specific customization, exosomes offer advantages over cell therapies, including improved safety, consistency, and lower immunogenicity (Keshtkar et al., 2018). These approaches may significantly improve outcomes and reduce amputation rates in DFU patients.

4.8.3 Nanotechnology and Smart Wound Dressings

Nanotechnologies and smart dressings are transforming diabetic foot ulcer (DFU) management by addressing delayed healing, impaired angiogenesis, and infection risk. Innovations like hydrogel-nanocomposites, polymeric nanofibers, and silver nanoparticles offer antimicrobial action, biosensor feedback, and controlled drug delivery, outperforming traditional dressings (Gupta et al., 2020). These dressings use nanomaterials to release agents such as antibiotics or growth factors in response to wound pH, temperature, or bacterial load (Wang et al., 2019). In DFUs, nanofiber scaffolds with agents like curcumin or insulin have enhanced collagen deposition and epithelialization (Shen et al., 2021). Additionally, biosensor-integrated dressings can monitor biomarkers to inform real-time treatment decisions (Pang et al., 2022). Despite their potential, challenges like cost, manufacturing complexity, and limited clinical validation hinder widespread use.

4.9 Challenges and Barriers in Wound Healing

Diabetic foot ulcers (DFUs) face complex barriers to healing due to interconnected local and systemic factors. Hyperglycemia prolongs inflammation and impairs leukocyte function, collagen synthesis, and angiogenesis, increasing infection risk (Brem & Tomic-Canic, 2007). Peripheral arterial disease limits oxygen and nutrient delivery, while neuropathy increases the risk of repeated trauma (Armstrong et al., 2017). Biofilms from multi-drug resistant organisms protect bacteria from immune responses and antibiotics, sustaining chronic infection (James et al., 2008). Psychosocial factors such as low socioeconomic status, poor adherence, and limited access to care also hinder healing (Bus & van Netten, 2016). These multilevel challenges highlight the need for comprehensive, stage-specific DFU care addressing both local wound and systemic health needs (Armstrong et al., 2001).

4.9.1 Patient Adherence and Psychosocial Factors

Treatment outcomes for diabetic foot ulcers (DFUs) are strongly influenced by patient adherence and psychosocial factors. Noncompliance with offloading, wound care, and glycemic control significantly increases the risk of poor healing and recurrence (Prompers et al., 2008). Many patients find offloading devices impractical, reducing their effectiveness (Bus et al., 2016a, 2016b). Psychosocial challenges like depression, isolation, and low health literacy also hinder consistent self-care (Vedhara et al., 2010). Among vulnerable populations, cultural beliefs, financial barriers, and limited access to care further impact adherence (Boulton, 2014). Addressing these barriers through education, psychological support, motivational interviewing, and culturally competent care can enhance outcomes and reduce complications (Bus et al., 2020a, 2020b).

4.9.2 Health System Limitations and Care Disparities

Chronic diabetic foot ulcer (DFU) outcomes are significantly affected by systemic healthcare inequities, especially for vulnerable and underrepresented populations. Limited access to specialized wound care services like podiatry and vascular surgery contributes to delayed diagnoses, poor management, and higher amputation rates (Lazzarini et al., 2018). Rural and disadvantaged populations often face transportation barriers and long wait times (Tan et al., 2022), while health literacy and insurance disparities further restrict timely care (Fitzpatrick et al., 2019). Racial and ethnic minorities, including Black and Hispanic patients, experience disproportionately high amputation rates due to systemic inequities in care delivery (Neville et al., 2009). Addressing these disparities requires policy reforms to expand telemedicine, culturally concordant care, and access to preventive health services (Lin et al., 2020a, 2020b).

4.9.3 Cost and Accessibility of Advanced Therapies

The adoption of advanced therapies for non-healing diabetic foot ulcers (DFUs)—such as growth factors, stem cell treatments, NPWT, and bioengineered skin—remains limited due to high costs and restricted access. While clinically effective, these treatments often lack reimbursement support and require specialized resources, making them less available in rural and low-resource settings (Armstrong et al., 2017; Hingorani et al., 2016). Even when viable, providers may avoid them due to exclusion from clinical guidelines and lack of payer coverage (Guest et al., 2018). These barriers exacerbate existing health disparities, underscoring the need for scalable models, faster regulatory pathways, and cost-effectiveness evaluations to improve accessibility and equity (Fig. 4.3).

For protection of Diabetic foot ulcer we have to wear clean and dry socks, do not walk in barefoot, wearing socks in bed, check the footwear before using, carefully clip to nails, sock feet in water and dry them carefully, moisturizer application, dry foot inspection, self surgery and treatment and diabetis management.

4.10 Future Directions and Research Gaps

Despite recent advances, significant research gaps remain in the treatment of non-healing diabetic foot ulcers (DFUs), affecting healing and limb preservation. Large, multicenter trials are needed to assess the long-term safety and efficacy of emerging therapies like gene editing, exosome-based treatments, and stem cell-derived products (Game et al., 2016). Progress is hindered by limited understanding of chronic inflammation, impaired angiogenesis, and biofilm formation in diabetic wounds

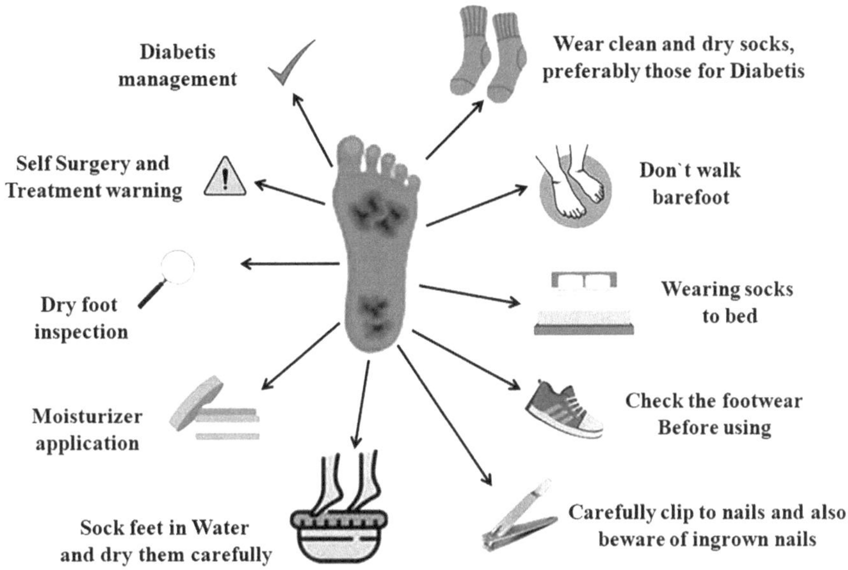

Fig. 4.3 Management of diabetic foot disease

(Eming et al., 2014). While precision medicine techniques show promise, their integration into DFU care is restricted by cost and accessibility (Falanga, 2012). Moreover, evidence on cost-effectiveness, demographic outcomes, and clinical guidelines for new therapies is lacking (Bus et al., 2020a). Future research must also address systemic and social health inequities to ensure equitable innovation.

4.10.1 Personalized Wound Care Approaches

Healing diabetic foot ulcers (DFUs) that do not respond to standard care requires individualized treatment tailored to patient-specific factors such as comorbidities, ulcer etiology, and adherence. Standardized approaches often fail due to variations in wound severity, vascular status, and patient health (Armstrong et al., 2017). Individualized care incorporates tools like risk stratification, biomarker profiling, and wound imaging to guide therapy (Sheehan et al., 2003). Patient data—such as HbA1c, neuropathy level, and diet—can inform the use of advanced therapies, offloading devices, and adjunctive options like hyperbaric oxygen (Bus et al., 2020a). Emerging technologies like AI and digital health platforms offer opportunities for improved surveillance, adherence, and clinical decision-making (Najafi et al., 2017). This personalized approach supports better resource use and long-term limb preservation.

4.10.2 Biomarker Discovery and Predictive Diagnostics

Predictive diagnostics and biomarker identification are advancing early detection and personalized treatment of non-healing diabetic foot ulcers (DFUs). Traditional assessments often miss molecular indicators of ulcer progression, delaying timely intervention (Game et al., 2016). Emerging technologies in proteomics, metabolomics, and genomics have identified biomarkers—such as growth factors, MMPs, and inflammatory cytokines (e.g., IL-6, TNF-α)—linked to chronic wound pathology (Serena et al., 2020). These markers can support point-of-care tools and predictive models to guide treatment based on healing potential (Wilkinson et al., 2020). Integration with imaging and AI platforms further enhances diagnostic accuracy (Yazdanpanah et al., 2018). However, challenges remain in validating biomarkers across diverse populations and translating findings into scalable clinical tools.

4.10.3 Translational Gaps from Bench to Bedside

Despite advances in experimental therapies for chronic diabetic foot ulcers (DFUs), a major gap remains between laboratory research and clinical application. Promising technologies—such as stem cells, gene therapies, growth factors, and nanotechnology—rarely translate into routine care (Hingorani et al., 2016). This gap stems from biological differences between animal models and humans, insufficient demographic testing, and challenges in evaluating safety and efficacy (Falanga, 2012). Regulatory hurdles, manufacturing complexity, and high trial costs further delay adoption (Lázaro-Martínez et al., 2021a, 2021b). Additionally, limited industry investment and weak collaboration among researchers, clinicians, and policymakers exacerbate the issue (Gottrup, 2012). Strengthening translational frameworks and interdisciplinary partnerships is essential for advancing clinical implementation.

4.11 Conclusion

Non-healing diabetic foot ulcers (DFUs) remain a major global health challenge, increasing morbidity, healthcare costs, and amputation risk. Their complex pathophysiology—driven by neuropathy, vascular disease, hyperglycemia, and systemic dysfunction—demands multifaceted, individualized care. While emerging therapies like stem cells, gene editing, exosome-based treatments, nanotechnology, and smart dressings show promise, barriers such as patient adherence, cost, limited availability, and the translational gap from lab to clinic hinder widespread adoption.

Personalized approaches, guided by biomarkers and risk stratification tools, are crucial for predicting healing outcomes and tailoring treatment. However, systemic inequities, regulatory hurdles, and lack of stakeholder incentives continue to delay implementation. Addressing these challenges requires healthcare policy reform, equitable access to advanced therapies, and integration of interdisciplinary teams—endocrinologists, vascular specialists, surgeons, and wound care nurses—into standardized care pathways.

Future priorities include large-scale, multicenter trials to validate innovative therapies and translational research frameworks that ensure real-world application. A shift toward integrated, patient-centered, and research-driven care is essential to improve healing rates, reduce amputations, and preserve limbs in people living with diabetes.

References

Abularrage, C. J., Conrad, M. F., Hackney, L. A., et al. (2018). Surveillance strategies for lower extremity bypass grafts. *Journal of Vascular Surgery, 68*(6), 1885–1892.

Adhikary, K., Banerjee, P., Barman, S., Bandyopadhyay, B., & Bagchi, D. (2024a, February). Nutritional aspects, chemistry profile, extraction techniques of lemongrass essential oil and it's physiological benefits. *Journal of the American Nutrition Association, 43*(2), 183–200. https://doi.org/10.1080/27697061.2023.2245435. Epub 2023 Aug 14. PMID: 37579058.

Adhikary, K., Ganguly, K., Chakrabarty S., Sarkar, R., Nag, R., Srivastava, S., Barman, S., Banerjee, P., Karak, P., Ashique, S., & Hussain, M. S. (2025, September 12). Understanding antimicrobial resistance: From mechanisms to public health implications. *Current Pharmaceutical Biotechnology*. https://doi.org/10.2174/0113892010406135250828050228. Epub ahead of print. PMID: 40947740.

Adhikary, K., Sarkar, R., Maity, S., Banerjee, I., Chatterjee, P., Bhattacharya, K., Ahuja, D., Sinha, N. K., & Maiti, R. (2024b). The underlying causes, treatment options of gut microbiota and food habits in type 2 diabetes mellitus: A narrative review. *Journal of Basic and Clinical Physiology and Pharmacology, 35*(3), 153–168. https://doi.org/10.1515/jbcpp-2024-0043. PMID: 38748886.

Adhikary, K., Sarkar, R., Maity, S., Sadhukhan, I., Sarkar, R., Ganguly, K., Barman, S., Maiti, R., Chakraborty, S., Chakraborty, T. R., Bagchi, D., & Banerjee, P. (2024). Immunomodulation of macrophages in diabetic wound individuals by structurally diverse bioactive phytochemicals. *Pharmaceuticals (Basel), 17*(10), 1294. https://doi.org/10.3390/ph17101294.PMID:39458935; PMCID:PMC11510503

Anitua, E., Sánchez, M., Orive, G., & Andía, I. (2015). Delivering growth factors for therapeutics. *Trends in Pharmacological Sciences, 29*(1), 37–41.

Armstrong, D. G., Boulton, A. J. M., & Bus, S. A. (2017). Diabetic foot ulcers and their recurrence. *New England Journal of Medicine, 376*(24), 2367–2375. https://doi.org/10.1056/NEJMra1615439

Armstrong, D. G., & Lavery, L. A. (2005). Negative pressure wound therapy after partial diabetic foot amputation: A multicentre, randomised controlled trial. *Lancet, 366*(9498), 1704–1710.

Armstrong, D. G., Lavery, L. A., Wu, S., & Boulton, A. J. M. (2001). Evaluation of removable and irremovable cast walkers in the healing of diabetic foot wounds: A randomized controlled trial. *Diabetes Care, 24*(6), 1019–1022. https://doi.org/10.2337/diacare.24.6.1019

Armstrong, D. G., Lavery, L. A., & Harkless, L. B. (2011). Validation of a diabetic wound classification system: The contribution of depth, infection, and ischemia to risk of amputation. *Diabetes Care, 21*(5), 855–859. https://doi.org/10.2337/diacare.21.5.855

Atter, W., McCollum, C. N., & Shandall, A. A. (2012). Reconstructive options for diabetic foot salvage. *International Wound Journal, 9*(4), 349–356.

Bakker, K., Apelqvist, J., & Schaper, N. C. (2016, January). International working group on the diabetic foot. Practical guidelines on the management and prevention of the diabetic foot 2015. *Diabetes/Metabolism Research and Reviews, 32*(Suppl 1), 7–15.

Bardill, J. R., Laughter, M. R., Stager, M., Liechty, K. W., Krebs, M. D., & Zgheib, C. (2022, January 15). Topical gel-based biomaterials for the treatment of diabetic foot ulcers. *Acta Biomaterialia, 138*, 73–91. https://doi.org/10.1016/j.actbio.2021.10.045. Epub 2021 Oct 30. PMID: 34728428; PMCID: PMC8738150.

Barrientos, S., Stojadinovic, O., Golinko, M. S., Brem, H., & Tomic-Canic, M. (2014). Growth factors and cytokines in wound healing. *Wound Repair Regen., 22*(5), 585–601.

Blome, E., Ayala, T. S., & Ennis, W. J. (2020). Gene therapy in diabetic wound healing. *Wound Repair and Regeneration, 28*(3), 247–254. https://doi.org/10.1111/wrr.12767

Blume, P. A., Walters, J., Payne, W., Ayala, J., & Lantis, J. (2008). Comparison of negative pressure wound therapy using vacuum-assisted closure with advanced moist wound therapy in the treatment of diabetic foot ulcers. *Diabetes Care, 31*(4), 631–636.

Bolton, L. L. (2019). *Ischemic foot ulcers in people with diabetes. Journal of Wound Care, 28*(3), 130–135. https://doi.org/10.12968/jowc.2019.28.3.130.

Boulton, A. J., Vileikyte, L., Ragnarson-Tennvall, G., & Apelqvist, J. (2005). The global burden of diabetic foot disease. *Lancet, 366*(9498), 1719–1724.

Boulton, A. J. M. (2014). The pathway to foot ulceration in diabetes. *Medical Clinics of North America, 97*(5), 775–790. https://doi.org/10.1016/j.mcna.2013.03.007

Brem, H., & Tomic-Canic, M. (2007). Cellular and molecular basis of wound healing in diabetes. *Journal of Clinical Investigation, 117*(5), 1219–1222. https://doi.org/10.1172/JCI32169

Briquez, P. S., Hubbell, J. A., & Martino, M. M. (2015). Extracellular matrix-inspired growth factor delivery systems for skin wound healing. *Advanced Wound Care, 4*(8), 479–489. https://doi.org/10.1089/wound.2014.0603

Brownrigg, J. R., Davey, J., Holt, P. J., et al. (2015). The association of ulceration of the foot with cardiovascular and all-cause mortality in patients with diabetes: A meta-analysis. *Diabetologia, 55*(11), 2906–2912.

Bus, S. A., & van Netten, J. J. (2016). A shift in priority in diabetic foot care and research: 75% of foot ulcers are preventable. *Diabetes/metabolism Research and Reviews, 32*(S1), 195–200. https://doi.org/10.1002/dmrr.2754

Bus, S. A., van Netten, J. J., Lavery, L. A., Monteiro-Soares, M., Rasmussen, A., Jubiz, Y., et al. (2016a). IWGDF guidance on the prevention of foot ulcers in at-risk patients with diabetes. *Diabetes/metabolism Research and Reviews, 32*(S1), 16–24. https://doi.org/10.1002/dmrr.2696

Bus, S. A., van Netten, J. J., Lavery, L. A., et al. (2016b). IWGDF guidance on the prevention of foot ulcers in at-risk patients with diabetes. *Diabetes/metabolism Research and Reviews, 32*(S1), 16–24.

Bus, S. A., van, Netten, J. J., Monteiro-, Soares, M., Lipsky, B. A., Schaper, N. C., & International Working Group on the Diabetic Foot. (2020a). Diabetic foot disease: From the evaluation of the "foot at risk" to the development of clinical guidelines. *Diabetes/metabolism Research and Reviews, 36*(S1), Article e3279. https://doi.org/10.1002/dmrr.3279

Bus, S. A., van Netten, J. J., Monteiro-Soares, M., Lipsky, B. A., Schaper, N. C., & IWGDF. (2020b). Guidelines on the prevention of foot ulcers in persons with diabetes. *Diabetes/Metabolism Research and Reviews, 36*(S1), e3269. https://doi.org/10.1002/dmrr.3269.

Chang, M., & Nguyen, T. T. (2021, March 2). Strategy for treatment of infected diabetic foot ulcers. *Accounts of Chemical Research, 54*(5), 1080–1093. https://doi.org/10.1021/acs.accounts.0c00864. Epub 2021 Feb 17. PMID: 33596041.

Conte, M. S., Bradbury, A. W., Kolh, P., et al. (2019). Global vascular guidelines on the management of chronic limb-threatening ischemia. *Journal of Vascular Surgery, 69*(6 Suppl), 3S-125S.

Conte, M. S., Bradbury, A. W., Kolh, P., White, J. V., Dick, F., Fitridge, R., et al. (2019). Global vascular guidelines on the management of chronic limb-threatening ischemia. *Journal of Vascular Surgery, 69*(6S). 3S–125S.e40. https://doi.org/10.1016/j.jvs.2019.02.016

Couturier, A., Calissi, C., Cracowski, J. L., Sigaudo-Roussel, D., Khouri, C., & Roustit, M. (2023, December). Mouse models of diabetes-related ulcers: a systematic review and network meta-analysis. *EBioMedicine, 98*, 104856. https://doi.org/10.1016/j.ebiom.2023.104856. Epub 2023 Oct 31. PMID: 38251464; PMCID: PMC10755106.

Dash, N. R., Dash, S. N., Routray, P., Mohapatra, S., & Mohapatra, P. C. (2021). Targeting nonhealing ulcers of lower extremity in human through autologous bone marrow-derived mesenchymal stem cells. *Regenenerative Therapy, 18*, 50–60. https://doi.org/10.1016/j.reth.2021.04.002

Deng, H., Li, B., Shen, Q., Zhang, C., Kuang, L., Chen, R., Wang, S., Ma, Z., & Li, G. (2023, April). Mechanisms of diabetic foot ulceration: A review. *Journal of Diabetes, 15*(4), 299–312. https://doi.org/10.1111/1753-0407.13372. Epub 2023 Mar 9. PMID: 36891783; PMCID: PMC10101842.

Driver, V. R., Lavery, L. A., Reyzelman, A. M., & Fitzgerald, R. H. (2015). A clinical trial of Integra Dermal Regeneration Template for diabetic foot ulcers. *Wound Repair Regeneration, 23*(6), 891–900.

Edmonds, M., Jeffcoate, W., Hinchliffe, R. J., & Bus, S. A. (2020). Current challenges and opportunities in the prevention and management of diabetic foot ulcers. *Diabetes/metabolism Research and Reviews, 36*(S1), Article e3241. https://doi.org/10.1002/dmrr.3241

Eming, S. A., Martin, P., & Tomic-Canic, M. (2014). Wound repair and regeneration: Mechanisms, signaling, and translation. *Science Translational Medicine, 6*(265), 265sr6. https://doi.org/10.1126/scitranslmed.3009337.

Faglia, E., Clerici, G., Caminiti, M., Quarantiello, A., Gino, M., & Morabito, A. (2006). Predicting the risk of major amputation in diabetic patients hospitalized for foot infection. *Diabetes Care, 29*(8), 1675–1680.

Faglia, E., Clerici, G., Caminiti, M., et al. (2012). Long-term prognosis of diabetic patients with critical limb ischemia: Comparison between surgical and percutaneous revascularization. *Diabetes Care, 35*(7), 1348–1354.

Falanga, V. (2005). Wound healing and its impairment in the diabetic foot. *The Lancet, 366*(9498), 1736–1743. https://doi.org/10.1016/S0140-6736(05)67700-8

Falanga, V. (2012). Wound healing and its impairment in the diabetic foot. *The Lancet, 366*(9498), 1736–1743. https://doi.org/10.1016/S0140-6736(05)67700-8

Farber, A., & Eberhardt, R. T. (2016). The current state of critical limb ischemia: A systematic review. *JAMA Surgery, 151*(11), 1070–1077.

Fernández-Montequín, J. I., Valenzuela-Silva, C. M., Díaz, O. G., Savigne, W., Sancho-Soutelo, N., Rivero-Fuentes, M. A., et al. (2009). Intralesional injections of recombinant human epidermal growth factor promote granulation and healing in advanced diabetic foot ulcers: Multicenter, randomized, placebo-controlled, double-blind study. *International Wound Journal, 6*(6), 432–443.

Fitzpatrick, T., Rosella, L. C., Calzavara, A., Petch, J., Pinto, A. D., Manson, H., & Goel, V. (2019). Looking beyond income and education: Socioeconomic status gradients among future high-cost users of health care. *American Journal of Preventive Medicine, 57*(1), 1–7. https://doi.org/10.1016/j.amepre.2019.02.016

Frykberg, R. G., Banks, J., Tierney, E., & Tallis, A. (2020). Offloading the diabetic foot ulcer: A systematic review and meta-analysis. *Advances in Wound Care, 9*(6), 298–308. https://doi.org/10.1089/wound.2019.1051

Gallagher, K. A., Liu, Z. J., & Xiao, M. (2024b). Microvascular dysfunction in diabetes: Implications for diabetic foot ulcers. *Diabetes Research and Clinical Practice, 205*, Article 110302. https://doi.org/10.1016/j.diabres.2023.110302

Gallagher, K. A., Mills, J. L., Armstrong, D. G., Conte, M. S., Kirsner, R. S., Minc, S. D., Plutzky, J., Southerland, K. W., & Tomic-Canic, M. (2024, January 23). American Heart Association Council on peripheral vascular disease; Council on cardiovascular and stroke nursing. Council on Clinical Cardiology; and Council on Lifestyle and Cardiometabolic Health. Current status and principles for the treatment and prevention of diabetic foot ulcers in the cardiovascular patient population: A scientific statement from the American Heart Association. *Circulation,*

149(4), e232-e253. https://doi.org/10.1161/CIR.0000000000001192. Epub 2023 Dec 14. PMID: 38095068; PMCID: PMC11067094.

Game, F. L., Apelqvist, J., Attinger, C., Hartemann, A., Hinchliffe, R. J., Löndahl, M., et al. (2016). IWGDF guidance on use of interventions to enhance the healing of chronic ulcers of the foot in diabetes. *Diabetes/metabolism Research and Reviews, 32*(Suppl 1), 75–83.

Game, F. L., Hinchliffe, R. J., Apelqvist, J., Armstrong, D. G., Bakker, K., Hartemann, A., et al. (2020a). A systematic review of interventions to enhance the healing of chronic ulcers of the foot in diabetes. *Diabetes/metabolism Research and Reviews, 32*(S1), 154–168. https://doi.org/10.1002/dmrr.2703

Game, F. L., & Jeffcoate, W. J. (2016). The role of growth factors in the healing of diabetic foot ulcers. *Diabetes/Metabolism Research and Reviews, 32*(Suppl 1), 128–134, 80–88. https://doi.org/10.1002/dmrr.2702

Game, F., Jeffcoate, W., Apelqvist, J., et al. (2020b). Specific guidelines for diabetic foot disease. *Diabetes/metabolism Research and Reviews, 36*(S1), Article e3260.

Gottrup, F. (2012). Optimizing wound treatment through health care structuring and professional education. *Wound Repair and Regeneration, 20*(2), 126–131. https://doi.org/10.1111/j.1524-475X.2012.00767.x

Guest, J. F., Fuller, G. W., Vowden, P., & Vowden, K. R. (2018). Diabetic foot ulcer management in clinical practice in the UK: Costs and outcomes. *International Wound Journal, 15*(1), 43–52. https://doi.org/10.1111/iwj.12816

Guo, Q., Ying, G., Jing, O., Zhang, Y., Liu, Y., Deng, M., & Long, S. (2023, May). Influencing factors for the recurrence of diabetic foot ulcers: A meta-analysis. *International Wound Journal, 20*(5), 1762–1775. https://doi.org/10.1111/iwj.14017. Epub 2022 Nov 17. PMID: 36385501; PMCID: PMC10088840.

Gupta, A., Kowalczuk, M., Heaselgrave, W., Britland, S. T., Martin, C., & Radecka, I. (2020). The production and application of hydrogels for wound management: A review. *European Polymer Journal, 134*, Article 109856. https://doi.org/10.1016/j.eurpolymj.2020.109856

Han, G., Ceilley, R., Kirsner, R. S., & Serena, T. (2012). Advanced skin substitutes and wound healing. *Wounds, 24*(11), 308–314.

Han, S. K., Kim, H. R., Kim, W. K., & Park, E. J. (2021). The use of mesenchymal stem cells in treatment of chronic nonhealing wounds: Current status and future prospects. *Plastic and Reconstructive Surgery, 148*(3), 657e–667e. https://doi.org/10.1097/PRS.0000000000008232

Heyboer, M., Milovanova, T. N., Wojtkowiak, J. W., et al. (2017). Hyperbaric oxygen therapy: Role in comprehensive wound care. *American Journal of Surgery, 214*(6), 1121–1126.

Hingorani, A., LaMuraglia, G. M., Henke, P., Meissner, M. H., Loretz, L., Zinszer, K. M., et al. (2016). The management of diabetic foot: A clinical practice guideline by the Society for Vascular Surgery in collaboration with the American Podiatric Medical Association and the Society for Vascular Medicine. *Journal of Vascular Surgery, 63*(2 Suppl), 3S-21S.

Huang, F., Lu, X., Yang, Y., Yang, Y., Li, Y., Kuai, L., Li, B., Dong, H., & Shi, J. (2023, January). Microenvironment-based diabetic foot ulcer nanomedicine. *Advanced Science (Weinh), 10*(2), e2203308. https://doi.org/10.1002/advs.202203308. Epub 2022 Nov 24. PMID: 36424137; PMCID: PMC9839871.

Iida, O., Takahara, M., Soga, Y., et al. (2013). Angiosome-directed angioplasty for critical limb ischemia: A randomized controlled trial. *Circulation: Cardiovascular Interventions, 6*(5), 545–553.

James, G. A., Swogger, E., Wolcott, R., Pulcini, E. D., Secor, P., Sestrich, J., Costerton, J. W., et al. (2008). Biofilms in chronic wounds. *Wound Repair and Regeneration, 16*(1), 37–44. https://doi.org/10.1111/j.1524-475X.2007.00321.x

Jeffcoate, W. J., Vileikyte, L., Boyko, E. J., Armstrong, D. G., & Boulton, A. J. M. (2018). Current challenges and opportunities in the prevention and management of diabetic foot ulcers. *Diabetes Care, 41*(4), 645–652. https://doi.org/10.2337/dc17-1836

Jeon, B. J., Choi, H. J., Kang, J. S., Tak, M. S., & Park, E. S. (2017, June). Comparison of five systems of classification of diabetic foot ulcers and predictive factors for amputation. *International*

Wound Journal, 14(3), 537–545. https://doi.org/10.1111/iwj.12642. Epub 2016 Oct 10. PMID: 27723246; PMCID: PMC7949506.

Keshtkar, S., Azarpira, N., & Ghahremani, M. H. (2018). Mesenchymal stem cell-derived extracellular vesicles: Novel frontiers in regenerative medicine. *Stem Cell Research & Therapy, 9*, 63. https://doi.org/10.1186/s13287-018-0791-7

Kirsner, R. S., Warriner, R. A., Michela, M., & Stojadinovic, A. (2012). Advanced biological therapies for diabetic foot ulcers. *Wound Repair Regen., 20*(6), 715–721.

Kranke, P., Bennett, M. H., Martyn-St James, M., Schnabel, A., Debus, S. E., & Weibel, S. (2015). Hyperbaric oxygen therapy for chronic wounds. *Cochrane Database of Systematic Reviews, 6*, CD004123.

Lavery, L. A., Armstrong, D. G., & Harkless, L. B. (1996, September–October). Classification of diabetic foot wounds. *The Journal of Foot and Ankle Surgery, 35*(6), 528–531.

Lavery, L. A., Davis, K. E., Berriman, S. J., Braun, L., Nichols, A., Kim, P. J., & Armstrong, D. G. (2020). WHS guidelines update: Diabetic foot ulcer treatment guidelines. *Wound Repair Regeneration, 28*(1), 1–20.

Lavery, L. A., Higgins, K. R., Lanctot, D. R., Constantinides, G. P., Zamorano, R. G., Athanasiou, K. A., et al. (2004). Home monitoring of foot skin temperatures to prevent ulceration. *Diabetes Care, 27*(11), 2642–2647. https://doi.org/10.2337/diacare.27.11.2642

Lavery, L. A., Peters, E. J. G., & Armstrong, D. G. (2007). What are the most effective interventions in preventing diabetic foot ulcers? *International Wound Journal, 4*(3), 248–252.

Lázaro-Martínez, J. L., Aragón-Sánchez, J., & García-Morales, E. (2014). Antibiotics versus conservative surgery for treating diabetic foot osteomyelitis: A randomized comparative trial. *Diabetes Care, 37*(3), 789–795.

Lázaro-Martínez, J. L., Aragón-Sánchez, J., & García-Morales, E. (2021a). Optimizing the use of negative pressure wound therapy for diabetic foot ulcers. *International Journal of Lower Extremity Wounds, 20*(1), 12–18. https://doi.org/10.1177/1534734620928125

Lázaro-Martínez, J. L., García-Álvarez, Y., García-Morales, E., Molines-Barroso, R. J., & Aragón-Sánchez, F. J. (2021b). Clinical effectiveness of advanced therapies in the management of diabetic foot ulcers: A systematic review. *Diabetes/metabolism Research and Reviews, 37*(8), Article e3453. https://doi.org/10.1002/dmrr.3453

Lazzarini, P. A., O'Rourke, S. R., Russell, A. W., Clark, D., & Kuys, S. S. (2018). Reduced incidence of foot-related hospitalisation and amputation amongst persons with diabetes in Queensland, Australia. *PLOS ONE, 13*(6), Article e0198301. https://doi.org/10.1371/journal.pone.0198301

Lazzarini, P. A., Pacella, R. E., Armstrong, D. G., & van Netten, J. J. (2019). Diabetes-related lower-extremity complications are a leading cause of the global burden of disability. *Diabetic Medicine, 36*(7), 856–863. https://doi.org/10.1111/dme.13958

Li, X., Xie, X., Lian, W., Shi, R., Han, S., Zhang, H., Wang, X., et al. (2019). Exosomes from adipose-derived stem cells promote diabetic chronic wound healing through SIRT3/SOD2. *Cells, 8*(8), 845. https://doi.org/10.3390/cells8080845

Li, Y., Ju, S., Li, X., Li, W., Zhou, S., Wang, G., Cai, Y., & Dong, Z. (2023). Characterization of the microenvironment of diabetic foot ulcers and potential drug identification based on scRNA-seq. *Front Endocrinology (Lausanne), 4*(13), Article 997880. https://doi.org/10.3389/fendo.2022.997880.PMID:36686438;PMCID:PMC9845942

Lin, C., Liu, J., & Sun, H. (2020a). Risk factors for lower extremity amputation in patients with diabetic foot ulcers: A meta-analysis. *PLoS ONE, 15*(9), Article e0239236. https://doi.org/10.1371/journal.pone.0239236.PMID:32936828;PMCID:PMC7494323

Lin, C. W., Armstrong, D. G., & Lavery, L. A. (2020b). Diabetic foot assessment: Importance of early vascular evaluation. *International Wound Journal, 17*(4), 989–995. https://doi.org/10.1111/iwj.13362

Lipsky, B. A., Berendt, A. R., Cornia, P. B., Pile, J. C., Peters, E. J., Armstrong, D. G., et al. (2012). 2012 Infectious Diseases Society of America clinical practice guideline for the diagnosis and treatment of diabetic foot infections. *Clinical Infectious Diseases, 54*(12), e132-173.

Lipsky, B. A., Senneville, E., Abbas, Z. G., Aragón-Sánchez, J., Diggle, M., Embil, J. M., et al. (2020a). IWGDF Guidelines on the diagnosis and treatment of foot infection in persons with diabetes. *Diabetes/metabolism Research and Reviews, 36*(S1), Article e3280. https://doi.org/10.1002/dmrr.3280

Lipsky, B. A., Senneville, E., Lauri, C., Joseph, W. S., Kavanagh, N., & Lázaro-Martínez, J. L. (2020b). Guidelines on the diagnosis and treatment of foot infection in persons with diabetes. *Clinical Infectious Diseases, 70*(3), 395–403. https://doi.org/10.1093/cid/ciz919

Liu, S., He, C. Z., Cai, Y. T., Xing, Q. P., Guo, Y. Z., & Chen, Z. L. (2017). Evaluation of negative-pressure wound therapy for patients with diabetic foot ulcers: Systematic review and meta-analysis. *Therapeutics and Clinical Risk Management, 13*, 533–544.

Löndahl, M., Fagher, K., Katzman, P., Nilsson, A., & Hammarlund, C. (2011). Wound healing, pain reduction, and quality of life after hyperbaric oxygen therapy in patients with diabetes and chronic foot ulcers. *Wound Repair and Regeneration, 19*(4), 447–458.

Löndahl, M., Katzman, P., Nilsson, A., & Hammarlund, C. (2010). Hyperbaric oxygen therapy facilitates healing of chronic foot ulcers in patients with diabetes. *Diabetes Care, 33*(5), 998–1003.

Luo, Y., Li, L., Zhao, P., Yang, C., & Zhang, J. (2022). Effectiveness of silver dressings in the treatment of diabetic foot ulcers: A systematic review and meta-analysis. *Journal of Wound Care, 31*(11), 979–986. https://doi.org/10.12968/jowc.2022.31.11.979. PMID: 36367799.

Luo, L., Xu, J., Chen, L., Zhou, D., & Xu, H. (2021). Advances in gene therapy for chronic wounds. *International Journal of Molecular Sciences, 22*(3), 1103. https://doi.org/10.3390/ijms22031103

Martínez-Gómez, D. A., Moreno-Ruíz, L. A., Cárdenas-Elizalde, M. R., González-González, J. G., & Villarreal-Pérez, J. Z. (2021). Management of diabetic foot ulcers with insulin: Pathophysiological bases and therapeutic perspectives. *Journal of Diabetes Research, 2021*, 5592704. https://doi.org/10.1155/2021/5592704

Martínez-Sánchez, A., Rodríguez-Godoy, R., Vega-Sánchez, R., Morera-Herrera, T., & Fernández-Montequín, J. I. (2019). Therapeutic effectiveness of human umbilical cord-derived growth factors in the management of chronic diabetic foot ulcers: A randomized controlled trial. *Diabetes Therapy, 10*(6), 2169–2179.

Mills, J. L., Armstrong, D. G., & Pomposelli, F. B. (2014). The Society for Vascular Surgery lower extremity threatened limb classification system: Risk stratification based on wound, ischemia, and foot infection (WIfI). *Journal of Vascular Surgery, 59*(1), 220–34.e1. https://doi.org/10.1016/j.jvs.2013.08.003

Mitra, A., Shahid, A., Kumari, S., Mukherjee, T., Pramanick, S., Mohanty, S., Ansari, M. A., Adhikary, K., Prabhakar, P. K., & Kesari, K. K. (2025). Optimizing wound healing: Insights from phytochemicals and advanced therapies. *Inflammopharmacology, 33*(7), 4009–4035. https://doi.org/10.1007/s10787-025-01806-x. Epub 2025 Jun 20 PMID: 40540111.

Najafi, B., Mohler, J., Grewal, G. S., Talal, T. K., Menzies, R. A., & Armstrong, D. G. (2017). An optical markerless system for daily foot monitoring in patients with diabetes. *Journal of Diabetes Science and Technology, 11*(3), 567–577. https://doi.org/10.1177/1932296817696847

Neville, R. F., Kayssi, A., Buescher, T., & Sadek, M. (2009). The impact of socioeconomic status on outcomes in diabetic patients with critical limb ischemia. *Journal of Vascular Surgery, 50*(S1), S43–S48. https://doi.org/10.1016/j.jvs.2009.06.003

Oni, D. (2020). Foot self-care experiences among patients with diabetes: A systematic review of qualitative studies. *Wound Management & Prevention, 66*(4), 16–25. https://doi.org/10.25270/wmp.2020.4.1625. PMID: 32294056.

Pang, Q., Lou, D., Li, S., Wang, G., Qiao, B., & Dong, J. (2022). Intelligent wound dressing with multifunctional properties for diabetic wound healing. *Advanced Functional Materials, 32*(10), 2109200. https://doi.org/10.1002/adfm.202109200

Pourkazemi, A., Ghanbari, A., Khojamli, M., Balo, H., Hemmati, H., Jafaryparvar, Z., & Motamed, B. (2020). Diabetic foot care: Knowledge and practice. *BMC Endocrine Disorders, 20*(1), 40. https://doi.org/10.1186/s12902-020-0512-y.PMID:32192488;PMCID:PMC7083045

Prompers, L., Huijberts, M., Apelqvist, J., Jude, E., Piaggesi, A., Bakker, K., Schaper, N., et al. (2008). High prevalence of ischemia, infection and serious comorbidity in patients with diabetic foot disease in Europe. *Diabetologia, 50*(1), 18–25. https://doi.org/10.1007/s00125-006-0491-1

Santema, T. B., Stoekenbroek, R. M., van Steekelenburg, M., et al. (2018). Hyperbaric oxygen therapy in the treatment of ischemic lower extremity ulcers in patients with diabetes: Results of the DAMO2CLES multicenter randomized clinical trial. *Diabetes Care, 41*(1), 112–119.

Schaper, N. C., Van Netten, J. J., Apelqvist, J., et al. (2020). IWGDF guidelines on the prevention and management of diabetic foot disease. *Diabetes/metabolism Research and Reviews, 36*(S1), Article e3265.

Serena, T. E., Gurtner, G. C., Ko, F., & Shang, Y. (2020). Novel diagnostic and therapeutic strategies for diabetic foot ulcers. *Diabetes/metabolism Research and Reviews, 36*(S1), Article e3278. https://doi.org/10.1002/dmrr.3278

Setacci, C., de Donato, G., Teraa, M., et al. (2014). Chapter IV: Treatment of critical limb ischemia. *European Journal of Vascular and Endovascular Surgery, 48*(S4), S70–S85.

Sheehan, P., Jones, P., Caselli, A., Giurini, J. M., & Veves, A. (2003). Percent change in wound area of diabetic foot ulcers over a 4-week period is a robust predictor of complete healing in a 12-week prospective trial. *Diabetes Care, 26*(6), 1879–1882. https://doi.org/10.2337/diacare.26.6.1879

Shen, S., Wu, Y., Liu, Y., Wu, D., & Li, J. (2021). Functional nanofibrous scaffolds for diabetic wound healing. *Frontiers in Chemistry, 9*, Article 706426. https://doi.org/10.3389/fchem.2021.706426

Singh, N., Armstrong, D. G., & Lipsky, B. A. (2005). Preventing foot ulcers in patients with diabetes. *JAMA, 293*(2), 217–228.

Snyder, R. J., & Cardinal, M. (2010). Differentiating diabetic foot ulcers: The role of wound assessment. *Wounds, 22*(4), 79–85.

Song, J., Liu, A., Liu, B., Huang, W., Jiang, Z., Bai, X., Hu, L., Zheng, S., Guo, S., Wu, J., & Chen, Q. (2022). Natural biologics accelerate healing of diabetic foot ulcers by regulating oxidative stress. *Frontiers in Bioscience (Landmark Ed), 27*(10), 285. https://doi.org/10.31083/j.fbl2710285. PMID: 36336859.

Sorber, R., & Abularrage, C. J. (2021). Diabetic foot ulcers: Epidemiology and the role of multidisciplinary care teams. *Seminars in Vascular Surgery, 34*(1), 47–53. https://doi.org/10.1053/j.semvascsurg.2021.02.006. Epub 2021 Feb 5 PMID: 33757635.

Tamir, E., Drexler, M., Vigler, N., Avisar, E., & Agar, G. (2020). Surgical offloading procedures for diabetic foot ulcers: A practical review. *Diabetic Foot Ankle, 11*(1), 1752067. https://doi.org/10.1080/2000625X.2020.1752067

Tan, T. W., Mustapha, B., Lansberg, M. G., Rymer, J. A., Lee, J. T., & Satiani, B. (2022). Access to care and the incidence of limb amputation in patients with peripheral artery disease. *Journal of Vascular Surgery, 75*(3), 987–995. https://doi.org/10.1016/j.jvs.2021.08.055

Tang, W. H., Zhao, Y. N., Cheng, Z. X., Xu, J. X., Zhang, Y., & Liu, X. M. (2024Jun). Risk factors for diabetic foot ulcers: A systematic review and meta-analysis. *Vascular., 32*(3), 661–669. https://doi.org/10.1177/17085381231154805. Epub 2023 Feb 5 PMID: 36740805.

Tesfaye, S., Boulton, A. J., Dyck, P. J., Freeman, R., Horowitz, M., Kempler, P., et al. (2010). Diabetic neuropathies: Update on definitions, diagnostic criteria, estimation of severity, and treatments. *Diabetes Care, 33*(10), 2285–2293.

Thackham, J. A., McElwain, D. L., & Long, R. J. (2008). The use of hyperbaric oxygen therapy to treat chronic wounds: A review. *Wound Repair and Regeneration, 16*(3), 321–330. https://doi.org/10.1111/j.1524-475X.2008.00372.x

van Netten, J. J., Price, P. E., Lavery, L. A., Monteiro-Soares, M., Rasmussen, A., Jubiz, Y., et al. (2020). Prevention of foot ulcers in the at-risk patient with diabetes: A systematic review. *Diabetes/metabolism Research and Reviews, 36*(S1), Article e3270. https://doi.org/10.1002/dmrr.3270

Vedhara, K., Dawe, K., Wetherell, M. A., Miles, J. N., Cullum, N., Dayan, C., & Weinman, J. (2010). Illness beliefs predict self-care behaviours in patients with diabetic foot ulcers: A prospective study. *Diabetes Research and Clinical Practice, 89*(2), 222–228. https://doi.org/10.1016/j.diabres.2010.03.017

Veves, A., Falanga, V., Armstrong, D. G., & Sabolinski, M. L. (2001). Graftskin, a human skin equivalent, is effective in the management of noninfected neuropathic diabetic foot ulcers: A prospective randomized multicenter clinical trial. *Diabetes Care, 24*(2), 290–295.

Wagner, F. W., Jr. (1981). The dysvascular foot: A system for diagnosis and treatment. *Foot & Ankle, 2*(2), 64–122.

Wang, C., Wang, C., Zhang, X., & Yu, X. (2019). Intelligent stimulus-responsive wound dressings for diabetic wound healing. *Journal of Materials Chemistry B, 7*(9), 1545–1561. https://doi.org/10.1039/C8TB02930B

Wilkinson, H. N., Hardman, M. J., & Sethi, S. (2020). The role of biomarkers in the diagnosis and prognosis of chronic wounds. *Wound Repair and Regeneration, 28*(5), 535–543. https://doi.org/10.1111/wrr.12779

Winters, C. L., Brigido, S. A., Liden, B. A., Simmons, M., Hartman, J. F., & Wright, M. L. (2016). A multicenter study involving the use of DermACELL in the treatment of chronic diabetic foot ulcers. *Wounds, 28*(3), 75–80.

Wu, S. C., Jensen, J. L., & Armstrong, D. G. (2018). Evaluation of the impact of a multidisciplinary limb preservation program on diabetic foot outcomes. *Journal of Vascular Surgery, 67*(2), 611–618.

Yazdanpanah, L., Nasiri, M., & Adarvishi, S. (2018). Literature review on the use of artificial intelligence for the diagnosis and treatment of diabetic foot ulcers. *International Journal of Endocrinology and Metabolism, 16*(4), Article e90335. https://doi.org/10.5812/ijem.90335

Zhang, Z., Zhang, W., Xu, Y., & Liu, D. (2022). Efficacy of hyperbaric oxygen therapy for diabetic foot ulcers: An updated systematic review and meta-analysis. *Asian Journal of Surgery, 45*(1), 68–78. https://doi.org/10.1016/j.asjsur.2021.07.047. Epub 2021 Aug 8 PMID: 34376365.

Zhao, L., Xu, D. B., Li, X. Y., et al. (2020). Efficacy of hyperbaric oxygen therapy in patients with diabetic foot ulcers: An updated systematic review and meta-analysis. *Diabetes/metabolism Research and Reviews, 36*(7), Article e3319.

Chapter 5
Eyes on the Future: Preventing Vision Loss and Retinopathy

Riya Sarkar, Rajat Kanti Ghosal, Koyel Banerjee, Pradipta Banerjee, and Rajkumar Maiti

Abstract Diabetic retinopathy (DR) continues to be a major global cause of irreversible blindness, impacting more than half of individuals living with diabetes. Currently, approximately 1.1 billion people worldwide experience some form of visual impairment, largely due to inadequate access to eye care services and assistive technologies, a number projected to escalate to 1.8 billion by 2050. Fortunately, the evolution of medical technologies, early screening programs, and the expanded use of anti-vascular endothelial growth factor (anti-VEGF) therapies have positioned diabetic retinopathy as one of the most preventable causes of blindness. Advancements in ophthalmic surgery such as corneal laser procedures, refractive surgeries like Laser-Assisted In Situ Keratomileusis (LASIK) and Photorefractive Keratectomy (PRK), minimally invasive glaucoma surgery (MIGS), and modern cataract techniques including phacoemulsification with advanced intraocular lenses (IOLs)—are collectively transforming vision care by offering permanent correction, faster recovery, improved visual outcomes, and effective long-term management of conditions like glaucoma through reduced intraocular pressure and optic nerve protection. To address the rising global demand for comprehensive eye care, the World Health Organization (WHO) promotes the Integrated People-Centred Eye Care (IPEC) framework. The aim of this chapter is to explore the current landscape and future directions in the prevention of vision loss, with a specific focus on diabetic retinopathy and other major causes of preventable blindness. It highlights the global

R. Sarkar · K. Banerjee
Department of Medical Laboratory Technology, Dr. B. C. Roy Academy of Professional Courses, Durgapur, India

R. K. Ghosal
Department of Bio-medical Sciences, School of Biosciences and Technology, Vellore Institute of Technology, Vellore, India

P. Banerjee
Department of Surgery, McGowan Institute for Regenerative Medicine, University of Pittsburgh, Pittsburgh, PA, USA

R. Maiti (✉)
Department of Physiology, Bankura Christian College, Bankura, India
e-mail: rajkumar@bankurachristiancollege.in

K. Adhikary et al. (eds.), *Healing Beyond Blood Sugar*,
https://doi.org/10.1007/978-981-95-8946-3_5

burden of visual impairment, the impact of emerging technologies, advancements in medical and surgical treatments, and the critical role of integrated healthcare systems and public–private partnership.

Keywords Vision therapy · Diabetic retinopathy · Integrated people centred eye care · Public–private partnership

5.1 Introduction

In every aspect and phase of our existence, vision—the most powerful sense—is essential. We often take eyesight for granted, yet without it, it is difficult to study, navigate, comprehend material, engage in school, and work. When the optic nerve and its operations are impacted by an eye problem, vision impairment results (Hutmacher, 2019). If they live for prolonged periods, everyone will eventually get more than one eye ailment that needs proper treatment. Near or distant vision impairment affects a minimum of 2.2 billion individuals worldwide. Nearly half of these instances, or at least 1 billion, include visual impairment that might have been avoided or has not yet been treated (Vashist et al., 2022).

Comparatively speaking, rates of untreated near-impaired vision are less than 10% in the wealthiest parts of North America, the Australian continent, the western part of Europe, and the Asia–Pacific, whereas they are projected to be over eighty percent in western, eastern, and central Africa below the Sahara (Eze et al., 2025). Ageing and an increased population are predicted to raise the likelihood that additional individuals may have visual impairments. To avoid irreversible impairment of vision, early detection and treatment are essential (Threatt et al., 2013). To avoid vision loss, get ophthalmologic care as soon as possible. One of the early signs of glaucoma might be a reduction in your field of vision. This illness frequently advances undetected until serious harm has been done. Disorders like conjunctivitis, dry eye disease, or more serious issues like scleritis can cause persistent redness. Consult if the redness doesn't go away with rest (Kalt et al., 2010).

Whether current vision or optimally corrected eyesight has been identified affects the occurrence of visual impairment. Nevertheless, this number rose significantly to 314 million people with V visual impairment when the frequency of improper refractive error correction was considered. This implies that an additional 153 million persons have vision impairment due to unchecked refractive errors alone. The varieties of retinal diseases, the risk variables associated with vision loss, and the latest developments in diagnostic methods for the general population will all be briefly covered in this chapter (Vashist et al., 2022).

5.2 Understanding Retinopathy

Retinopathy is a general term for conditions where the retina—the light-sensitive layer at the back of the eye—becomes damaged, most often due to underlying vascular or systemic causes. When retinal blood vessels leak, grow abnormally, or fail to deliver adequate oxygen, retinal structure and function can be compromised, potentially leading to vision loss or even blindness (Rivera et al., 2011).

5.2.1 Pathophysiology of Retinopathy

Diabetic retinopathy develops as a consequence of chronic hyperglycemia, which initiates a series of metabolic and vascular abnormalities in the retina. Prolonged hyperglycemia activates the polyol pathway, increases advanced glycation end-products (AGEs), and enhances oxidative stress and inflammation. These changes cause pericyte loss, basement membrane thickening, and endothelial cell dysfunction, ultimately leading to breakdown of the blood-retinal barrier. Capillary non-perfusion and ischemia stimulate upregulation of vascular endothelial growth factor (VEGF) and other pro-angiogenic mediators, resulting in abnormal neovascularisation. Additionally, chronic low-grade inflammation, leukostasis, and microglial activation contribute to neuronal apoptosis and progressive retinal neurodegeneration. Together, these processes drive the transition from non-proliferative retinopathy (microaneurysms, haemorrhages, exudates) to proliferative stages characterised by pathological angiogenesis and vision-threatening complications (Kusuhara et al., 2018).

5.3 Types of Retinopathy

5.3.1 Diabetic Retinopathy

Diabetic retinopathy (DR) is a microvascular complication of diabetes and the leading cause of preventable blindness in working-age adults. Chronic hyperglycemia induces structural and functional alterations in the retinal vasculature, including pericyte apoptosis, basement membrane thickening, and endothelial dysfunction. These changes lead to capillary occlusion, microaneurysm formation, vascular leakage, and ischemia. Progression of ischemia stimulates overexpression of VEGF, driving neovascularization and proliferative disease. In addition to vascular injury, retinal neurodegeneration, oxidative stress, and low-grade inflammation play critical roles in the pathogenesis of DR. Clinically, DR is categorized into non-proliferative and proliferative stages, with diabetic macular edema (DME) as a vision-threatening manifestation that may occur at any stage (Vujosevic et al., 2020).

5.3.2 Hypertensive Retinopathy

Hypertensive retinopathy refers to the spectrum of retinal microvascular changes caused by chronic systemic hypertension. Elevated blood pressure induces vasoconstriction, increased vascular permeability, and structural remodeling of retinal arterioles. Early changes include generalized and focal arteriolar narrowing, arteriovenous crossing changes (arteriovenous nicking), and arteriolar wall thickening. With sustained hypertension, endothelial dysfunction and breakdown of the blood-retinal barrier result in hemorrhages, cotton-wool spots, and hard exudates. In advanced stages, malignant hypertension leads to optic disc edema and exudative retinal detachment. The severity of retinopathy correlates with both the duration and level of hypertension, and it serves as a marker of systemic vascular damage and cardiovascular risk (Wong & Mitchell, 2004).

5.3.3 Retinopathy of Prematurity

Retinopathy of prematurity (ROP) is a vasoproliferative retinal disorder that occurs in premature and low-birth-weight infants due to incomplete retinal vascularisation. Exposure to supplemental oxygen and fluctuating oxygen levels after preterm birth disrupt normal angiogenesis, leading to delayed vessel growth and subsequent retinal ischemia. The ischemic retina upregulates VEGF and insulin-like growth factor-1 (IGF-1), resulting in abnormal neovascularization at the junction of vascular and avascular retina. These fragile new vessels may regress spontaneously or progress to fibrovascular proliferation, vitreous haemorrhage, and tractional retinal detachment, causing irreversible blindness. ROP is staged (I–V) based on the International Classification, ranging from mild peripheral changes to total retinal detachment. Early screening and timely treatment with laser photocoagulation or intravitreal anti-VEGF therapy are crucial for preventing vision loss (Dammann et al., 2023).

5.3.4 Radiation and Other Forms

Radiation Retinopathy is a delayed microangiopathy that develops months to years after ocular or periocular radiation therapy, commonly seen in patients treated for ocular tumors, head and neck cancers. Ionizing radiation damages endothelial cells and pericytes, leading to capillary non-perfusion, microaneurysms, telangiectasia, and macular edema. Clinically, it resembles diabetic retinopathy, with hemorrhages, cotton-wool spots, and neovascularization, and may progress to vision-threatening complications (Sahoo et al., 2021).

Other Forms of Retinopathy include retinopathy associated with systemic conditions such as sickle cell disease (sickle cell retinopathy), anaemia, autoimmune disorders, or infections. These conditions cause ischemic or proliferative retinal changes due to altered blood rheology, vascular occlusion, or immune-mediated injury. Toxic retinopathy may also occur secondary to drugs (e.g., chloroquine, hydroxychloroquine), while traumatic retinopathy can result from mechanical or blast injuries (Heckenlively & Ferreyra, 2008).

Together, these non-diabetic, non-hypertensive retinopathies highlight the retina's vulnerability to diverse vascular, metabolic, and environmental insults.

5.4 Risk Factors for Vision Loss and Retinopathy

The development and progression of retinopathy, as well as the risk of vision loss, are influenced by a combination of systemic, ocular, and environmental factors (Lee et al., 2015).

- **Metabolic risk factors** such as poor glycemic control, longer duration of diabetes, hypertension, dyslipidemia, and obesity significantly increase the risk of diabetic retinopathy and macular oedema.
- **Vascular risk factors** like chronic hypertension and atherosclerosis accelerate microvascular damage, while prematurity and oxygen therapy are key determinants in retinopathy of prematurity.
- **Treatment-related factors**, including exposure to ionizing radiation or use of retinotoxic drugs (e.g., chloroquine, tamoxifen), can also precipitate retinopathy.
- **Lifestyle and demographic factors** such as smoking, anemia, pregnancy, and genetic predisposition contribute to susceptibility and severity. Early identification and control of these risk factors are critical in reducing the burden of vision-threatening retinopathy.

5.4.1 Systemic Conditions

Several systemic conditions predispose to the development or progression of retinopathy through microvascular and metabolic dysfunction. Diabetes mellitus is the leading cause, where chronic hyperglycemia induces endothelial injury, pericyte loss, and ischemia, resulting in diabetic retinopathy. Systemic hypertension contributes via arteriolar narrowing, vascular leakage, and ischemic changes that manifest as hypertensive retinopathy. Renal disease and dyslipidemia further accelerate retinal microangiopathy by altering vascular homeostasis. Hematological disorders such as sickle cell disease and severe anemia impair blood rheology and oxygen delivery, producing ischemic and proliferative retinopathy. Autoimmune diseases (e.g., lupus, sarcoidosis) and infectious conditions (e.g., HIV, tuberculosis, syphilis) can also cause secondary retinopathy through immune-mediated or inflammatory pathways. These systemic associations highlight the retina as a sensitive marker of generalized vascular health (Di Marco et al., 2022).

5.4.2 *Age and Genetic Predisposition*

5.4.2.1 Age

It is an important determinant in the onset and severity of retinopathy. In diabetic retinopathy, increasing age and longer duration of diabetes markedly elevate the risk of microvascular damage and vision-threatening complications. In retinopathy of prematurity, by contrast, younger gestational age and very low birth weight are strong risk factors due to incomplete retinal vascular development (Kwinta & Pietrzyk, 2007).

5.4.2.2 Genetic

Genetic predisposition also plays a crucial role, as polymorphisms in genes regulating angiogenesis (e.g., VEGF, IGF-1), oxidative stress pathways, and inflammatory mediators have been linked to increased susceptibility and progression of retinopathy. Family history and ethnic background further influence disease risk, suggesting a heritable component. Together, age-related vulnerability and genetic susceptibility act synergistically with systemic and environmental factors to determine the onset, progression, and severity of vision loss from retinopathy (Kwinta & Pietrzyk, 2007).

5.4.2.3 Lifestyle and Environmental Factors

Lifestyle and environmental determinants significantly influence the risk and progression of retinopathy (Beulens et al., 2022).

- Smoking is strongly associated with oxidative stress, endothelial dysfunction, and worsening of both diabetic and hypertensive retinopathy.
- Poor diet rich in saturated fats and low in antioxidants contributes to metabolic dysregulation, while physical inactivity exacerbates obesity, insulin resistance, and vascular injury.
- Alcohol consumption and psychological stress are additional modifiers linked to systemic vascular damage.
- Environmental factorssuch as excessive oxygen exposure in preterm infants (leading to retinopathy of prematurity), chronic exposure to ionizing radiation, and air pollution (through inflammatory and oxidative pathways) have also been implicated.

Collectively, these modifiable factors interact with systemic conditions and genetic susceptibility, highlighting the importance of preventive lifestyle interventions in reducing the burden of vision-threatening retinopathy.

5.4.3 Socioeconomic and Access-Related Barriers

Socioeconomic status and healthcare access strongly influence the risk, detection, and management of retinopathy. Individuals from low-income or rural backgrounds often face limited access to ophthalmic screening, delayed diagnosis, and inadequate treatment facilities. High treatment costs, lack of insurance coverage, and competing financial priorities frequently prevent timely interventions such as laser therapy, anti-VEGF injections, or surgery. Educational barriers contribute to poor awareness of retinopathy symptoms and the importance of regular eye examinations, especially in patients with diabetes or hypertension. Geographic disparities, including shortage of trained specialists and inadequate infrastructure in resource-limited regions, further exacerbate the burden. Collectively, these barriers result in higher rates of advanced disease and irreversible vision loss in disadvantaged populations (Ravindranath et al., 2023).

5.5 Clinical Presentation and Diagnosis

5.5.1 Symptoms and Early Warning Signs

Some of our crucial systems are our eyes, and finding problems early can mean the difference between keeping your vision sound and having damage that can't be fixed. Although many eye conditions are quiet in their initial phases, we can seek prompt medical assistance by being aware of small changes (Miller & Hanumunthadu, 2022).

5.5.2 Vision Impairing

A detached retina may require prompt medical attention, and rapid or gradual vision impairment may be a sign of diabetic retinopathy, cataracts, glaucoma, or another underlying issue (Miller & Hanumunthadu, 2022).

5.5.3 Ocular Pain or Uneasiness

Chronic discomfort around or within the eye is abnormal and might be an indication of corneal abrasions, glaucoma, or infections like uveitis. It must be evaluated right once if there is erythema or sensitisation to light (Miller & Hanumanth, 2022).

5.5.4 Light Rays and Floating Objects

Even if they are normal occasionally, a rapid rise in floating debris or light flashes may be a sign of a retinal rupture or detachment. To avoid vision loss, get ophthalmologic care as soon as possible (Miller & Hanumanth, 2022).

5.5.5 Diagnostic Tools and Imaging Modalities

For medical systems across the world, the rising incidence of diabetes and associated complications—particularly diabetes mellitus—presents a serious problem. Diagnostic patterns are changing because of technological developments like artificial intelligence, smartphone-based photography, and teleophthalmology. Broad field photography is being influenced by imaging techniques such as Colour Fundus Imaging, FFA-based OCT, and OCT Angiography. Although incorporating these methods into healthcare settings is advised, the Slit-Lamp Biomicroscope (SLB) is still essential for referral and treatment choices. Due to their high cost, successful countrywide testing initiatives for DR are uncommon (Saleh et al., 2022).

5.5.6 The Study of Ophthalmology

By using cutting-edge imagery and technology to deliver medical care remotely, teleophthalmology proves to be an affordable option. Its effectiveness in remote visits is supported by research, which shows that it has a high level of specificity and sensitivity for identifying retinopathy and efficiently triaging patients according to the severity of the disease screening grade, freeing up eye specialists to concentrate more on treatments. For example, teleophthalmology showed encouraging results in evaluating retinal pictures for DR during the recent three-year research with 1646 patients, reaching an average resolution of ninety percent and a precision of 84.6%, respectively (Wong & Hyman, 2008).

5.5.7 Cinematography in the Widefield and Ultra-Widefield Conditions

For the past thirty years, the seven-field imaging procedure has been considered the norm for DR detection and classification in clinical studies. However, it only involves 34.0% of the cornea, and it requires time, solid fixation, and considerable patient cooperation. In order to detect and categorise DR, ultra-wide field photography provides a thorough picture regarding the cornea, capturing up to 80.0%, or approximately 200 °C, of the retina in a single shot. It improves speed and convenience by enabling retinal scanning without pupil dilation, particularly for those with impaired cataracts. Clarus and Optos Ultra-Widefield Colour (UWF-C) cameras exhibited a lower percentage of ungradable pictures but showed high agreement with the Conventional Seven-Field approach for DR identification and staging severity (Kąpa et al., 2024).

5.5.8 Data Mining and Intelligent Systems in DR

Ophthalmological diagnosis is undergoing a revolution because of recent developments in artificial intelligence (AI) and machine learning (ML), especially in the detection and screening of diabetic retinal disease. AI helps ophthalmologists better comprehend radiological and medical information by simulating human cognitive processes. By learning from large datasets, deep learning algorithms—such as Convolutional Neural Network (CNNs)—achieve exceptional accuracy and hold promise for more effective and dependable DR screening techniques.

The FDA has authorised AI-powered tabletop devices for the detection and categorisation of DR. Even in the absence of a steady internet connection, AI systems have demonstrated promise for doing distant, extensive DR checks. For a thorough evaluation of diabetic retinal disease, researchers are investigating the integration of AI with imaging modalities such as OCT, Optical Coherence Tomography Angiography (OCTA), Fluorescein Angiography (FA), Ultra-Widefield Imaging (UWFI), and portable cameras. Due to quicker exams and instantaneous findings, AI screening has resulted in excellent patient satisfaction and improved attendance at follow-up appointments. These developments demonstrate how AI and ML may improve patient outcomes and alter healthcare (Kąpa et al., 2024).

Although there is a lot of promise for improving screening accuracy and efficiency, using artificial intelligence and deep learning in DR diagnosis has drawbacks. If training is done on big datasets that are not representative of varied populations, biases may be introduced. Artificial intelligence systems may perform worse in real-world situations that differ from training data. Access to AI technology may be restricted by the high upfront costs of implementation (Kąpa et al., 2024).

5.5.9 The Use of Nanotechnology

The benchmark screening method in DR, cerebral examination using fluorescent dye angiography, has also made use of nanotechnology. Using extensively branched synthetic polyethyleneimine nanoparticles (PEI-NHAc-FS) to deliver intravenous fluorescence salt (FS) decreases the dye's biological absorption and subsequent retention in the body while preserving optical performance on par with free FS.

The secret to postponing the start of DR is to identify and treat hypoxia before it causes retinal neovascularisation. DR has been successfully prevented by inhibitors of the hypoxia-induced factor-1 (HIF-1), which stimulates the production of growth factors, including PDGF and VEGF. Traditionally given by regular intraocular injections, two of these inhibitors—doxorubicin and daunorubicin—have low water volatility and accumulate on the retina's surface (Kąpa et al., 2024) (Fig. 5.1).

5.5.10 Techniques of Ocular Scanning

Capturing the retinal picture using the proper medical imaging modality is the initial stage in developing any artificial intelligence algorithm for the identification, diagnosis, and classification of retinal illnesses, as seen in Fig. 5.1. The detection and treatment of AMD, or age-related macular degeneration, and diabetic retinopathy have been enhanced by developments in retinal imaging. Figure 5.2 provides an overview of the medical imaging modalities utilised for DR and AMD detection, diagnosis, and staging. The traditional imaging method for AMD is fundus fluorescein angiography (FFA), which is an effective tool for determining the condition's existence and severity. Nowadays, a lot of people employ optical coherence tomography (OCT) to diagnose neovascular lesions early and to determine the reduction criteria for anti-vascular endothelium growth component therapy (anti-VEGF).

Since the vessels of the retina are the area of the retina most impacted in diabetic eyes, FFA is now regarded as the gold standard method for evaluating it. Early identification of DR is made possible by visual coherence tomography angiography (OCTA), which can identify small alterations in the vessels in the retina before the onset of retinopathy's clinical symptoms. It can also assist in monitoring for DR in groups that are at risk. During this part, we will go over the different techniques regarding DR as well as AMD identification and management. We will describe the subtypes and subdivisions of each modality and provide a thorough example of how to use each medium for AMD and DR initial identification and diagnosis (Saleh et al., 2022).

5.5.11 Fundoscopy

A fundoscopy is a straightforward examination in which a medical professional look into your eyes using magnification instruments with a light attached. It is frequently included in standard medical examinations. Additionally, it's frequently used in the diagnosis of diseases, wounds, and several other situations.

The word "fundus," which refers to the inside rear border of our eye in medicine, is where the term originates. Since an eyepiece is one of the instruments most frequently used for fundoscopy, the procedure is also frequently referred to as eye surgery (Corr, 2023).

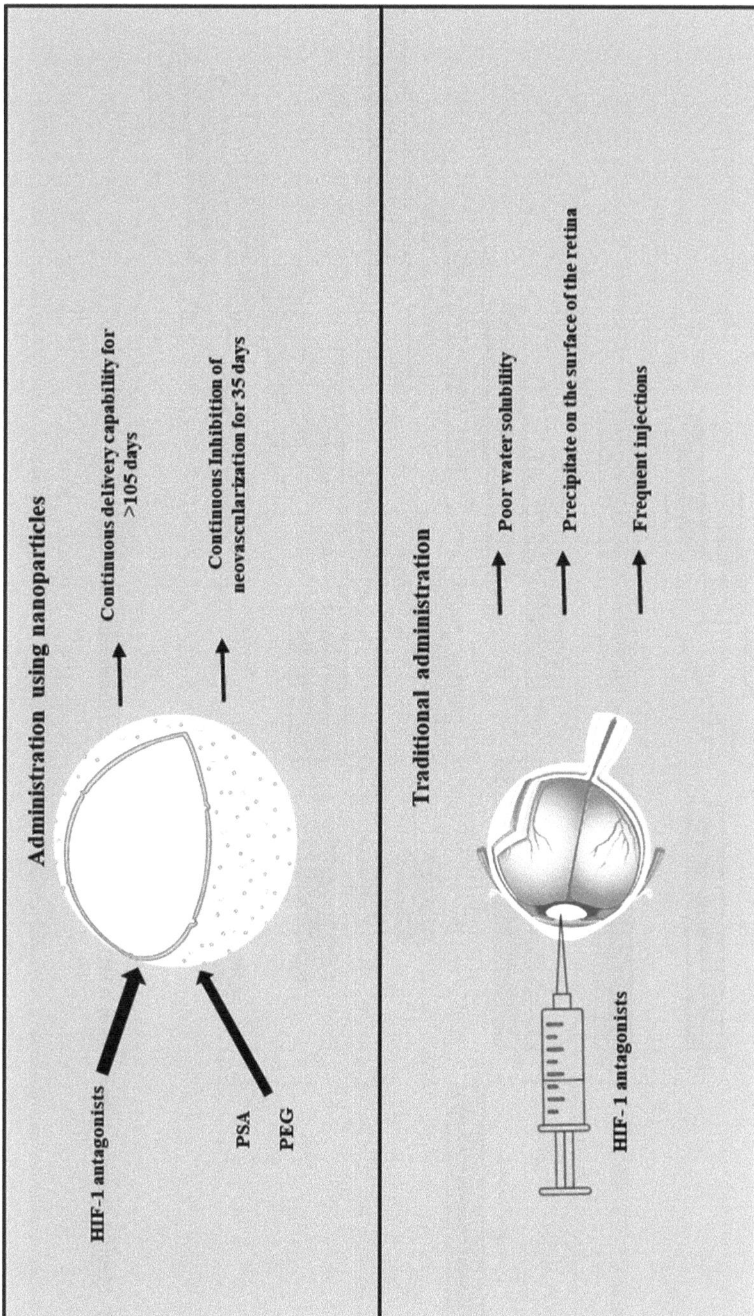

Fig. 5.1 Contrasting the application of HIF-1 antagonists

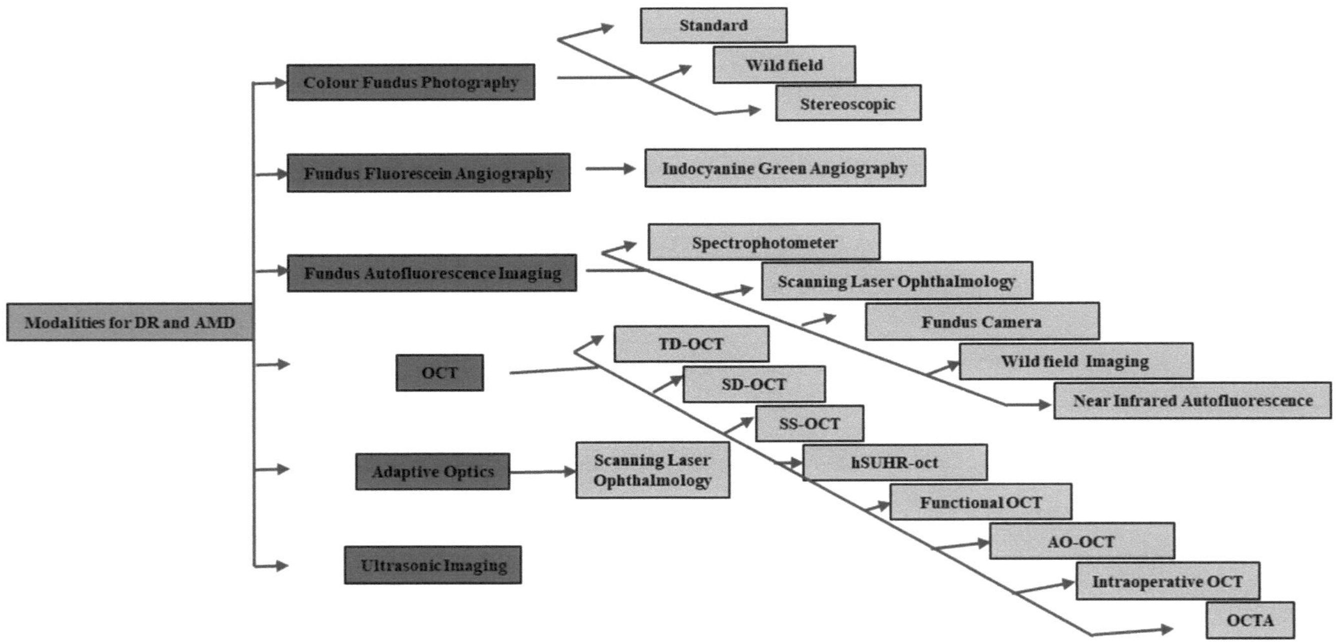

Fig. 5.2 Medical imaging techniques for AMD, including DR evaluation, treatment, and identification

A healthcare professional can do one of two forms of fundoscopy, each requiring a different device.

- Ophthalmoscopy done directly. This kind makes use of a portable gadget with a mounted light and a single magnifying window. Through the magnifying glass, the light aligns and aims at the object you're attempting to observe. Your healthcare professional will sit standing in front of us, grasping this gadget in their hand, and gaze directly into your eye via the magnified window.
- Ophthalmoscopy using indirect means. A cylindrical frame with a viewing strip at the front, which the provider may see, using one or both eyes, is frequently used for this sort of device. Additionally, the physician will place a portable condensing lens directly on the outside of our eye. Your doctor can see the back of your eye more clearly and with greater magnification if you angle that condensing lens. The healthcare professional can additionally observe this in three dimensions if they're using both eyes.

5.5.12 Optical Coherence Tomography (OCT)

Because of their similar operating principles, OCT and medical ultrasonography are frequently compared. Waves are sent to the tissue being examined by both medical imaging modalities, and the tissue structure reflects the waves. By analysing the back-reflected pulses and calculating their delay, the extent of the reflections may be ascertained. Near-infrared light, which is used in OCT, travels far more quickly than ultrasound. Since it is impossible to measure the back-reflected waves' delays directly, an analogous measurement is employed. A portion of the light is supplied to a control arm of known length, while another component is aimed at the sample via an interferometer (Aumann et al., 2019).

5.5.13 Ocular Impairment Tomography, OCT Angiography, and UWF Fluorescein Angiography

Current technological advancements allow users to overcome the restricted field of vision (FOV), which can lead to an erroneous measurement of the extent of DR. This is made possible by the introduction of UWF fluorescein-based angioplasty (FA), OCT, and OCTA. When it comes to advanced DR assessment and retinal neovascularisation (NV) detection, FA is the benchmark. Pathology detection and diagnostic efficiency are increased when UWF imaging and FA are combined. OCTA is recognised for non-invasive evaluation of diabetic microvascular characteristics, including NV, despite the possibility of adverse effects. Research utilising widefield OCTA (WF-OCTA) showed that PDR detection has a 95.0% sensitivity. In the time-based areas where they are more common, WF-OCTA found 93% of NV elsewhere (NVE).

Furthermore, WF-OCTA recognised 72.0% of the total NVEs that were visible on UWF-FA inside the scope of view. These findings demonstrate the effectiveness of the WF-OCTA test in PDR identification, which is consistent with DR evaluation and is consistent with those of previous research (Aumann et al., 2019).

Recent advances in artificial intelligence and machine learning (AI) are revolutionising ophthalmological diagnostics, particularly in detecting and screening diabetic retinal disease (DR). AI helps eye specialists better comprehend radiological and medical information by simulating how humans think. Deep learning algorithms, including CNNs, excel in accuracy by learning from vast datasets, promising more efficient and reliable DR screening methods (Aumann et al., 2019).

5.5.14 AI and Teleophthalmology Advances

The FDA has approved a number of AI-powered tabletop devices that have exceptional DR detection and categorisation capabilities. As of 2023, for example, a renowned team previously IDx-DR exceeded strict human grader requirements with an acceptance rate of 87.2% and a precision of 90.7%. With intensities of 94.6% and 92.7% and particularities of 85.9% and 92.4% for mtmDR and retinal DR, respectively, the EyeArt system automatically identifies more-than-mild and eye-threatening DR. Although there is a lot of promise for improving screening accuracy and efficiency, using AI and DL for DR diagnosis has drawbacks. Biases may be introduced by relying too heavily on training datasets, AI algorithms may perform worse in real-world situations that vary from the training set, and the high upfront expenses of deploying AI technology may restrict its use. Despite automated evaluations, image quality is still an issue, and cybersecurity threats need to be addressed to safeguard patient information (Olawade et al., 2025).

5.6 Strategies for Prevention

5.6.1 Primary Prevention (Lifestyle, Screening)

Digital ocular cameras have revolutionised DR screening, and several communities with low to middle incomes are now using them. This issue covers the many camera varieties and the factors to consider when selecting one, as well as practical advice on the best way to take high-quality retinal photos, how to save and manage pictures of the retina, and how to take care of the camera.

Following their acquisition, the retinal pictures are analysed for indications of DR and ranked using the selected classification system, which establishes whether the patient requires a referral to the eye centre for additional testing by a doctor of optics. An eye doctor or a qualified grader may grade, based on the DR curriculum and circumstances. Most settings today teach allied health professionals and even non-medical workers how to evaluate retinal pictures because of the sheer volume of images that require grading. Through computerised evaluation of retinal pictures, artificial intelligence technology, which has advanced quickly in the field of DR over the past ten years, offers new ways to help in the delivery of DR programs. The International Clinical Diabetic Retinopathy (ICDR) intensity scale is used by many DR grading platforms that are sold commercially (Mwangi & Bascaran, 2023).

5.6.2 Secondary Prevention (Monitoring and Early Intervention)

Reducing vision loss requires early identification of diabetes-related retinopathy. Frequent tests can detect the illness early on, enabling prompt treatment and management.

5.6.2.1 Advantages of Frequent Diabetic Patient Screening

Frequent diabetic retinopathy screenings provide several advantages, such as:

- Early diabetic retinopathy identification and treatment
- Lower risk of disease development.
- Better standard of life.

5.6.2.2 Fluorescein Angiography

An intrusive imaging method that shows the retina's blood vessels using a dye. Utilising Cutting-Edge Technology to Identify Diabetic Retinopathy.

Diagnosing diabetic retinopathy is becoming easier with the use of advanced technologies like ML, or machine learning, and artificial intelligence (AI). Large datasets may be analysed by these tools, which can also spot trends that human therapists would miss.

5.6.2.3 Tertiary Prevention (Managing Complications and Disability)

A person's everyday life is usually greatly and permanently impacted by visual impairment, also known as low vision (caused by DR), a form of blurred vision that cannot be further repaired with conventional spectacles, contact lenses, medical therapy, or surgery. As a tertiary preventive measure, low vision rehabilitation techniques aim to maximise the residual vision in people with visual impairments. These types of exercises can lessen eye strain, increase contrast sensitivity, and improve visual function. Vision rehabilitation exercises can be very helpful for DR patients in preserving visual acuity and adjusting to alterations in vision.

A person's ability to focus in low-light illumination and identify objects against varied backgrounds can be enhanced via contrast sensitivity training, which entails differentiating between different contrast levels. Daily tasks that are difficult for DR patients to complete, such as writing, reading, and facial recognition, can be greatly enhanced by this assistance. Individuals can read and do intricate activities more easily with the help of extendable devices and portable or standing magnifying glasses that expand text and pictures (Rák et al., 2025).

5.6.3 Community-Based Prevention Programs

The availability of specialised funds and personnel resources to recognise and address ocular and sight health concerns and to maintain a focus on initiatives to enhance eyesight health over time is a basic concern for municipal and state public health organisations. Even major health departments find it difficult to satisfy the considerable capacity (i.e., funds, appropriate personnel, and a properly qualified workforce) needed to provide every aspect of anticipated services pertaining to public health. An already difficult situation is made worse by increased statutory requirements and unrelenting public demand for services. According to a paper, Ph.Ds are today confronted with "declining public spending, ongoing assaults from adversaries (including affected sectors and opposition political parties), restricted authority in politics, and competitors abusing their responsibilities." Additionally, there are differences in the degree of freedom that municipalities and state governments have when using federal grant funding (for example, block grants offer wide guidelines for expenditure choices, whereas category focus grants often give state and regional governments less discretion).

Consequently, the growing demand is not adequately addressed or funded by other, more traditional public health programs, such as promoting wellness, inspection, and development of policies, which include tracking fundamental societal and environmental factors, as well as eye and vision problems. According to some research, a significant and disproportionate share of public health funding is allocated to ensuring and connecting people to health care services, at the expense of agencies' capacity to provide other essential amenities. Eye and vision health are not usually included in national public health target lists; therefore, programmatic attention may be limited (Twa, 2017).

5.7 Treatment Approaches

5.7.1 *Pharmacological Therapies*

Persons using progressive Diabetic Retinopathy (PDR) have demonstrated improvements in clarity of vision and a reduction in radial retinal field loss when treated with anti-VEGF medication (ranibizumab). Compared to PRP, this therapy also had fewer DME patients and a lower requirement for vitrectomy. Comparing intravitreal anti-VEGF therapy to PRP, studies have demonstrated reductions in retinal disease Severity scores, as well as a decreased risk of cataracts and DME. PRP and aflibercept were examined for patients having PDR without DME in the Medical Effectiveness and Mechanical Evaluation of Aflibercept in the Treatment for Proliferation Diabetes Retinopathy (CLARITY) experiment. However, in real-world settings, ranibizumab's efficacy is not maintained after 24 months.

Steroid treatment is used to treat diffuse oedema in the macula, which is crucial for the development of diabetic macular oedema (DME). Steroids have an anti-inflammatory effect that helps downregulate pro-inflammatory and pro-angiogenic mediators, which are essential for DME development. Topical corticosteroid treatments are preferred for DME due to their potential side effects. There are several options for administering steroids, including intravitreal injection, subtenon injection, and dexamethasone intravitreal implant (DEX). For many years, intravitreal triamcinolone acetonide injections (IVTA) have been a crucial part of the treatment of DME, leading to notable improvements in visual acuity and macular thickness. Nevertheless, several injections are necessary to sustain its effectiveness because of its brief duration of action. DME patients are also treated with subtenon acetonide triamcinolone injection (STTA) (Tomita et al., 2021).

5.7.2 *Laser Therapy*

Four associated risk factors for blurred vision in DR were found by the diabetic retinal disease study (DRS); eyes having three or more warning signs were deemed "at high risk." Pan-retinal photocoagulation (PRP) is regarded as a crucial therapeutic method, and laser therapy for DR has been developed for several decades. Only 1% of individuals and 4% of eyeballs suffer from serious vision loss within five years after a photocoagulation procedure, and PRP lowers the chance of severe blindness in DR by as much as fifty per cent. To solve these issues, the structure of the scan laser was created, which improves the reduction of the nerve fibre layer and lowers inflammatory cytokines and discomfort. Nevertheless, compared to traditional PRP, the pattern scanning laser has a low safety margin, is susceptible to cloudy media, and has been shown to increase the incidence of corneal, iris, and neovascular glaucoma. For individuals with NPDR, targeted ocular pigmentation (TRP) has been utilised to reduce the rate at which PDR progresses. To apply navigated pattern PRP to NPAs in a targeted manner, the guided pattern laser navigated laser photocoagulator (NAVILAS) was created. To find the optimal course of treatment for DR, further research is required, and a luminescence angiogram (FA) is required to detect NPAs (Tomita et al., 2021).

5.7.3 Surgical Interventions (Vitrectomy)

Surgery is necessary for PDR patients who have tractional retinal detachment near the retina, haemorrhaging retinal detachment, or thick and recurring vitreous haemorrhage. A retinal transplant is a surgical procedure used to treat conditions affecting the optic nerve and aqueous. Specialists remove the vitreous during the procedure and replace it with a different solution. If there is a retinal tear or NPA, light coagulation is required to reattach the retina. The longer a retinal detachment lasts in PDR patients, the more difficult it is to regain eyesight because macular photoreceptor function deteriorates. The advancement of wide-angle viewing devices and small-incision vitrectomy techniques has led to enhanced vitreoretinal operations in recent years. Because vitrectomy is less intrusive and safer thanks to these procedures, individuals with PDR may benefit from an earlier vitrectomy if they have macula dragging because of fibrovascular tissue covering the macula. For DME with an inner retinal barrier or thicker rear retinal cortex with vitreous traction, a vitrectomy has been shown to enhance visual acuity. When the results of retinal photocoagulation and medication therapy, like steroids and anti-VEGF, were unsatisfactory, vitreoretinal surgery can potentially be explored as an option for treatment. DME can be treated via posterior vitreous separation and internal restricting membrane peeling. The return of macular fluid with the corneal membrane may result from the inner restricting membrane acting as a framework for proliferative myofibroblasts. Following vitrectomy for DME, 496 eyes had increased visual acuity over the long term, which was like the effects of anti-VEGF treatment. Twelve months following therapy, vitrectomy reduced central macular thickness more significantly than intravitreal triamcinolone acetonide (IVTA), but there was no statistically significant improvement in visual acuity. After six months, vitrectomy was found to be morphologically more effective than grid laser therapy, but there was no discernible change in visual function. Furthermore, morphology and visual function did not significantly change after a year. However, it has been shown that the outlook of sight after in-vitro removal for DME, absent macular traction, was unaffected by its existence or the absence of an inner limiting membrane separation. The efficacy of the cystotomy procedure for long-term morphological and functional reductions of refractory cyst-like macular oedema related to DR (Tomita et al., 2021).

5.7.4 Emerging Therapies and Innovations

5.7.4.1 In DR, Fenofibrate is Utilised as Therapy

In the United States, fenofibrate, which acts as a peroxisome proliferator-activated receptor alpha (PPARα) antagonist, has been used since 1998 to treat those with metabolic syndrome and dyslipidaemia. It is a possible treatment for metabolic syndrome since it has been demonstrated to lower levels of free fatty acids and boost the production of omega-3 fatty acids and high-density lipid cholesterol. Fenofibrate's ability to prevent DR has also been demonstrated in animal experiments; in diabetic db/db mice, oral fenofibrate acid therapy reduced neuronal cell death and preserved rhythmic potentials. In hypertensive mouse retinas, oral treatment also reduced neuroinflammation and cellular oxidative stress. Fenofibrate is not strongly advised for use in individuals with severe renal impairment; nevertheless, because of its effects on elevated blood creatinine levels, which raises questions regarding possible harm to renal function. Scientists are trying to create more effective treatments for PPARα activation.

5.7.4.2 In DR, Pema Fibrate Medication

Kowa Corporation, Ltd. has created Pema fibrate, an active PPARα modulator, as a less hazardous substitute for fenofibrate. According to clinical research conducted in Japan, Pema fibrate raises serum creatinine levels and enhances liver function, making it a safer choice forindividuals with serious kidney problems. Pemafibrate may be utilised as a medication to treat diabetes and retinopathy, according to experimental animal research.

In diabetic mice, oral Pema fibrate therapy ameliorates poor endothelial function, raises the blood level of fibroblast growth factor 21 (FGF21), and decreases plasma levels of lipids and vasoconstrictive eicosanoids. In diabetic rats, it also guards against retinal neovascularisation and retinal dysfunction brought on by diabetes. A phase 3 randomised controlled study is now being conducted to see whether methyl cellulose is helpful for metabolic issues and whether it may be utilised for the management of retinal diseases, such as DR (Tomita et al., 2021).

5.8 Technological and Research Advances

5.8.1 Role of Artificial Intelligence in Early Detection

Every facet of healthcare is changing due to AI, and vision treatment is no exception. As science develops, AI has emerged as a potent ally in accelerating the detection of serious eye disorders that may cause blindness if treatment is not received. AI is now enabling the earlier diagnosis of ocular and visual nerve problems because of its accuracy, speed, and capacity to learn from large volumes of data (Shuet al., 2024).

5.8.2 Genetic and Molecular Therapies

A novel treatment for hereditary retinal disorders brought on by mutations in certain genes is gene therapy. Progressive vision loss and, frequently, blindness are the results of these conditions, which include retinal pigmentation, Leber congenital amaurosis at birth (LCA), and achromatopsia. Gene therapy's fundamental idea is to repair genetic defects and restore regular cell function by introducing functioning copies of damaged genes into afflicted cells. The use of viruses called adeno-associated viruses (AAVs) as vectors to introduce genes that treat into retinal cell lines is one of the most important advancements in genetic treatment for optometry. AAVs are favoured due to their low sensitivity and efficient transduction of retinal cells (Pei et al., 2024).

5.8.3 Advances in Retinal Imaging

Chronic retinal conditions, glaucoma, high blood pressure, and cataracts are just a few of the ophthalmic and systemic conditions for which retinal photography has become an essential diagnostic and treatment tool. These illnesses are the primary causes of avoidable blindness and frequently act as warning signs for other illnesses, including metabolic and cardiovascular diseases. To avoid permanent harm, early identification and prompt intervention are crucial. However, traditional diagnostic techniques, including fundus imaging, are still restricted since they need specialised supplies, expensive prices, and expert interpretation. To overcome these obstacles, this research uses developments in artificial intelligence and image processing to create an automated retinal diagnosis system (Fenner et al., 2018; Kulkarni & Deshpande, 2019).

5.8.4 Novel Drug Delivery Systems

Novel drug delivery methods are of great interest because of the shortcomings of the present pharmacological and surgical treatments for DR. The capacity of intraocular medication delivery to produce focused, long-lasting therapeutic benefits with less systemic adverse effects has drawn particular interest. Innovations in ocular systems for drug delivery are covered in this section, with an emphasis on sustained release systems and methods that utilise nanotechnology (Al-Qaysi et al., 2023).

5.8.5 Techniques Based on Nanotechnology

Compared to traditional drug administration techniques, systems based on nanotechnology provide several benefits, such as improved bioavailability, controlled absorption, and targeted distribution to the retina. For the therapy of DR, nanoparticles such as liposomes, polymer nanoparticles, and micro-emulsions are being investigated. Both hydrodynamic and lipophilic medications may be encapsulated by these nanocarriers, enabling the passage of a variety of treatments to the eye. The ability of tiny carrier molecules to penetrate the blood-retinal barrier (BRB), something that is frequently weakened in DR, is one of their main advantages. Drugs can be administered straight to the retina via nanoparticles, increasing therapeutic effectiveness and local dosage (Campbell & Humphries, 2014).

5.8.6 Mechanisms of Sustained Release

By delivering medications over long periods of time, sustained release devices reduce the need for frequent injections and increase patient compliance. These systems, which may discharge therapeutic chemicals gradually over weeks or months, comprise hydrogels, polymers that degrade, and implanted devices. The intramuscular implant, which delivers medication to the retina under regulated conditions, is one of the most extensively researched sustained-release methods in DR (Adak et al., 2025).

5.9 Policy, Advocacy, and Public Health Perspectives

5.9.1 National and Global Eye Health Initiatives

The WHO has placed strong emphasis on eye health as a global priority. In 2013, its 194 member states adopted the *Universal Eye Health: Global Action Plan 2014–2019 (GAP)*, which aimed to cut preventable vision loss by 25% by 2019. At that time, an estimated 285 million people worldwide were visually impaired, including about 39 million who were blind. Most cases were linked to cataracts and uncorrected refractive errors—both conditions that are largely treatable.

The GAP followed earlier initiatives such as *VISION 2020: The Right to Sight,* launched in 1999 by WHO and the International Agency for the Prevention of Blindness (IAPB). These programs urged countries to improve cataract surgery services, expand access to affordable spectacles, and prepare for the rising burden of chronic eye conditions like glaucoma, age-related macular degeneration (AMD), and diabetic retinopathy (DR). Unlike cataracts, these conditions cannot be cured but can be managed with timely detection and ongoing care.

Many nations have aligned their efforts with these global goals. For instance, India's *National Programme for Control of Blindness and Visual Impairment (NPCBVI)* is one of the world's largest public eye health initiatives, providing millions of free cataract surgeries, DR screenings, and corrective glasses. In the UK, the *NHS Diabetic Eye Screening Programme (DESP)* ensures annual retinal exams for all individuals with diabetes aged 12 and above, enabling early identification and treatment of DR before it causes vision loss (Gupta & Kocur, 2014).

The GAP also called for a broader health systems approach, focusing on six areas: service delivery, health workforce, health information, access to technologies, financing, and governance. Even in high-income countries like Canada, challenges remain—such as ensuring equal access to care for underserved communities and coping with the rising burden of chronic eye disease in an ageing population.

Another core objective was evidence-based advocacy through better data collection. Tracking the prevalence of vision loss, cataract surgical rates, and uptake of screening programs helps countries identify gaps and measure real progress. Beyond treatment, the GAP encouraged development of rehabilitation and low-vision services, as well as partnerships across sectors like education and social welfare (Abdulhussein & Hussein, 2022).

5.9.2 Integrating Eye Care into Primary Health Services

Integrated care refers to aligning patient-centered strategies across the health system, and it is crucial for reducing diabetes-related vision loss. The WHO Global Action Plan calls for decentralizing eye services and embedding them within primary health care (PHC). However, a major challenge is the shortage and uneven distribution of trained eye health professionals, especially in low-resource regions such as sub-Saharan Africa.

Debates continue between vertical programs, which target a single disease like blindness prevention, and horizontal models that integrate care more broadly into PHC. In practice, most countries adopt a hybrid approach depending on local needs. For example, the UK's NHS pursued integration to improve efficiency, though outcomes vary—often showing the greatest benefit for patients with complex conditions.

In India, home to nearly 20% of the world's blind population, integrating primary eye care (PEC) into PHC has improved access in underserved communities. Still, barriers such as staff shortages, weak coordination, and poor infrastructure persist. Similar challenges are seen in Tanzania and across sub-Saharan Africa, where trained PHC workers often lose motivation without ongoing specialist support and resources.

Successful integration relies on three key considerations: desirability (will it add value?), feasibility (can PHC workers deliver effectively?), and timing (does the system have capacity?). While integration is not a universal solution, strengthening PEC within PHC—supported by task-shifting, teleophthalmology, and robust referral systems—can significantly improve access, reduce late-stage blindness, and empower communities (Maseko et al., 2021).

5.9.3 Cost-Effectiveness of Screening and Prevention

Early detection, accurate diagnosis, and timely treatment of DR can prevent most diabetes-related vision loss and are widely recommended by professional bodies such as the American Academy of Ophthalmology, which advises annual retinal examinations. Despite this, only about half of people with diabetes in developed countries undergo yearly screening, and rates are likely even lower in developing regions due to poor awareness, limited access, and geographic barriers.

Screening for DR is consistently shown to be cost-effective. Health economic analyses demonstrate that early interventions save quality-adjusted life years (QALYs), reduce productivity loss, and lower long-term treatment costs. Comparative studies suggest that systematic or universal screening is more effective than opportunistic detection, while targeted screening may be appropriate for high-risk populations. Extending intervals to every 2 years in low-risk patients can further improve cost-effectiveness without compromising safety.

Teleophthalmology has emerged as one of the most scalable and cost-effective solutions. Studies from the United States, Canada, Singapore, India, Brazil, and South Africa confirm that remote fundus photography with AI or specialist grading not only improves detection but also reduces travel costs, enhances patient satisfaction, and saves healthcare systems millions of dollars annually. For example, in Singapore, universal teleophthalmology screening could save an estimated $21.6 million over a lifetime, while in rural India and South Africa, it remains cost-effective even with partial uptake.

Although telemedicine requires initial investment, falling equipment costs, cloud-based storage, smartphone-enabled fundus photography, and automated image analysis continue to increase efficiency and sustainability. Overall, integrating DR screening into primary care with teleophthalmology is both clinically effective and economically sound, particularly for underserved populations (Avidor et al., 2020; Javitt & Aiello, 1996).

5.9.4 Emerging Technologies in DR Screening and Management

New imaging and digital health tools are transforming DR care. Ultrawide-field cameras and OCT-A improve early detection and allow precise monitoring, including response to anti-VEGF therapy. Portable and smartphone-based fundus photography expands access in low-resource settings, while AI-assisted telescreening enables

Table 5.1 Emerging technologies for DR screening and management (Pearce & Sivaprasad, 2020)

Technology	Key benefit	Main limitation
Ultrawide-Field (UWF) imaging	Captures up to 200 °C of retina in a single shot; detects peripheral lesions linked to progression; reduces ungradable images by > 80%	High equipment cost; limited availability in low-resource settings
Optical coherence tomography angiography (OCT-A)	Non-invasive visualization of retinal microvasculature; early detection of ischemia and neovascularization	Still being validated for large-scale screening; requires expensive equipment
Portable and smartphone-based fundus cameras	Affordable, user-friendly, comparable accuracy to standard imaging; ideal for rural areas	Variable image quality; requires good operator training
Telescreening programs	Expands access via mobile units and cloud-based grading; proven cost-effective; increases screening uptake	Needs reliable internet, infrastructure, and referral pathways
AI-assisted image analysis	FDA-approved tools (e.g., IDx-DR) achieve $\geq$ 80% sensitivity/specificity; reduces specialist workload	Requires large, diverse datasets for accuracy; regulatory and ethical considerations

mass, cost-effective screening and timely referral. Collectively, these advances strengthen both **screening** and **management**, improving outcomes and resource efficiency, Table 5.1 describes the screening and management of these technologies (Fenner et al., 2018).

5.10 Future Directions

5.10.1 Personalized Medicine in Retinopathy

Diabetic retinopathy (DR), once viewed primarily as a microvascular complication of diabetes, is now recognized as a multifactorial disease involving both vascular and neurodegenerative processes. Persistent hyperglycemia triggers oxidative stress, accumulation of advanced glycation end products, inflammation, and VEGF-driven angiogenesis, alongside genetic and epigenetic influences. This complexity contributes to disease heterogeneity and highlights the need for tailored therapeutic strategies.

Advances in *omics* technologies—genomics, proteomics, and metabolomics—have enabled the identification of DR phenotypes with distinct molecular profiles and progression risks. Such stratification paves the way for personalized medicine, where treatment is matched to individual characteristics, improving efficacy and minimizing adverse effects. For example, tailoring anti-VEGF therapy or laser treatment to patient-specific biomarkers can reduce treatment burden and enhance visual outcomes.

Artificial intelligence (AI) adds a further dimension to personalization. Deep learning models trained on large datasets of retinal images have achieved diagnostic accuracy rates above 90%, with sensitivities and specificities often exceeding 94%. Beyond automated screening, AI can integrate clinical and systemic factors—such as diabetes duration, HbA1c trends, renal function, and retinal vascular morphology—to guide individualized management. AI-driven telemedicine platforms also expand access to specialized DR care in underserved regions, offering earlier diagnosis and intervention to reduce preventable vision loss.

While challenges remain—such as standardizing molecular and imaging data, addressing costs, and ensuring equitable access—personalized medicine, supported by AI, holds the potential to revolutionize DR management and shift care from generalized treatment to patient-specific strategies (Chondrozoumakis et al., 2025; Jin et al., 2025).

5.10.2 Global Challenges and Opportunities

The global rise in diabetes has led to an increasing prevalence of DR, posing significant challenges to healthcare systems worldwide. Limited access to trained eyecare professionals, particularly in rural and underserved regions, results in delayed diagnosis and treatment. Screening programs remain inconsistent, with disparities in methodology and coverage between countries. Financial and infrastructural constraints, along with technological barriers such as image quality and grading expertise, further hinder effective DR management. Additionally, gaps in public awareness reduce patient engagement in regular screening and timely interventions, contributing to preventable vision loss.

Despite these challenges, substantial opportunities exist to mitigate the global burden of DR. Advances in imaging technology, including ultra-wide-field fundus photography and artificial intelligence-assisted screening, enable earlier and more accurate detection. Telemedicine initiatives and mobile eye clinics can extend services to remote populations, improving access and follow-up care. Standardized screening protocols and international disease severity classifications facilitate efficient communication and management. Public health campaigns promoting awareness and adherence to diabetes care can enhance patient participation, while policy support, including national screening programs and funding initiatives, can reduce the socioeconomic impact of DR. Furthermore, ongoing research and international collaboration offer prospects for personalized interventions and cost-effective strategies to combat DR globally (Sivaprasad et al., 2023).

5.10.3 Vision 2030: Who and Global Action Plan

- WHO aligns with the **UN 2030 Agenda for Sustainable Development**, emphasizing eye health as part of global health equity.
- **WHA73.4 (2020)** on *Integrated People-Centred Eye Care (IPEC)* marked a key milestone.

5.10.4 Global 2030 Eye Care Targets

- **Cataract surgery (eCSC)**: Increase coverage by 30% by 2030 (aim for universal coverage if already $\geq$ 70%).
- **Refractive error correction (eREC)**: Increase coverage by 40% by 2030 (aim for universal coverage if already $\geq$ 60%).

5.10.5 Diabetic Retinopathy in Vision 2030

- DR affects **30–40% of diabetics;** > 100 million people globally.
- Advances in **screening, imaging (OCT), laser (PRP, PASCAL), anti-VEGF, and surgery** have reduced vision loss.

5.10.6 In Sight Strategy (IAPB)

Goal: **eliminate preventable sight loss** and ensure universal access to eye care.

5.10.7 Three Pillars

- **Elevate**eye health as a social and economic issue.
- **Integrate** eye health into wider health systems (IPEC).
- **Activate** public demand and market change (campaigns, partnerships, affordable products) (Stern et al., 2024; Tan & Wong, 2023).

5.11 Conclusion

Vision is one of the most vital senses, and its preservation demands a proactive and comprehensive approach. Retinopathy and other causes of vision loss are largely preventable through timely screening, early diagnosis, risk factor modification, and equitable access to care. Advances in medical therapy, technology, and patient education provide powerful tools to safeguard sight, but their success depends on awareness, collaboration, and commitment across healthcare systems and communities. By keeping our focus on prevention, we can ensure that future generations enjoy not only longer lives but also lives enriched with clear and lasting vision.

CRediT Authorship Contribution Statement Riya Sarkar, Rajat Kanti Ghosal and Koyel Banerjee, Writing review & editing, Writing-original draft. Pradipta Banerjee and Rajkumar Maiti, Reviewing, editing & supervision.

Declarations Competing Interests The authors declare no competing interests.

References

Abdulhussein, D., & Abdul, H. M. (2022). WHO Vision 2020: Have we done it? *Neuroophthalmology, 46*(6), 331–339. https://doi.org/10.1080/09286586.2022.2127784

Adak, S., Jadhav, V. S., & Khatri, D. K. (2025). Emerging innovations in ophthalmic drug delivery for diabetic retinopathy: A translational perspective. *Drug Delivery and Translational Research, 20*, 1–32.

Al-Qaysi, Z. K., Beadham, I. G., Schwikkard, S. L., Bear, J. C., Al-Kinani, A. A., & Alany, R. G. (2023). Sustained release ocular drug delivery systems for glaucoma therapy. *Expert Opinion on Drug Delivery, 20*(7), 905–919.

Aumann, S., Donner, S., Fischer, J., & Müller, F. (2019). Optical coherence tomography (OCT): Principle and technical realization. *High Resolution Imaging in Microscopy and Ophthalmology: New Frontiers in Biomedical Optics, 14*, 59–85.

Avidor, D., Loewenstein, A., Waisbourd, M., & Nutman, A. (2020). Cost-effectiveness of diabetic retinopathy screening programs using telemedicine: A systematic review. *Cost Effectiveness and Resource Allocation, 18*(16), 1–12. https://doi.org/10.1186/s12962-020-00213-3

Beulens, J. W., Pinho, M. G., Abreu, T. C., den Braver, N. R., Lam, T. M., Huss, A., Vlaanderen, J., Sonnenschein, T., Siddiqui, N. Z., Yuan, Z., & Kerckhoffs, J. (2022). Environmental risk factors of type 2 diabetes—An exposome approach. *Diabetologia, 65*(2), 263–274.

Campbell, M., & Humphries, P. (2014, January 23). The blood-retina barrier: Tight junctions and barrier modulation. In *Biology and regulation of blood-tissue barriers* (pp. 70–84). Springer.

Chondrozoumakis, G., Chatzimichail, E., Habra, O., Vounotrypidis, E., Papanas, N., Gatzioufas, Z., & Panos, G. D. (2025). Retinal biomarkers in diabetic retinopathy: From early detection to personalized treatment. *Journal of Clinical Medicine, 14*(4), 1343.

Corr, R. H. (2023). Fundoscopy in the smartphone age: Current ophthalmoscopy methods in neurology. *Arquivos De Neuro-Psiquiatria, 81*(05), 502–509.

Dammann, O., Hartnett, M. E., & Stahl, A. (2023). Retinopathy of prematurity. *Developmental Medicine & Child Neurology, 65*(5), 625–631.

Di Marco, E., Aiello, F., Lombardo, M., Di Marino, M., Missiroli, F., Mancino, R., Ricci, F., Nucci, C., Noce, A., Di Daniele, N., & Cesareo, M. (2022). A literature review of hypertensive retinopathy: Systemic correlations and new technologies. *European Review for Medical and Pharmacological Sciences, 26*(18), 6424–6443.

Eze, G. C., Chukwunonye, C. R., & Onah, E. S. (2025). Prevalence and causes of blindness among eye patients seen in a state tertiary hospital in Enugu, Nigeria. *Journal of Medical Research and Surgery, 6*(3), 92–99.

Fenner, B. J., Wong, R. L., Lam, W. C., Tan, G. S., & Cheung, G. C. (2018). Advances in retinal imaging and applications in diabetic retinopathy screening: A review. *Ophthalmology and Therapy, 7*(2), 333–346.

Gupta, N., & Kocur, I. (2014). Chronic eye disease and the WHO universal eye health global action plan 2014–2019. *Canadian Journal of Ophthalmology, 49*(5), 403–404.

Heckenlively, J. R., & Ferreyra, H. A. (2008, April). Autoimmune retinopathy: A review and summary. In *Seminars in immunopathology, 30* (2), 127–134.

Hutmacher, F. (2019). Why is there so much more research on vision than on any other sensory modality? *Frontiers in Psychology, 4*(10), Article 481030.

Javitt, J. C., & Aiello, L. P. (1996). Cost-effectiveness of detecting and treating diabetic retinopathy. *Annals of Internal Medicine, 125*(11), 860–867. https://doi.org/10.7326/0003-4819-125-11-199612010-00020

Jin, K., Yu, H., Wei, W., & Grzybowski, A. (2025). Editorial: Personalized medicine of diabetes retinopathy: From bench to bedside. *Frontiers in Endocrinology (Lausanne), 16*, 1597332. https://doi.org/10.3389/fendo.2025.1597332

Kalt, W., Hanneken, A., Milbury, P., & Tremblay, F. (2010). Recent research on polyphenolics in vision and eye health. *Journal of Agricultural and Food Chemistry, 58*(7), 4001–4007.

Kąpa, M., Koryciarz, I., Kustosik, N., Jurowski, P., & Pniakowska, Z. (2024). Modern approach to diabetic retinopathy diagnostics. *Diagnostics, 14*(17), 1846.

Kulkarni, S., & Deshpande, C. R. (2019). Recent advances in retinal imaging and diagnostics. *Community Eye Health, 32*(107), S9.

Kusuhara, S., Fukushima, Y., Ogura, S., Inoue, N., & Uemura, A. (2018). Pathophysiology of diabetic retinopathy: The old and the new. *Diabetes & Metabolism Journal, 42*(5), 364.

Kwinta, P., & Pietrzyk, J. J. (2007). Retinopathy of prematurity: Is genetic predisposition an important risk factor? *Expert Review of Ophthalmology, 2*(2), 275–283.

Lee, R., Wong, T. Y., & Sabanayagam, C. (2015). Epidemiology of diabetic retinopathy, diabetic macular edema and related vision loss. *Eye and Vision, 2*(1), 1715.

Maseko, S. N., van Staden, D., & Mhlongo, E. M. (2021). The rising burden of diabetes-related blindness: A case for integration of primary eye care into primary health care in Eswatini. *Healthcare (Basel), 9*(7), 835. https://doi.org/10.3390/healthcare9070835

Miller, J. R., & Hanumunthadu, D. (2022). Inflammatory eye disease: An overview of clinical presentation and management. *Clinical Medicine, 22*(2), 100–103.

Mwangi, N., & Bascaran, C. (2023). Preventing vision loss due to diabetic retinopathy. *Community Eye Health, 36*(119), 1.

Olawade, D. B., Weerasinghe, K., Mathugamage, M. D., Odetayo, A., Aderinto, N., Teke, J., & Boussios, S. (2025). Enhancing ophthalmic diagnosis and treatment with artificial intelligence. *Medicina, 61*(3), 433.

Pearce, E., & Sivaprasad, S. (2020). A review of advancements and evidence gaps in diabetic retinopathy screening models. *Clinical Ophthalmology, 14*, 3285–3296. https://doi.org/10.2147/OPTH.S267521

Pei, X., & Huang, D., & Li, Z. (2019). Genetic insights and emerging therapeutics in diabetic retinopathy: from molecular pathways to personalized medicine. *Frontiers in Genetics, 15*, 1416924.32.

Rák, T., Kovács-Valasek, A., Pöstyéni, E., Gábriel, R., & Csutak, A. (2025). Low vision rehabilitation and eye exercises: A comprehensive guide to tertiary prevention of diabetic retinopathy. *Life, 15*(6), 857.

Ravindranath, R., Bernstein, I. A., Fernandez, K. S., Ludwig, C. A., & Wang, S. Y. (2023). Social determinants of health and perceived barriers to care in diabetic retinopathy screening. *JAMA Ophthalmology, 141*(12), 1161–1171.

Rivera, J. C., Sapieha, P., Joyal, J. S., Duhamel, F., Shao, Z., Sitaras, N., Picard, E., Zhou, E., Lachapelle, P., & Chemtob, S. (2011). Understanding retinopathy of prematurity: Update on pathogenesis. *Neonatology, 100*(4), 343–353.

Sahoo, N. K., Ranjan, R., Tyagi, M., Agrawal, H., & Reddy, S. (2021). Radiation retinopathy: Detection and management strategies. *Clinical Ophthalmology, 8*, 3797–3809.

Saleh, G. A., Batouty, N. M., Haggag, S., Elnakib, A., Khalifa, F., Taher, F., Mohamed, M. A., Farag, R., Sandhu, H., Sewelam, A., & El-Baz, A. (2022). The role of medical image modalities and

AI in the early detection, diagnosis and grading of retinal diseases: A survey. *Bioengineering, 9*(8), 366.
Shu, Q., Pang, J., Liu, Z., Liang, X., Chen, M., Tao, Z., Liu, Q., Guo, Y., Yang, X., Ding, J., & Chen, R. (2024). Artificial Intelligence for early detection of pediatric eye diseases using mobile photos. *JAMA Network Open, 7*(8), e2425124.
Sivaprasad, S., Sen, S., & Cunha-Vaz, J. (2023). Perspectives of diabetic retinopathy—Challenges and opportunities. *Eye, 37*(11), 2183–2191. https://doi.org/10.1038/s41433-022-02384-0
Stern, J., Yasmin, S., Qureshi, M. B., & Bourne, R. (2024). 2030 In Sight: The future of global eye health. *Eye, 38*(11), 1979–1980. https://doi.org/10.1038/s41433-023-02815-2
Tan, T. E., & Wong, T. Y. (2023). Diabetic retinopathy: Looking forward to 2030. *Frontiers in Endocrinology, 9*(13), 1077669. https://doi.org/10.3389/fendo.2022.1077669
Threatt, J., Williamson, J. F., Huynh, K., Davis, R. M., & Hermayer, K. (2013). Ocular disease, knowledge and technology applications in patients with diabetes. *The American Journal of the Medical Sciences, 345*(4), 266–270.
Tomita, Y., Lee, D., Tsubota, K., Negishi, K., & Kurihara, T. (2021). Updates on the current treatments for diabetic retinopathy and possibility of future oral therapy. *Journal of Clinical Medicine, 10*(20), 4666.
Twa, M. D. (2017). Making eye health a population imperative: A question of priorities. *Optometry and Vision Science, 94*(4), 443.
Vashist, P., Senjam, S. S., Gupta, V., Gupta, N., Shamanna, B. R., Wadhwani, M., Shukla, P., Manna, S., Yadav, S., & Bharadwaj, A. (2022). Blindness and visual impairment and their causes in India: Results of a nationally representative survey. *PLoS One, 17*(7), Article e0271736.
Vujosevic, S., Aldington, S. J., Silva, P., Hernández, C., Scanlon, P., Peto, T., & Simó, R. (2020). Screening for diabetic retinopathy: New perspectives and challenges. *The Lancet Diabetes & Endocrinology, 8*(4), 337–347.
Wong, T. Y., & Hyman, L. (2008). Population-based studies in ophthalmology. *American Journal of Ophthalmology, 146*(5), 656–663.
Wong, T. Y., & Mitchell, P. (2004). Hypertensive retinopathy. *New England Journal of Medicine, 351*(22), 2310–2317.

Chapter 6
When the Kidney Fail: Navigating Nephropathy and Dialysis

Arijit Mondal, Ishita Sil, Nirjhar Duttagupta, Suddhasattya Dey, and Sabina Yasmin

Abstract Renal impairment is caused by nephropathy and nephrotoxicity, both of which have a major impact on the world's healthcare system. Numerous kidney disorders, each with unique pathophysiological mechanisms and clinical presentations, are included in the category of nephropathy. These include glomerulonephritis, diabetic nephropathy, hypertensive nephropathy, and polycystic kidney disease. To investigate the viewpoints of haemodialysis patients, a qualitative methodology was employed. An metropolitan teaching hospital's outpatient haemodialysis clinic served as the site of one-on-one, in-person, semi-structured interviews. Relying mainly on biomarkers for disease diagnosis and monitoring, accurate assessment of chronic kidney disease (CKD) in older adults is vital for prompt intervention and therapy. Systemic inflammation, metabolic alterations, and drug use are widespread within this populace and can drastically modify biomarkers such serum creatinine, estimated glomerular filtration rate and albuminuria. On the other hand early innovators like Willem Kolff and Belding Scribner developed dialysis, which led to a number of significant shifts in the economics, epidemiology, and morality of renal failure treatment. But even though dialysis services, especially haemodialysis, have rapidly expanded, especially in nations with high incomes, genuine focused on patients advancement is moving more slowly now. Similar to haemodialysis, cardiovascular events account for over half of all PD deaths, and there is a lot of interest in figuring out what modality-specific factors lead to these events. Important discoveries emphasize the

A. Mondal · S. Dey (✉)
Department of Pharmacy, IQ City Institute of Pharmaceutical Sciences, Durgapur, West Bengal, India
e-mail: kuntal.kuni@gmail.com

I. Sil
Department of Pharmacy, JIS University, Kolkata, West Bengal, India

N. Duttagupta
Department of Pharmacy, Bengal College of Pharmaceutical Technology, Dubrajpur, West Bengal, India

S. Yasmin (✉)
Department of Pharmaceutical Chemistry, College of Pharmacy, King Khalid University, Abha, Saudi Arabia
e-mail: sahussain@kku.edu.sa

K. Adhikary et al. (eds.), *Healing Beyond Blood Sugar*,
https://doi.org/10.1007/978-981-95-8946-3_6

significance of averting nephrotoxic substances associated with medical and environmental settings, the necessity of careful monitoring of renal function, and the significance of early diagnosis by biomarkers.

Keywords Nephropathy · Nephrotoxicity · Glomerulonephritis · Polycystic kidney disease

6.1 Introduction: The Global Burden of Renal Impairment

6.1.1 Overview of Nephropathy and Nephrotoxicity

Silent and modest, the human kidney is responsible for some of the most important functions of the body, including waste removal, blood pressure maintenance, fluid balance regulation, and metabolic harmony. However, there are significant repercussions when this essential organ fails. Diseases and disorders of the kidneys and urinary tissues are examples of changes to the urinary system. A urinary tract infection, an infection of the lower urinary structures, is one of the most prevalent pathologic conditions of the urinary system that many individuals will experience at some point in their lives. End-stage renal disease (ESRD), also known as renal failure or kidney failure, is a medical illness characterized by the kidneys' capacity to filter waste products from the blood being diminished to less than 15% of normal levels (Institute of Diabetes & Digestive and Kidney Diseases, https://www.niddk.nih.gov/health-information/kidney-disease/kidney-failure). Kidney stones and other urinary system obstructions are also somewhat prevalent. Numerous systemic diseases or problems of the kidneys itself can compromise renal function. The kidneys are directly connected to all other organ systems because they filter blood. Consequently, acute or chronic renal insults might be fatal. As children get older and mature, the prevalence and nature of renal and urinary tract illnesses change; congenital abnormalities may be a part of newborn disorders. Since the kidney and urinary tissues are still developing in children, renal failure may present with different processes and symptoms than those observed in adults (Craft et al., 2019).

Acute kidney failure may result from hemolytic uremic syndrome, hypotension, urinary tract obstruction, certain medications, and rhabdomyolysis. Diabetes, hypertension, nephrotic syndrome, and polycystic kidney disease are conditions that can lead to chronic kidney failure. Acute failure is frequently recognized by a combination of elevated serum creatinine levels and diminished urine output. A glomerular filtration rate (GFR) below 15 or the requirement for renal replacement therapy are the principal criteria for diagnosing chronic renal failure. Furthermore, it is analogous to stage 5 chronic renal disease (Guevara & Borello, 2013). For example, Chronic hyperglycemia and glucose intolerance brought on by compromised insulin action and/or secretion are hallmarks of diabetes. Most diabetic patients in both rich and developing nations suffer from micro- and macro-diabetic chronic vascular problems. Diabetic nephropathy, retinopathy, and neuropathy are among the microvascular problems that cause a great deal of morbidity in this patient population. The most frequent cause of death for diabetic individuals is macrovascular complications, which include peripheral vascular disease, ischemic stroke, and accelerated coronary heart disease (Sagoo & Gnudi, 2020).

Renal impairment is caused by nephropathy and nephrotoxicity, both of which have a major impact on the world's healthcare system. Numerous kidney disorders, each with unique pathophysiological mechanisms and clinical presentations, are included in the category of nephropathy. These encompass glomerulonephritis, diabetic nephropathy, hypertensive nephropathy, and polycystic kidney disease. If neglected, nephrotoxicity, often caused by pharmaceuticals or environmental toxins, may lead to acute kidney injury (AKI) or chronic kidney disease (CKD). Effective kidney injury prevention and treatment depend on an understanding of the underlying mechanisms and risk factors. Even though each of these subjects has been extensively studied, there is still a lack of comprehensive understanding about the various pathophysiological processes, the significance of early detection, and the best techniques to treat nephropathy and nephrotoxicity (Javed et al., 2025).

6.1.2 Impact on Global Healthcare Systems

The nephrotoxicity of Aristolochia was not addressed seriously until 1964, when a Chinese physician by the name of Songhan Wu reported two patients who had experienced acute renal failure as a result of consuming excessive amounts of Aristolochiamanshuriensis. A team of Belgian researchers revealed in the early 1990s that a subset of young female patients had interstitial renal fibrosis that was progressing quickly (Vanherweghem et al., 1993; Zhou et al., 2023). Chronic kidney disease (CKD) impacts around 753 million individuals globally, leading to over one million deaths annually, predominantly attributable to hypertension, diabetes, and glomerulonephritis (Chronic Kidney Disease, 2025). The financial burden is significant: annual expenses per patient increase sharply from approximately $3060 in early-stage chronic kidney disease to over $57300 for hemodialysis and $75,300 for transplant procedures (Jha et al., 2023). In the face of this challenge, artificial intelligence is emerging as a formidable ally. AI-driven predictive algorithms, like those developed by Fresenius Medical Care, can identify dialysis patients susceptible to hospitalization, facilitating prompt interventions and minimizing expensive stays (Preciado et al., 2019). Table 6.1 is showing the impact of nephrotoxicity on global healthcare system in a precise way.

Table 6.1 Impact of nephrotoxicity on global healthcare system

Impact area	Evidence/data	Implications for healthcare systems
Prevalence/burden	Chronic kidney disease (CKD) impacts between 8 and 14% of the global population; diabetic nephropathy accounted for roughly 107.6 million common cases in 2021 (Jha et al., 2023)	A significant volume of patients exerts continuous pressure on diagnostic, monitoring, and therapeutic services; strategic planning for increasing incidence is needed
Mortality and disability	In 2021, there were around 477,300 deaths globally attributed to diabetic nephropathy, resulting in around 11.28 million disability-adjusted life years (DALYs) lost due to the condition (Zhang et al., 2021). The death rate of dialysis patients is comparable to that of specific malignancies	Elevated mortality and morbidity result in less productive life, heightened demand for comorbidity treatment (particularly cardiovascular disease), and increased strain on palliative and end-of-life care
Economic costs	The direct expenditures per patient increase markedly with the advancement of chronic kidney disease (CKD) stages: Stage G3a approximately \$3060, hemodialysis around \$57334 annually, and the first year post-kidney transplant approximately \$75,326. Additionally, the expenses associated with CKD Stage 4 and 5 are up to four times greater than those in previous stages	Significant strain on national health budgets; resource distribution predominantly favors severe chronic kidney disease or renal replacement therapy; opportunity costs in other health sectors; necessity for cost containment
Healthcare access and inequity	Numerous low-income or lower-middle-income nations have restricted access to renal replacement therapy; certain countries are unable to offer hemodialysis, peritoneal dialysis, or transplantation to all those in need. The density of nephrologists exhibits significant variation between low-income and high-income regions	Disparities in survival and outcomes; ethical, policy, and financial ramifications; necessity to enhance capacity and infrastructure; global health priority must encompass chronic kidney disease (CKD)
Quality of life and indirect costs	The Health Related Quality of Life (HRQoL) declines with advancement: typical EuroQoL 5D scores approximate 0.80 to 0.86 in early chronic kidney disease (CKD), decreasing to around 0.73 to 0.79 in stages 4 and 5. Moreover, the loss of productivity and social expenses, including work loss and caregiver strain, are significant	Both direct medical expenses and indirect costs, including employment loss and caregiving, intensify the social burden; governments must account for these factors when formulating chronic kidney disease care and prevention strategies

6.2 Understanding Nephropathy: Types and Pathophysiology

6.2.1 Glomerulonephritis

Glomerulonephritis [GN] includes various disorders that induce glomerular inflammation and damage via a combination of immune-mediated processes, host factors, and environmental stimuli, including infections. Glomerulonephritis may occur exclusively in the kidneys or as part of a systemic condition, with manifestations varying from chronic, largely asymptomatic hematuria to acute renal failure (Zhang et al., 2021). Glomerulonephritis comprises a collection of renal illnesses marked by inflammation of the glomeruli, the small capillary networks crucial for blood filtration. This inflammation, typically resulting from immune-mediated injury to the glomerular basement membrane, mesangium, or capillary endothelium, impairs the kidneys' ability to filter blood. This may result in symptoms such as hematuria, proteinuria, and azotemia (Zhang et al., 2021). Clinically, it may present quickly, as observed in post-streptococcal glomerulonephritis subsequent to infection, or chronically, progressively impairing renal function over the years. Patients may exhibit symptoms that include cola-colored or frothy urine, hypertension, edema, nausea, and malaise. In extreme situations, such rapidly progressive glomerulonephritis, the decline in kidney function is very fast, and immediate action is needed. If glomerulonephritis is not promptly diagnosed and treated, it may progress to chronic kidney disease or end-stage renal failure, necessitating dialysis or transplantation for the patient. Knowing its many causes, many ways it can show up, and how serious it can be is important for directing successful therapy and keeping the kidneys healthy (Keskinyan et al., 2023). The rising aging population has led to a higher prevalence of acute glomerulonephritis in elderly people, attributed to elevated incidences of endocarditis linked to the continued use of intravenous medications and cardiac devices. Consequently, this illness affects both young children and old persons. Acute glomerulonephritis primarily results from soft tissue infections, especially beta-hemolytic streptococcal pharyngitis in infants, known as acute post-streptococcal glomerulonephritis. Consistent with previous studies, we noted that the highest prevalence and incidence rates were recorded in children. The initial increase in age-standardized prevalence and incidence was observed in the 10 to 14 age group, succeeded by a decline in younger individuals, and by a slight fluctuation in the older demographic (Glomerulonephritis | National Kidney Foundation, https://www.kidney.org/kidney-topics/glomerulonephritis). Presently, GN is mostly classified according to histological lesion patterns, encompassing both primary and secondary forms, along with numerous potential diagnoses for each category. Historical factors influence the classification of glomerulonephritis [GN], particularly the evolution of kidney biopsy techniques and the ability of light microscopy to discern patterns of glomerular injury, predominantly based on variations in cellular composition, deposits, and matrix proteins in distinct regions of the glomerulus (Guo et al., 2021). A kidney biopsy verifies the diagnosis of glomerulonephritis, elucidates immunological activity, and assesses the extent of irreversible damage. A kidney-centric viewpoint has hindered the progress of conceptual frameworks for illness classification. This technique has had a minimal influence on comprehending the regulation of aberrant immune processes that trigger and sustain glomerulonephritis by generating nephritogenic humoral and cellular immune effectors outside the kidney (Romagnani et al., 2023).

6.2.2 Diabetic Nephropathy

Diabetic nephropathy (DN) is a common and severe complication of diabetes mellitus (DM), associated with increased morbidity and mortality in diabetic patients. In the United States, the population of diabetic persons commencing treatment for end-stage renal disease (ESRD) increased significantly from over 40,000 in 2000 to over 50,000 in 2014. In China, the incidence and prevalence of diabetic nephropathy have markedly increased during the past decade. The estimated number of diabetic patients with chronic kidney disease (CKD) in China is 24.3 million. The worldwide incidence of diabetes is rapidly escalating, especially in developing countries. The escalating prevalence of diabetes is expected to result in a concomitant rise in the occurrence of diabetic nephropathy, unless there is immediate improvement in clinical preventative strategies (Bajema et al., 2018). Diabetic nephropathy (DN) refers to a distinct kidney condition directly associated with chronic diabetes, often corroborated by histological irregularities. Diabetic nephropathy (DN) is a diverse illness characterized by albuminuria and/or a reduction in estimated glomerular filtration rate (eGFR) in patients with diabetes. The American Diabetes Association (ADA) defines pathological albuminuria as an albumin-to-creatinine ratio (ACR) over 30 mg/g. In type 1 diabetes mellitus (T1DM), diabetic nephropathy (DN) is rarely detected within the first decade of the disease; nevertheless, its incidence increases between 10 and 20 years post-diagnosis, reaching up to 3% annually (Samsu, 2021). Diabetic nephropathy (DN), a microvascular consequence of diabetes, results in renal impairment and is the most common complication of type 2 diabetes mellitus. It is the principal cause of end-stage renal disease worldwide, associated with considerable morbidity and mortality. It manifests in approximately 40% of individuals with diabetes a decade post-diagnosis of type 2 diabetes mellitus. Stage 4 diabetic nephropathy (DN) is characterized by persistent albuminuria, indicated by an albuminuria excretion rate surpassing 300 mg/d or 200 μg/min, assessed at least twice within a three to six-month period, alongside a progressive reduction in glomerular filtration rate (GFR), often associated with increased blood pressure, ultimately leading to end-stage renal disease (Pelle et al., 2022).

6.2.3 Hypertensive Nephropathy

A global epidemic of chronic kidney disease [CKD] prevails; hypertensive nephropathy ranks second to diabetes as a primary cause of advancing CKD. Due to the increasing morbidity, mortality, and expenses associated with end-stage renal disease [ESRD], there is an urgent necessity for novel therapeutic strategies to effectively reduce albuminuria, manage blood pressure, and delay the progression of hypertensive nephropathy to ESRD. The prudent use of renin–angiotensin–aldosterone system [RAAS] inhibitors and the achievement of blood pressure targets are crucial for reducing cardiovascular and renal outcomes (Thipsawat, 2021). Hypertensive nephropathy denotes the gradual deterioration of renal function resulting from chronic hypertension. Chronic hypertension damages small renal vasculature, leading to arteriolar hyalinosis, myointimal hyperplasia, and constriction of small arteries and arterioles. This vascular remodeling diminishes renal perfusion, resulting in glomerular ischemia and subsequent glomerular sclerosis. Certain nephrons experience hyperfiltration as a compensatory mechanism, which paradoxically exacerbates damage and results in increased glomerulosclerosis and podocyte depletion. Tubulointerstitial damage, marked by tubular atrophy and interstitial fibrosis, occurs following vascular injury and ischemia, leading to a decline in renal function. The renin–angiotensin–aldosterone system [RAAS] facilitates vasoconstriction, fibrosis, and inflammation (Hart & Bakris, 2010). Histologically, benign nephrosclerosis is characterized by hyaline arteriosclerosis, glomerular tuft collapse, wrinkled basement membranes, and interstitial fibrosis; in contrast, malignant hypertension leads to more severe lesions, including fibrinoid necrosis and hyperplastic alterations in arterioles (Seccia et al., 2017). Therapeutic goals emphasize strict blood pressure control, often utilizing renin-angiotensin system antagonists [ACE inhibitors or ARBs], alongside lifestyle modifications such as sodium restriction, weight management, and monitoring for proteinuria and decreased glomerular filtration rate. Effective therapy may significantly decelerate the progression of end-stage renal disease, and in rare cases, renal function may be partially restored (Wang et al., 2013). Hypertensive renal disease has become the third most common cause of chronic renal failure in patients receiving dialysis. In the elderly population, chronic renal insufficiency is the primary cause of hypertensive renal disease, hypertension nephropathy may develop in hypertension patients with severe renal alterations after 5–10 years of the condition. This discovery has mostly been evidenced in vascular pathology, ischemic glomerular alterations, and acute tubular interstitial damage. This study analyzed 47 renal biopsy instances without significant problems. All patients' blood pressure normalized. Furthermore, 41 instances exhibited a 24-h urine protein ratio of less than 150 mg, 10 patients experienced minor renal impairment, and eight patients had a serum creatinine level that normalized. Only one instance of severe renal impairment was noted, and the renal function of this patient did not significantly improve after treatment (Seccia et al., 2017).

6.2.4 Polycystic Kidney Disease

Polycystic Kidney Disease (PKD) is a hereditary disorder characterized by the progressive formation of many fluid-filled cysts in the kidneys. These cysts cause renal tissue enlargement and progressive degradation of functioning nephrons, ultimately impairing the kidney's ability to filter waste and regulate fluid and electrolyte balance. There are two principal inherited types: autosomal dominant polycystic kidney disease (ADPKD), the more common variation typically manifesting in maturity (ages 30–40), and autosomal recessive polycystic kidney disease (ARPKD), which is rarer yet more severe, with symptoms often apparent in infancy or even prenatally (Hypertensive Nephropathy: Causes, Symptoms, & Treatment Options [Internet], https://thekingsleyclinic.com/resources/hypertensive-nephropathy-causes-symptoms-and-treatment-options/). The pathophysiology entails abnormalities in genes including PKD1, PKD2, and PKHD1, which impair proper tubule formation and function. These mutations disrupt cellular signaling, specifically concerning primary cilia and the regulation of epithelial cell proliferation and fluid secretion, resulting in cyst development (Medicine et al., 2020). Clinically, patients may initially exhibit no symptoms. As cysts increase, symptoms like flank or abdominal pain, hypertension, hematuria, urinary tract infections, nephrolithiasis, and abdominal distension may manifest. Additional extra-renal symptoms may include hepatic cysts, vascular anomalies [such as cerebral aneurysms], and cardiac valve disorders (Hypertensive Nephropathy: Causes, Symptoms, & Treatment Options [Internet], https://thekingsleyclinic.com/resources/hypertensive-nephropathy-causes-symptoms-and-treatment-options/). Diagnosis primarily relies on imaging techniques [ultrasound, CT, MRI], whereas genetic testing is utilized in certain cases. Although a cure is unavailable, management focuses on decelerating disease progression and mitigating consequences by stringent blood pressure regulation, infection and pain management, lifestyle alterations, and, in late cases, dialysis or transplantation. Recent treatment advancements, such as medicines that influence intracellular signaling, exemplified by tolvaptan, demonstrate potential in altering disease progression (Wilson, 2004).

6.3 The Role of Biomarkers in Chronic Kidney Disease [CKD]

6.3.1 Importance in Diagnosis and Monitoring

Chronic kidney disease (CKD) is characterized by diminished kidney function, indicated by a glomerular filtration rate (GFR) below 60 mL/min/1.73 m^2 and/or the existence of renal impairment persisting for a minimum of 3 months. Chronic Kidney Disease (CKD) is acknowledged as a concealed epidemic, constituting a significant public health issue that impacts 13.4% of the adult population and results in 1.2

million fatalities annually (National Kidney Foundation. https://www.kidney.org/kidney-topics/polycystic-kidney-disease). A biomarker is a quantifiable sign of normal or disease-related biological processes, or reactions to therapeutic interventions. In chronic kidney disease [CKD], there may be indicators in the blood, urine, or tissue that reflect kidney function, damage, or inflammation. Standard markers comprise eGFR [estimated glomerular filtration rate, calculated from serum creatinine and, at times, cystatin C] and proteinuria/albuminuria [particularly the urine albumin-to-creatinine ratio, UACR]. These are beneficial yet possess restrictions. A significant concern is that renal impairment frequently manifests prior to a decline in eGFR or the emergence of proteinuria. Consequently, there exists a latent phase in early chronic kidney disease during which damage occurs, however present diagnostic methods lack sensitivity (Mizdrak et al., 2022).

- Conventional metrics such as serum creatinine/eGFR and proteinuria typically exhibit abnormalities only when significant renal impairment has transpired. Biomarkers, such as injury markers, can indicate harm at an early stage. NGAL and KIM-1 work as biomarkers of tubular injury, but cystatin C is minimally affected by muscle mass, offering a more accurate functional evaluation across diverse populations (Lopez-Giacoman & Madero, 2015).
- Biomarkers, including certain urine miRNAs, exhibit excellent sensitivity and specificity in diagnosing chronic kidney disease (CKD), potentially detecting the ailment before the emergence of overt albuminuria or a reduction in estimated glomerular filtration rate (eGFR). Biomarker panels or combinations [injury + functional + structural] typically exceed the efficacy of individual standard tests (Alobaidi, 2025).
- Certain biomarkers, such as urinary miRNAs and damage markers, can be assessed in urine, which is less invasive than procedures like biopsy. Biomarkers can specify the affected region of the nephron [glomerular, tubular, interstitial] and show the presence of inflammation, oxidative stress, or fibrosis, rather than merely identifying "kidney disease." This aids in differential diagnosis and therapeutic planning (GantsetsegGarmaa et al., 2024).
- Specific biomarkers assessed at diagnosis can aid in forecasting the progression rate of CKD, the probability of complications, and cardiovascular risk, among other factors. This enables clinicians to promptly identify high-risk patients and implement more assertive interventions.
- MicroRNAs, especially those present in urine, are emerging as diagnostic tools. A recent comprehensive study and meta-analysis demonstrated favorable pooled sensitivity and specificity for several miRNAs in differentiating chronic kidney disease from non-chronic kidney disease. Additional contemporary biomarkers under investigation encompass ADMA, SDMA, and uromodulin, which may enhance diagnostic accuracy.

6.3.2 Challenges in Older Adults Due to Systemic Inflammation, Metabolic Alterations, and Drug Use

Aging leads to a state termed "inflammaging," marked by chronic low-grade systemic inflammation that heightens vulnerability to many diseases. It exacerbates results in renal disease. Chronic renal disease is closely linked to inflammation. The systemic inflammatory response index (SIRI), comprising lymphocyte, neutrophil, and monocyte counts, has shown a favorable correlation with the prevalence of chronic kidney disease (CKD). An link has been identified between the condition and the systemic immune–inflammation index (SII), which encompasses lymphocyte, neutrophil, and platelet counts (Li et al., 2024a; Rysz et al., 2017). Moreover, inflammation diminishes healing mechanisms [e.g., following acute injury] to a greater extent in elderly kidneys. They have diminished resiliency. The structural and functional reserves, including the number of nephrons and regenerating capability, are reduced (Li et al., 2024b).

Substance use among older adults—polypharmacy, nephrotoxic substances, and modified pharmacokinetics resulting from diminished renal clearance and inflammation—presents significant dangers. Pharmaceuticals eliminated by the kidneys or liver may accumulate; inflammatory conditions might modify medication metabolism and distribution, complicating dosage adjustments. Biomarkers indicative of tubular injury, such as NGAL and KIM 1, may enhance the early identification of drug-induced damage; however, their specificity is compromised in older patients with chronic kidney disease due to the effects of inflammation and metabolic disorders.

Integrating biomarker utilization in older CKD populations necessitates recognition of interacting confounders—systemic inflammation, metabolic disturbances, and pharmacological exposure—to prevent the overestimation or underestimation of renal injury, misclassification of disease stage, or oversight of early deterioration.

6.3.3 Key Biomarkers: Serum Creatinine, Estimated Glomerular Filtration Rate [eGFR], Albuminuria

Serum creatinine, estimated glomerular filtration rate (eGFR), and albuminuria are essential indicators in the evaluation of chronic kidney disease (CKD). Serum creatinine levels reflect renal function, while eGFR approximates glomerular filtration rate. Albuminuria indicates renal dysfunction by detecting elevated albumin concentrations in urine. These markers collectively aid in the diagnosis, staging, and monitoring of chronic renal disease progression. Table 6.2 includes additional biomarkers and their corresponding details.

Table 6.2 Biomarkers and their details

Biomarker	What it reflects/why useful	Limitations/issues
Creatinine [serum]	Conventional indicator of renal function. Simple and extensively utilized	Determined by muscle mass, age, sex, and food; lacks sensitivity for early injury (Mizdrak et al., 2022)
Cystatin C	Superior than creatinine in certain instances; less reliant on muscle mass. When combined with creatinine, it yields improved estimations of eGFR	Higher cost; potential limitations in availability; challenges with standardization
Albuminuria/Uacr	Indicator of glomerular injury; manifests before to some other functional deteriorations. Robust predictor of chronic kidney disease progression and cardiovascular risk	Variability, such as that caused by hydration and activity, necessitates repeated measurements; not all cases of chronic kidney disease have significant albuminuria
Ngal [Urine/Plasma]	Tubular damage biomarker; increases promptly, highly sensitive (Lopez-Giacoman & Madero, 2015)	Issues of specificity; variability among assays; expense
Kim-1	Another tubular injury biomarker; valuable for differentiating damage (Mizdrak et al., 2022)	Identical constraints as previously mentioned
Fibroblast growth Factor-23 [Fgf-23], Supar, Adma Etc	Consider additional factors: mineral metabolism, inflammation, and endothelial dysfunction; they might assist in risk classification (GantsetsegGarmaa et al., 2024)	Some remain experimental; standardization and extensive cohort validations are absent
Inflammatory Markers [Il-6, Il-1, Etc.]	Indicate the inflammatory condition associated with progression and cardiovascular risk. Can monitor advancement	Low specificity; may be raised due to numerous factors; less informative in isolation; inter-individual variability

6.4 Patient Perspectives: Insights from Hemodialysis Patients

6.4.1 Qualitative Methodology and Study Design

This study employed a qualitative descriptive/phenomenological methodology to investigate patient perspectives on long-term maintenance hemodialysis. The objective is to comprehend the meanings, challenges, needs, and coping techniques derived from the lived experiences of patients, rather than to assess or quantify those experiences. A qualitative design was employed to investigate the demands of hemodialysis patients from their viewpoints through semi-structured telephone interviews and thematic data analysis. This design was considered the most suitable method for the current study as it examines experiences and occurrences from the perspective of the participants when limited information exists regarding the subject under investigation (Gupta et al., 2024).

Data Collection

Method: Semi-structured, in-depth interviews employing an interview guide featuring open-ended questions. Topics may encompass: daily routines, bodily symptoms [fatigue, pain, side effects], emotional experiences [anxiety, depression, identity], social interactions and roles, financial burdens, coping techniques, and expectations from healthcare providers.

Alternative or supplementary methods: Incorporate focus groups to investigate collective experiences; conduct observations during dialysis sessions if practicable; utilize patient diaries or notebooks to document daily variations.

Procedure: Secure ethical approval. Upon obtaining consent, interviews [about 45–60 min] are audio-recorded, and field notes are documented. Verbatim transcription, translation if necessary.

Data Analysis

Employ thematic analysis or inductive content analysis to discern patterns, themes, and subthemes. The "Exploring the Needs" study included thematic analysis (Gupta et al., 2024).

A descriptive phenomenological method may be utilized to clarify the fundamental structures of experience. The study titled "The Lived Experiences of Patients Undergoing Hemodialysis with the Concept of Care" employed a descriptive phenomenological design (Almutary et al., 2023).

Steps for analysis: Acquaintance: peruse transcripts multiple times.

Open coding: a method of line-by-line coding to produce preliminary codes.

Classifying codes into themes and subthemes.

Examining themes, articulating their definitions, and correlating them with research inquiries.

Reflexivity: the researcher contemplates biases and assumptions.

Utilize qualitative software [e.g., NVivo, MAXQDA] if accessible to facilitate organization.

Rigor/Reliability

Credibility: member checking [participants reviewing significant results], peer debriefing.

Transferability: comprehensive, detailed account of context and participants' backgrounds.

Reliability: a comprehensive audit trail of coding decisions and established protocols.

Confirmability: reflexivity and triangulation [utilization of diverse data sources, methodologies, or analysts].

Ethical Considerations

Informed consent, confidentiality, and voluntary participation.

Address sensitive topics [emotional discomfort] by preparing a plan for referral or support if necessary. Guaranteeing anonymity in quotations.

6.4.2 *Findings from Semi-Structured Interviews in an Urban Teaching Hospital*

Semi-structured interviews with haemodialysis patients in urban hospitals or comparable clinical environments uncover a diverse array of lived experiences, emphasizing several domains—physical, psychological, social, economic, and existential. Principal conclusions derived from the investigations encompass:

1. **Physical Burden and Fatigue**: Patients consistently report severe weariness during and following dialysis sessions, which restricts their ability to do everyday tasks. This is associated with symptoms like discomfort, cramps, sleep problems, and overall malaise. These physical limitations affect daily routines, roles, and perceptions of life quality (Gupta et al., 2024).
2. **Psychological & Emotional Impact**: Anxiety, despair, and a profound sense of loss of control or identity manifest prominently. Patients express concerns regarding disease advancement, reliance, and ambiguity about the future. Emotional stress is intensified by recurrent hospital visits and interruptions to daily life. Certain research indicate that adaption transpires with time; nonetheless, emotional support from healthcare personnel is frequently perceived as inadequate.
3. **Social Role Changes & Need for Family Support**: Dialysis frequently modifies familial responsibilities and social engagement. Patients report an inability to perform job, caregiving, or social roles as they formerly did. Assistance from family members is essential for emotional, logistical, and financial support; yet, patients sometimes experience feelings of isolation or alterations in their relationships.
4. **Economic Strain & Access Constraints**: Cost is a persistent motif. Research from India and Saudi Arabia indicates that patients are transitioning to more affordable dialysis centers, decreasing session frequency owing to fiscal limitations, incurring personal expenditures, losing employment capacity, and expressing concerns regarding long-term affordability. Urban environments

exhibit significant disparities in the accessibility and expense of services (Shahgholian & Yousefi, 2018).

5. **Adaptation & Coping Strategies**: Patients adopt several coping strategies, including modifying daily routines, depending on social and familial support, emphasizing relaxation, and occasionally recognizing dialysis as essential. Religious or spiritual convictions may contribute to the maintenance of hope (Elias et al., 2022).
6. **Gaps in Support Services**: Across research, there is a perception of inadequate support, particularly in psychological, emotional, and social domains. Patients express a demand for enhanced communication with healthcare personnel, counseling services, increased information, and psychological interventions. Additionally, there is heterogeneity in service quality and discrepancies in the presentation or comprehension of treatment alternatives.

6.4.3 *Patient Experiences and Challenges*

Qualitative research involving hemodialysis patients repeatedly indicates that the treatment experience is beset by multifaceted challenges—physical, emotional, social, and economic. A study of young patients [ages 18 to 45] in China revealed that physical symptoms, including exhaustion, dizziness, and dry mouth, coexisted with depression, low self-esteem, and challenges in social adjustment, such as work obstacles and conflicts in role identification (Ogwang et al., 2023).

Patients at Kiruddu National Referral Hospital in Uganda characterized hemodialysis as essential for survival, although they also expressed mental turmoil, physical constraints, and reliance on family for financial and logistical assistance. Adaptation was observed, but subsequent to significant mental distress (Elias et al., 2022).

In Iran, interviews for a research on hope among ESRD patients indicated that threats to hope include the cumulative load of medical symptoms, social isolation, economic hardships, and occupational constraints. Notwithstanding this, positive coping mechanisms [spirituality, familial support, psychological methods] surfaced as significant mitigating resources (Rao et al., 2025).

A meta-synthesis of young and middle-aged patients worldwide indicated that several individuals experience disruptions in their daily routines, face financial burdens due to extended treatment, encounter negative emotions, and have unmet needs for psychological, social, and informational support.

6.5 Historical Milestones in Dialysis Development

6.5.1 *Contributions of Willem Kolff and Belding Scribner*

Willem Johan "Pim" Kolff [1911–2009] is esteemed as the progenitor of artificial organs, particularly for his groundbreaking contributions to the creation of the first effective clinically utilized dialysis equipment. In the Netherlands during World War II, Kolff constructed a spinning drum kidney, known as a "artificial kidney," with cellulose tubing [cellophane], hardwood drums, and a custom pump system. Although his first 15 patients did not survive, in September 1945, his 16th patient, a 67-year-old woman in uremic coma from acute renal failure, recovered after 11 h of dialysis (Rambod et al., 2023). This initial accomplishment confirmed that therapeutic hemodialysis could effectively treat acute renal failure. Subsequent to the war, Kolff bequeathed his prototypes to hospitals in the United States and elsewhere, and his devices [e.g., the Kolff Brigham machine] established the groundwork for global acute renal support (Haemodialysis was first used successfully in, https://historyofnephrology.org/hd/haemodialysis-was-first-used-successfully-in-1945).

Nevertheless, those initial devices were not intended for prolonged maintenance dialysis in chronic renal failure. This paradigm shift is primarily due to Belding H. Scribner. In 1960, at the University of Washington, Scribner, alongside Wayne Quinton and surgeon David Dillard, devised the Scribner shunt—an external arteriovenous Teflon shunt facilitating indwelling access between an artery and a vein in the forearm. This technology enabled repeated dialysis access without necessitating new vascular operations for each session (Sharma et al., 2024). The initial patient with this shunt, Clyde Shields, survived for eleven years while on dialysis.

Subsequent to the development of the Scribner Shunt, several significant advancements occurred: the establishment in 1962 of the inaugural outpatient/community dialysis center [Seattle Artificial Kidney Center], which rendered chronic dialysis outside hospital environments viable; enhancements in access, dialysate formulation, home dialysis, peritoneal dialysis, and the optimization of dialysis efficacy and complication management (Blagg, 2011).

Kolff's invention facilitated the treatment of acute kidney failure, whereas Scribner's inventions permitted continuous, repeated dialysis, converting end-stage renal disease from a nearly certain fatal prognosis to a controllable condition. Their collaborative efforts established the technological and organizational framework for contemporary hemodialysis care (Haemodialysis was first used successfully in, https://historyofnephrology.org/hd/haemodialysis-was-first-used-successfully-in-1945).

6.5.2 Evolution of Dialysis Techniques

Dialysis has significantly advanced from its primitive origins, propelled by technological breakthroughs, improved vascular access, and a focus on patient-centered care. The initial human dialysis endeavors originated with Georg Haas in 1924, who employed external cannulas [artery and vein] for acute situations. Mechanical dialysis progressed with Willem Kolff's artificial kidney in the 1940s, solidifying hemodialysis as a viable treatment (Our History | Dialysis, Research | Northwest Kidney Centers, https://www.nwkidney.org/about-us/our-history).

A significant innovation in chronic care occurred in the 1960s with the development of the autologous arteriovenous fistula [AVF] by Brescia, Cimino, and associates [1966], which continues to be the benchmark for long-term vascular access owing to its durability and reduced infection risk (Hassanein et al., 2025). Subcutaneous grafts utilizing synthetic materials [e.g., PTFE] and tunneled central venous catheters subsequently enhanced patient options when arteriovenous fistulas were impractical.

Recently, the discipline has shifted focus towards improving patient quality of life using portable and wearable dialysis equipment. The "Wearable Artificial Kidney" [WAK] signifies a significant advancement in the provision of prolonged and continuous dialysis beyond traditional clinical environments. Preliminary human trials of WAK demonstrated encouraging solute removal and hemodynamic stability during 24-h therapy (Mishler, 2009). Furthermore, peritoneal dialysis has experienced advancements, including automated, continuous flow, and wearable PD devices, while dialysis consumables and membranes have become increasingly biocompatible and efficient (Gura et al., 2016).

6.5.3 Economic, Epidemiological, and Ethical Implications

Dialysis, particularly maintenance hemodialysis, places considerable financial strain on patients, healthcare systems, and nations. In India, the expense for each hemodialysis session in a private hospital, encompassing both direct and indirect charges, was approximately INR 4500, with a significant chunk paid out of pocket, rendering long-term therapy prohibitive for many individuals (Bazaev, 2020). In Ethiopia, the costs for patients with End-Stage Renal Disease (ESRD) were high, causing many individuals to miss treatment sessions or essential medications due to financial constraints (Suja et al., 2012). Comparative analyses across modalities indicate that home dialysis and peritoneal dialysis are generally more cost-effective under various scenarios. A "PD first" policy in Thailand has superior cost usefulness compared to "HD first" from both public and governmental viewpoints, however cost thresholds are significant (Assanatham et al., 2022).

From an epidemiological perspective, the escalating incidence of chronic kidney disease [CKD] and resultant end-stage renal disease [ESRD] results in heightened

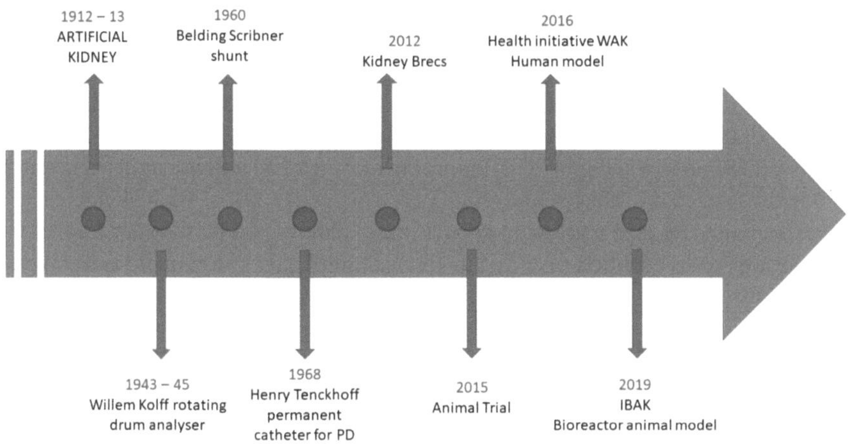

Fig. 6.1 Developments of dialysis

demand for dialysis. Low- and middle-income nations are particularly impacted, experiencing limited access and elevated mortality rates due to the unavailability or unaffordability of renal replacement medication (Mushi et al., 2015).

Ethically, numerous issues emerge: equity of access [wealth, geography, insurance], fairness in modality selection [patients frequently unable to afford home dialysis despite its advantages], transparency regarding costs, and the responsibility of health systems to equilibrate resource allocation [dialysis versus prevention versus transplantation]. Policy considerations emphasize that cost reduction must not undermine safety or quality of care, while ethical frameworks advocate for the provision of dialysis services based on necessity rather than just on financial capability. Figure 6.1 is graphically showing the developments of dylasis.

6.6 Current Challenges in Dialysis Services

6.6.1 Expansion in High-Income Countries

High-income countries [HICs] encounter distinct obstacles as dialysis services grow to accommodate rising demand. Demographic changes, resource limitations, and patient-centered care challenges are exerting increasing pressure on healthcare systems.

Increasing Demand and Aging Populations

The aging population is a significant catalyst for the necessity of expansion. Japan faces a significant challenge due to its rapidly aging population; the anticipated incidence of dialysis patients is estimated to rise by roughly 12.8% from 2012 [approximately 36,590 individuals] to 2025 [approximately 41,270 individuals], particularly among those aged 85 years and beyond (Wakasugi et al., 2015). With the increase in life expectancy, there is a growing population of elderly people who are fragile and have various comorbidities, resulting in greater complexity of treatment and elevated expenditures (Hyodo et al., 2025).

Rising Costs and Economic Strain

Dialysis unfairly allocates a significant percentage of healthcare spending, especially in high-income countries. In Japan, dialysis patients constitute 0.275% of the population, although they account for around 3.4% of total medical expenditures only through outpatient maintenance dialysis. Expenses escalate for elderly people experiencing frailty, hospitalizations, and concomitant conditions. Consequently, maintaining growth without jeopardizing the quality of care presents a difficulty.

Workforce & Infrastructure Constraints

Even in high-income countries, there exist shortages or misallocations of specialized personnel, including nephrologists, dialysis nurses, and vascular access specialists (Chen et al., 2024). Moreover, substantial fixed expenses associated with dialysis facilities, machinery, consumables, and maintenance pose obstacles to expansion while upholding quality standards.

Unequal Access & Modality Mix

Expansion by itself does not ensure equity. Home dialysis [peritoneal or home hemodialysis] is underutilized in numerous high-income countries due to preferences or disincentives among patients, providers, or systems. Geographic inequities persist, as remote or rural communities encounter access difficulties despite a generally high capacity (Yongphiphatwong et al., 2025).

Sustainability and Quality

During expansion, maintaining quality is essential—dialysis adequacy, infection control, vascular access integrity, patient outcomes, and quality of life. Unsupervised resource scaling poses a risk of inconsistency. Technologies, reimbursement methods, and policy frameworks must facilitate both expansion and sustainability.

6.6.2 *Slower Progress in Patient-Centred Advancements*

Notwithstanding the increasing acknowledgment of the significance of patient-centered care in dialysis, advancements have been inconsistent and more gradual than anticipated by numerous stakeholders. A study entitled Advances in Human Centered Care to Address Contemporary Unmet Needs in Chronic Dialysis noted that, despite the rising frailty and multimorbidity among patients, traditional hospital haemodialysis practices have remained unchanged for the past thirty years, with minimal implementation of human-centered care models (Jayanti & Rangan, 2024).

A qualitative case study from Canada revealed that while patients prefer more personalized care, existing hemodialysis services are structured according to provider priorities, emphasizing metabolic and dialysis objectives over comprehensive well-being. Numerous patients encounter disjointed care and inadequate consideration of their beliefs, values, or living situations (Lewis et al., 2019).

Nephrologists indicate that shared decision-making remains problematic: patients frequently encounter modality options but are subtly influenced by providers; their involvement in ongoing care [e.g., concerning lifestyle, scheduling, symptom management] is limited by systemic constraints and policies. The impetus to standardize targets [such as dialysis frequency, fistula-first rules, and billing incentives] may constrain customization to individual requirements (Andersen-Hollekim et al., 2021).

Furthermore, self-management assistance is inadequately developed: patients indicate challenges in obtaining longitudinal, comprehensible instructional resources in formats that align with their literacy levels or lifestyles. Communication obstacles endure between healthcare providers and patients regarding acceptable trade-offs [e.g., convenience against clinical advantages] (Lin & Hwang, 2020).

6.6.3 Modality-Specific Factors Influencing Outcomes

A crucial element is residual renal function [RRF]: peritoneal dialysis [PD] generally maintains RRF for a longer duration than standard intermittent hemodialysis [HD], which correlates with enhanced fluid equilibrium, reduced cardiovascular problems, and higher survival rates, especially during the first treatment phase. A study examining cardiovascular outcomes in hemodialysis (HD) versus peritoneal dialysis (PD) indicated that patients undergoing PD demonstrated a greater residual urine volume, which acts as a protective factor against cardiovascular disease (CVD) (Refaat et al., 2016).

An further significant influence is patient comorbidities and age. An extensive registry research in Australia and New Zealand demonstrated that mortality disparities between peritoneal dialysis [PD] and hemodialysis [HD] are significantly influenced by age and comorbidity burden: PD shown a diminished death rate within the first 90 days among patients; however, after one year, the advantage fluctuated according to patient characteristics (McDonald et al., 2009). A study in southern China revealed that younger patients with congestive heart failure exhibited improved survival rates with peritoneal dialysis [PD], while older age groups shown a survival advantage with hemodialysis [HD] (He et al., 2022).

Quality of life (QoL) signifies a certain outcome associated with a modality. Meta-analyses comparing quality of life in hemodialysis (HD) and peritoneal dialysis (PD) reveal that PD patients often report enhanced outcomes in treatment satisfaction, flexibility, autonomy, and social well-being; in contrast, HD patients may exhibit superior physical functioning or support, depending on the specific study and local context (Zazzeroni et al., 2017).

Ultimately, elements such as modality-specific technical challenges [e.g., access difficulties in hemodialysis, peritoneal membrane longevity in peritoneal dialysis] and iron management [varying requirements and strategies in hemodialysis versus peritoneal dialysis] also affect outcomes. The administration methods, dosages, and frequency of iron vary by modality, potentially influencing anemia management, patient complaints, and death rates (van Lieshout et al., 2024).

6.7 Cardiovascular Complications in Dialysis Patients

6.7.1 Prevalence and Impact on Mortality

Cardiovascular disease (CVD) continues to be the primary cause of morbidity and mortality among dialysis patients, with its prevalence and risk much surpassing that of the general population. In patients undergoing hemodialysis [HD] or peritoneal dialysis [PD], left ventricular hypertrophy [LVH] impacts roughly 70–75% of persons, with clinical heart failure and coronary artery disease also prevalent (Foley et al., 1998).

Epidemiological studies estimate cardiovascular death rates to be between 9 to 14% annually in dialysis groups. A cross-sectional study with a two-year follow-up involving HD patients indicated an annual cardiovascular death rate of approximately 8.5% and an overall mortality rate of about 13.7% (Petrović & Stojimirović, 2008). A separate analysis indicated that cardiovascular disease constitutes up to 40% of fatalities among dialysis users worldwide (Jegatheesan et al., 2017).

Numerous conventional risk factors—hypertension, diabetes, dyslipidemia, and a sedentary lifestyle—are significantly frequent in dialysis populations. In the CORDIAL study conducted in Brazil, among 1215 hemodialysis patients, hypertension was observed in around 87.5%, dyslipidemia in about 84.7%, sedentary lifestyles in roughly 73.1%, tobacco usage in around 53.7%, and diabetes in approximately 35.8% (Burmeister et al., 2014).

Nontraditional risk factors significantly contribute: fluid overload, anemia, aberrant mineral bone metabolism, inflammation, oxidative stress, and exposure to uremic toxins. Research indicates that the decline of residual kidney function, frequent volume fluctuations during hemodialysis, and the bioincompatibility of dialysis materials elevate cardiovascular risk (Jegatheesan et al., 2017).

The repercussions are grave: patients on dialysis often perish not only from infections or metabolic complications but also from heart failure, sudden cardiac death, myocardial infarction, and arrhythmias. Their risk of cardiovascular death is 10—20 times greater than that of age-, gender-, and race-matched controls from the general population (Foley et al., 1998).

6.7.2 *Differences Between Hemodialysis and Peritoneal Dialysis*

Recent studies indicate modality-specific disparities in cardiovascular risk between patients undergoing hemodialysis and those receiving peritoneal dialysis. A substantial Taiwanese cohort of newly diagnosed end-stage renal disease (ESRD) patients without a history of cardiovascular disease indicated that individuals undergoing hemodialysis (HD) exhibited a markedly increased risk of new-onset congestive heart failure (CHF) relative to those receiving peritoneal dialysis (PD) (adjusted hazard ratio $\approx$ 1.29; 95% confidence interval: 1.13–1.47), particularly within the initial year of dialysis. Nonetheless, there was no substantial disparity in the risk of ischemic heart disease between the two modalities (Wang et al., 2016).

A recent meta-analysis of 28 studies comparing cardiovascular disease (CVD) events revealed that atrial fibrillation (RR ~ 1.29), congestive heart failure (CHF) (RR ~ 1.23), and peripheral arterial disease (RR ~ 1.13) were more prevalent in hemodialysis (HD) patients than in peritoneal dialysis (PD) patients. Notably, whereas cardiovascular disease [CVD] events were more frequent, cardiovascular mortality was relatively lower in hemodialysis [HD] compared to peritoneal dialysis [PD]. Relative risk is roughly 0.89; 95% confidence interval: 0.828 to 0.960 (Ng et al., 2021).

Additional observations indicate that peritoneal dialysis [PD] may prolong residual renal function, facilitating fluid equilibrium and alleviating cardiac stress. In contrast, hemodialysis [HD] patients experience significant fluid shifts, frequent blood pressure variations, and potentially greater cardiac burden associated with vascular access [e.g., arteriovenous fistula effects], This may result in an increased prevalence of congestive heart failure [CHF] and atrial arrhythmias (Ng et al., 2021).

Additional observations indicate that peritoneal dialysis [PD] may prolong residual renal function, facilitating fluid equilibrium and alleviating cardiac stress. In contrast, hemodialysis [HD] patients experience significant fluid shifts, frequent blood pressure variations, and potentially greater cardiac burden associated with vascular access [e.g., arteriovenous fistula effects], This may result in an increased prevalence of congestive heart failure [CHF] and atrial arrhythmias.

6.7.3 Strategies for Risk Assessment and Management

Effective management of cardiovascular disease [CVD] in dialysis patients necessitates thorough risk evaluation and specific interventions. A recent study underscores the importance of customizing cardiovascular risk assessment by integrating both conventional risk variables [hypertension, diabetes, dyslipidemia, smoking] and non-conventional factors [fluid overload, inflammation, mineral bone disease, uremic toxins].

Risk assessment procedures encompass the systematic monitoring of biomarkers [e.g., C-reactive protein, hemoglobin A1c], evaluation of volume status, and analysis of residual renal function. Exercise testing and cardiac rehabilitation programs, according to dialysis status, are recommended to evaluate functional capability and identify subclinical cardiovascular disease (Perone et al., 2025).

Effective management necessitates meticulous fluid and volume regulation—minimizing interdialytic weight gain, maximizing dry weight, and preventing excessive ultrafiltration volumes during hemodialysis to alleviate cardiac stress. Management of blood pressure, glucose levels [in diabetics], lipid profiles, and treatment of anemia are essential modifiable components.

Considerations about dialysis modalities are significant: the utilization of biocompatible membranes, high-flux dialyzers, and perhaps convective therapies such as hemodiafiltration may mitigate inflammatory burden and cardiovascular mortality, however clear randomized controlled trial evidence is absent for certain procedures.

Holistic care models that incorporate patient education, lifestyle modifications [nutrition, physical activity, smoking cessation], and multidisciplinary teams [nephrologists, cardiologists, nurses, dietitians] are increasingly regarded as essential for mitigating cardiovascular morbidity and mortality in this high-risk population (Li et al., 2024).

6.8 Preventing Nephrotoxicity: Medical and Environmental Considerations

6.8.1 Identification of Nephrotoxic Substances

Nephrotoxicity denotes renal impairment induced by chemicals, pharmaceuticals, or environmental substances. The prompt recognition of nephrotoxic agents is essential for preventing acute kidney damage [AKI] and for averting the advancement to chronic kidney disease [CKD].

Types of Nephrotoxic Agents

Pharmaceuticals: Common medical nephrotoxins include non-steroidal anti-inflammatory medications [NSAIDs], certain antibiotics [e.g., aminoglycosides], chemotherapeutic medicines, immunosuppressants, and radiographic contrast media.

Patient factors, such as pre-existing kidney disease, comorbidities, age, and dehydration, along with pharmacological features, including dosage, duration, administration method, and potential for accumulation, affect risk (Popović et al., 2016).

Environmental chemicals and heavy metals: Exposure to metals including cadmium [Cd], lead [Pb], mercury [Hg], arsenic [As], and silica has been shown to cause proximal tubular damage and serve as early indications of renal impairment (Pócsi et al., 2022).

Mixtures and environmental pollutants: Real-world exposure frequently entails combinations of substances—metallic alloys in drinking water, industrial contaminants, electronic waste, and agrochemicals—rather than isolated agents. Such mixes frequently exhibit additive or synergistic nephrotoxic effects.

Biomarkers and Detection

- Conventional indicators such as serum creatinine and blood urea nitrogen [BUN] exhibit limited sensitivity and reflect alterations only when damage is significantly progressed. More sensitive biomarkers are progressively employed to identify early injury:
- KIM-1, NGAL, and N-acetyl β-D-glucosaminidase are urine or serum biomarkers that facilitate the early identification of proximal tubular damage.
- Cystatin C is effective for identifying alterations in GFR prior to creatinine in some contexts (Al-Naimi et al., 2019).

Mechanisms & Risk Stratification

Network biology methodologies have elucidated the interactions between nephrotoxic agents and kidney-specific pathways [e.g., apoptosis, oxidative stress, AGEs RAGE signaling] as well as gene networks linked to nephrotoxic disorders (Xi et al., 2023). Risk stratification entails the amalgamation of exposure history [occupational, environmental, substance use], patient susceptibility [age, baseline renal function, comorbidities], and preliminary biomarker or imaging indicators of harm.

Implications

Comprehending nephrotoxic chemicals from both medical [pharmaceutical] and environmental origins, together with identifying them through more sensitive biomarkers, facilitates preventative interventions [minimizing or avoiding exposure], legislative initiatives, regulatory supervision, and clinical surveillance. Timely identification has demonstrated efficacy in reversing or alleviating damage, particularly when exposures are curtailed or diminished (Uber & Sutherland, 2020).

6.8.2 Importance of Early Detection and Monitoring

Nephrotoxicity, whether induced by pharmaceuticals, environmental toxins, or occupational exposures, frequently advances insidiously until substantial renal impairment has transpired. Conventional markers, like serum creatinine and blood urea nitrogen (BUN), are delayed indications, increasing only after significant nephron loss or functional deterioration (Redahan & Murray, 2017).

Timely identification by sensitive biomarkers or functional assessments can provide intervention before to irreversible harm. Research indicates that biomarkers such as KIM-1 (Kidney Injury Molecule 1), NGAL (Neutrophil Gelatinase Associated Lipocalin), Cystatin C, and IL-18 exhibit significant elevations prior to the increase in serum creatinine in contexts such as drug-induced acute kidney injury (e.g., platinum-based chemotherapy) and in animal models of nephrotoxicity (Abdelsalam et al., 2018).

In environmental contexts, preliminary indicators of glomerular or tubular injury, such as albuminuria, β2 microglobulin, NAG, enzymes, or low molecular weight proteinuria, aid in detecting subclinical damage from heavy metals or chemical exposures before the development of overt chronic kidney disease (CKD) (Bernard & Lauwerys, 1989).

Monitoring of at-risk populations—patients receiving nephrotoxic drugs, persons with pre-existing chronic kidney disease, the elderly, or those with considerable environmental exposure—is crucial. Timely intervention [dose modification, medication replacement, exposure minimization] informed by early indicators facilitates the maintenance of renal function, diminishes morbidity, and mitigates the advancement to end-stage renal disease [ESRD]. Therefore, the integration of early detection techniques into clinical and public health practices is essential for nephroprotection (Wu & Huang, 2018).

6.8.3 Preventive Measures and Patient Education

Preventing nephrotoxicity necessitates a dual approach: the implementation of clinical preventive interventions and the empowerment of individuals through education. Clinical measures encompass utilizing safer or non-nephrotoxic alternatives when feasible, modifying drug dosages according to baseline renal function, ensuring sufficient hydration before, during, and after exposure [e.g., with contrast agents or cisplatin], and monitoring for early indicators of renal injury through biomarkers [serum creatinine, BUN, and emerging markers] (Sari, 2019). Particular consensus comments [e.g., on cisplatin administration] underscore the reduction of concomitant nephrotoxins, pre- and post-hydration, and the utilization of antioxidants when suitable (Ashrafi et al., 2022).

Environmental preventive measures encompass minimizing exposure to heavy metals [lead, cadmium, arsenic] by interventions in drinking water, food safety, air pollution management, and occupational safety protocols (Sabath & Robles-Osorio, 2012).

Patient education is essential. Essential educational content encompasses: awareness of nephrotoxic drugs [prescription, over-the-counter, herbal products]; strategies for maintaining hydration; identification of early symptoms of kidney injury; significance of regular kidney function monitoring; avoidance of harmful agent combinations; lifestyle modifications [diet, reduction of excessive salt intake, limitation of exposure to environmental toxins] (Naik & Jeedi, 2025).

Involving patients in shared decision-making, employing culturally sensitive communication, and utilizing educational materials customized to literacy, language, and risk profiles improve adherence and efficacy.

Preventive therapeutic management combined with patient education establishes a foundation for diminishing the occurrence or progression of nephrotoxicity in both medical and environmental contexts. Figure 6.2 is showing the general prevention of nephropathy and nephrotoxicity.

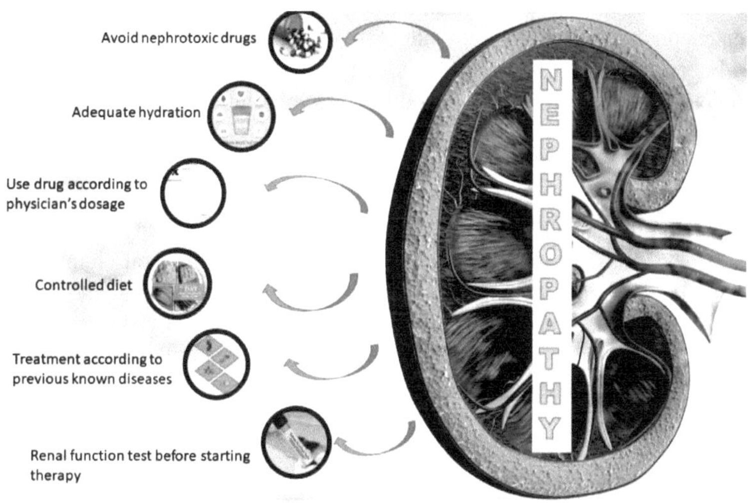

Fig. 6.2 General Preventive factors of nephropathy and nephrotoxicity

6.9 Conclusion: Navigating the Future of Nephropathy and Dialysis

6.9.1 Emphasis on Early Diagnosis and Intervention

The progression of chronic kidney disease [CKD], nephropathy, and the ensuing requirement for dialysis can be substantially altered with timely diagnosis and intervention. Recent studies reveal that chronic kidney disease (CKD) is frequently underrecognized in its first stages—typically asymptomatic—leading individuals to seek medical attention only after significant renal function decline, hence limiting treatment options.

The advancement of chronic kidney disease [CKD], nephropathy, and the subsequent necessity for dialysis can be significantly modified with prompt identification and intervention. Recent studies indicate that chronic kidney disease (CKD) is often underdiagnosed in its first stages—usually asymptomatic—resulting in patients pursuing treatment only after considerable renal function deterioration, hence constraining therapeutic alternatives (Mutatiri et al., 2024).

Intervention in early chronic kidney disease promotes the implementation of lifestyle modifications [diet, blood pressure regulation, glycemic control], pharmacotherapy [RAS inhibitors, SGLT2 inhibitors], and the management of anemia and mineral bone disorders, all of which aid in delaying the decline of renal function (Mutatiri et al., 2024).

In the future, health systems must emphasize awareness, accessibility to screening and diagnostics, continuous monitoring, and prompt referral channels. Integrating early diagnosis into primary care, enhancing patient education, and utilizing predictive analytics can transform the approach from reactive dialysis initiation to proactive preservation of kidney health. This method enhances individual patient results and may significantly alleviate the societal burden of dialysis.

6.9.2 Integrating Patient Perspectives into Care

Incorporating patient perspectives into nephropathy and dialysis care is increasingly acknowledged as vital for boosting results, improving patient satisfaction, and matching therapy with the priorities of individuals impacted. Research indicates that patient involvement—via shared decision-making, information transfer, and care planning—is an essential element of patient-centered dialysis care. In "Patient Participation in Dialysis Care: A Qualitative Study," both patients and professionals highlighted that involvement varies from information exchange to active participation in treatment decisions and self-management activities (Årestedt et al., 2019).

Nephrologists have asserted that patient-centered outcomes must be expressly specified by patients' preferences and objectives, including well-being, symptom load, and their personal definitions of "success" beyond laboratory results. Nonetheless, obstacles encompass systemic pressures, absence of measurement instruments, and a predominant emphasis on biochemical objectives (Tong et al., 2017).

Home-based and person-centered care interventions present promising models: a scoping analysis revealed that patient-centered interventions in home dialysis improved patients' capacity to engage in decision-making about modality, treatment delivery, and illness management. Research, including Patient Centered Care Could Improve Quality of Life and Survival, indicates that adjusting drugs based on patient-reported outcomes (PROs), nutritional status, and thorough evaluations may improve quality of life and potentially elevate survival rates (Tong et al., 2017).

Health systems should routinely integrate patient perspectives by utilizing patient-reported outcomes [PROs], shared decision-making frameworks, accessible data, and individualized treatment objectives. This transition may facilitate the alignment of professional priorities with patient values, thereby fostering care that is both medically effective and significant to patients' lives.

6.9.3 Future Directions in Research and Clinical Practice

Recent research indicates various possible avenues for enhancing nephropathy prevention, management, and dialysis practices. A vital area is precision medicine and molecular phenotyping. The integration of transcriptomic, proteomic, metabolomic, and lipidomic data in diabetic kidney disease (DKD) facilitates the identification of disease subtypes that may exhibit varying therapeutic responses to SGLT2 inhibitors, non-steroidal mineralocorticoid receptor antagonists, and endothelin A receptor antagonists (Innovations in Dialysis: Transforming Kidney Care for a Healthier Future, https://www.alliedacademies.org/articles/innovations-in-dialysis-transforming-kidney-care-for-a-healthier-future-31547.html?utm_source=chatgpt.com).

Technological innovation in dialysis encompasses the development of wearable and portable equipment, online hemodiafiltration, remote monitoring, and real-time data analytics, all aimed at enhancing patient comfort, alleviating treatment burden, and improving outcomes (Li & Padman, 2025).

Comprehensive data and artificial intelligence hold much promise; the amalgamation of electronic medical records, claims data, and biomarkers with machine learning may improve the forecasting of progression to end-stage renal disease (ESRD) and aid in improving the timing and method of dialysis (Li & Padman, 2025).

Moreover, interdisciplinary and integrated care models—encompassing nephrology, primary care, cardiology, nutrition, and patient education—are increasingly essential to manage comorbidities, cardiovascular risk, and enhance quality of life. Clinical trials focused on patient-reported outcomes, in addition to biochemical measures, are crucial.

In clinical practice, the introduction of early diagnostic programs, screening of high-risk individuals, utilization of biomarkers for earlier identification, and provision of flexible, patient-centered treatment choices [such as home dialysis and hybrid modes] are essential. These future prospects indicate a transition from reactive care to proactive, personalized techniques aimed at diminishing disease burden, enhancing survival, and improving the quality of life for patients with CKD and those undergoing dialysis.

References

Abdelsalam, M., Elmorsy, E., Abdelwahab, H., Algohary, O., Naguib, M., El Wahab, A. A., et al. (2018). Urinary biomarkers for early detection of platinum based drugs induced nephrotoxicity. *BMC Nephrology, 19*(1), 219.

Almutary, H., Al-ghamdi, R., Miajan, Z., Alharbi, A., Badokhon, R., Alharazi, R., et al. (2023) Exploring the needs of patients undergoing hemodialysis: A qualitative study. *Cureus, 15*(12), e50076.2023

Al-Naimi, M. S., Rasheed, H. A., Hussien, N. R., Al-Kuraishy, H. M., & Al-Gareeb, A. I. (2019). Nephrotoxicity: Role and significance of renal biomarkers in the early detection of acute renal injury. *Journal of Advanced Pharmaceutical Technology & Research, 10*(3), 95.

Alobaidi, S. (2025). Emerging biomarkers and advanced diagnostics in chronic kidney disease: Early detection through multi-omics and AI. *Diagnostics (Basel), 15*(10), 1225.

Andersen-Hollekim, T., Landstad, B. J., Solbjør, M., Kvangarsnes, M., & Hole, T. (2021, February 16). Nephrologists' experiences with patient participation when long-term dialysis is required. *BMC Nephrology, 22*(1).

Årestedt, L., Martinsson, C., Hjelm, C., Uhlin, F., & Eldh, A. C. (2019). Patient participation in dialysis care—A qualitative study of patients' and health professionals' perspectives. *Health Expectations, 22*(6), 1285–1293.

Artificial Intelligence in Kidney Disease: A Comprehensive Study and Directions for Future Research.

Ashrafi, F., Mortazavi, M., & Nematbakhsh, M. (2022). The prevention of Cisplatin-induced nephrotoxicity: A general consensus statement of a group of oncologist-hematologists, adult and pediatric nephrologists, radiation oncologists, clinical pathologists, clinical pharmacologists, and renal physiologists on cisplatin therapy in cancer patients. *International Journal of Preventive Medicine, 13*, 21.

Assanatham, M., Pattanaprateep, O., Chuasuwan, A., Vareesangthip, K., Supasyndh, O., Lumpaopong, A., et al. (2022). Economic evaluation of peritoneal dialysis and hemodialysis in Thai population with End-stage Kidney Disease. *BMC Health Services Research, 22*(1), 1384.

Bajema, I. M., Wilhelmus, S., Alpers, C. E., Bruijn, J. A., Colvin, R. B., Cook, H. T., et al. (2018). Revision of the International Society of Nephrology/Renal Pathology Society classification for lupus nephritis: Clarification of definitions, and modified National Institutes of Health activity and chronicity indices. *Kidney International, 93*(4), 789–796.

Bazaev, N. A. (2020). Wearable artificial kidney Renart-PD. *BioMedical Engineering, 54*(2), 83–87.

Bernard, A., & Lauwerys, R. (1989). Epidemiological application of early markers of nephrotoxicity. *Toxicology Letters, 46*(1–3), 293–306.

Blagg, C. R. (2011). The 50th anniversary of long-term hemodialysis: University of Washington Hospital, March 9th, 1960. *Journal of Nephrology, 24*(Suppl 17), S84-88.

Burmeister, J. E., Mosmann, C. B., Costa, V. B., Saraiva, R. T., Grandi, R. R., Bastos, J. P., et al. (2014). Prevalence of cardiovascular risk factors in hemodialysis patients—The CORDIAL study. *Arquivos Brasileiros De Cardiologia, 102*(5), 473–480.

Chen, T., Sun, X., Tsuei, S., Yang, R., Yip, W., & Fu, H. (2024, December 21). Care for end-stage kidney disease in China: progress, challenges, and recommendations. *The Lancet Regional Health—Western Pacific, 54*, 101268–101268. Available from: https://www.thelancet.com/journals/lanwpc/article/PIIS2666-6065(24)00262-1/fulltext

Chronic Kidney Disease. (2025). *Wikipedia* [Internet]. https://en.wikipedia.org/w/index.php?title=Chronic_kidney_disease&oldid=1308982936

Craft, J., Gordon, C., Tiziani, A., Huether, S. E., Mccance, K. L., Brashers, V. L., et al. (2019). *Understanding pathophysiology—ANZ adaptation* (3rd ed.). Mosby.

Elias, M. A., Van Damme, W., & Wouters, E. (2022). Accessibility and quality of haemodialysis services in an urban setting in South India: A qualitative multiperspective study. *British Medical Journal Open, 12*(2), Article e052525.

Foley, R. N., Parfrey, P. S., & Sarnak, M. J. (1998). Epidemiology of cardiovascular disease in chronic renal disease. *Journal of the American Society of Nephrology, 9*(12 Suppl), S16-23.

GantsetsegGarmaa, N. R., TamásKói, N. U., Gergő, Kleiner D., et al. (2024). Panel miRNAs are potential diagnostic markers for chronic kidney diseases: a systematic review and meta-analysis. *BMC Nephrology, 13*(25), 1.

Glomerulonephritis | National Kidney Foundation. https://www.kidney.org/kidney-topics/glomerulonephritis

Guevara, B. A., & Borello, A. (2013). Guevara e-book by alfonso-borello - EPUB, 9781301324729.

Guo, Q., Wu, S., Xu, C., Wang, J., & Chen, J. (2021). Global disease burden from acute glomerulonephritis 1990–2019. *Kidney International Reports, 6*(8), 2212–2217.

Gupta, S., Mandal, S., Banerjee, K., Almarshood, H., Pushpakumar, S. B., & Sen, U. (2024). Complex pathophysiology of acute kidney injury (AKI) in aging: Epigenetic regulation, matrix remodeling, and the healing effects of H2S. *Biomolecules, 14*(9), 1165.

Gura, V., Rivara, M. B., Bieber, S., Munshi, R., Smith, N. C., Linke, L., et al. (2016). *A wearable artificial kidney for patients with end-stage renal disease*. American Society for Clinical Investigation. https://insight.jci.org/articles/view/86397/sd/1?utm_source=chatgpt.com

Haemodialysis was first used successfully in 1945. *History of Nephrology*. https://historyofnephrology.org/hd/haemodialysis-was-first-used-successfully-in-1945

Hart, P. D., & Bakris, G. L. (2010). Hypertensive nephropathy: Prevention and treatment recommendations. *Expert Opinion on Pharmacotherapy, 11*(16), 2675–2686.

Hassanein, M., Radhakrishnan, Y., Hernandez Garcilazo, N., Khor, S. Y., Norouzi, S., Anvari, E., et al. (2025). Global hemodialysis vascular access care: Three decades of evolution*. *The Journal of Vascular Access, 26*(1), 5–14.

He, Z., Liang, H., Huang, J., Zhang, D., Ma, H., Lin, J, et al. (2022, October 17). Impact of dialysis modality choice on the survival of end-stage renal disease patients with congestive heart failure in southern China: A retrospective cohort study, 9.

Hyodo, T., Hirawa, N., Kuragano, T., Takemoto, Y., Urabe, S., Adiya, S., et al. (2025, January 6). The present status of dialysis patients in Asian countries as of 2022 from a medical economic point of view. *Renal Replacement Therapy, 11*(1).

Hypertensive Nephropathy: Causes, Symptoms, and Treatment Options [Internet]. *The Kingsley Clinic*. https://thekingsleyclinic.com/resources/hypertensive-nephropathy-causes-symptoms-and-treatment-options/

Innovations in Dialysis: Transforming Kidney Care for a Healthier Future [Internet]. https://www.alliedacademies.org/articles/innovations-in-dialysis-transforming-kidney-care-for-a-healthier-future-31547.html?utm_source=chatgpt.com

Javed, A., Mahmood, T., Tiwari, R., Ahsan, F., Ansari, V. A., Bano, S., et al. (2025). Navigating nephropathy and nephrotoxicity: Understanding pathophysiology unveiling clinical manifestations, and exploring treatment approaches. *Journal of Basic and Clinical Physiology and Pharmacology, 36*(2–3), 69–93.

Jayanti, S., & Rangan, G. K. (2024). Advances in human-centered care to address contemporary unmet needs in chronic dialysis. *International Journal of Nephrology Renovascular Disease, 17*, 91–104.

Jegatheesan, D., Yang, W., Krishnasamy, R., Hawley, C., Johnson, D. W., Jegatheesan, D., et al. (2017). Cardiovascular disease in dialysis patients. In *Aspects in dialysis* [Internet]. IntechOpen [cited 2025 Sep 24]. https://www.intechopen.com/chapters/56689

Jha, V., Al-Ghamdi, S. M. G., Li, G., Wu, M. S., Stafylas, P., Retat, L., et al. (2023). Global economic burden associated with chronic kidney disease: A pragmatic review of medical costs for the inside CKD research programme. *Advances in Therapy, 40*(10), 4405–4420.

John Hopkins Medicine. Polycystic Kidney Disease [Internet]. Johns Hopkins Medicine. (2020). https://www.hopkinsmedicine.org/health/conditions-and-diseases/polycystic-kidney-disease

Keskinyan, V. S., Lattanza, B., & Reid-Adam, J. (2023). Glomerulonephritis. *Pediatrics in Review, 44*(9), 498–512.

Lewis, R. A., Benzies, K. M., MacRae, J., Thomas, C., & Tonelli, M. (2019). An exploratory study of person-centered care in a large urban hemodialysis program in Canada using a qualitative case-study methodology. *Canadian Journal of Kidney Health and Disease, 1*(6), 2054358119871539.

Li, L., Chen, K., Wen, C., Ma, X., & Huang, L. (2024). Association between systemic immune-inflammation index and chronic kidney disease: A population-based study. *PLoS ONE, 19*(2), e0292646-e292656.

Li, X., Cui, L., & Xu, H. (2024a). Association between systemic inflammation response index and chronic kidney disease: A population-based study. *Front Endocrinology (Lausanne), 15*, 1329256.

Li, Y., & Padman, R. (2025). *Enhancing end stage renal disease outcome prediction: A multi-sourced data-driven approach [Internet].* http://arxiv.org/abs/2410.01859

Li, Z., Song, L., Hua, R., Xia, F., Hu, D., Luo, Z., et al. (2024, May 30). Knowledge, attitudes, and practices toward cardiovascular complications among end-stage renal disease patients undergoing maintenance hemodialysis. BMC Public Health, *24*(1).

Limonte, C. P., Kretzler, M., Pennathur, S., Pop-Busui, R., & de Boer, I. H. (2022). Present and future directions in diabetic kidney disease. *Journal of Diabetes and Its Complications, 36*(12), Article 108357.

Lin, C. C., & Hwang, S. J. (2020). Patient-centered self-management in patients with chronic kidney disease: Challenges and implications. *International Journal of Environmental Research and Public Health, 17*(24), 9443.

Lopez-Giacoman, S., & Madero, M. (2015). Biomarkers in chronic kidney disease, from kidney function to kidney damage. *World Journal of Nephrology, 4*(1), 57–73.

Masakane, I., Ito, M., Tanida, H., & Nawano, T. (2023). Patient-centered care could improve quality of life and survival of dialysis patients: Dialysis prescription and daily practice. *Blood Purification, 52*(Suppl 1), 44–55.

McDonald, S. P., Marshall, M. R., Johnson, D. W., & Polkinghorne, K. R. (2009). Relationship between dialysis modality and mortality. *Journal of the American Society of Nephrology, 20*(1), 155–163.

Mishler, R. (2009). Autologous arteriovenous fistula creation by nephrologists. *Advances in Chronic Kidney Disease, 16*(5), 321–328.

Mizdrak, M., Kumrić, M., Kurir, T. T., & Božić, J. (2022). Emerging biomarkers for early detection of chronic kidney disease. *Journal of Personalized Medicine, 12*(4), 548.

Mushi, L., Marschall, P., Fleßa, S. (2015, June 15). The cost of dialysis in low and middle-income countries: a systematic review. *BMC Health Services Research [Internet], 15*(1). https://www.ncbi.nlm.nih.gov/pmc/articles/PMC4642658/

Mutatiri, C., Ratsch, A., McGrail, M., Venuthurupalli, S. K., & Chennakesavan, S. K. (2024). Primary and specialist care interaction and referral patterns for individuals with chronic kidney disease: A narrative review. *BMC Nephrology., 25*(1), 149.

Naik, R. S., & Jeedi, N. M. (2025). Mechanisms, risk factors and preventive measures associated with drug-induced nephrotoxicity: Review article. *Journal of Pharma Insights and Research, 3*(3), 028–035.

National Institute of Diabetes and Digestive and Kidney Diseases. *Kidney failure—NIDDK*. https://www.niddk.nih.gov/health-information/kidney-disease/kidney-failure

Ng, C. H., Ong, Z. H., Sran, H. K., & Wee, T. B. (2021). Comparison of cardiovascular mortality in hemodialysis versus peritoneal dialysis. *International Urology and Nephrology, 53*(7), 1363–1371.

Ogwang, A. J., Murungi, E. B., Vallence, N., & Esther, B. (2023). Lived experiences of patients on hemodialysis treatment at Kiruddu National Referral Hospital: A phenomenological study. *Patient Related Outcome Measures, 13*(14), 393–408.

Our History | Dialysis, Research | Northwest Kidney Centers. https://www.nwkidney.org/about-us/our-history

Pelle, M. C., Provenzano, M., Busutti, M., Porcu, C. V., Zaffina, I., Stanga, L., et al. (2022). Up-date on diabetic nephropathy. *Life, 12*(8), 1202.

Perone, F., Bernardi, M., Loguercio, M., Jacoangeli, F., Velardi, S., Metsovitis, T., et al. (2025). Cardiovascular disease risk assessment, exercise training, and management of complications in patients with chronic kidney disease. *International Journal of Cardiology Cardiovascular Risk and Prevention, 6*(25), Article 200386.

Petrović, D., & Stojimirović, B. (2008). Cardiovascular morbidity and mortality in patients treated with hemodialysis–epidemiological analysis. *Vojnosanitetski Pregled, 65*(12), 893–900.

Pócsi, I., Dockrell, M. E., & Price, R. G. (2022). Nephrotoxic biomarkers with specific indications for metallic pollutants: Implications for environmental health. *Biomark Insights, 17*, 11772719221111882.

Polycystic kidney disease (PKD)—Symptoms, causes, treatment | National Kidney Foundation. https://www.kidney.org/kidney-topics/polycystic-kidney-disease

Popović, B., Šutić, I., & Marković, N. B. (2016). Nephrotoxic drugs. *Acta Medica Croatica, 70*(4–5), 309–314.

Preciado, P., Zhang, H., Thijssen, S., Kooman, J. P., Van Der Sande, F. M., & Kotanko, P. (2019). All-cause mortality in relation to changes in relative blood volume during hemodialysis. *Nephrology Dialysis Transplantation, 34*(8), 1401–1408.

Rambod, M., Pasyar, N., & Parviniannasab, A. M. (2023). A qualitative study on hope in Iranian end stage renal disease patients undergoing hemodialysis. *BMC Nephrology, 24*(1), 281.

Rao, H., Guo, Y., Qiu, L., & Ren, X. (2025). Exploring health challenges and coping strategies in young patients undergoing maintenance hemodialysis: A qualitative study. *BMC Nephrology, 26*(1), 378.

Redahan, L., & Murray, P. T. (2017). Biomarkers of drug-induced kidney injury. *Current Opinion in Critical Care, 23*(6), 463–469.

Refaat, H., Sany, D., Mohab, A., & Ezzat, H. (2016). Comparing dialysis modality and cardiovascular mortality in patients on hemodialysis and peritoneal dialysis. *Advances in Peritoneal Dialysis, 32*, 22–31.

Renalyx launches India's first indigenous AI based smart hemodialysis machine, makes renal care accessible and affordable. *Mumbai News—The Times of India*.

Reynolds M, *DeepMind's new AI predicts kidney injury two days before it happens*. Wired.

Romagnani, P., Kitching, A. R., Leung, N., & Anders, H. J. (2023). The five types of glomerulonephritis classified by pathogenesis, activity and chronicity (GN-AC). *Nephrology Dialysis Transplantation, 1*(38, Supplement_2), ii3–10.

Rysz, J., Gluba-Brzózka, A., Franczyk, B., Jabłonowski, Z., & Ciałkowska-Rysz, A. (2017). Novel biomarkers in the diagnosis of chronic kidney disease and the prediction of its outcome. *International Journal of Molecular Sciences, 18*(8), 1702.

Sabath, E., & Robles-Osorio, M. L. (2012). Renal health and the environment: Heavy metal nephrotoxicity. *Nefrología, 32*(3), 279–286.

Sagoo, M. K, & Gnudi, L. (2020). Diabetic nephropathy: An overview. In L. Gnudi & D. A. Long (Eds.), *Diabetic nephropathy* (pp. 3–7). Springer US (Methods in Molecular Biology; vol. 2067).

Samsu, N. (2021). Diabetic nephropathy: Challenges in pathogenesis, diagnosis, and treatment. *BioMed Research International, 2021*(1), 1497449.

Sari, A. (2019). Nephrotoxic effects of drugs. In *Poisoning in the modern world—New tricks for an old dog?* [Internet]. IntechOpen. https://www.intechopen.com/chapters/65306

Seccia, T. M., Caroccia, B., & Calò, L. A. (2017). Hypertensive nephropathy. Moving from classic to emerging pathogenetic mechanisms. *Journal of Hypertension, 35*(2), 205–212.

Shahgholian, N., & Yousefi, H. (2018). The lived experiences of patients undergoing hemodialysis with the concept of care: A phenomenological study. *BMC Nephrology., 19*(1), 338.

Sharma, N., Khav, E., Elahmadi, A., Ong, J., & Parag, S. (2024). Dr. Willem Kolff: The father of the artificial kidney. *Cureus, 16*(9), e69098.

Suja, A., Anju, R., Anju, V., Neethu, J., Peeyush, P., & Saraswathy, R. (2012). Economic evaluation of end stage renal disease patients undergoing hemodialysis. *Journal of Pharmacy and Bioallied Sciences, 4*(2), 107–111.

Thipsawat, S. (2021). Early detection of diabetic nephropathy in patient with type 2 diabetes mellitus: A review of the literature. *Diabetes & Vascular Disease Research, 18*(6), 14791641211058856.

Tong, A., Winkelmayer, W. C., Wheeler, D. C., van Biesen, W., Tugwell, P., Manns, B., et al. (2017). Nephrologists' perspectives on defining and applying patient-centered outcomes in hemodialysis. *Clinical Journal of the American Society of Nephrology, 12*(3), 454–466.

Uber, A. M., & Sutherland, S. M. (2020). Nephrotoxins and nephrotoxic acute kidney injury. *Pediatric Nephrology(Berlin, Germany), 35*(10), 1825–1833.

van Lieshout, T. S., Klerks, A. K., Mahic, O., Vernooij, R. W. M., Eisenga, M. F., van Jaarsveld, B. C., et al. (2021). Comparative iron management in hemodialysis and peritoneal dialysis patients: A systematic review. *Front Nephrology, 4*. https://doi.org/10.3389/fneph.2024.1488758/full

Vanherweghem, J. L., Depierreux, M., Tielemans, C., Abramowicz, D., Dratwa, M., Jadoul, M., et al. (1993). Rapidly progressive interstitial renal fibrosis in young women: Association with slimming regimen including Chinese herbs. *Lancet, 341*(8842), 387–391.

Wakasugi, M., Kazama, J. J., & Narita, I. (2015). Anticipated increase in the number of patients who require dialysis treatment among the aging population of Japan. *Therapeutic Apheresis and Dialysis, 19*(3), 201–206.

Wang, I. K., Lu, C. Y., Lin, C. L., Liang, C. C., Yen, T. H., Liu, Y. L., et al. (2016). Comparison of the risk of de novo cardiovascular disease between hemodialysis and peritoneal dialysis in patients with end-stage renal disease. *International Journal of Cardiology, 1*(218), 219–224.

Wang, X. C., Liu, C. H., Chen, Y. J., Wu, Y., Yang, L. S., Liu, H. M., et al. (2013). Clinical and pathological analysis of the kidney in patients with hypertensive nephropathy. *Experimental and Therapeutic Medicine, 6*(5), 1243–1246.

Wilson, P. D. (2004). Polycystic kidney disease: New understanding in the pathogenesis. *International Journal of Biochemistry & Cell Biology, 36*(10), 1868–1873.

Wu, H., & Huang, J. (2018). *Drug-induced nephrotoxicity: Pathogenic mechanisms, biomarkers and prevention strategies*. http://eurekaselect.com; https://eurekaselect.com/article/86766

Xi, K., Zhang, M., Li, M., Tang, Q., Zhao, Q., & Chen, W. (2023). Unveiling the mechanisms of nephrotoxicity caused by nephrotoxic compounds using toxicological network analysis. *Molecular Therapy Nucleic Acids, 10*(34), Article 102075.

Yongphiphatwong, N., Teerawattananon, Y., Supapol, P., Pandejpong, D., Chuanchaiyakul, T, Sutawong J., et al. (2025, April 1). The way home: a scoping review of public health interventions to increase the utilization of home dialysis in chronic kidney disease patients. *BMC Nephrology, 26*(1).

Zazzeroni, L., Pasquinelli, G., Nanni, E., Cremonini, V., & Rubbi, I. (2017). Comparison of Quality of Life in Patients Undergoing Hemodialysis and Peritoneal Dialysis: A Systematic Review and Meta-Analysis. *Kidney & Blood Pressure Research [Internet], 42*(4), 717–727. https://www.ncbi.nlm.nih.gov/pubmed/29049991

Zhang, L., Jiang, L., Xu, R., Zhang, X., Zhang, B., & Yue, R. (2021). Epidemiological research on diabetic nephropathy at global, regional, and national levels from 1990 to 2021: An analysis derived from the global burden of disease 2021 study. *Front Endocrinology*.

Zhou, Q., Jiang, L., Su, T., Liu, G., & Yang, L. (2023). Overview of aristolochic acid nephropathy: An update. *Kidney Research and Clinical Practice, 42*(5), 579–590.

Chapter 7
The Body-Brain Connection: Cognitive Decline and Mental Health

Abhishek Ambawatiya, Ritu Dahiya, Sarasa Meenakshi, Mamta Bishnoi, Sirajudheen Anwar, Krishna Murti, Md. Abubakar, and Nitesh Kumar

Abstract The complex two-way relationship between the body and brain is crucial for maintaining mental health and cognitive function. Problems with physiological systems can lead to cognitive decline, anxiety, depression, and neurodegenerative disorders. This review examines the neurobiological mechanisms that support this connection, encompassing the nervous, endocrine, and immune systems, as well as the gut-brain axis and the hypothalamic–pituitary–adrenal (HPA) axis. This chapter examines the primary causes of cognitive impairment, including ageing, chronic inflammation, hormonal imbalances, lifestyle factors (such as diet, exercise, and sleep), and chronic stress. It also talks about how these things are related to diseases like Alzheimer's, Parkinson's, and vascular dementia. Mental health disorders are conceptualised as having physiological origins, affected by systemic inflammation, metabolic dysregulation, and pain. In contrast, interventions such as physical activity, mindfulness, pharmacotherapy, and non-pharmacological therapies (e.g., cognitive training and neuromodulation) exhibit potential for alleviating these effects. Future directions emphasise individualised medicine, new technologies (such as AI-driven

A. Ambawatiya · Md. Abubakar (✉) · N. Kumar (✉)
Department of Pharmacology and Toxicology, National Institute of Pharmaceutical Education and Research (NIPER), Hajipur, India
e-mail: mdabuabakr731@gmail.com

N. Kumar
e-mail: nitesh.kumar04@niperhajipur.ac.in

R. Dahiya
School of Pharmacy, Lingaya's Vidyapeeth (Deemed to be University), Faridabad, India

S. Meenakshi · K. Murti
Department of Pharmacy Practice, National Institute of Pharmaceutical Education and Research, Hajipur, India

M. Bishnoi
Department of Pharmacy, School of Medical and Allied Science, Galgotias University, Greater Noida, India

S. Anwar
Department of Pharmacology and Toxicology, College of Pharmacy, University of Hail, Hail, Saudi Arabia

K. Adhikary et al. (eds.), *Healing Beyond Blood Sugar*,
https://doi.org/10.1007/978-981-95-8946-3_7

biomarkers and brain-computer interfaces), and strategies to maintain brain health in the long term. This chapter emphasises the necessity for comprehensive interventions that focus on body-brain synergy to avert cognitive decline and bolster mental resilience by promoting an integrative, multimodal approach.

Keywords Body-brain connection · Cognitive decline · Mental health · HPA axis · Neuroinflammation · Gut-brain axis · Lifestyle interventions · Personalized medicine

7.1 Introduction to the Body-Brain Connection

7.1.1 Body-Brain Connection

The body and brain function as a single integrated system, continuously exchanging information, rather than operating separately as isolated entities. All the body's vital systems, including the nervous, endocrine, immune, and other organs and tissues, are interrelated with the brain for their dynamic communication exchanges (Buzsáki, 2023). In this sense, we can say that all cognitive, emotional, behavioural, and sensory activities reflect biological origins and have a biological impact; similarly, every motor or physiological activity affects the way we think and feel. The autonomic nervous system (ANS) regulates all vital activities that facilitate the control of respiration, heart rate, digestion, and a range of stress responses (Thompson et al., 2020). The endocrine system also serves as a bridge between the brain. The brain, especially the hypothalamus, controls hormone secretion that influences sleep, mood, cognition, behaviour, and energy. The systems create a feedback mechanism through which the brain sends signals, and the body responds accordingly, and vice versa (McEwen, 1999).

For example, when you become stressed, the brain activates the hypothalamic–pituitary–adrenal (HPA) axis to release cortisol and adrenaline. It helps to regulate how the body reacts to stress and prepares the body for fight, flight, or freeze. In this axis, corticotropin-releasing hormone, adrenocorticotropic hormone and cortisol hormone send feedback signals, and this negative feedback loop ensures hormone balance and recovery after stress. The HPA axis acts as the communication connection between mind and body, converting psychological stress into hormonal signals that affect physical health and emotional well-being (Sharan and Vellapandian, 2024). Such a type of feedback system between body and brain represents a continuous exchange of information between the physiology and psychology of the whole person.

7.1.1.1 The Bidirectional Information Flow

Information passed between the body and brain is bidirectional; in that it flows both ways:

- **Top-down communication** occurs when the brain actively takes part to regulate various vital systems via sending signals, e.g., controlling respiration, cardiac rate, hormone secretion, and muscle movement.
- **Bottom-up communication** is the reverse of the above cycle; in this body's physiologic activities, sensory and chemical signals are sent to the brain, and accordingly, the brain sends signals to the body, such as hunger-thirst signals, pain-inflammation, sensations from the gut, and immune responses.

7.1.1.2 Main Systems Involved in the Body-Brain Connection

Multiple biological systems facilitate this ongoing communication:

The nervous system

The central nervous system (CNS), the control centre of the body, coordinates all voluntary and involuntary actions. It consists of two main parts: the brain and the spinal cord. The brain is a complex organ composed of the cerebrum, cerebellum, brainstem, and diencephalon. The spinal cord is made of long, thin bundles of nerve fibres. CNS receives information, interprets it, and sends signals to muscles and glands to produce movement or reactions. CNS closely works with PNS, which transmits signals back and forth to the body. The PNS hosts the autonomic nervous system (ANS), which is essential for the body's involuntary functions. The ANS is further divided into two branches: the sympathetic nervous system (SNS) and the parasympathetic nervous system (PNS) (Thau et al., 2022).

The endocrine system

The endocrine system is a network of glands that releases chemical messengers known as hormones. These hormones are released into the bloodstream and regulate various body functions, including growth, metabolism, reproduction, and mood, through the actions of cortisol, adrenaline, serotonin, and dopamine, among others. This system works slowly and continuously, unlike the nervous system (Campbell & Jialal, 2022). Major endocrine glands are hypothalamus (releases CRH, TRH, and GnRH), pituitary gland (GH, TSH, ACTH, LH, and FSH), pineal glans (Melatonin), Thyroid Gland (T4, T3, and Calcitonin) Parathyroid (PTH), adrenal gland (cortisol, adrenaline, and aldosterone), pancreas (insulin, and glucagon), Gonads (estrogen, progesterone, and testosterone) and thymus (Thymosin) (Ring, 2025). Regulation of metabolism, growth and development, reproduction, response to stress, Homeostasis, mood and behavioural control are a few key functions of the endocrine system.

The immune system

The immune system and the brain work together to maintain overall health and balance, a process known as homeostasis. The vagus nerve plays a crucial role in connecting the brain to major organs, as well as in communicating between the body and the central nervous system. Any inflammation or infection signals are sent to the brain via the vagus nerve, and the brain activates anti-inflammatory pathways, known as the inflammatory reflex (Bonaz et al., 2017).

The gut–brain axis

The gut due to the presence of the enteric nervous system (ENS) which is a complex network of embedded neurones within the walls of the digestive tract, referred to as the "second brain," It is through the ENS that the gut communicates with the brain directly using the vagus nerve, sending messages about digestion, nutrient balance, and the composition of gut microbes (Pediatric Neurogastroenterology, 2022). The gut microbiome (the trillions of bacteria that populate the intestines) produces neurotransmitters such as serotonin and dopamine that, in turn, influence mood, memory and emotional regulation (Mhanna et al., 2023). Recent advancements in neuroscience, psychoneuroimmunology, and mind–body medicine have made the body–brain connection measurable and observable. For example, functional MRI (fMRI) scans show that emotions are "not only in the head," but run through complex networks that involve the brainstem, heart, and viscera. Research also indicates quantitative benefits of mind–body practices such as mindfulness, breathwork, and exercise on neuroplasticity and immune function (Jiménez & Mills, 2012). As shown in Fig. 7.1

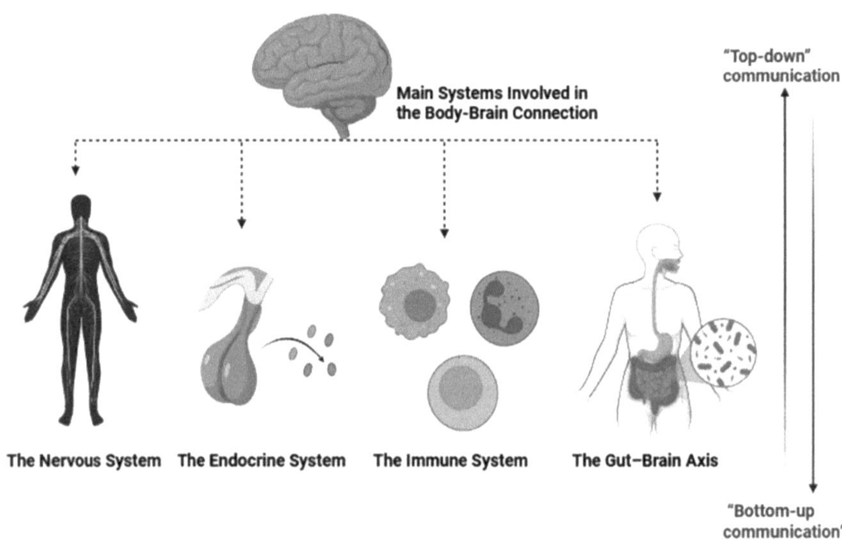

Fig. 7.1 The diagram illustrates the key biological systems that mediate communication between the body and the brain, including the nervous system, endocrine system, immune system, and the gut–brain axis. These systems enable bidirectional signaling—"top-down" communication from the brain to regulate bodily functions, and "bottom-up" communication from the body to influence brain activity and mental states

7.1.2 *Importance of Understanding Cognitive and Mental Health Interactions*

The connection between mind and body is not only structural but functional and experiential. It is crucial to understand the physiological state of the brain and body in relation to cognitive states, as well as how cognitive states influence physiological responses, to advance mental health care, education, and human performance (Renoir et al., 2013). Mental states and cognitive processes are not separate systems; they are part of the same neurobiological system, with overlapping dimensions. Every emotional change we experience impacts the way we think. Every cognitive state we access (such as stress, optimism, and concentration) causes a physiological state change in our body (Salzman & Fusi, 2010).

7.1.2.1 The Interplay of Cognition and Emotion

Cognition and emotion are inextricably linked, forming the very essence of the human experience. Cognition includes mechanisms such as attention, memory, perception, and problem-solving. Emotion can also influence motivation, decision-making, and interpretations of actions (Tyng et al., 2017).

A substantial body of evidence emerged in neuroscience showing that the two processes, cognition and emotion, are reliant on shared anatomical structures. For example, the amygdala (involved in emotional processing) and the prefrontal cortex (involved in executive control) are never disconnected (Okon-Singer et al., 2015). In other words, they are assumed to be exchanging information constantly. This complex interchange between cognition and emotion occurs effortlessly and, in a desirable state, so that a person can think clearly, modulate behaviour/emotions, and adaptively respond to challenges in their life (Liu et al., 2009). However, if this is damaged in some way (i.e., stress, trauma, hormonal imbalance), emotional reactions can hinder the cognitive processes, often resulting in anxiety, impulsivity, and a general fatigue of cognitive resources (Eslinger et al., 2021).

So, the complexity of this interaction shows that mental health is a neural harmony between emotional processing and cognitive systems.

7.1.2.2 Cognitive Health as Part of Mental Well-Being

Across the lifespan, mental and cognitive health exists in a dynamic, reciprocal relationship.

Cognitive activities such as attention, memory, learning, decision-making, and problem-solving form the base of mental health, as these also decide how effectively a person can perceive, interpret, and respond to their environment (Gautam et al., 2024). For example:

- Sleep is essential for neural repair, memory consolidation, and emotional regulation. Sleep deprivation disrupts the prefrontal cortex and heightens amygdala activity.
- Nutritional deficits, such as low levels of omega-3 fatty acids, iron, amino acids or B-vitamins, limit the synthesis of neurotransmitters serotonin and dopamine, leading to mood instability, fatigue, and cognitive dullness.
- Sedentary lifestyles reduce blood flow and oxygen supply to the brain by slowing the metabolism of the brain and are associated with depression, anxiety, and cognitive decline.

On the other hand, regular physical activity, adequate sleep, balanced nutrition, mindfulness, meditation, and cognitive training all contribute to improved clarity of thought and emotional modulation. Thus, maintaining physical brain health through a balanced diet, regular exercise, and stress management is essential for preserving both cognitive performance and emotional stability. Aspects of cognitive health emphasize that the physical health of the brain is a significant contributor, if not the primary contributor, to maintaining mental health (Calderone et al., 2024).

7.1.2.3 Mental Health and Cognitive Decline

Across the lifespan, mental and cognitive health are interconnected. Disruptions in emotional well-being can impair thinking, memory, and attention, while declines in cognitive performance can intensify feelings of sadness, anxiety, or frustration (McManus et al., 2022). Some examples are:

Individuals with chronic anxiety often experience difficulties with working memory, attention, and decision-making. This happens because hyperactivation of the amygdala, the brain's fear center, continuously signals the prefrontal cortex. As a result, cognitive resources are drained, leading to poor concentration and reduced problem-solving ability (Dehdar & Raoufy, 2023). In older adults, neurodegenerative diseases such as Alzheimer's disease or parkinson's disease not only impair memory, attention, and reasoning but also produce emotional symptoms like apathy, irritability, or depression (Mortby et al., 2022).

The connection between thoughts, emotions, and physical health is a biological reality, not just a psychological concept (Ohrnberger et al., 2017) Stress triggers the hypothalamic–pituitary–adrenal (HPA) axis, leading to increased cortisol levels, a higher heart rate, and elevated blood pressure. Chronic stress can impair immunity, digestion, and even brain structure over time. Physical states, such as illnesses like thyroid disorders or chronic pain, can affect the mind and influence mood and cognitive clarity. Nutritional deficiencies and poor sleep can impair neurotransmitter production, resulting in reduced cognitive efficiency and emotional resilience. In short, the mind and body form an integrated system, providing a more comprehensive understanding of what it means to be healthy and mentally strong (Yaribeygi et al., 2017).

7.2 Mechanisms Linking Body and Brain

The intricate interplay between the brain and body is fundamentally governed by the interactive functions of the nervous, endocrine, and immune systems, collectively forming what is often referred to as the neuro-endocrine-immune (NEI) network (Eslinger et al., 2021). This integrated system is crucial for maintaining physiological balance and influencing mental health and cognitive processes. Psychological stress can activate the nervous system, which in turn influences the endocrine and immune systems, leading to or exacerbating conditions such as skin diseases. Understanding these complex interactions is critical for developing holistic approaches to health. For instance, interventions focusing on adjusting cognition and emotion, psychoeducation, and family-focused therapy can address mental health issues arising from a disordered limbic system, which is influenced by factors like inflammation, genetic background, and environmental stressors (Daëron, 2022).

7.2.1 The Nervous System's Function

The nervous system functions as the body's primary communication network, facilitating rapid adaptation to both internal and external stimuli through its intricate relay of information between the brain, spinal cord, and the rest of the body. Beyond its role in general communication, the nervous system actively participates in modulating attentional processes and emotional states. Anxiety, for example, can significantly impair the neural suppression of known distractor features during visual search tasks.

7.2.1.1 Central and Peripheral Systems

These protective systems are made up of two central functions:

The central nervous system (CNS) is primarily made up of the brain and spinal cord. Its purpose is to process information, make decisions, and have to do with higher-order, cognitive, and emotional functions (Thau et al., 2022).

The peripheral nervous system (PNS) connects the CNS to the remainder of the body, carrying signals to and from muscles, organs, and glands. The PNS is made of the autonomic nervous system ANS, which is responsible for involuntary bodily functions, such as heart rate, digestion, and breathing (Shoykhet & Structure, 2011). The ANS consists of at least two divisions:

- The sympathetic nervous system (SNS) is responsible for the "fight or flight" response to stress, getting the body prepared for a stressful or dangerous situation or another stressor.
- The parasympathetic nervous system (PNS) supports the body's "rest and digest" functions (e.g., recovery, repair, energy conservation).

A healthy balance between these two systems supports emotional regulation and overall physical well-being. Chronic stress keeps the SNS triggered, and the PNS downregulated, which can result in neuromotor dysfunction (i.e., anxiety), sleep disruption, and decline in immune health, particularly in long-term chronic stressors (Weissman & Mendes, 2021).

7.2.1.2 The Brain as a Regulator of the Body

Through sensory feedback, the brain continuously assesses the internal environment of the body and makes adjustments to its functions to maintain a stable internal state, known as homeostasis. For instance, as body temperature increases, the brain elicits physiological responses to cool the body. Similarly, a decrease in energy levels triggers hunger sensations in the brain. Several brain structures hold an essential place in linking the body and mind:

- The hypothalamus responds with hormonal responses, regulates hunger levels, maintains body temperature, and elicits responses to stress.
- The amygdala processes emotional stress responses, such as fear and pleasure.
- The prefrontal cortex is involved in considering options for making a decision, emotional regulation, and responding to and relieving stress.

Together, these brain structures form a dynamic feedback loop where physiological sensations modulate emotional and cognitive states, while mental states influence physiological activity.

7.2.2 Hormonal Influences on Cognition and Mood

Hormones are released by the endocrine glands into the bloodstream to act as chemical messengers. They control energy levels, metabolism, growth, and mood. Hormones act throughout the body, and thus, they are an essential link between the brain and other parts of the body (Campbell & Jialal, 2022).

7.2.2.1 The Endocrine System and the HPA Axis

One of the most significant links between the body and the brain is the hypothalamic–pituitary–adrenal (HPA) axis, which regulates the body's response to stress.

When you experience a stressor, the hypothalamus releases corticotropin-releasing hormone (CRH), which prompts the secretion of adrenocorticotropic hormone (ACTH) from the pituitary gland. ACTH signals the adrenal glands to release cortisol, the primary stress hormone (Kageyama et al., 2021). Cortisol increases alertness and energy in the short term, which helps the body cope with stressors. When cortisol levels are high for long periods of time, it begins to damage the brain, specifically the hippocampus, which plays a role in memory and likely contributes to mental health issues such as anxiety, depression, and mental fatigue (Knezevic et al., 2023).

7.2.2.2 Sex Hormones and Brain Function

Hormones such as estrogen, progesterone and testosterone also affect mood and cognition.

- Estrogen supports serotonin production and protects brain cells, which helps stabilize moods and maintain sharper memory.
- Progesterone fosters relaxation and calm but may cause irritability and/or fatigue if in excess or imbalance.
- Testosterone boosts motivation, confidence and energy, but high levels may foster increased aggression and impulse levels.

Hormonal fluctuations, particularly those occurring during significant life stages such as puberty, pregnancy, and menopause, exert a profound influence on emotional stabilization and cognitive performance through their intricate interactions within the neuro-endocrine-immune (NEI) network. These changes highlight the bidirectional communication between the endocrine system and the nervous system, affecting various brain functions and contributing to psychological and cognitive alterations.

7.2.2.3 Thyroid and Metabolic Hormones

The thyroid gland plays a vital role in regulating the body's metabolic rate through the production of thyroxine (T4) and triiodothyronine (T3) hormones. When thyroid hormone levels are insufficient (hypothyroidism), the body's metabolism slows down, leading to symptoms such as fatigue, slowed thinking, poor concentration, and depressive mood (Nuguru et al., 2022). Conversely, excess thyroid hormone production (hyperthyroidism) accelerates metabolic processes and can lead to anxiety, nervousness, restlessness, and insomnia. Elevated T_3 and T_4 levels overstimulate the central nervous system, increasing heart rate, irritability, and emotional sensitivity.

7.2.3 *Inflammation and Its Impact on Mental Health*

Inflammation has emerged as a significant factor in the pathophysiology of various mental health conditions, including depression and anxiety. Research over the past two decades has established a strong association between elevated inflammatory markers and psychiatric disorders, suggesting that inflammation is not merely a consequence but potentially a contributing cause of these conditions (Skaper et al., 2018).

7.2.3.1 The Immune System–Brain Connection

A key mechanism underlying the immune system-brain connection in mental health involves the activation of glial cells—specifically astrocytes and microglia—within the central nervous system (CNS). When activated, these cells release a cascade of pro-inflammatory cytokines, such as tumour necrosis factor-alpha (TNF-α), interleukin-1 beta (IL-1β), and interleukin-6 (IL-6) (Bhol et al., 2024). However, when the immune system remains overactive, an increased permeability of the blood–brain barrier (BBB) is triggered by stress, a poor diet, lack of sleep, or infection, or systemic inflammatory mediators like interferon-alpha (IFN-α), which interfere with neurotransmitter function and neural connectivity.

Research shows that elevated levels of immune cells in the BBB lead to activation of glial cells and amplify the inflammatory response, resulting in neuronal damage and dysfunction. These inflammatory markers, including C-reactive protein (CRP), tumour necrosis factor-alpha (TNF-α), and interleukin-6 (IL-6), are associated with depression, fatigue, and cognitive decline. A more recently investigated biomarker, the C-reactive protein to lymphocyte ratio (CLR), has also been associated with depression and anxiety in diverse populations. These findings underscore the importance of considering the immune system's role in brain health and mental well-being, paving the way for more targeted and holistic treatment approaches for psychiatric disorders—this field of study is known as psychoneuroimmunology (Paganin & Signorini, 2024).

7.2.3.2 Stress and Inflammation

Stress is a well-established modulator of immune function, often leading to an upregulation of pro-inflammatory pathways. This intricate connection involves a complex interplay of neural, endocrine, and immune mechanisms. Under acute stress, the body typically mounts a "fight or flight" response, involving the rapid release of hormones such as cortisol and catecholamines. Stress activates the HPA axis, leading to the release of glucocorticoids like cortisol. While glucocorticoids initially have anti-inflammatory effects, chronic exposure can lead to glucocorticoid receptor insensitivity, resulting in a paradoxical pro-inflammatory state. This dysregulation contributes to persistent inflammation. This can create a feedback loop: stress causes inflammation, and inflammation in turn worsens mood and increases stress sensitivity. Breaking this cycle is essential for mental well-being.

7.2.3.3 Reducing Inflammation to Protect Mental Health

Several lifestyle factors help lower inflammation and support healthy brain function:

- Regular exercise reduces inflammatory markers and boosts endorphins.

- Balanced nutrition, especially diets rich in omega-3 fatty acids, antioxidants, and fibre, supports gut health and reduces inflammation.
- Adequate sleep allows the body to repair and regulate immune activity.
- Mindfulness and relaxation techniques lower stress hormones and reduce inflammatory responses.

7.3 Cognitive Decline: Causes and Contributors

A gradual decline in intellectual abilities, including memory, reasoning, attention, and problem-solving, characterizes cognitive decline. While mild cognitive change is often considered a regular part of ageing, pathological cognitive decline can lead to debilitating disorders such as dementia and Alzheimer's disease. Recognizing biological, psychological, and lifestyle factors related to cognitive decline is essential in developing preventive and therapeutic approaches (Colita et al., 2024).

7.3.1 Ageing and Neurodegenerative Diseases

Ageing is influenced by cellular stress, immune system alterations, and mitochondrial dysfunction, which collectively contribute to accelerated ageing and age-related diseases. Ageing leads to a decline in body functions and age-related diseases, for example, Alzheimer's disease, which adversely affects human health and longevity. Key biological mechanisms linking ageing to neurodegeneration include DNA damage and repair deficiencies, oxidative stress, reduced neurogenesis, telomere shortening, cellular senescence, neuronal death, synaptic pruning, and decreased plasticity. With age, the hippocampus, a crucial component in learning and memory, becomes significantly smaller, leading to slower processing speeds and increased memory lapses (Marzola et al., 2023).

Neurodegenerative diseases, such as Alzheimer's disease (AD), Parkinson's disease (PD), Huntington's disease (HD), and amyotrophic lateral sclerosis (ALS), and vascular dementia, are characterized by the accumulation of misfolded and aggregated proteins, such as amyloid-beta (Aβ) and tau in AD, α-synuclein in PD, and mutant huntingtin (mHTT) in HD. They are amplified by the brain's innate immune response to pathological protein aggregates and cellular debris. Activated microglia and astrocytes, while initially protective, can become chronically activated, releasing neurotoxic substances that perpetuate a cycle of inflammation and neuronal damage, thereby accelerating disease progression. Key genetic risk factors include mutations in the *APP*, *PSEN1*, and *PSEN2* genes for early-onset AD, and the *APOE4* allele for late-onset AD. PD is defined by the loss of dopamine-producing neurons and α-synuclein pathology, resulting in its characteristic motor deficits (Abyadeh et al., 2023).

Oxidative stress and mitochondrial dysfunction also contribute to the acceleration of neuronal ageing. Reactive oxygen species (ROS) impair neuronal integrity and cause damage to lipids, proteins, and DNA. Likewise, neuroinflammation is caused by activated microglia and astrocytes, secreting cytokines including IL-1β and TNF-α, resulting in synaptic loss and neuronal apoptosis (Jurcău et al., 2022).

7.3.2 Lifestyle Factors: Diet, Exercise, and Sleep

Lifestyle factors have a profound impact on brain health and brain ageing. Recent studies have revealed that behaviours that can be modified, such as diet, physical activity level, and sleep quality, can alter cognitive patterns.

Dietary habits can either favour or guard against cognitive decline. Diets considered protective in the context of cognitive decline include antioxidants, omega-3 fatty acids, vitamins (B12, D, and E), and polyphenols, such as those found in the Mediterranean diet, which help preserve neuronal health by diminishing oxidative stress and inflammation (Johnstone et al., 2025). Conversely, higher consumption of saturated fats, refined sugars, and processed foods can increase the risk of insulin resistance, vascular dysfunction, and neuroinflammation, all of which can affect cognitive function. Nutritional deficiencies have been linked to memory loss and neural abnormalities, including defects in the vitamin B complex and omega-3 fatty acids.

Regular exercise of the cardiovascular system enhances cerebral blood flow, promotes neurogenesis (the development of new neurons), and increases the expression of BDNF (brain-derived neurotrophic factor). Regular exercise, also known as physical activity, releases the body's endorphins and growth factors, which can enhance and promote synaptic plasticity. Aerobic exercise (walking, swimming, or cycling), even for a short period of time, improved executive function and memory in older adults suffering from mild cognitive changes (Romero Garavito et al., 2025).

Sleep, often an overlooked lifestyle factor, is critical to memory consolidation and the maintenance of synaptic homeostasis and function. During deep sleep, the brain clears metabolic waste products of neural energy use (including amyloid beta) from the interstitial space to the glymphatic system. Sleep loss and chronic sleep deprivation can lead to conditions that disrupt sleep architecture, which are significantly associated with cognitive decline (Erum & Dam, 2019).

7.3.3 Chronic Stress and Cognitive Impairment

Chronic stress significantly contributes to cognitive decline through several neuroendocrine, inflammatory, and structural mechanisms. Chronic activation of the hypothalamic–pituitary–adrenal (HPA) axis increases cortisol levels, which can lead to damage of the hippocampal neurons, inhibition of neurogenesis, and impairment in synaptic functioning. Elevated cortisol levels also negatively impact glucose uptake and cerebral blood flow, leading to reductions in cognitive efficiency (Knezevic et al., 2023).

Chronic stress also initiates neuroinflammation with the activation of microglia and increasing tonic levels of pro-inflammatory cytokines that impact neurotransmitter signalling and plasticity, facilitating depressive and anxious behaviours leading to further cognitive declines. In addition to HPA axis dysregulation and neuroinflammation, chronic stress alters the dopamine and serotonin systems, both of which are known to have key roles in motivation, learning and emotional regulation (Sălcudean et al., 2025).

Neuroimaging studies have shown that chronic psychological stress is associated with synaptogenesis in the hippocampus (hippocampal shrinkage), hyperactivity of the amygdala, and impaired functionality of the prefrontal cortex, all of which are pharmacologically and physiologically linked to disturbances in memory, attention, and decision-making. Lastly, chronic stress contributes to the acceleration of telomere shortening (a marker of cellular ageing), thereby increasing susceptibility to neurodegenerative disorders (Ben-Zion et al., 2023).

7.4 Mental Health and Its Physical Roots

Physical processes that take place throughout the body are closely related to mental health, which is often thought of as being solely psychological. The brain never operates in isolation; it is constantly interacting with hormones, organ systems, immunological reactions, and metabolic processes. According to recent scientific discoveries, physical health conditions, including systemic inflammation, chronic pain, and gut microbiota imbalance, can significantly affect mental and emotional wellness. The gut-brain axis, physical illnesses, and chronic pain are the three main physical components of mental health that are examined in this chapter.

7.4.1 The Gut-Brain Axis and Mental Well-Being

The gut-brain axis is a complex, two-way communication system that links the central nervous system (CNS) with the gastrointestinal (GI) tract via neurological, hormonal, and immunological pathways. The vagus nerve, enteric nervous system (ENS), and gut bacteria are at the core of this interaction and have an impact on behaviour, emotions, and cognitive functions (Ashique et al., 2024).

The gut microbiome, comprising trillions of bacteria, fungi, and viruses, produces a range of neuroactive compounds that regulate mood and anxiety, including serotonin, dopamine, and gamma-aminobutyric acid (GABA). Surprisingly, about 90% of the serotonin in the body is produced in the gut. A disorder known as dysbiosis, characterized by an imbalance in the composition of gut bacteria, can alter these neurochemical levels. Anxiety, despair, and mood changes may follow from this (Dezfouli et al., 2025). Intestinal inflammation signals also impact mental health. Bacterial endotoxins, such as lipopolysaccharides (LPS), can enter the systemic circulation and cause inflammation in the brain when the intestinal barrier becomes compromised, allowing it to become "leaky." Cognitive impairment and depressive symptoms have been associated with elevated levels of cytokines.

Additionally, through the hypothalamic–pituitary–adrenal (HPA) axis, the gut microbiome regulates stress responses. A balanced microbiome maintains standard cortisol control, while stress reactivity is increased by dysbiosis. By re-establishing microbial balance and reducing inflammation, probiotic and prebiotic treatments, collectively referred to as psychobiotics, have demonstrated promise in elevating mood and reducing anxiety.

7.4.2 Physical Health Conditions and Their Psychological Effects

Chronic medical disorders and physical ailments have a significant impact on mental health and frequently produce a biopsychosocial feedback loop. In addition to affecting the body, diseases, including diabetes, heart disease, thyroid issues, and autoimmune diseases, also change the chemistry of the brain and how emotions are controlled. For example, depression is closely linked to diabetes mellitus. Hyperglycemia damages neurotransmitter function and neuroplasticity by inducing oxidative stress and neuroinflammation (Wan et al., 2021). Moreover, emotions of exhaustion and pessimism are exacerbated by the psychological strain of managing a chronic illness. Similarly, cognitive impairments and depressive symptoms are caused by cardiovascular disease (CVD), which alters cerebral perfusion and oxygenation. According to the "vascular depression" theory, people may be more susceptible to depression if they have microvascular damage in areas of the brain that control emotions, such as the amygdala and prefrontal cortex (Do et al., 2010).

Systemic inflammation and cytokine dysregulation are associated with mood swings in autoimmune diseases, such as lupus and multiple sclerosis. Chronic immune activation affects neurotransmitter systems, such as glutamate and serotonin, leading to fatigue, irritability, and cognitive decline. Furthermore, the psychological stress of having a chronic illness can exacerbate physical symptoms, creating a vicious cycle. The stigma, lifestyle limitations, and uncertainty about how the disease may progress heighten symptoms of anxiety and sadness (Bruno et al., 2020).

By attending to patients' physical and emotional needs, integrated care models which combine medical and psychological support have shown improved outcomes.

7.4.3 The Role of Chronic Pain in Mental Health Disorders

A physical and psychological ailment, chronic pain is defined as pain that persists for longer than three months or longer than the normal healing time of regular tissue repair. In addition to interfering with day-to-day activities, it also alters the neuronal circuits that control mood and perception, which frequently results in anxiety, depression, and disturbed sleep (Stretanski et al., 2025).

According to neuroimaging research, chronic pain alters activity in the amygdala, prefrontal cortex, and anterior cingulate cortex—regions crucial for mood regulation. Central sensitization, a condition in which the nervous system becomes hypersensitive and intensifies both physical and mental distress, is triggered by the ongoing stimulation of pain pathways (Martucci & MacKey, 2018).

Neurotransmitters, including serotonin and norepinephrine, which are also linked to mood disorders, are dysregulated in chronic pain biochemically. Antidepressants, especially serotonin-norepinephrine reuptake inhibitors (SNRIs), are frequently used to treat chronic pain disorders, which can explain this overlap (Marks et al., 2009). The psychological repercussions of chronic pain, such as helplessness, social disengagement, and lack of purpose, can contribute to the deterioration of mental health. Pain-related sleep deprivation raises emotional reactivity and weakens coping mechanisms. Additionally, there are biological factors like inflammation, neuroplastic changes, and hyperactivity of the HPA axis that are shared by depression and chronic pain (Brandt et al., 2022). A multimodal approach that includes medication, cognitive-behavioural therapy (CBT), physical rehabilitation, and mindfulness-based therapies is required to manage chronic pain effectively. When the psychological and physical components of pain are addressed, both function and quality of life are restored (Table 7.1.1).

7.5 Interventions for Cognitive and Mental Health

Through the body-brain connection, cognitive and mental health interventions are gaining increasing recognition as essential for maintaining psychological well-being and brain function. Multifaceted treatments, including exercise, diet, cognitive training, and mind–body techniques, support neural resilience and emotional control (Al Sager et al., 2024). Regular physical activity enhances cerebral perfusion, stimulates neurogenesis and synaptic plasticity, and modulates stress and inflammatory pathways, ultimately leading to improved cognitive performance. Lifestyle choices, such as diet (e.g., high sugar, high fat, or Mediterranean diet), physical activity, smoking, alcohol consumption, and socioeconomic status, profoundly influence the risk and progression of neurodegenerative diseases, thereby supporting cognitive processes and mood stability (Bryce et al., 2024). Mind–body practices, encompassing physical activity, a balanced diet, cognitive training, adequate sleep, and mindfulness meditation, are crucial for disease management and prevention. These

Table 7.1.1 Mechanistic pathways connecting the body–brain axis to cognitive and emotional dysregulation.

Mechanism	Biological description	Impact on cognitive function	Associated mental health outcomes	Clinical implications
Oxidative stress	Imbalance between ROS generation and antioxidant defense mechanisms	Causes neuronal damage, DNA oxidation, and synaptic dysfunction	Accelerated ageing, cognitive impairment, and neuropsychiatric disorders	Antioxidant therapy (vitamin E, polyphenols),
Genetic mutations	Mutations in genes regulating amyloid metabolism, synaptic plasticity, or neurotransmitter pathways	Alters neuronal survival and synaptic integrity	Alzheimer's disease, Parkinson's disease, and schizophrenia	Gene therapy, personalized medicine approaches
Cerebrovascular damage	Reduced cerebral blood flow and endothelial dysfunction	Limits nutrient and oxygen supply to neurons	Vascular dementia, stroke-related cognitive decline	Antihypertensive therapy, neuroprotective strategies
Accumulation of pathological Proteins	Aggregation of amyloid-β, tau, or α-synuclein in neural tissues	Interferes with neuronal communication and synaptic health	Alzheimer's disease, Parkinson's disease, dementia	Immunotherapy, aggregation inhibitors
Neurotransmitter dysfunction	Altered dopamine, serotonin, or acetylcholine signaling	Impairs attention, memory, and mood regulation	Depression, schizophrenia, ADHD, dementia	Neurotransmitter-targeted pharmacotherapy
Neuroinflammation	Chronic activation of microglia and astrocytes leads to the release of pro-inflammatory cytokines (IL-1β, TNF-α, IL-6)	Impairs neuronal signaling and promotes neurodegeneration	Depression, Alzheimer's disease, and anxiety disorders	Anti-inflammatory agents, lifestyle modulation, and immunomodulators

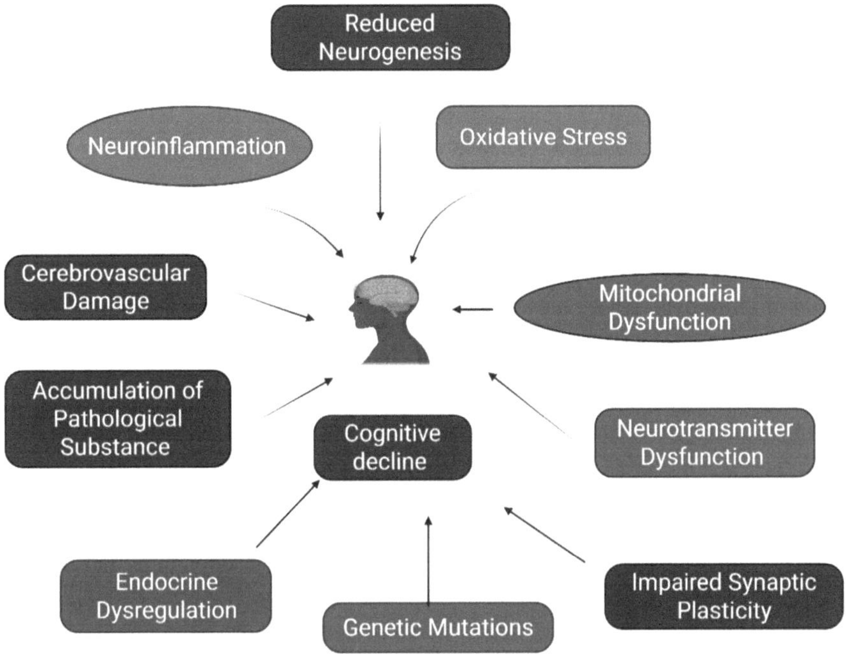

Fig. 7.2 Molecular and cellular cascades linking body physiology to brain dysfunction

practices can modify disease risk factors by enhancing cortical connectivity and regulating stress-related neuroendocrine activity, thereby improving attentional control and emotional balance. By activating both physiological and psychological systems, these therapies enhance the bidirectional relationship between the body and brain, providing a holistic approach to preserving cognitive health and mental well-being throughout the lifespan (Castellano-Tejedor & Cencerrado, 2024) (Fig. 7.2).

7.5.1 Physical Activity as a Cognitive and Mood Enhancer

Physical activity plays a critical role in enhancing cognitive function and mood, with multiple studies highlighting its benefits:

Improvement in cognitive function: Regular physical activity is recognized for enhancing cognitive abilities, including memory and thinking skills. It can indirectly enhance cognition by improving mood, sleep, and reducing stress and anxiety.

Mood Enhancement: Exercise is a scientifically verified mood booster, known to decrease symptoms of both depression and anxiety. This effect is attributed mainly to the increase in endorphin levels—neurotransmitters that promote well-being.

Stress and Anxiety Reduction: Engaging in regular physical activity can significantly help manage stress and anxiety. The production of neurotransmitters such as dopamine and serotonin during physical activity contributes to this stress-relieving effect (de Costa & Moreira-Almeida, 2025). Physical activity increases blood flow and oxygen delivery to the brain, supporting its functions, including cognition, concentration, and memory, and also promotes neuroplasticity, the brain's ability to form new neural connections. This process enhances cognitive functions such as learning and memory and improves overall brain health, particularly in the hippocampus. Exercise stimulates the release of neurotransmitters such as serotonin and dopamine, which play a crucial role in regulating mood, motivation, and focus. These "feel-good" chemicals help to reduce symptoms of depression and anxiety, leading to improved emotional well-being. These mental health benefits stem from improved synaptic plasticity and the upregulation of neurotrophic factors, such as brain-derived neurotrophic factor (BDNF) and insulin-like growth factor-1 (IGF-1) (Crandon et al., 2025).

Additionally, exercise improves metabolic health, lowers oxidative stress, and regulates systemic and central inflammatory processes—all of which support the preservation of brain integrity and cognitive resilience. By controlling the hypothalamic–pituitary–adrenal (HPA) axis, reducing stress-related cortisol release, and promoting the balance of neurotransmitters such as serotonin, dopamine, and gamma-aminobutyric acid (GABA), which are essential for emotional regulation, physical activity significantly improves mood in ways that extend beyond cognition (Ekelund et al., 2025). When considered as a whole, these physiological and neurochemical changes underscore the dual function of exercise as both a mood stabilizer and a cognitive enhancer, rendering it a crucial non-pharmacological intervention in preventive and therapeutic approaches for mental health disorders and cognitive impairment.

7.5.2 Nutritional Approaches to Support Brain Health

Apart from overall undernutrition, a lack of specific nutrients can have lasting effects on brain development. During pregnancy, essential nutrients such as protein, iron, copper, zinc, iodine, folate, and essential fatty acids are crucial for the proper development and function of the nervous system. Breastfeeding supports cognitive development through the combined effects of breast milk's nutrient and bioactive composition, as well as the sensory, emotional, and bonding experiences it provides. Polyunsaturated fatty acids (PUFAs) play a crucial role in maintaining the structural integrity and regulating the function of neurons, endothelial cells, and glial cells within the brain. Among them, the omega-3 fatty acids eicosapentaenoic acid (EPA) and docosahexaenoic acid (DHA), vitamins (such as B-complex, D, and E), and polyphenols modulate neurotransmission, attenuate neuroinflammation, enhance mitochondrial function, and promote neuronal survival and neurogenesis, thereby facilitating cognitive processes, including memory, attention, and executive function (Garfinkel & Eccleston, 2025).

Additionally, nutritional approaches influence oxidative stress and neuroinflammatory pathways, which are key factors in the development of neurodegenerative diseases and age-related cognitive decline. Additionally, following general brain-healthy dietary patterns, such as the Mediterranean, MIND, or DASH-type diets, is linked to lower rates of cognitive decline and improvements in mood and emotional regulation, most likely through synergistic effects on metabolic regulation, neurotrophic support, and vascular health (Genovese et al., 2024). Personalized nutritional strategies are crucial for maintaining mental and cognitive health, as new research suggests that gut-brain axis regulation and nutrient-gene interactions may have additional implications (Gkintoni et al., 2025). Taken together, our results highlight the potential of focused and comprehensive nutritional strategies as effective, non-pharmacological therapies for maintaining cognitive performance and enhancing psychological well-being.

7.5.3 Mind–body Practices: Meditation, Yoga, and Mindfulness

Yoga is a comprehensive lifestyle integrating ethical principles, physical exercise, breath regulation, and meditative practices, undertaken with mindfulness and intentionality. These practical interventions aim to enhance cognitive function and mental health through the body–brain connection. These practices promote neuroplasticity, enhance functional and structural connectivity in brain regions involved in attention, executive function, and emotional regulation, and modify stress-related neuroendocrine activity, as evidenced by scientific studies including systematic reviews, meta-analyses, and neuroimaging studies (Goldberg, 2025). Frequent meditation, yoga, or mindfulness exercises can lower cortisol levels, improve autonomic regulation, and reduce the hyperactivity of the hypothalamic–pituitary–adrenal (HPA) axis, all of which can lessen the adverse cognitive and emotional effects of long-term stress. Additionally, these treatments affect neurotransmitter systems, including as dopamine, serotonin, and gamma-aminobutyric acid (GABA), which support cognitive flexibility, attentional control, and mood stabilization (Guzman-Holst et al., 2025). Additionally, mind–body techniques enhance neurotrophic factors, including brain-derived neurotrophic factor (BDNF), which supports synaptic plasticity and neuronal survival, and reduces systemic inflammation and oxidative stress, both of which are linked to neurodegeneration and age-related cognitive decline (Halkiopoulos & Gkintoni, 2025).

Together, meditation, yoga, and mindfulness act as powerful non-pharmacological approaches that enhance body–brain connectivity and support cognitive, emotional, and mental health.

The Role of medical and therapeutic approaches

Researchers have shown that body aging and brain aging are correlated; aging of one organ system accelerates the aging of another, so addressing cognitive decline and mental health, considering the body–brain connection, is significant for mitigating disease progression and for understanding the health promotion strategies and treatment approaches from purely symptomatic treatments to disease-modifying strategies (Maderthaner & Edwards, 2025). Pharmacological interventions, including cholinesterase inhibitors for AD and levodopa for PD, NMDA receptor modulators, stem cell therapy, Immunotherapy, Incretin-based therapies, gene therapy, and emerging disease-modifying agents, all help to stabilize neurotransmitter function, reduce excitotoxicity, and slow the progression of neurodegenerative processes (Hallion et al., 2024). Complementing pharmacotherapy, therapeutic approaches such as cognitive rehabilitation, psychotherapy, and structured behavioural interventions target neurocognitive and psychosocial mechanisms by enhancing compensatory cognitive strategies, emotional regulation, and adaptive functioning (Li et al., 2024).

Additionally, integrative medical strategies can target the root causes through efficient self-regulation, enabling the body to self-organize and maintain stability, balance, and overall health within the disease continuum. These neurostimulation techniques and precision medicine approaches have shown promise in modulating neural circuits, promoting synaptic plasticity, and improving mood and cognitive outcomes (Haque & Dutta, 2025). Many randomized controlled trials indicate that the body, as indexed by high-frequency heart rate variability (HF-HRV), and the brain, as indexed by midline anterior cingulate cortex (ACC) theta power, work in correlation to regulate brain and body dysfunction and imbalance, ameliorate symptoms, and treat disorders. Collectively, these medical and therapeutic modalities operate synergistically to preserve neuronal integrity, reduce symptom burden, and support mental well-being, emphasizing the importance of a multidisciplinary approach in maintaining body–brain health across the lifespan (Jadeja & Dudhat, 2025).

7.5.4 Pharmacological Interventions for Cognitive and Mental Health

Pharmacological interventions help to manage neurodegenerative and neuropsychiatric conditions linked to dysregulation of the body–brain connection. Current therapeutic strategies target neurotransmitter systems, neuroinflammation, and synaptic dysfunction to treat the root cause of these receptors, thereby preserving cognitive performance and emotional stability (Magomedova & Fatima, 2025). Acetylcholinesterase inhibitors Razadyne (approved in 2001), donepezil hydrochloride, rivastigmine tartrate, galantamine hydrobromide and NMDA receptor antagonists (memantine hydrochloride) remain symptomatic approved pharmacological options for AD and related dementias, functioning via preserving acetylcholine (Ach) level in the synapse, enhancing cholinergic transmission and regulating glutamatergic excitotoxicity, respectively (Mou et al., 2024). These agents provide modest improvements in cognition and functional ability, but have limitations as they are unable to stop or reverse the progression of the disease and behavioural changes. Antidepressants, especially selective serotonin reuptake inhibitors (SSRIs) and serotonin-norepinephrine reuptake inhibitors (SNRIs), are essential for regulating mood, lowering depressive symptoms, and indirectly improving cognitive function by restoring neurochemical imbalances and reducing stress-related neurotoxicity (Nevoit et al., 2025).

Recent developments focus on neuroprotective and disease-modifying medications, such as anti-tau therapies and anti-amyloid monoclonal antibodies (e.g., lecanemab and aducanumab), which aim to reduce the accumulation of pathogenic proteins and neuronal death. To improve neuronal survival and synaptic repair, pharmacological regulation of neurotrophic pathways, mitochondrial function, and oxidative stress is also being studied (Pujari, 2023). To maximize neuronal resilience and cognitive efficiency, the complementary use of nootropics, neurostimulants, and metabolic regulators is also being investigated. Together, these pharmacological strategies seek to alter fundamental disease mechanisms in addition to symptom relief, highlighting the developing precision-based paradigm in the treatment of mental health issues and cognitive decline (Ramos et al., 2024).

7.5.5 Cognitive Behavioural Therapy (CBT) and Other Psychotherapies

CBT plays a significant role in improving cognitive and emotional functioning by taking a differential treatment approach by considering interindividual differences within the context of the body–brain connection, particularly in depression, anxiety, or stress-related disorders (Ruiz-Ranz & Asín-Izquierdo, 2025). CBT adopts an evidence-based toolbox, on the principle that maladaptive thoughts and behaviours contribute to psychological distress and cognitive dysfunction; thus, allowing for the systematic integration of treatment modules to promote adaptive coping and enhance cognitive flexibility (Sammons et al., 2024). CBT conditions adopt the German standard CBT manual for depression, including psychoeducation, cognitive restructuring, and behaviour activation, measurable neuroplastic changes in brain regions associated with emotion regulation, which support its efficacy in enhancing both cognitive control and mood stability. By focusing on emotional awareness, stress resilience, and interpersonal functioning, various psychotherapy modalities, such as mindfulness-based cognitive therapy (MBCT), acceptance and commitment therapy (ACT), and interpersonal therapy (IPT), can enhance cognitive behavioural therapy (CBT) (Sandoval et al., 2025).

Together, these methods lessen psychological distress, ease symptoms of anxiety and depression, and enhance executive performance by modifying brain networks related to self-regulation and attention. All things considered, CBT and related psychotherapies offer evidence-based, non-pharmacological techniques that improve neural adaptability, emotional stability, and general cognitive function, making them

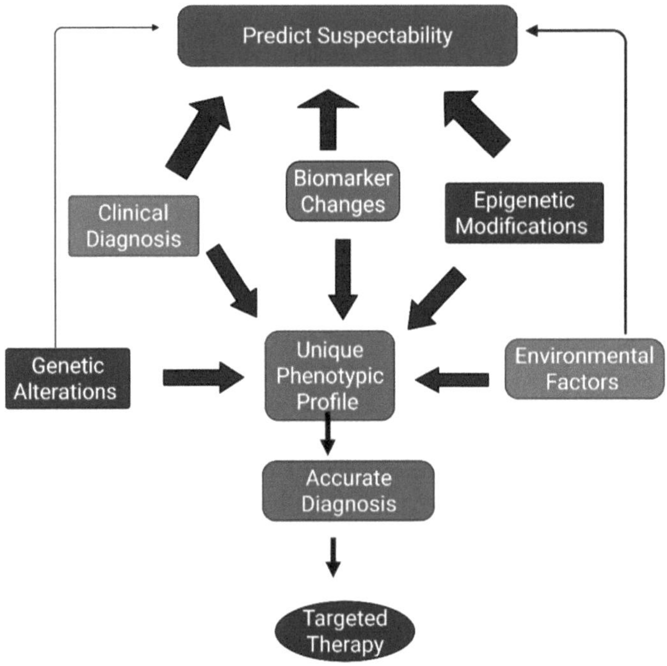

Fig. 7.3 Integrative framework of genetic, epigenetic, and environmental determinants in cognitive decline

essential parts of all-encompassing treatments for mental health conditions and cognitive decline (Schmidt et al., 2025) (Fig. 7.3).

7.5.6 Integrative Medicine and Holistic Approaches

It is increasingly recognized as a multifaceted framework for cognitive and mental health, simultaneously integrating physiological, psychological, and environmental determinants (Sharma et al., 2024). These approaches combine conventional methods with complementary strategies, including botanicals, dietary supplements, mind–body interventions, lifestyle modifications, non-invasive neuromodulation, and optimization of sleep and stress management techniques. According to recent literature, integrative interventions have the potential to modify disease rather than relieve symptoms by simultaneously modulating multiple pathophysiological mechanisms, such as neuroinflammation, oxidative stress, mitochondrial dysfunction, tau and amyloid pathology, vascular insufficiency, and cholinergic deficits (Ţenea-Cojan Ştefăniţă et al., 2025).

Evidence suggests that specific herbal agents and botanical extracts exhibit neuroprotective effects in preclinical and limited clinical trials; however, their translational applicability is limited by factors such as variability in study design, inconsistent bioavailability, the absence of standardization in herbal formulations, and potential interactions with conventional pharmacotherapies (Tropea & Giacometti, 2025). Various lifestyle components, such as a balanced diet, regular physical activity, social/cognitive engagement, and good sleep, provide beneficial results when synergistically embedded among neural, immune, metabolic, and endocrine systems within integrative models. Integrative care approaches emphasize not only the patient's recovery but also the caregiver's health and quality of life, acknowledging the profound interconnection between the two (Verdonk et al., 2025).

7.6 Future Directions in Body-Brain Research

It points toward increasingly integrative, multimodal, and precision-oriented approaches (Shimko & James, 2025).

- First, there is a growing focus on new biomarkers, especially blood-based markers (e.g., phosphorylated tau variants, neurofilament light chain, GFAP) and inflammatory cytokines, which can more sensitively and less invasively identify early pathological processes and predict the progression of neuropsychiatric symptoms and cognitive decline (Udeh-Momoh et al., 2025).
- Second, advanced functional connectivity and brain network analyses by using resting-state fMRI, EEG/MEG, and graph theory are increasingly used to identify early disruptions in brain neuronal connectivity before cognitive deficits appear, allowing timely planning of interventions (Vettriselvan et al., 2025).
- Third, innovative clinical models such as "brain health services" or next-generation memory clinics combine biomarker testing, lifestyle coaching, digital tools and technologies, and preventive therapies to slow disease progression and provide personalize treatment (Yu et al., 2025).
- Fourth, it is still crucial to separate the interactions between various pathogenic elements, such as neuroinflammation, vascular dysfunction, amyloid/tau pathology, and lymphatic clearance: To elucidate causative pathways and the best targets for intervention, investigations integrating imaging, fluid biomarkers, and physiological data are necessary (Zeng & Lo, 2025).

These approaches collectively suggest that to maintain body-brain health, future research should focus on multimodal biomarkers, early diagnosis, tailored therapies, and digitally enhanced preventive models.

7.6.1 Emerging Technologies in Neuroscience

Emerging advancements in neuroscience are revolutionizing how we map, modulate, and analyse the brain's structure and function with the help of novel tools and technologies with high spatial, temporal, and mechanistic precision (Ambretti et al., 2025). Key advances include brain-computer interfaces (BCIs) and multimodal decoding algorithms, which fuse signals across EEG, fMRI, ECoG, and other modalities via machine learning to interpret neural activity with fine granularity and control external devices directly from neural states (Chudy et al., 2025). Complementing neuromorphic engineering (e.g. Spintronic devices) seeks to mimic biological neural computation at low power and in a hardware substrate, enabling more "brain-like" processing in artificial systems and potential closed-loop neuromodulation.

Advances in molecular and genetic tools, including optogenetics, chemogenetics, and gene editing (e.g., CRISPR), enable the precise manipulation of cell populations to probe causal links in brain networks and test interventions at the molecular level. Furthermore, artificial intelligence (AI) and large foundation models are being leveraged to analyze multimodal, high-dimensional neuroscience data (imaging, genomics, electrophysiology) for biomarker discovery, predictive modeling, and simulation of brain systems (Fakorede et al., 2025). Finally, wearables and ambient sensors (e.g., portable neuroimaging, mobile EEG, biosensors) are enabling the continuous monitoring of brain–body states outside the laboratory, facilitating real-time assessments of cognitive and affective dynamics in everyday life. Together, these technologies are converging toward a future in which behavioural, physiological, and neural data streams are integrated to deliver precision diagnostics and dynamically adaptive interventions in cognitive and mental health (Froom, 2025).

7.6.2 Personalized Medicine for Cognitive and Mental Health

Personalized medicine for cognitive and mental health represents a transformative approach that aims to improve how diagnoses and treatments are tailored, ensuring they more accurately capture and respond to each person's unique health profile, encompassing biological, genetic, and lifestyle factors. Recent research on neurodegenerative and psychiatric illnesses has shown that early diagnosis and stratification of cognitive decline are made possible by integrating multi-omics data (genomics, proteome, metabolomics), neuroimaging, and digital biomarkers (Hawke et al., 2024). When compared to traditional therapies, personalized interventions that address neurovascular variables, inflammatory and metabolic dysfunctions, and genetic predispositions (such as APOE variations) have demonstrated superior cognitive outcomes. Similar frameworks are used in mental health by precision psychiatry, which uses biomarker-guided models to optimize psychopharmacology and psychotherapy and predict treatment response. AI and machine learning are increasingly being used to analyze complex datasets and generate personalized treatment recommendations (Kelly et al., 2024). Progress toward personalized brain healthcare is both promising and challenging, as the availability of inconsistent data, high costs, and limited large-scale studies hinders its widespread use. Future work focuses on integrating biological, behavioural, and environmental information to create more adaptive and preventive care for personalized medicine.

7.6.3 Preventive Strategies for Long-Term Brain Health

Preventive strategies for long-term brain health emphasize early, multidomain interventions that target modifiable risk factors across the life course to delay or prevent cognitive decline and associated mental health disorders (Kostović, 2025). Current evidence indicates that adopting healthy lifestyle behaviours—such as regular physical activity, balanced nutrition, adequate sleep, and avoidance of smoking and excessive alcohol—during midlife significantly attenuates the risk of neurodegeneration later. Multidomain approaches that combine diet, exercise, cognitive stimulation, and cardiovascular risk management show promise in maintaining cognitive function, with emerging mechanistic data indicating reductions in oxidative stress and neuroinflammatory markers, improved vascular function, and enhanced synaptic plasticity (Lawrence et al., 2024). Subjective cognitive decline and preclinical populations are important target groups for preventive actions. In addition, public health initiatives and "brain health services" (specialized programs for risk screening, personalised risk communication, and tailored preventive plans) are being developed to scale these interventions. Despite encouraging findings, gaps remain in long-term follow-up studies, standardized outcome measures, equitable access, and demonstrable cost-effectiveness (Liu et al., 2024).

7.7 Conclusion

Over the past few decades, evidence has been accumulating to highlight the interconnectedness of body and brain systems. The literature reviewed that physiological, metabolic, vascular, immunological, and lifestyle aspects are correlated with cognitive decline and deterioration of mental health (Lo & Zeng, 2025). This review integrates evidence that physical activity, nutrition, mind–body interventions, pharmacological and psychotherapeutic approaches, non-pharmacological therapies, and precision strategies collectively point toward a multipronged, systems-level framework for maintaining brain health (Lo et al., 2024). Research has shown that, despite single therapy, multimodal, personalized, and early preventive strategies offer the most significant promise for improving outcomes. Future research should focus on long-term studies that incorporate robust cohort studies, combining genetic and brain imaging data with digital tools, and design flexible, personalized treatments that can adapt to individualized interventions (Olawade et al., 2024). In the conclusion, turning the idea of body–brain synergy into real, practical solutions that protect memory, boost mental strength, and support healthy aging will require linking scientific understanding with practical, scalable action.

7.7.1 Key Takeaways

The link between the body and brain illustrates how profoundly our physical health, metabolism, circulation, immunity, and daily habits impact our thoughts and emotions. Studies reveal that combining exercise, good nutrition, mindfulness, medication, and therapy in a personalized manner can work together more effectively to support brain health and emotional well-being (Wang et al., 2024). Early intervention and precision-guided strategies based on genetic, biomarker, and lifestyle profiling can help prevent cognitive decline and promote mental health. Advanced neuroimaging, wearable monitoring, digital phenotyping, and multi-omic biomarkers are examples of emerging technologies that are improving early detection, real-time monitoring, and tailored intervention. Large-scale longitudinal studies, standardized outcomes, and the inclusion of diverse groups remain essential for validating efficacy and translating mechanistic insights into scalable clinical practice, despite advancements (Wester et al., 2025). Collectively, these findings highlight the importance of holistic, personalized, and proactive approaches in promoting long-term cognitive and mental health.

7.7.2 Encouraging a Holistic Approach to Health

In order to maximize brain function and mental well-being, a holistic approach to health stresses the integration of physical, nutritional, cognitive, emotional, and social domains. Evidence from recent studies suggests that interventions targeting various lifestyle aspects—such as regular exercise, a balanced diet, mind–body techniques, stress reduction, and social interaction—act in concert to maintain emotional and cognitive resilience (Yıldız Karaahmet et al., 2025). Holistic strategies recognise that the body and brain influence each other, indicating a bidirectional relationship where enhanced metabolic, vascular, and immune function, associated with improved cognitive and emotional regulation, contributes to overall physiological stability (Zeng et al., 2025). In addition to reducing the risk of cognitive decline, adopting individualized, multimodal, and preventative strategies within a holistic framework also enhances adaptive coping, quality of life, and long-term mental health. A forward-thinking paradigm for long-term brain-body wellbeing is represented by incorporating such all-encompassing approaches into clinical practice and public health campaigns (Chen et al., 2024).

7.8 Availability of Data

None.

Acknowledgements We would like to thank the infrastructure and fellowship support to Md. Abubakar and were extended by the Department of Pharmaceuticals, Ministry of Chemicals and Fertilizers, Government of India, NIPER HAJIPUR. We also extend our gratitude to Ritu Dahiya from the School of Pharmacy, Lingaya's Vidyapeeth (Deemed to be a University), Faridabad, Haryana, India, and Dr. Nitesh Kumar for their support and guidance in executing this work plan. All figures have been made using www.Biorander.com, and grammar corrections have been made using www.Grammarly.com in this manuscript.

Author Contribution **Abhishek Ambawatiya** and **Ritu Dahiya** were involved in the conceptualization, writing of the original draft, mechanistic insight, input on critical points, editing; **Sarasa Meenakshi** and **Mamta Bishnoi** for manuscript editing, and figure preparation; **Sirajudheen Anwar, Krishna Murti** for manuscript reviewing, and editing, **Md. Abubakar and Dr. Nitesh Kumar** was involved in the conceptualization, manuscript writing, reviewing, conceptualization of figures and approved the version to be published.

Funding None.

Conflict of Interest None.

References

Abyadeh, M., Gupta, V., Paulo, J. A., Mahmoudabad, A. G., Shadfar, S., Mirshahvaladi, S., et al. (2023). Amyloid-beta and tau protein beyond Alzheimer's disease. *Neural Regeneration Research, 19*(6), 1262.

Al Sager, A., Goodman, S. H., Jeong, J., Bain, P. A., & Ahun, M. N. (2024). Effects of multi-component parenting and parental mental health interventions on early childhood development and parent outcomes: A systematic review and meta-analysis. *Lancet Child Adolesc Health, 8*(9), 656–669.

Ambretti, A., Monacis, D., Forte, P., Morsanuto, S., Savoia, T., D'Anna, C., et al. (2025). Future perspectives for physical education in primary school to promote innovative co-planning practices. *Journal of Inclusive Methodology and Technology in Learning and Teaching, 5*(1).

Ashique, S., Mohanto, S., Ahmed, M. G., Mishra, N., Garg, A., Chellappan, D. K., et al. (2024). Gut-brain axis: A cutting-edge approach to target neurological disorders and potential synbiotic application. *Heliyon, 10*(13), Article e34092.

Ben-Zion, Z., Korem, N., Fine, N. B., Katz, S., Siddhanta, M., Funaro, M. C., et al. (2023). Structural neuroimaging of hippocampus and Amygdala subregions in posttraumatic stress disorder: A scoping review. *Biological Psychiatry Global Open Science, 4*(1), 120.

Bhol, N. K., Bhanjadeo, M. M., Singh, A. K., Dash, U. C., Ojha, R. R., Majhi, S., et al. (2024). The interplay between cytokines, inflammation, and antioxidants: Mechanistic insights and therapeutic potentials of various antioxidants and anti-cytokine compounds. *Biomedicine & Pharmacotherapy, 178*, Article 117177.

Bonaz, B., Sinniger, V., & Pellissier, S. (2017, November). The vagus nerve in the neuro-immune axis: Implications in the pathology of the gastrointestinal tract. *Frontiers in Immunology, 8*.

Brandt, L., Liu, S., Heim, C., & Heinz, A. (2022). The effects of social isolation stress and discrimination on mental health. *Translational Psychiatry, 12*(1), 398.

Bruno, A., Dolcetti, E., Rizzo, F. R., Fresegna, D., Musella, A., Gentile, A., et al. (2020). Inflammation-associated synaptic alterations as shared threads in depression and multiple sclerosis. *Frontiers in Cellular Neuroscience, 14*, 169.

Bryce, S., Cheng, N., Dalton, A., Ojinnaka, A., Stainton, A., Zbukvic, I., et al. (2024). Cognitive health treatment priorities and preferences among young people with mental illness: The your mind, your choice survey. *Early Intervention in Psychiatry, 18*(2), 94–101.

Buzsáki, G. (2023). Cognition from the body-brain partnership: Exaptation of memory. *Annual Review of Neuroscience, 46*, 191–210 (annualreviews.org).

Calderone, A., Latella, D., Impellizzeri, F., de Pasquale, P., Famà, F., Quartarone, A., et al. (2024, November). Neurobiological changes induced by mindfulness and meditation: A systematic review. *Biomedicines, 12*(11), 2613.

Campbell, M., & Jialal, I. (2022, September). *Physiology, endocrine hormones*. StatPearls.

Castellano-Tejedor, C., & Cencerrado, A. (2024). Gamification for mental health and health psychology: Insights at the first quarter mark of the 21st century. *International Journal of Environmental Research and Public Health, 21*(8), 990.

Chen, T., Dai, Y., Hu, C., Lin, Z., Wang, S., Yang, J., et al. (2024). Cellular and molecular mechanisms of the blood–brain barrier dysfunction in neurodegenerative diseases. *Fluids Barriers CNS, 21*(1), 60.

Chudy, D., Vuletić, V., & Raguž, M. (2025). Deep brain stimulation-clinical experience, indications, and future perspectives. *Rad Hrvatske Akademije Znanosti i Umjetnosti. Medicinske Znanosti, 567*(70–71), 139.

Colita, E., Mateescu, V. O., Olaru, D. G., & Popa-Wagner, A. (2024). Cognitive decline in ageing and disease: Risk factors, genetics and treatments. *Current Health Sciences Journal, 50*(2), 170.

de Costa, M. A., & Moreira-Almeida, A. (2025). The mind-brain problem: Ethical and clinical implications for psychiatry. *Int Rev Psychiatry*, 1–13.

Crandon, T., Vivian, E., Jach, M., Rantanen, L., Quek, H., Lupton, M., et al. (2025). Wildfires and brain health: A physiological and psychological interplay. Available SSRN 5531418.

Daëron, M. (2022). The immune system as a system of relations. *Frontiers in Immunology, 13*, Article 984678.

Dehdar, K., & Raoufy, M. R. (2023). Brain structural and functional alterations related to anxiety in allergic asthma. *Brain Research Bulletin, 202*, Article 110727.

Dezfouli, M. A., Rashidi, S. K., Yazdanfar, N., Khalili, H., Goudarzi, M., Saadi A, et al. (2025). The emerging roles of neuroactive components produced by gut microbiota. *Molecular Biology Reports, 52*(1).

Do, D. P., Beam Dowd, J., Ranjit, N., House, J. S., & Kaplan, G. A. (2010). Hopelessness, depression, and early markers of endothelial dysfunction in U.S. adults. *Biopsychosocial Science and Medicine, 72*(7), 613–619.

Ekelund, R., Holmström, S., Gustafsson, H., Ivarsson, A., Lundqvist, C., & Stenling, A. (2025). Interventions for improving mental health in athletes: A scoping review. *International Review of Sport and Exercise Psychology, 18*(1), 503–538.

Van Erum, J., Van Dam, D., & De Deyn, P. P. (2019). Alzheimer's disease: Neurotransmitters of the sleep-wake cycle. *Neuroscience & Biobehavioral Reviews, 105*, 72–80.

Eslinger, P. J., Anders, S., Ballarini, T., Boutros, S., Krach, S., Mayer, A. V., et al. (2021). The neuroscience of social feelings: Mechanisms of adaptive social functioning. *Neuroscience and Biobehavioral Reviews, 128*, 592–620.

Fakorede, S., Alkhameys, F., Liao, K., Martin, L., & Devos, H. (2025). Neural evidence for attentional resource allocation to postural control using body brain imaging. *Behavioural Brain Research*, 115716.

Froom, V. (2025). *Future directions of AI & machine consciousness: Exploring minds without flesh in a technological age*. 2gay Publishing.

Garfinkel, S. N., & Eccleston, C. (2025). Interoception and pain: Body–mind integration, rupture, and repair. *Pain, 166*(7), 1470–1474.

Gautam, S., Jain, A., Chaudhary, J., Gautam, M., Gaur, M., Grover, S. (2024). Concept of mental health and mental well-being, it's determinants and coping strategies. *Indian Journal of Psychiatry, 66*(Suppl 2), S231.

Genovese, L. A., Riva, G., & Di, L. D. (2024). Beyond chronic pain exploring body-brain interaction to understand and treat chronic pain conditions. *Cyberpsychology, Behavior, and Social Networking, 27*(7), 518–520.

Gkintoni, E., Vassilopoulos, S. P., & Nikolaou, G. (2025). Mindfulness-based cognitive therapy in clinical practice: A systematic review of neurocognitive outcomes and applications for mental health and well-being. *Journal of Clinical Medicine, 14*(5), 1703.

Goldberg, G. (2025). *The body-brain connection: Evidence-based ways to reduce anxiety, boost engagement, and increase comprehension across classrooms*. Corwin Press.

Guzman-Holst, C., Streckfuss Davis, R., Andrews, J. L., & Foulkes, L. (2025). Scoping review: Potential harm from school-based group mental health interventions. *Child and Adolescent Mental Health, 30*(3), 208–222.

Halkiopoulos, C., & Gkintoni, E. (2025). The role of machine learning in AR/VR-based cognitive therapies: A systematic review for mental health disorders. *Electronics, 14*(6).

Hallion, L. S., Hsu, K. J., & Schleider, J. L. (2024). Cognitive training for mental health problems. *Nature Mental Health, 2*(1), 17–24.

Haque, S., & Dutta, P. (2025). The heart-brain axis in the context of cardiovascular disease. *Physiology*.@@@@

Hawke, L. D., Nguyen, A. T. P., Wang, W., Brown, E. E., Xu, D., Deuville, S., et al. (2024). Systematic review of interventions for mental health, cognition and psychological well-being in long COVID. *BMJ Mental Health, 27*(1).

Jadeja, Y., & Dudhat, K. (2025). Advancements in the brain chip technology: Current landscape and future prospects. *Analytical & Bioanalytical Electrochemistry, 17*(2), 85–134.

Jiménez, J. A., & Mills, P. J. (2012, January). Behavioral medicine. *Encyclopedia of human behavior* (2nd ed., pp. 311–318).

Johnstone, A. M., Albanese, E., Crabtree, D. R., Dalile, B., Grabrucker, S., Gregory, J. M., et al. (2025). Consensus statement on exploring the Nexus between nutrition, brain health and dementia prevention. *Nutrition & Metabolism (London), 22*(1), 82.

Jurcău, M. C., Andronie-Cioara, F. L., Jurcău, A., Marcu, F., Ţiţ, D. M., Paşcalău, N., et al. (2022). The link between oxidative stress, mitochondrial dysfunction and neuroinflammation in the pathophysiology of Alzheimer's disease: Therapeutic implications and future perspectives. *Antioxidants, 11*(11), 2167.

Kageyama, K., Iwasaki, Y., & Daimon, M. (2021). Hypothalamic regulation of corticotropin-releasing factor under stress and stress resilience. *International Journal of Molecular Sciences, 22*(22), 12242.

Kelly, C., Trumpff, C., Acosta, C., Assuras, S., Baker, J., Basarrate, S., et al. (2024). A platform to map the mind–mitochondria connection and the hallmarks of psychobiology: The MiSBIE study. *Trends in Endocrinology and Metabolism, 35*(10), 884–901.

Knezevic, E., Nenic, K., Milanovic, V., & Knezevic, N. N. (2023). The role of cortisol in chronic stress, neurodegenerative diseases, and psychological disorders. *Cells, 12*(23), 2726.

Kostović, I. (2025). Symposium: "Newer Insights in Brain Research." *Rad Hrvatske Akademije Znanosti i Umjetnosti. Medicinske Znanosti, 567*(70–71), 109.

Lawrence, H. R., Schneider, R. A., Rubin, S. B., Matarić, M. J., McDuff, D. J., & Bell, M. J. (2024). The opportunities and risks of large language models in mental health. *MIR Mental Health, 11*(1), Article e59479.

Li, Z., Li, J., Kong, J., Li, Z., Wang, R., & Jiang, F. (2024). Adolescent mental health interventions: A narrative review of the positive effects of physical activity and implementation strategies. *Frontiers in Psychology, 15*, 1433698.

Liu, C., Liang, X., & Sit, C. H. P. (2024). Physical activity and mental health in children and adolescents with neurodevelopmental disorders: A systematic review and meta-analysis. *JAMA Pediatrics, 178*(3), 247–257.

Liu, Y., Fu, Q. F., & Fu, X. L. (2009). The interaction between cognition and emotion. *Chinese Science Bulletin, 54*(22), 4102–4116.
Lo, C. H., & Zeng, J. (2025). TNF as a mediator of metabolic inflammation and body-brain interaction in obesity-driven neuroinflammation and neurodegeneration. *Ageing Research Reviews*, 102891.
Lo, H. K. Y., Fong, T. K. H., Cheung, T., Ngan, S. T. J., Lui, W. Y. V., Chan, W. C., et al. (2024). Enhanced cognition and modulation of brain connectivity in mild neurocognitive disorder: The promise of transcranial pulse stimulation. *Biomedicines, 12*(9), 2081.
Maderthaner, L., & Edwards, M. J. (2025). Mind-body integration in brain health. *Clinical and Translational Neuroscience, 9*(3), 37.
Magomedova, A., & Fatima, G. (2025). Mental health and well-being in the modern era: A comprehensive review of challenges and interventions. *Cureus, 17*(1).
Marks, D. M., Shah, M. J., Patkar, A. A., Masand, P. S., Park, G. Y., & Pae, C. U. (2009). Serotonin-norepinephrine reuptake inhibitors for pain control: Premise and promise. *Current Neuropharmacology, 7*(4), 331.
Martucci, K. T., & MacKey, S. C. (2018). Neuroimaging of pain: Human evidence and clinical relevance of central nervous system processes and modulation. *Anesthesiology, 128*(6), 1241.
Marzola, P., Melzer, T., Pavesi, E., Gil-Mohapel, J., Brocardo, P. S. (2023). Exploring the role of neuroplasticity in development, aging, and neurodegeneration. *Brain Science, 13*(12), 1610.
McEwen, B. S. (1999). Endocrine effects on the brain and their relationship to behavior.
McManus, E., Haroon, H., Duncan, N. W., Elliott, R., & Muhlert, N. (2022). The effects of stress across the lifespan on the brain, cognition and mental health: A UK biobank study. *Neurobiology of Stress, 18*, Article 100447.
Mhanna, A., Martini, N., Hmaydoosh, G., Hamwi, G., Jarjanazi, M., Zaifah, G., et al. (2023). The correlation between gut microbiota and both neurotransmitters and mental disorders: A narrative review. *Medicine (Baltimore), 103*(5), Article e37114.
Mortby, M. E., Adler, L., Agüera-Ortiz, L., Bateman, D. R., Brodaty, H., Cantillon, M., et al. (2022). Apathy as a treatment target in Alzheimer's disease: Implications for clinical trials. *The American Journal of Geriatric Psychiatry, 30*(2), 119–147.
Mou, Y. K., Song, X. Y., Wang, H. R., Wang, Y., Liu, W. C., Yang, T., et al. (2024). Understanding the nose–brain axis and its role in related diseases: A conceptual review. *Neurobiology of Diseases, 202*, Article 106690.
Pediatric Neurogastroenterology. (2022). Pediatr Neurogastroenterol.
Nevoit, G., Poderiene, K., Potyazhenko, M., Mintser, O., Jarusevicius, G., & Vainoras, A. (2025). The concept of biophotonic signaling in the human body and brain: Rationale problems and directions. *Frontiers in Systems Neuroscience, 19*, 1597329.
Nuguru, S. P., Rachakonda, S., Sripathi, S., Khan, M. I., Patel, N., & Meda, R. T. (2022Aug). Hypothyroidism and depression: A narrative review. *Cureus, 14*(8), Article e28201.
Ohrnberger, J., Fichera, E., & Sutton, M. (2017). The relationship between physical and mental health: A mediation analysis. *Social Science and Medicine, 195*, 42–49.
Okon-Singer, H., Hendler, T., Pessoa, L., & Shackman, A. J. (2015). The neurobiology of emotion-cognition interactions: Fundamental questions and strategies for future research. *Frontiers in Human Neuroscience, 9*, 126667.
Olawade, D. B., Wada, O. Z., Odetayo, A., David-Olawade, A. C., Asaolu, F., & Eberhardt, J. (2024). Enhancing mental health with Artificial Intelligence: Current trends and future prospects. *Journal of Medicine, Surgery, and Public Health, 3*, Article 100099.
Sharan, P., & Vellapandian, C. (2024, August). Hypothalamic-Pituitary-Adrenal (HPA) Axis: Unveiling the potential mechanisms involved in stress-induced Alzheimer's disease and depression. *Cureus, 16*(8), e67595.
Paganin, W., & Signorini, S. (2024). Inflammatory biomarkers in depression: Scoping review. *Bjpsych Open, 10*(5), Article e165.
Pujari, V. (2020). The relationship between behavior and brain network. *Idea, 6*(7).

Ramos, G., Hernandez-Ramos, R., Taylor, M., & Schueller, S. M. (2024). State of the science: Using digital mental health interventions to extend the impact of psychological services. *Behavior Therapy, 55*(6), 1364–1379.
Renoir, T., Hasebe, K., & Gray, L. (2013). Mind and body: How the health of the body impacts on neuropsychiatry. *Frontiers in Pharmacology, 4*, 158.
Ring, M. (2025Oct). An integrative approach to HPA axis dysfunction: From recognition to recovery. *American Journal of Medicine, 138*(10), 1451–1463.
Romero Garavito, A., Díaz Martínez, V., Juárez Cortés, E., Negrete Díaz, J. V., & Montilla Rodríguez, L. M. (2025). Impact of physical exercise on the regulation of brain-derived neurotrophic factor in people with neurodegenerative diseases. *Frontiers in Neurology, 15*, 1505879.
Ruiz-Ranz, E., & Asín-Izquierdo, I. (2025). Physical activity, exercise, and mental health of healthy adolescents: A review of the last 5 years. *Sports Medicine and Health Science, 7*(3), 161–172.
Sălcudean, A., Bodo, C. R., Popovici, R. A., Cozma, M. M., Păcurar, M., Crăciun, R. E., et al. (2025). Neuroinflammation—A crucial factor in the pathophysiology of depression—A comprehensive review. *Biomolecules, 15*(4), 502.
Salzman, C. D., & Fusi, S. (2010). Emotion, cognition, and mental state representation in Amygdala and prefrontal cortex. *Annual Review of Neuroscience, 33*, 173.
Sammons, M., Popescu, M. C., Chi, J., Liberles, S. D., Gogolla, N., & Rolls, A. (2024). Brain-body physiology: Local, reflex, and central communication. *Cell, 187*(21), 5877–5890.
Sandoval, H., Ibáñez, B., Contreras, M., Troncoso, F., Castro, F. O., Caamaño, D., et al. (2025). Extracellular vesicles from preeclampsia disrupt the blood-brain barrier by reducing CLDN5. *Arteriosclerosis, Thrombosis, and Vascular Biology, 45*(2), 298–311.
Schmidt, U. H., Claudino, A., Fernández-Aranda, F., Giel, K. E., Griffiths, J., Hay, P. J., et al. (2025). The current clinical approach to feeding and eating disorders aimed to increase personalization of management. *World Psychiatry, 24*(1), 4–31.
Sharma, A., Rushton, K., Lin, I. W., Nguyen, T., & Althoff, T. (2024). Facilitating self-guided mental health interventions through human-language model interaction: A case study of cognitive restructuring. In *Proceedings of the 2024 CHI Conference on Human Factors in Computing Systems* (pp. 1–29).
Shimko, G. A., & James, K. H. (2025). The relationship between motor development and ADHD: A critical review and future directions. *Behavioral Sciences (Basel), 15*(5), 576.
Shoykhet, M., & Clark, R. S. B. (2011). Structure, function, and development of the nervous system. *Pediatric critical care* (pp. 783–804).
Skaper, S. D., Facci, L., Zusso, M., & Giusti, P. (2018). An inflammation-centric view of neurological disease: Beyond the neuron. *Frontiers in Cellular Neuroscience, 12*, 72.
Stretanski, M. F., Kopitnik, N. L., Matha, A., & Conermann, T. (2025). Chronic pain. *Chronic diseases: An encyclopedia of causes, effects, and treatments* (Vol. 1 A-H/Vol. 2 I-Z, pp. 599–601).
Țenea-Cojan, T., Dinescu, V. C., Gheorman, V., Dragne, I. G., Gheorman, V., Forțofoiu, M. C., et al. (2025). Exploring multidisciplinary approaches to comorbid psychiatric and medical disorders: A scoping review. *Life, 15*(2), 251.
Thau, L., Reddy, V., & Anatomy, S. P. (2022, October). Central nervous system. *BMJ, 1*(4293), 478–478.
Thompson, J. W. G., Kosofsky, B., Dhamala, E., & Duggan, R. (2020). Electrophysiology monitoring. *Biomarkers Trauma Brain Injury*, 113–142.
Tropea, D., & Giacometti, E. (2025). *Brain-body connections.*
Tyng, C. M., Amin, H.U., Saad, M. N. M., & Malik, A. S. (2017, August). The influences of emotion on learning and memory. *Frontiers in Psychology, 8*, 1454.
Udeh-Momoh, C. T., Migeot, J., Blackmon, K., Mielke, M. M., Melloni, M., Cox, L., et al. (2025). Resilience and brain health in global populations. *Nature Medicine*, 1–14.
Verdonk, C., Ajijola, O. A., & Khalsa, S. S. (2025). Toward a multidisciplinary neurobiology of interoception and mental health. *Current Opinion in Neurobiology, 94*, Article 103084.

Vettriselvan, R., Velmurugan, P. R., Varshney, K. R., EP, J., & Deepika, R. (2025). Health impacts of smartphone and internet addictions across age groups: Physical and mental health across generations. *Impacts of digital technologies across generations* (pp. 187–210). IGI Global Scientific Publishing.
Wan, J., Chua, E. Y. C., Soon, W. S. W., Xie, Y., & Tang, W. E. (2021). The impact of a mental health service on chronic disease management in primary care. *Singapore Medical Journal, 62*(5), 235.
Wang, S., Zhou, S., Han, Z., Yu, B., Xu, Y., Lin, Y., et al. (2024). From gut to brain: Understanding the role of microbiota in inflammatory bowel disease. *Frontiers in Immunology, 15*, 1384270.
Weissman, D. G., & Mendes, W. B. (2021). Correlation of sympathetic and parasympathetic nervous system activity during rest and acute stress tasks. *International Journal of Psychophysiology, 162*, 60.
Wester, R. A., Steinbrenner, T., Hanraths, S., Ehrenthal, J. C., Iovoli, F., Fritz, J., et al. (2025). Practices of personalized treatment selection among German psychotherapists: A preregistered mixed methods study. *Psychotherapy Research*, 1–14.
Yaribeygi, H., Panahi, Y., Sahraei, H., Johnston, T. P., & Sahebkar, A. (2017). The impact of stress on body function: A review. *EXCLI Journal, 16*, 1057.
Yıldız Karaahmet, A., Bilgiç, F. Ş, Yılmaz, T., & Shafaati, L. S. (2025). The effects of cognitive interventions on quality of life in infertile women: A meta-analysis of randomized controlled trials. *Journal of Psychosomatic Obstetrics and Gynecology, 46*(1), 2560828.
Yu, T., Wang, Z., Chen, Y., Xiang, Y., Wu, M., Zhang, M., et al. (2025). Blood–brain barrier (BBB) dysfunction in CNS diseases: Paying attention to pericytes. *CNS Neuroscience & Therapeutics, 31*(5), Article e70422.
Zeng, J., & Lo, C. H. (2025). Lipid metabolism dysregulation in obesity-related diseases and neurodegeneration. *Frontiers in endocrinology* (Vol. 16, pp. 1564003). Frontiers Media.
Zeng, J., Cheong, L. Y. T., & Lo, C. H. (2025). Therapeutic targeting of obesity-induced neuroinflammation and neurodegeneration. *Front Endocrinol (Lausanne), 15*, 1456948.

Chapter 8
Movement Matters: Musculoskeletal Disorders and Mobility Solutions

Subhankari Prasad Chakraborty and Mokhtar Rejili

Abstract Diabetes mellitus is well known for vascular, renal, ophthalmic, and neuropathic complications. Musculoskeletal health refers to the performance of locomotor system, involving muscles, bones, joints and adjacent connective tissues. Musculoskeletal impairments consist of more than 150 different diseases or conditions that affect the system. Such impairments are categorized by the impairments of bones, muscles, joints, ligaments, nerves, disc, tendons and adjacent connective tissues that lead to temporary or lifelong disorders. Musculoskeletal disorders are characterized by pain and limitations in mobility and dexterity, and reducing the individual's ability to work, lower levels of well being and reduced ability to participate in society. Many of these musculoskeletal complications are underdiagnosed, under-managed, yet contribute substantially to disability, impair physical activity, and thereby form a vicious cycle. The risk of musculoskeletal disorders (MSDs) can be reduced by incorporating few changes in daily routine like stretching, posture adjusting, and using ergonomic tools. This work systematically examines: (1) the epidemiology and types of musculoskeletal disorders seen in diabetes; (2) the pathophysiological mechanisms linking hyperglycemia and other metabolic derangements to musculoskeletal pathology; (3) impact on mobility, function, and quality of life; (4) current and emerging solutions like therapeutic, rehabilitative, technological to prevent or mitigate MSDs; and (5) gaps in research, recommendations for integrating musculoskeletal care into diabetic management: healing beyond blood sugar.

Keywords Diabetes · Musculoskeletal disorder · Bone deformity · Myopathies · Rehabilitation

---

S. P. Chakraborty (✉)
Department of Physiology, Ramananda College, Bishnupur, Bankura, India
e-mail: subhankariprasad@gmail.com

M. Rejili
Department of Biology, College of Sciences, Imam Mohammad Ibn Saud Islamic University (IMSIU), Riyadh, Saudi Arabia
e-mail: msrejili@imamu.edu.sa

K. Adhikary et al. (eds.), *Healing Beyond Blood Sugar*,
https://doi.org/10.1007/978-981-95-8946-3_8

8.1 Introduction

Diabetes mellitus (DM) affects hundreds of millions globally considering the complications of microvascular (retinopathy, nephropathy, neuropathy) and macrovascular (cardiovascular disease, peripheral arterial disease). However, less visible but still impactful are musculoskeletal complications. Musculoskeletal complication includes connective tissue stiffening, tendinopathies, joint motion loss, arthropathies, soft tissue thickening, etc. Although these are often non-fatal, but they significantly impair the function, activity, and quality of life, and thereby contributing to morbidity, healthcare burden, and indirectly worsening metabolic control. The concept "Healing Beyond Blood Sugar" is crucial that managing diabetes through controlling glucose levels and to preserve or restore mobility of bones, joints, muscles, tendons, and feet.

8.1.1 Overview of Diabetes

Diabetes, a metabolic disorder, is caused by resistance to insulin, either as a result of insufficient insulin secretion and function, or both. Diabetes affected 463 million people in 2019 and will affect 700 million by 2045 in the world. It is mainly characterized by high blood glucose level; known as hyperglycemia. The decreased function of insulin on target organs also causes the abnormal metabolism of carbohydrate, protein and fat. Diabetes affects all organs and systems of the human body. Chronic hyperglycemia is associated with long-term dysfunction of the heart, blood vessels, eyes, kidneys, nervous system and musculoskeletal system (Liane, 2023). Current research has suggested that diabetes has an important role in the development of several conditions such as adhesive capsulitis of the glenohumeral joint (AC), stenosing flexor tenosynovitis of the finger (SfTf), calcific tendinitis (Chammas et al., 1995; Crispin & Alcocer-Varela, 2003; Griggs et al., 1995; Lequesne et al., 1977). Diabetes itself does not cause such disorders, but it can be a predisposing factor (Balci et al., 1999). Recent studies explores the etiopathophysiology behind its predisposition towards the development of musculoskeletal disorders in diabetic patients, as well as increased severity of pain and functional impairment and inferior treatment efficacy (Fitzgibbons & Weiss, 2008; Salek et al., 2010; Vance et al., 2012).

8.1.2 Overview of Musculoskeletal Health

Musculoskeletal health denotes the performance of locomotor system including integral muscles, bones, joints and adjacent connective tissues. Musculoskeletal impairments include more than 150 different diseases/conditions that affect the locomotor system, and are characterized by the impairments of muscles, bones, joints and adjacent connective tissues that lead to temporary or lifelong restrictions in function and participation. Musculoskeletal conditions are described by pain and restrictions in mobility that reduces the ability of work and participate in society. Musculoskeletal conditions are relevant from childhood to older age, ranges from sudden arise (like fractures, sprains and strains, associated with pain and limitations in functioning) or long term conditions (like chronic primary low back pain and osteoarthritis) (Cieza et al., 2021). Musculoskeletal conditions include conditions that affect:

Joints: osteoarthritis, rheumatoid arthritis, psoriatic arthritis, gout, spondyloarthritis;

Bones: osteoporosis, osteopenia and associated fragility fractures, traumatic fractures;

Muscles: sarcopenia

Multiple body areas or systems: regional (back and neck pain) and widespread (fibromyalgia) pain, inflammatory diseases such as connective tissue diseases and vasculitis.

Musculoskeletal conditions are the highest contributor to global need for rehabilitation (Williams et al., 2018).

8.1.3 *Scope and Purpose of This Chapter*

This chapter will focus on the discussion of diabetes associated musculoskeletal disorders (MSDs) and mobility solution in form of musculoskeletal complications such as frozen shoulder, carpal tunnel syndrome, diabetic cheiroarthropathy, Charcot joint; pharmacological, physical therapy and surgical interventions to combat it; and preventive strategies. The purpose of this chapter is to promote early detection, educate healthcare providers, and raise awareness about musculoskeletal complications during diabetes.

8.2 Epidemiology and Types of Musculoskeletal Disorders in Diabetes Mellitus

8.2.1 *Prevalence*

Musculoskeletal disorders are common in diabetic populations, often co-existing, and some have modifiable risk factors or amenable to intervention. Multiple studies show high prevalence of MSDs disorders in people with diabetes. A systematic review reported that overall prevalence of MSDs among diabetic patients is about 58.15%; and hand was the most commonly affected area (almost 33.05%), followed by the shoulder (Kaka et al., 2019). A cross-sectional study from Turkey dealing with 702 diabetic patients reported that 45.9% had one or more MSDs (Choi et al., 2022). In Egypt, about 53% among Type 2 diabetics had MSDs (Edis et al., 2025). A cross-sectional study from Morocco reveals that 34.4% of diabetic patients are associated with had one or more MSDs; osteoarthritis (OA), hand disorders, shoulder

Table 8.1 Prevalence of musculoskeletal disorders with or without diabetes mellitus (Choi et al., 2022; Majjad et al., 2018)

Musculoskeletal disorder	With diabetes (%)	Without diabetes (%)
Adhesive capsulitis	11–30	2–10
Limited joint mobility	8–50	0–26
Dupuytren's contracture	20–63	5–10
Carpel tunnel syndrome	11–16	2–5
Flexor tenosynovitis	10–12	< 1
Diffuse idiophatic sheletal hyperostosis	13–50	2–15

capsulitis (Majjad et al., 2018). These results vary depending on age, type of diabetes, duration, glycemic control, presence of complications, and the definitions used. The prevalence of musculoskeletal disorders with or without diabetes mellitus is summerized in Table 8.1.

8.2.2 *Types of Musculoskeletal Disorders in Diabetes Mellitus*

Diabetic patients experienced a variety of MSDs. Common MSDs in diabetes are summarized below:

Limited Joint Mobility (LJM): Sometimes called diabetic cheiroarthropathy. Symptoms include stiffening of hand joints, thickening of skin, "prayer sign" or "tabletop sign" (Radwan et al., 2017).

Adhesive capsulitis of the shoulder: Also known as frozen shoulder. Symptoms include pain, stiffness, reduced motion and restricted shoulder movements (Mueller, 2016).

Carpal Tunnel Syndrome (CTS): Also called as tenosynovitis, Dupuytren's contracture. Symptoms include compressive neuropathy due to connective tissue changes and swelling (Choi et al., 2022).

Charcot joint: Also known as neuropathic arthropathy: It includes severe and destructive joint changes in feet with neuropathy (Eitner & Wildemann, 2021).

Dupuytren's contracture: It is the thickening and contracture of palmar fascia (Choi et al., 2022).

Trigger finger: Involves tenosynovitis, flexor issues in hand tendons (Hussain et al., 2025).

Charcot arthropathy: Commonly known as diabetic foot complications: It is not only the ulceration and infection, but also changes in bone, joint mobility in foot/ankle (Choi et al., 2022).

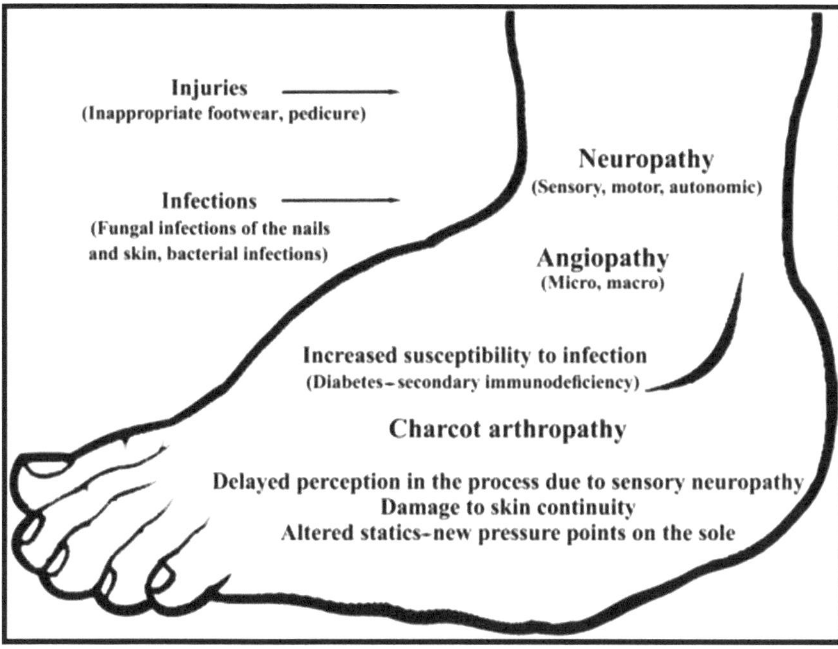

Fig. 8.1 Musculoskeletal disorders associated with diabetes mellitus

Osteoarthritis: It is especially weight-bearing at joints (knee, hip). Obesity often aggravates as risk factor (Majjad et al., 2018).

Bone changes: Osteoporosis, increased risk of fractures, especially with neuropathy is found in type 1 diabetics due to impaired bone density and delayed fracture healing (Monteiro et al., 2018).

Muscle-related issues: Muscle cramps, diabetic muscle infarction, reduced muscle mass (sarcopenia) (Radwan et al., 2017) (Fig. 8.1).

8.2.3 Risk Factors and Associated Variables in Musculoskeletal Disorders in Diabetes Mellitus

Some of the factors associated with higher prevalence or severity of MSDs:

Duration of diabetes: Longer period of diabetes correlates with more MSDs (Choi et al., 2022).

Glycemic control: Poor control of HbA1c is associated with certain disorders like adhesive capsulitis, Dupuytren's, CTS (Choi et al., 2022).

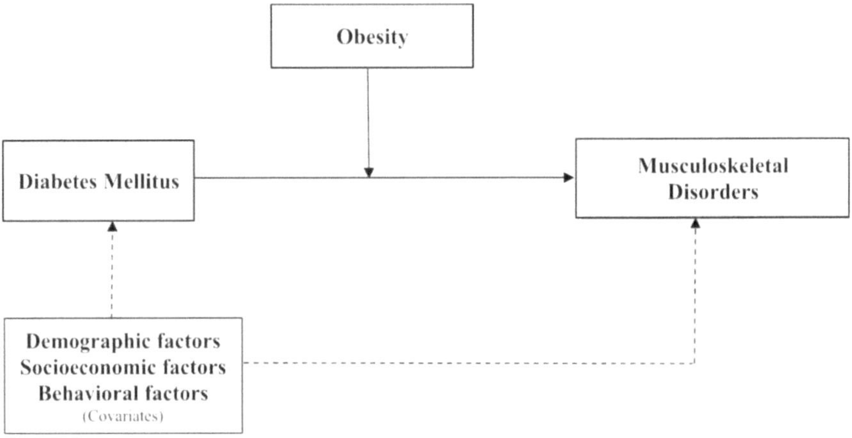

Fig. 8.2 Role of obesity and diabetes for prognosis of musculoskeletal disorders

Obesity: Overweight contributes mechanical load and amplifies joint stress (Majjad et al., 2018) (Fig. 8.2).

Microvascular complications: Neuropathy and retinopathy has strong association with MSDs (Choi et al., 2022).

Age and gender: Old aged female are often at higher risk of shoulder, hand disorders (Majjad et al., 2018).

Dyslipidemia: Studies reported that dyslipidemia and other metabolic derangements is associated with MSDs to some extent (Majjad et al., 2018).

8.3 Pathophysiology of Musculoskeletal Disorders in Diabetes Mellitus

8.3.1 Hyperglycemia, Advanced Glycation End Products (AGEs)

High blood glucose level leads to the non-enzymatic glycation of proteins and lipids to form AGEs. AGEs accumulate in collagen and other connective tissue proteins. Such accumulation causes cross-linking, stiffening of tendons, ligaments, joint capsules, skin and reduces elasticity and joint mobility (Sozen et al., 2018). AGEs-RAGE (receptor for advanced glycation end-products) axis induces oxidative stress, inflammation, and worsened tissue damage (Kaka et al., 2019).

8.3.2 Microvascular and Macrovascular Changes

Diabetes causes endothelial dysfunction, thickening of capillary basement membrane and reduces perfusion in the microcirculation to connective tissues, tendons, joint capsules and skin. Tissue repairing is impaired due to decline perfusion of microcirculation that makes the slowly healing of minor injuries (Choi et al., 2022). In diabetes, impairments of mobility can precede macrovascular complications and contribute to hospitalizations. Microangiopathy and peripheral arterial disease also reduces the blood supply to musculoskeletal tissues; results of impairment of tissue repairing that contributes to ischemic changes and delayed the healing process (Eitner & Wildemann, 2021).

8.3.3 Neuropathy

Peripheral neuropathy leads to impaired proprioception, altered gait, muscle weakness and reduced protective sensation. The foot and ankle joints loose feedback. The patient may involuntarily overuse or misuse the joints and leading to deformities. Neuropathy can also reduce the pain perception and reflexes that causes the downward protective feedback mechanism (Radwan et al., 2017).

8.3.4 Connective Tissue and Skin Changes

Increased collagen deposition causes the thickening of peri-articular soft tissues, glycosylation of structural proteins; result of changes in tendon, ligament and capsular tissues. The stiffness of skin reduces the mobility and increases the risk of cracking (Hussain et al., 2025; Radwan et al., 2017).

8.3.5 Inflammation, Oxidative Stress and Altered Cellular Signalling

Chronic low-grade inflammation elevates the levels of cytokines (e.g., IL-6, TNF-α) and reactive oxygen species that causes oxidative stress and amplify tissue damage. This state also develops the insulin resistance in muscle; changes the insulin-like growth factor (IGF) signalling and ultimately altered bone turnover (Radwan et al., 2017).

8.3.6 *Obesity, Mechanical Load and Sedentary Life Style*

Obesity or excess body weight increases the mechanical loads on joints (knees, hips, spine) and accelerates the osteoarthritis. Reduced physical activity may lead to muscle weakness and poor joint stability. Behaviour of sedentary life style is associated with reduced joint lubrication, muscle atrophy, and meagre coordination and balance (Sozen et al., 2018).

8.3.7 *Hormonal and Bone Metabolism Alterations*

Bone metabolism is altered in type 1 and type 2 diabetes. Decreased bone mineral density is associated in type 1 diabetes; whereas in type 2, bone density remains normal or slightly increases but the quality of bone is inferior that rises the risk of fracture. Certain anti-diabetic medicine like thiazolidinediones has adverse effects on bone (Radwan et al., 2017).

8.4 Impact on Mobility, Function and Quality of Life

MSDs interfere with mobility and overall physical function in following ways:

8.4.1 *Effect on Activities of Daily Living (ADLs)*

Pain, joint stiffness, loss of flexibility in hands, shoulders and ankles reduces the daily living tasks like dressing, feeding, standing, walking, balancing and personal hygiene. Such complications increase the risk of falling and fractures. Shoulder problems interfere with overhead reaching (Monteiro et al., 2023; Weatherall et al., 2024).

8.4.2 *Gait, Locomotion, and Walking Mechanics*

Reduce mobility of ankle-foot joint, muscle weakness and altered plantar pressures due to pre-ulcerative changes leads to altered gait, slower walking, fear of walking and rises the risk of fall and fracture (Monteiro et al., 2023).

8.4.3 *Pain, Psychological Impacts and Participation*

Chronic pain of osteoarthritis, tendon disorders and neuropathic pain reduces the day-to-day physical activity. Psychological changes like depression, fear reduces the mobility as well as participation in work and social life (Weatherall et al., 2024).

8.4.4 *Downward Spiral Effects*

Decrease physical mobility reduces the physical activity; result of weight gain that leads to obesity and insulin resistance and hampers the glycemic control (Monteiro et al., 2023).

8.5 Mobility Solutions and Therapeutic Strategies

To heal beyond blood sugar, interventions must address by not only metabolic control but also the mobility, structure and function of musculoskeletal system. Some strategies with promising potential are summarized below (Weatherall et al., 2024).

8.5.1 *Medical and Pharmacological Interventions*

Glycemic control: Strict control of blood glucose level lowers the HbA1c which helps to reduce AGE formation and protect and preserve the connective tissue. Higher HbA1c is associated with MSDs (Choi et al., 2022).

Anti-inflammatory agents: NSAIDs are used for the pain management in neuropathy and corticosteroid injections are preferred for local tendon or joint inflammation in adhesive capsulitis (Sozen et al., 2018).

Disease-modifying agents for bone health: Co-morbidities of MSDs such as dyslipidemia, obesity should be controlled. Bisphosphonates and vitamin D supplementation is preferred for the treatment of osteoporosis or osteopenia (Browne et al., 2001).

8.5.2 *Physical Therapy, Exercise Therapies and Rehabilitation*

Flexibility and Range of Motion (ROM) Exercises: Regular passive stretching and joint mobilization for shoulders, hands and ankle to get benefit of frozen shoulder and limited joint mobility (Majjad et al., 2018).

Strength training: It supports joint stability especially intrinsic and extrinsic foot muscles and improves the muscle mass, supports joints, helps gait and balance (Monteiro et al., 2023).

Low impact cardiovascular exercise: Walking, cycling, and swimming as weight management aid and to improve circulation by maintaining mobility while minimizing joint stress (Monteiro et al., 2018).

Weight loss / body composition management: By reducing mechanical load (Radwan et al., 2017).

Balance and proprioceptive exercises: to reduce the risk of fall (especially with neuropathy) (Sartor et al., 2014) (Fig. 8.3).

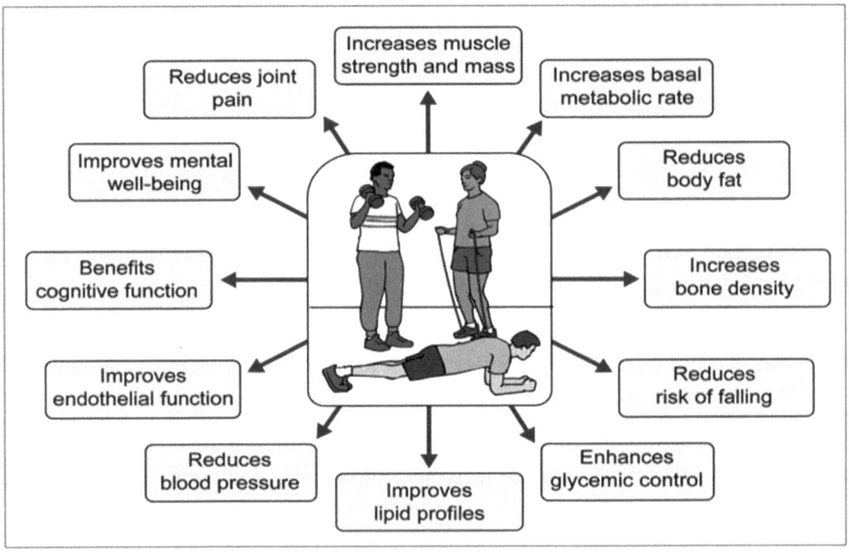

Fig. 8.3 Functions of musculoskeletal exercise to overcome musculoskeletal impairments in diabetes

8.5.3 Orthotics, Physiotherapy and Manual Therapy

Foot orthoses/special footwear: Offloading devices for high plantar pressure areas, especially in diabetic foot risk, plantar pressure offloading, preventing ulcers and reducing foot/ankle joint strain (Browne et al., 2001).

Hand splints, braces: Used for CTS, trigger finger, wrist support, custom insoles, and footwear t to reduce plantar pressures (Browne et al., 2001).

Physiotherapy: Get relief form pain, improving joint function (e.g. for adhesive capsulitis), includes stretching and mobilization (Majjad et al., 2018).

Assistive mobility supports: Walkers, canes where joint pain or neurological deficits interfere with gait (Weatherall et al., 2024).

8.5.4 Emerging and Technological Solutions

AI-driven offloading prescription: Based on patient biomechanics, Artificial Intelligence (AI) is used for diabetic foot for designing customized insoles/footwear to prevent ulcer (Weatherall et al., 2024).

Tele-rehabilitation: For guided exercise and engagement (Kaka et al., 2019).

Mobile/digital health interventions: To monitor mobility and support adherence to exercise regimens (Yom-Tov et al., 2017).

8.5.5 Surgical or Interventional Approaches

Corticosteroid injections are preferred for severe adhesive capsulitis or tendon inflammation. For dupuytren's contracture, surgery or minimally invasive procedures is approached. For Charcot arthropathy, not only restriction of body weight, immobilization, off-loading, but also sometimes surgical reconstruction is advised (Eitner & Wildemann, 2021).

8.5.6 Lifestyle, Foot Care and Education

Weight reduction is key to reduce mechanical stress on joints. Daily inspection, proper foot hygiene and footwear, and management of minor foot injuries in foots is advised. Patient education and behaviour change regarding consistent exercise and reduction of sedentary time is encouraged. Early screening of MSDs including joint mobility checks, hand function, foot/ankle screening at routine diabetic check-up is recommended (Monteiro et al., 2023).

8.6 Challenges, Gaps and Future Directions

- More longitudinal studies are required to clarify temporal relationships between hyperglycemia, gender, age, metabolic control and MSDs.
- The access of mobility-preserving interventions (such as physiotherapy, orthoses, advanced footwear) is limited to low-resource settings due to cost, awareness and infrastructure barriers.
- More research regarding the development of novel technologies like wearable sensors, remote monitoring; personalized devices to combat with MSDs during glycemia need to be investigated.
- Research for understanding the bone quality and the role of bone health in type 1 and type 2 diabetes need to be explored.

8.7 Recommendations

To achieve "Healing Beyond Blood Sugar," the following recommendation are to be considered:

- Routine musculoskeletal screening including hand mobility, shoulder range, foot/ankle assessment, neuropathy, vascular checks and questionnaires for pain, stiffness for diabetic patient.
- Education for patient regarding movement, flexibility, joint care, exercises at home, joint protection and weight management.
- Multidisciplinary care teams iIncluding physiotherapists, podiatrists, occupational therapists and orthopedists within diabetic care clinic.
- Tailored exercise rehabilitation programs with low-impact aerobic strength, flexibility, balance training and orthoses as needed.
- Use of technological aids like sensors, smart walkers, tele-rehab, AI for custom orthoses and remote monitoring.
- Research priorities for cost-effective longitudinal cohort studies for tracking musculoskeletal function in diabetes, before and after interventions.
- Insurance coverage of physiotherapy, orthotics and rehab by health systems.

8.8 Summary and Conclusion

Musculoskeletal disorders are incredibly common among diabetic patient. They affect hands, shoulders, joints of lower limbs, connective tissues; contribute to failure of mobility, decrease muscle strength, damage bones, and decrease the quality of life via reducing physical activity. Such impairments, thereby worsening the metabolic outcomes in a vicious cycle. Healing beyond blood sugar implies a holistic approach, addressing metabolic control and functional health. It requires proactive attention to musculoskeletal health: early screening, good glycemic and metabolic control, patient education, lifestyle modification (exercise, weight management), physical therapy, orthotic and surgical interventions, and the use of modern emerging technological solutions for monitoring and personalized interventions. This holistic care approach not only improves the mobility and reduces pain, but also supports better health, quality of life, and long-term outcomes in diabetic patient.

References

Balci, N., Balci, M. K., & Tuzuner, S. (1999). Shoulder adhesive capsulitis and shoulder range of motion in type II diabetes mellitus: Association with diabetic complications. *Journal of Diabetes and Its Complications, 13*(3), 135–140. https://doi.org/10.1016/s1056-8727(99)00037-9

Browne, D. L., McCrae, F. C., & Shaw, K. M. (2001). Musculoskeletal diseases in diabetes. *Practical Diabetes, 18*(2), 62–64.

Chammas, M., Bousquet, P., Renard, E., Poirier, J. L., Jaffiol, C., & Allieu, Y. (1995). Dupuytren's disease, carpal tunnel syndrome, trigger finger, and diabetes mellitus. *The Journal of Hand Surgery, 20*(1), 109–114. https://doi.org/10.1016/S0363-5023(05)80068-1

Choi, J. H., Kim, H. R., & Song, K. H. (2022). Musculoskeletal complications in patients with diabetes mellitus. *The Korean Journal of Internal Medicine, 37*(6), 1099–1110. https://doi.org/10.3904/kjim.2022.168

Cieza, A., Causey, K., Kamenov, K., Hanson, S. W., Chatterji, S., & Vos, T. (2021). Global estimates of the need for rehabilitation based on the Global Burden of Disease study 2019: A systematic analysis for the Global Burden of Disease Study 2019. *The Lancet, 396*(10267), 2006–2017. https://doi.org/10.1016/S0140-6736(20)32340-0

Crispin, J. C., & Alcocer-Varela, J. (2003). Rheumatologic manifestations of diabetes mellitus. *The American Journal of Medicine, 114*(9), 753–757. https://doi.org/10.1016/s0002-9343(03)00140-2

Edis, P., Ozdemir, N., & Hekimsoy, Z. (2025). The musculoskeletal disorders in diabetic patients and the evaluation of their relationship with metabolic parameters and microvascular complications. *Acta Endocrinol (Buchar), 20*(2), 136–142. https://doi.org/10.4183/aeb.2024.136

Eitner, A., & Wildemann, B. (2021). Diabetes-osteoarthritis and joint pain. *Bone and Joint Research, 10*(5), 307–309. https://doi.org/10.1302/2046-3758.105

Fitzgibbons, P. G., & Weiss, A. P. (2008). Hand manifestations of diabetes mellitus. *Journal of Hand Surgery, 33*(5), 771–775. https://doi.org/10.1016/j.jhsa.2008.01.038

Griggs, S. M., Weiss, A. P., Lane, L. B., Schwenker, C., Akelman, E., & Sachar, K. (1995). Treatment of trigger finger in patients with diabetes mellitus. *The Journal of Hand Surgery, 20*(5), 787–789. https://doi.org/10.1016/S0363-5023(05)80432-0

Hussain, S., Irfan, M., Khan, M., Khan, M. K., Awan, S. K., Raza, S. S., Adil, A. N. K., & Varrassi, G. (2025). From glycemia to grip: A comprehensive review of musculoskeletal complications in diabetic patients. *The Cureus Journal of Medical Sciences, 17*(8), Article e90838. https://doi.org/10.7759/cureus.90838

Kaka, B., Maharaj, S. S., & Fatoye, F. (2019). Prevalence of musculoskeletal disorders in patients with diabetes mellitus: A systematic review and meta-analysis. *Journal of Back and Musculoskeletal Rehabilitation, 32*(2), 223–235. https://doi.org/10.3233/BMR-171086

Lequesne, M., Dang, N., Bensasson, M., & Mery, C. (1977). Increased association of diabetes mellitus with capsulitis of the shoulder and shoulder-hand syndrome. *Scandinavian Journal of Rheumatology., 6*(1), 53–56. PMID: 66744.

Liane, O. A. (2023). Global, regional, and national burden of diabetes from 1990 to 2021, with projections of prevalence to 2050: A systematic analysis for the Global Burden of Disease Study 2021. *The Lancet, 402*(10397), 203–234. https://doi.org/10.1016/S0140-6736(25)00053-4

Majjad, A., Errahali, Y., Toufik, H., Djossou, J., Ghassem, M. A., Kasouati, J., & Maghraoui, A. E. (2018). Musculoskeletal disorders in patients with diabetes mellitus: A Cross-Sectional Study. *International journal of rheumatology*. https://doi.org/10.1155/2018/3839872

Monteiro, R. L., Drechsel, T. J., Ferreira, J. S. S. P., Zippenfennig, C., & Sacco, I. C. N. (2023). Potential predictive effect of mechanical properties of the plantar skin and superficial soft tissue, and vibration perception on plantar loading during gait in individuals with diabetes. *BMC Musculoskeletal Disorder, 24*(1), 712. https://doi.org/10.1186/s12891-023-06851-7

Monteiro, R. L., Sartor, C. D., Ferreira, J. S. S. P., Dantas, M. G. B., Bus, S. A., & Sacco, I. C. N. (2018). Protocol for evaluating the effects of a foot-ankle therapeutic exercise program on daily activity, foot-ankle functionality, and biomechanics in people with diabetic polyneuropathy: A randomized controlled trial. *BMC Musculoskeletal Disorder, 19*(1), 400. https://doi.org/10.1186/s12891-018-2323-0

Mueller, M. J. (2016). Musculoskeletal impairments are often unrecognized and underappreciated complications from diabetes. *Physical Therapy, 96*(12), 1861–1864. https://doi.org/10.2522/ptj.20160326

Radwan, A., Arafa, O., Ahmed, A., & Abd-El Mageed, S. (2017). Musculoskeletal disorders in type 2 diabetes mellitus. *Sohag Medical Journal, 21*(3), 255–260. https://doi.org/10.21608/smj.2017.39739

Salek, A. K., Mamun, M. A., Haque, M. A., Mannan, M., Ali, E., Islam, S., Rizvi, A. N., Chowdhury, A. Z., Islam, J., Rahman, M. H., & Ferdous, C. (2010). Serum triglyceride level in type 2 diabetes mellitus patients with or without frozen shoulder. *Bangladesh Medical Research Council Bulletin, 36*(2), 64–67. https://doi.org/10.3329/bmrcb.v36i2.6990

Sartor, C. D., Hasue, R. H., Cacciari, L. P., Butugan, M. K., Watari, R., Passaro, A. C., Giacomozzi, C., & Sacco, I. C. (2014). Effects of strengthening, stretching and functional training on foot function in patients with diabetic neuropathy: Results of a randomized controlled trial. *BMC Musculoskeletal Disorder, 15*, 137. https://doi.org/10.1186/1471-2474-15-137

Sozen, T., Başaran, N. Ç., Tınazlı, M., & Ozışık, L. (2018). Musculoskeletal problems in diabetes mellitus. *European Journal of Rheumatology, 5*(4), 258–265. https://doi.org/10.5152/eurjrheum.2018.18044

Vance, M. C., Tucker, J. J., & Harness, N. G. (2012). The association of hemoglobin A1c with the prevalence of stenosing flexor tenosynovitis. *The Journal of Hand Surgery, 37*(9), 1765–1769. https://doi.org/10.1016/j.jhsa.2012.06.007

Weatherall, T., Avsar, P., Nugent, L., Moore, Z., McDermott, J. H., Sreenan, S., Wilson, H., McEvoy, N. L., Derwin, R., Chadwick, P., & Patton, D. (2024). The impact of machine learning on the prediction of diabetic foot ulcers—A systematic review. *Journal Tissue Viability, 33*(4), 853–863. https://doi.org/10.1016/j.jtv.2024.07.004

Williams, A., Kamper, S. J., Wiggers, J. H., O'Brien, K. M., Lee, H., Wolfenden, L., Yoong, S. L., Robson, E., McAuley, J. H., Hartvigsen, J., & Williams, C. M. (2018). Musculoskeletal conditions may increase the risk of chronic disease: A systematic review and meta-analysis of cohort studies. *BMC Medicine, 16*(1), 167. https://doi.org/10.1186/s12916-018-1151-2

Yom-Tov, E., Feraru, G., Kozdoba, M., Mannor, S., Tennenholtz, M., & Hochberg, I. (2017). Encouraging physical activity in patients with diabetes: Intervention using a reinforcement learning system. *Journal of Medical Internet Research, 19*(10), Article e338. https://doi.org/10.2196/jmir.7994

Chapter 9
Breaking the Stigma: Addressing Sexual Dysfunction and Intimacy in Diabetes

Dibya Pal, Riya Sarkar, Sangita Das, Mounir Trabelsi, and Debidas Ghosh

Abstract Living with diabetes brings many physical and emotional challenges, and one of the most overlooked challenges is its impact on sexual health and intimacy. People with diabetes both men and women often experience sexual problems like erectile dysfunction, vaginal dryness, decreased desire for mating, painful intercourse and loss of libido. These issues don't just affect the body; they also take a toll on emotional well-being and relationships. Because of stigma and embarrassment, many people suffer in silence and thinking they are alone in this struggle. This chapter shines a light on the connection between diabetes and sexual dysfunction by explaining how changes in blood glucose levels, nerve damage, hormonal imbalances, and mental stress, it focuses on the emotional side of living with these problems. Open conversations with partners and healthcare providers are key to breaking the silence and finding support. This chapter also focuses on a kinder, more understanding approach from both society and the medical community. Sexual health should be a normal part of diabetes care, not something hidden away. By creating safe spaces for dialogue and providing proper treatment along with counselling, we can help people with diabetes to increase their quality adjusted life years. This chapter is an alarming call to break the stigma, emphasizing that intimacy, trust, and connection remain vital regardless of the health challenges someone may face in diabetes.

Keywords Diabetes · Counselling · Sexual dysfunction · Quality adjusted life years · Stigma

D. Pal
Department of Bio-Medical Laboratory Science and Management, Molecular Medicine, Nutrigenomics and Public Health Research Laboratory, Vidyasagar University, Paschim Midnapore, India

R. Sarkar · S. Das
Department of Medical Laboratory Technology, Dr. B. C. Roy Engineering College, Durgapur, India

M. Trabelsi
Faculty of Medicine Sousse, University of Sousse Tunisia, Sousse, Tunisia

D. Ghosh (✉)
Debra Thana Sahid Kshudiram Smriti Mahavidyalaya, Paschim Midnapore, India
e-mail: debidasghosh999@gmail.com

K. Adhikary et al. (eds.), *Healing Beyond Blood Sugar*,
https://doi.org/10.1007/978-981-95-8946-3_9

9.1 Introduction

9.1.1 The Hidden Impact of Diabetes on Sexual Health

Sexual health is often regarded as a private matter, but in reality, it is an integral part of overall well-being. For people living with diabetes, however, this important dimension of life is frequently overlooked, remained hidden behind stigma and silence. The sexual complications of diabetes are not isolated problems; there are closely tied to the same vascular and neurological processes that drive other diabetic complications. Yet, because they remain hidden behind stigma and silence, they are often overlooked, leaving many to suffer quietly (Fig. 9.1).

Sexual dysfunction (SD) has strong impact on emotional health, intimacy and self-esteem. In men, erectile dysfunction (ED) is the most frequent sexual complication and about 75% of men with persistent diabetes experience ED (Isidro, 2012).

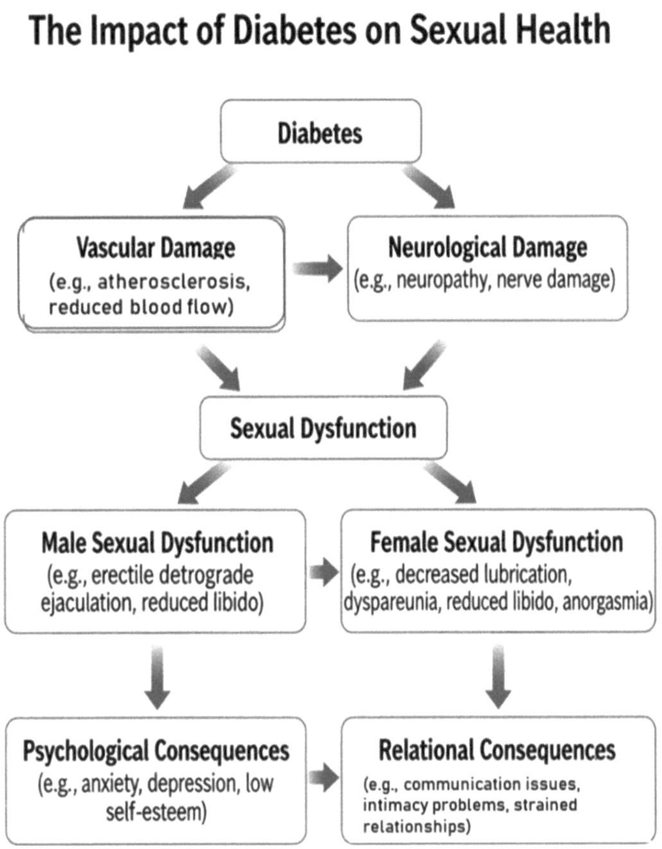

Fig. 9.1 Diabetes associated sexual dysfunction

The reasons are heterogenous: chronic hyperglycemia damages small blood vessels and nerves, impairs nitric oxide (NO) availability, and disrupts normal vascular relaxation. Beyond being a barrier to intimacy, ED has deeper clinical significance. It is increasingly recognized as an early warning sign of cardiovascular disease, a sentinel marker of endothelial dysfunction (An et al., 2025). Thus, ignoring ED in diabetes is not only detrimental to quality of life but may also delay the detection of serious systemic disease.

For women, the landscape of SD is more complex and unfortunately less well studied. Female sexual dysfunction (FSD) encompasses a wide spectrum of difficulties: reduced libido, impaired arousal, vaginal dryness due to decreased lubrication, challenges in achieving orgasm, and dyspareunia (painful intercourse). Estimates suggest that between 50 and 70% of women with diabetes face some form of FSD, with type 2 diabetes (T2D) showing particularly high prevalence (Derosa et al., 2023). Biological mechanisms like as fluctuating estrogen levels, reduced genital blood flow from vascular damage, and diabetic neuropathy—interfere with normal sexual responses. However, the issue extends beyond biology. Women with diabetes-related FSD often report greater emotional distress, anxiety, and diminished quality of life compared to those without sexual problems (Rogoznica et al., 2023). The lack of attention to female sexual health in clinical care further increase their suffering that creates a cycle of neglect and silence.

The hidden impact of such complications is profound. Men may struggle with feelings of inadequacy or loss of masculinity, while women may feel unattractive or disconnected from their bodies. These insecurities ripple outward into relationships. Partners, lacking understanding, may misinterpret the withdrawal from intimacy as rejection, disinterest, or even infidelity.

In this way, SD in diabetes acts as a silent disruptor. It affects intimacy, destabilizes emotional bonds, and diminishes psychological well-being. Unlike visible complications of diabetes that command urgent medical attention, sexual health problems remain in the shadows, quietly hampering quality of life and straining relationships. Recognizing this hidden burden is the first step toward breaking the silence and restoring both physical and emotional health for individuals and couples living with diabetes.

9.1.2 Why Sexual Dysfunction Is Often Ignored?

Although SD is one of the most common complications of diabetes, not discussed in both clinical practice and social discourse. This silence is not accidental, it is reinforced by a combination of cultural, psychological, and medical factors that make conversations about intimacy difficult, uncomfortable, or simply invisible.

Social and Cultural Stigma

In many parts of the world, sexuality is still treated as a taboo subject. Talking about intimate problems, especially in public or medical settings, is seen as shameful or inappropriate. This silence is even more noticeable among women, who may feel bound by traditional gender roles that discourage open discussions about desire, pleasure, or intimacy. The cultural message, often unspoken, is that sexual problems are not important enough to be voiced, an attitude that leaves countless individuals to suffer in isolation.

Clinical Oversight and Discomfort

Healthcare providers themselves often play a role in perpetuating this neglect. In busy clinical settings, physicians tend to focus on complications considered "life-threatening," such as cardiovascular disease, kidney dysfunction, or retinopathy. While these are undeniably critical, sexual health is frequently sidelined, viewed as less urgent or even irrelevant. Moreover, many healthcare professionals lack training in sexual medicine. They may feel uncomfortable initiating conversations about intimacy, worry about offending patients, or believe that patients would not want to discuss such sensitive topics. This discomfort creates a mutual silence, patients wait for doctors to ask, while doctors assume patients will speak up if the issue is important. As a result, the subject never come to surface.

Normalization and Misconceptions

Another major barrier is the widespread belief that SD is simply a normal part of aging. Patients may attribute declining sexual desire or performance to "getting older," while physicians may adopt the same view, dismissing concerns without proper check-ups. This normalization delays recognition and prevents timely intervention. In reality, while aging can bring changes in sexual function, the dysfunction associated with diabetes is pathological and often treatable. By writing it off as "natural," both patients and service providers neglect this issue.

Psychological Barriers

The burden of diabetes like constant blood glucose monitoring, dietary restrictions, and fear of complications already weighs heavily on patients. Adding sexual difficulties to the mix often brings feelings of guilt, inadequacy, or hopelessness. Depression and anxiety are both common in diabetes and serve as amplifiers of SD: they not only worsen performance and desire but also discourage individuals from seeking help (Kalra et al., 2018).

The Cost of Ignoring SD

The consequences of this silence are far-reaching. For men, erectile dysfunction is not just a sexual problem but can be a hidden indicator of vascular disease, meaning opportunities for early detection of heart problems may be missed. For women, unresolved dysfunction often leads to emotional withdrawal, loneliness, and a sense of invisibility.

Recent studies highlight how profoundly intertwined sexual health is with mental health and diabetes outcomes. For instance, in women with type 1 diabetes (T1D), depression has been shown to be a stronger predictor of SD than vascular complications themselves, torching the psychological weight of this issue. In men, poor glycemic control strongly correlates with erectile and orgasmic difficulties, revealing how closely everyday diabetes management intersects with sexual well-being (Meamar et al., 2025).

9.1.3 *Breaking the Silence*

Breaking the silence means this field is valid and diabetic care should be practice and compassionate by information collection through open ended question asking, safe and private space for discussion with empathies and support couples. In diabetic care, sexual health is discussed at least level though it has immerse impact on self-confidence, relationship and emotional well-being. Health care professionals frequently untouch the conversation about sexual health as this is considered as unimportant, untreatable and shameful. The truth is that it is a treatable consequence in diabetes.

9.2 Understanding Diabetes and Its Systemic Complications

9.2.1 *Overview of T1D and T2D*

Type 1 diabetes can develop at any age of human life cycle though it is primarily noted in below 20 years age group. It happens when the pancreas stops making insulin because the insulin-producing beta cells are destroyed or no longer function properly. People living with T1D need daily insulin injections to keep their blood sugar levels within a healthy range. While the exact cause is still not fully known, researchers believe it arises from a combination of genetic predisposition and environmental triggers (Kumar et al., 2020).

Type 2 diabetes is the most common type of diabetes. Although it typically develops in adulthood, the growing rates of obesity and inactive lifestyles mean that more teenagers and young adults are now being affected, sometimes first showing signs as prediabetes. In T2D, the body's fat, muscle, and liver cells don't respond the way they should to insulin, called insulin resistance. When this happens, sugar can't enter the cells to be used for energy and instead starts accumulation in the blood. This resistance doesn't appear all at once; it gradually develops over time (Eberle & Stichling, 2021).

9.2.2 *Pathophysiology of Diabetes and Sexual Health*

The development of diabetes is complex, with no single cause driving the disease. When it comes to ED and FSD in people with diabetes, several biological changes are thought to play a role. These include the buildup of harmful molecules called advanced glycation end-products (AGEs), higher levels of oxygen free radicals, hormonal imbalance and reduced production of NO. Other contributing factors include changes in endothelin receptor activity, structural alterations in tissues, overactivation of the RhoA/Rho-kinase pathway, selective damage to NO-dependent nerves, and problems with signaling pathways such as the cGMP-dependent kinase-1 (PKG-1). Together, these changes interfere with normal reproductive function (Morano, 2003).

9.2.3 *Oxidative Stress and Its Role in Diabetic Complications*

Oxidative stress, caused by abnormal metabolism, is a key factor in the development of diabetes and its complications. High blood sugar (hyperglycemia) and elevated blood fats (hyperlipemia) trigger the body to produce excessive reactive oxygen species (ROS). This happens through increased activity in the mitochondria, enhanced activity of enzymes like NADPH oxidase, and other processes that promote oxidative damage such as the protein kinase C pathway, the hexosamine and polyol pathways, and the formation of AGEs. Together, these changes intensify oxidative stress, contributing to the progression of diabetes and its related health problems.

9.2.3.1 Impact on Endocrine and Nervous Systems

Sexual dysfunction is common in people with diabetes and often underreported. In men with diabetes the prevalence of ED is markedly higher than in non-diabetic peers (estimates ~35–75% depending on age and diabetes duration); women with diabetes also have elevated rates of decreased desire, arousal/lubrication problems, pain and orgasmic difficulties, although studies in women are fewer and findings more heterogeneous.

Nervous system also affected and develop neuropath both in peripheral and autonomic nervous system:

- **Peripheral somatic neuropathy**: Small-fiber and large-fiber peripheral neuropathy can reduce genital sensation (penile shaft, clitoris, vulva), impairing arousal, orgasm, and tactile sexual response. Sensory loss also contributes to sexual pain in some women.
- **Autonomic neuropathy**: Damage to parasympathetic and sympathetic fibers that mediate erection, lubrication, ejaculation and orgasm, principal mechanism linking diabetes to SD. Autonomic dysfunction reduces neurogenic NO release and impairs smooth-muscle relaxation in corpora cavernosa (men) and vaginal blood flow (women), producing poor erection/lubrication and delayed or absent orgasm. Cardiac autonomic neuropathy often coexists and signals generalized autonomic involvement.

9.2.3.2 Vascular/Endothelial Dysfunctions (Crossing Nervous and Endocrine Roles)

Chronic hyperglycaemia, dyslipidaemia and inflammation accelerate macro- and microvascular diseases; endothelial dysfunction lowers NO bioavailability, worsens penile blood inflow and genital tissue perfusion, and contributes to vaginal dryness and dyspareunia. Vascular disease often coexists with neuropathy and amplifies SD.

9.2.3.3 Endocrine (Hormonal) Alterations

- **Hypogonadism/low testosterone (men):** Men with T2D frequently have lower total and free testosterone, linked to reduced libido, energy, and erectile capacity. Insulin resistance, obesity, and chronic inflammation are implicated mechanisms. Testosterone deficiency also worsens mood and can compound sexual problems.
- **Women—complex hormonal milieu:** Diabetes interacts with sex steroids, SHBG, and possibly ovarian function; however, in women the strongest drivers of SD are often mixed (vascular/neuropathic + psychological), and the hormonal links are less straightforward than in men. Thyroid dysfunction, hyperprolactinaemia and medication effects (e.g., antidepressants, some antihypertensives) also affect sexual function in both sexes (Begum et al., 2024).

9.2.3.4 Central Nervous System/Neurochemical and Psychosocial Pathways

Diabetes is associated with higher rates of depression and anxiety; these conditions and some psychotropic medications suppress libido and sexual response. Central insulin resistance and metabolic inflammation may alter neurotransmitter systems (dopamine, serotonin, NO pathways) that regulate sexual desire and reward. Cognition, body image and partner dynamics also mediate intimacy and sexual satisfaction (Begum et al., 2024).

9.2.4 Quality Adjusted Life Years (QALYs): A Broader Health Metric

Sexual dysfunctionmainly ED in men and FSD in women are highly prevalent in people with diabetes and substantially reduces health-related quality of life (HRQoL) and intimate relationships. This makes SD, valid target for QALY-based cost-utility assessment alongside other diabetes complications. QALYs are widely used by health technology assessment agencies to compare interventions across conditions; incorporating SD into QALY calculations allows policymakers to compare the value of SD treatments (medical, behavioral, device/surgical) with other diabetes interventions (Augustovski et al., 2017).

9.2.5 *Disability Adjusted Life Years (DALYs) and Impact of Diabetes*

Diabetes mellitus is now one of the leading global causes of DALYs, with the Global Burden of Disease study estimating 67 million DALYs in 2019, more than double the 1990 figure. DALYs from diabetes arise from both years of life lost due to premature mortality (mainly cardiovascular and renal complications) and years lived with disability from complications such as neuropathy, retinopathy, amputations, and kidney failure. While high-income countries see a greater proportion of years lived with disability (YLD) due to longer survival with diabetes, low- and middle-income countries carry higher years of life lost (YLL) due to poor access to care. The DALY framework highlights the urgent need for prevention, early detection, and comprehensive management of diabetes to curb its growing impact on global health (Kitaw et al., 2024).

9.3 Sexual Dysfunction in Diabetic Men and Women

9.3.1 *International and National Scenario of Diabetes Induced Sexual Dysfunctions*

Globally, SD has emerged as one of the most prevalent yet under-recognized complications of diabetes. In men, ED affects nearly 40–70% of those with diabetes, with prevalence rising sharply in T2D and with advancing age or poor glycemic control. In women, the burden is equally concerning. Studies from Europe, North America, and Asia indicate that 20–80% of women with diabetes suffer from some form of FSD, including reduced libido, poor arousal, and dyspareunia (Rogoznica et al., 2023). Unlike ED, FSD has been historically neglected in research, yet evidence clearly links it to neuropathy, microvascular complications, hormonal imbalance, and psychological distress. Health systems worldwide are slowly recognizing the importance of this issue. The American Diabetes Association (ADA) Standards of Care 2025 now explicitly recommend screening for ED in men with diabetes or prediabetes, while also emphasizing sexual health as a part of quality-of-life assessment (ADA, 2025). Similarly, the International Diabetes Federation (IDF) has advocated for integrating discussions on sexual health into patient education and routine care (IDF, 2008). These developments mark a global shift—from silence and stigma to proactive recognition of SD as a legitimate and treatable complication of diabetes.

In India, where the burden of diabetes is among the highest in the world, the prevalence of SD mirrors global trends. A 2025 meta-analysis reported that over 60% of Indian men with T2D suffer from ED, with many cases being moderate to severe (Rana et al., 2025). Smaller clinical studies across states have consistently shown prevalence rates ranging from 55% to nearly 70% (Langer et al., 2019; Talwar & Talwar, 2021). Among women, although data are more limited, available studies suggest a comparably high prevalence of FSD, especially in domains of desire, lubrication, and orgasmic difficulties. Despite this heavy burden, the issue often goes unnoticed in routine care because of cultural taboos, patient hesitancy, and lack of physician training. Encouragingly, professional guidelines in India are beginning to address this gap. On the public health front, the National Programme for Prevention and Control of Cancer, Diabetes, Cardiovascular Diseases and Stroke (NPCDCS, now NP-NCD) provides a nationwide framework for diabetes screening and care. While SD is not yet specifically included in program checklists, this platform offers an opportunity to integrate sexual health assessment into diabetes management at the primary-care level. As India faces a rising tide of diabetes, addressing its sexual complications is crucial not only for physical and reproductive health but also for mental well-being, marital harmony, and overall quality of life.

9.3.2 *Erectile Dysfunction in Men with Diabetes*

Erectile dysfunction in diabetic men arises from complex disturbances at the vascular, neuronal, hormonal, and cellular levels, all converging on the impairment of NO-mediated smooth muscle relaxation in the corpus cavernosum. The disruptions are multifactorial: chronic hyperglycemia, oxidative stress, mitochondrial injury, endothelial dysfunction, neuropathy, and hormonal imbalances each contribute to the pathology.

Endothelial Dysfunction and NO–cGMP Pathway Suppression

In healthy men, sexual stimulation activates non-adrenergic non-cholinergic (NANC) neurons and endothelial cells, leading to NO release. It diffuses into smooth muscle cells and binds soluble guanylyl cyclase (sGC), producing cyclic GMP (cGMP). Elevated cGMP activates protein kinase G (PKG), which lowers intracellular Ca^{2+} via phosphorylation of ion channels and pumps, causing cavernosal smooth muscle relaxation and penile erection (Yafi et al., 2016).

Diabetes-induced disruption

- AGEs bind to their receptor (RAGE) on endothelial cells. This activates NF-κB signaling, upregulating inflammatory cytokines and adhesion molecules.
- AGEs also enhance NADPH oxidase activity, generating superoxide radicals (O_2^-). Superoxide directly inactivates NO, forming peroxynitrite ($ONOO^-$), which nitrates tyrosine residues of proteins, damaging eNOS and sGC.

- Endothelial Nitric Oxide Synthase (eNOS) becomes "uncoupled" due to oxidation of its cofactor tetrahydrobiopterin (BH_4). Instead of producing NO, uncoupled eNOS generates additional ROS, worsening oxidative stress.
- Downregulation of eNOS and sGC expression reduces cGMP synthesis, resulting in diminished cavernosal smooth muscle relaxation (Singh et al., 2014).

Oxidative Stress and Mitochondrial Dysfunction

- In hyperglycemia, excessive glucose flux into the mitochondrial electron transport chain leads to overproduction of superoxide.
- Superoxide reacts with NO, forming peroxynitrite, which nitrates and inactivates mitochondrial proteins, impairing oxidative phosphorylation.
- Mitochondrial permeability transition pore (mPTP) opening and release of cytochrome c activate caspase-9 and caspase-3, initiating apoptosis of endothelial and smooth muscle cells.
- Protein kinase C (PKC) activation by diacylglycerol (DAG) contributes to vascular dysfunction by increasing endothelin-1 (vasoconstrictor) and decreasing prostacyclin (vasodilator).
- Ultimately, oxidative stress shifts the penile tissue microenvironment toward vasoconstriction, endothelial cell death, and reduced vasodilatory capacity (Pal et al., 2024).

Diabetic Neuropathy and Neural NO Deficiency

- Excess glucose is reduced to sorbitol by aldose reductase, consuming NADPH. Depletion of NADPH lowers glutathione regeneration, weakening antioxidant defenses and worsening oxidative stress in peripheral nerves.
- Sorbitol accumulation leads to osmotic injury, demyelination, and axonal degeneration in autonomic and sensory fibers.
- Neuronal Nitric Oxide Synthase (nNOS) expression in cavernous nerves is downregulated, reducing neuronal NO release during sexual stimulation.
- Neurotrophic factors, such as NGF (nerve growth factor), are suppressed in diabetes, further impairing nerve regeneration.
- Impaired neural signaling to cavernosal smooth muscle, weakening initiation of erection (Singh et al., 2014).

Hormonal Dysregulation: Hypogonadism in Diabetes

- Insulin resistance and hyperinsulinemia interfere with the hypothalamic–pituitary–gonadal (HPG) axis.
- High insulin and leptin levels blunt pulsatile GnRH secretion from the hypothalamus, lowering LH release from the pituitary.
- Reduced LH impairs Leydig cell steroidogenesis, decreasing testosterone levels (Pal et al., 2024).
- Inflammation and oxidative stress further suppress Leydig cell function by damaging mitochondrial steroidogenic acute regulatory protein (StAR) and cytochrome P450 side-chain cleavage enzyme (P450scc), both essential for testosterone biosynthesis.

- Low testosterone decreases expression of PDE5 and NO synthases, making penile tissue less responsive to vasodilatory stimuli.
- This creates a vicious cycle: low testosterone worsens endothelial and neural NO deficiency, while ED itself further reduces testosterone through hypogonadal–obesity–ED syndrome.

Inflammatory Signaling and Tissue Remodeling

- NF-κB pathway activation by hyperglycemia and AGEs promotes transcription of TNF-α, IL-6, and ICAM-1.
- These cytokines cause endothelial apoptosis, promote vascular adhesion, and recruit inflammatory cells.
- Chronic inflammation triggers TGF-β/Smad signaling, stimulating deposition of collagen and extracellular matrix in cavernosal tissue.
- Over time, smooth muscle cells are replaced by fibrotic tissue, decreasing penile elasticity and compliance.
- Apoptotic markers (Bax upregulation, Bcl-2 downregulation, cytochrome c release, caspase-3 activation) confirm programmed cell death in cavernosal smooth muscle under diabetic conditions (Pal et al., 2024).

9.3.3 *Female Sexual Dysfunctions*

While male sexual problems are well-documented, FSD in diabetes is comparatively under-recognized, though equally impactful. Women with diabetes may experience multiple interrelated issues that affect arousal, lubrication, orgasm, and overall sexual satisfaction.

9.3.3.1 Vaginal Dryness, Dyspareunia, and Low Arousal

Vaginal dryness is a frequent complaint among diabetic women and is mainly attributable to vascular and neuropathic changes. Reduced genital blood flow, compounded by impaired autonomic nerve function, leads to insufficient lubrication during sexual activity. This dryness often causes dyspareunia (painful intercourse), which discourages sexual intimacy and contributes to avoidance of sexual activity.

Low arousal is another consequence, partly linked to poor vascular responsiveness but also to reduced sensory input due to neuropathy. The cumulative effect is a significant decline in sexual pleasure and satisfaction.

9.3.3.2 Hormonal Changes and Vaginal Infections

Hormonal disturbances in diabetic women further aggravate SD. Poorly controlled diabetes can disrupt estrogen and androgen balance, both of which are essential for maintaining sexual drive and vaginal health. Declining estrogen levels—particularly in peri- and post-menopausal diabetic women—contribute to thinning of the vaginal mucosa, loss of elasticity, and greater susceptibility to microtrauma during intercourse.

Furthermore, chronic hyperglycemia increases susceptibility to recurrent vaginal and urinary tract infections, which not only cause discomfort but also result in sexual avoidance due to fear of pain or worsening symptoms.

9.3.4 Decreased Libido and Sexual Dissatisfaction in Men and Women

Sexual desire or libido is influenced by complex interactions between hormones, vascular health, neurological function, and psychological well-being. In diabetes, disturbances in these areas commonly culminate in reduced libido and dissatisfaction with sexual experiences.

9.3.4.1 Testosterone Deficiency in Men

Testosterone is crucial for male libido and erectile physiology. Men with diabetes especially those with T2D, commonly present with hypogonadism characterized by reduced serum testosterone levels. Insulin resistance and obesity, frequently coexisting with diabetes, contribute to suppression of gonadal function through increased aromatization of testosterone to estrogen and altered hypothalamic-pituitary signaling.

Low testosterone not only reduces sexual desire but also worsens erectile dysfunction by decreasing penile smooth muscle integrity and responsiveness to NO. Fatigue, loss of muscle mass, and depressive symptoms further impair overall sexual well-being.

9.3.4.2 Estrogen and Androgen Changes in Women

In women, estrogen deficiency particularly after menopause is a significant determinant of low libido. However, diabetic women may also experience reduced androgen levels, which play a critical role in sexual desire and responsiveness. Declining androgen activity leads to diminished clitoral sensitivity, reduced arousal, and less intense orgasms.

Combined with vascular and neuropathic factors, these hormonal imbalances substantially impair sexual satisfaction, making the problem multifactorial and complex to treat.

9.3.5 Sexual Health Across the Lifespan in Diabetic Patients

Sexual health challenges in diabetes vary across different stages of life. In younger patients, reproductive concerns may dominate, with fears of infertility, pregnancy complications, and reduced sexual confidence. Adolescents and young adults with T1D may also struggle with self-image and reluctance to engage in relationships due to their chronic condition.

In middle-aged patients, the combination of metabolic syndrome, obesity, and diabetes-related complications markedly increases the risk of SD. This stage is often complicated by psychosocial stressors such as work-life pressures, marital strain, and caregiving responsibilities.

In older adults, age-related hormonal decline, cardiovascular complications, and multiple co-morbidities compound the adverse impact of diabetes on sexual function. Moreover, sexual health in the elderly is often overlooked in clinical practice, despite evidence that intimacy remains important for quality of life in this population.

9.3.6 Sexual Dysfunction and Intimacy in Diabetes—Role of Hormones

Hormones are fundamental regulators of sexual health, and their dysregulation in diabetes contributes significantly to impaired intimacy. In men, testosterone deficiency disrupts libido, erectile function, and overall sexual confidence. In women, reduced estrogen and androgen levels impair vaginal health, lubrication, and arousal. Dysregulated insulin and leptin signaling, frequently observed in metabolic syndrome, also interact with reproductive hormones and modulate sexual desire indirectly.

The hormonal impact of diabetes extends beyond the biological dimension into relational intimacy. Sexual dissatisfaction can strain partnerships, leading to reduced emotional closeness and communication gaps. Fear of failure, performance anxiety, and reduced self-image, all linked to hormonal disturbances, create barriers to healthy intimacy.

9.4 Psychological, Emotional, and Relationship Effects

9.4.1 Depression, Anxiety, and Self-Esteem Issues

Diabetes-Related Distress and Self-Esteem: A survey of 255 diabetic patients found that diabetes distress—a chronic emotional burden tied to daily disease management—negatively predicted both self-management and self-esteem, particularly more so in type 1 than T2D. Among older adults in Mexico, 11.5% experienced low self-esteem, and around 25.5% had symptoms of depression. Low self-esteem was linked to poorer self-care behaviors (notably diet and exercise), even after controlling for other factors (Kaiser & Mehboob, 2020).

Depression, Anxiety and Emotional Burden: A comprehensive review reports that approximately 41% of people with diabetes experience poor psychological well-being, with depression and anxiety being twice as common in those with T2D. Depression increases risk for developing diabetes and vice versa.

A qualitative focus-group study among women with T2D revealed themes of depression, anxiety, anger, driven by disease changes, caregiving roles, and relationship pressures—indicating that these emotional states deeply affect quality of life (Penckofer et al., 2007).

9.4.2 The Emotional Toll on Couples and Relationships

Diabetes is often experienced as a "we-disease", where partners share daily responsibilities. Over one-third of partners experience significant emotional stress. Blood sugar fluctuations, mood swings, and treatment-related stress often reduce sexual intimacy, affecting relationship satisfaction.

9.4.3 Isolation and Internalized Shame

A concept analysis revealed that people with diabetes may withdraw socially due to fear of judgment, dietary restrictions interfering with social life, or emotional distress—leading to isolation, reduced self-efficacy, poor glycaemic control, delayed healing, and ultimately, worse disease outcomes (Lin et al., 2024).

A qualitative study of adults with T2D identified a four-stage process: encountering negative experiences → reevaluating self → reconstructing identity → and balancing social roles. Those internalizing stigma develop low self-worth and reduce social participation, which undermines treatment adherence (Kato et al., 2016).

A cross-sectional study of 209 patients found that higher self-stigma predicted poorer engagement in self-care behaviors, independently of self-efficacy or depression. Internalized shame was a major barrier to self-management (Lin et al., 2022).

9.4.4 *Sexual Identity and Body Image Concerns*

A qualitative study of women with diabetes identified "negative sexual self-evaluation" as a major barrier to sexual life many reported feeling physically and emotionally unattractive due to living with diabetes. Many women worried about medical devices interfering in intimacy about 50% of insulin pump users reported that the pump interfered with their sexual relationships, contributing to feelings of embarrassment and lowered body image (Hoorsan et al., 2022).

In a controlled comparison, women with T2D reported significantly lower sexual desire, lubrication, orgasmic capacity, and overall satisfaction compared to healthy controls; in contrast, T1D had little or no such impact. Men with diabetes report decreased erotic drive, diminished sexual arousal, and dissatisfaction, often linked to changes in sexual attitudes and body image distortions, even when marital adjustment was unaffected (Schiavi et al., 1995).

9.5 The Role of Stigma and Silence

Sexual dysfunction are regular among people both men and women but speaking about sexuality and intimacy remain remarkable challenges because of deeply rooted culture and societal taboos. These taboos hamper open communication between patients and healthcare professionals that effect diagnosis, treatment and quality of life.

9.5.1 *Cultural and Societal Taboos Surrounding Sexuality*

Sexual health is one of the major stigmatized and neglected perspective in human wellbeing, basically in the condition of chronic disease like diabetes. In many culture basically in rural areas or conservative societies, sexuality is viewed as a private or even shameful topic.

Silence regarding sexuality is passing from generation to generation, people grow up without proper sexual education and in diabetic people, this silence set off dangerous as neuropathy, vascular changes and hormonal imbalances and effect individual sexual health. Cultural and societal taboos regarding sexuality promote a way of silence, stiffness and lack effective communication, diagnosis and manage SD in people suffering from diabetes.

9.5.2 Gender Disparities in Discussion and Diagnosis

For deep rooted gender principals, provider biases, different healthcare interaction practices encourage in remarkable disparities among the men and women in addressing and managing sexual complications in clinical settings. All clinical research and studies about SD in diabetes has being focused only on men basically regarding ED, it is considered as a medical condition with a comprehensive physiological mechanism that making it continuous concealed, studied and treated. But in case of FSD that caused low libido, vaginal dryness, anorgasmia or dyspareunia are less discussed or barely researched and lay aside as psychosomatic or subordinate to emotional distress. This disparities may be because of inappropriate substantiate diagnostic equipment for women, complex and combined nature of female sexual function or for societal discomfort around female sexuality etc. Women are less comfortable to discussed about sexual complications due to shame or fear of being judged or any other reason, but men can be more likely to look for medical advice whenever they experiencing erectile dysfunction, as it is well recognized and has pharmacologic treatment options. Hence, gender disparities needs a gender-sensitive viewpoint that gives a equal screening, diagnosis, treatment and education that is crucial for wellbeing of individual and to overcome SD especially in diabetic patients.

9.5.3 Embarrassment in Clinical Settings

Many people feel uncomfortable in conversations regarding sexual problems because of fear of belief that sexual concerns are not a topic for medical consultations. Healthcare professionals also feel embarrassment or disquiet when addressing sexual health basically when the lack formal training in sexual health communication, gender, culture, or age gap between professionals and patients, or for lack of privacy. The reciprocal discomfort among patient and healthcare professional lead to unrecognizing of SD, patient dissatisfaction, poor quality of life from unsolved intimacy issue. Healthcare professionals needs to received communication training to confidently and thoughtfully discussed about sexual health, clinic should ensure privacy, enough consultation time, a non-judgemental atmosphere to overcome embarrassment in clinical settings.

9.5.4 *Misconception About Diabetes and Sexual Dysfunctions*

There are various misconception regarding diabetes and SD. One of the major misconceptions about sexual problems are separate to diabetes but in reality diabetes can caused neuropathy that effect arousal and orgasm, vascular issues formed ED in men and reduced genital blood flow in women, hormonal imbalances etc.

People and healthcare professionals only concentrate on men and ED and neglect the detrimental impact on women. There was a misconception that controlling blood sugar can fixed SD complications, while glycemic control is important but it does not alter SD once nerve damaged is occurred. For the management of SD need medication (e.g., inhibitors, lubricants), hormonal therapy, psychosexual counselling etc.

9.6 Barriers to Diagnosis and Treatment

9.6.1 *Patient Hesitation and Lack of Disclosure*

A survey of 595 diabetic patients revealed that 53.8% reported sexual problems, but only 9.9% had ever been asked about them by their physician. Merely 6.3% of women and 15.3% of men had ever raised the issue voluntarily. Lack of clinician training and discomfort—combined with societal stigma—were key impediments. Additionally, many diabetes guidelines (including ADA's) omit routine sexual health assessment at initial or follow-up visits, reinforcing the invisibility of these concerns in clinical care. In qualitative focus groups of women with T2D, themes like guilt, embarrassment, and shame dominated discussions of intimacy. Sexual dysfunction often remains invisible because women feel uncomfortable disclosing it even in clinical settings (Sarkadi & Rosenqvist, 2003).

9.6.2 *Inadequate Sexual Health Training among Healthcare Providers*

Many clinicians lack training, confidence and systems to ask about sexual function or intimacy so SD in people with diabetes remains under-diagnosed and under-treated.

Factors Contributing to Inadequate Sexual Health Training among Healthcare Providers:

- Multiple studies report that a large majority of clinicians cite insufficient training in sexual history taking and sexual-health care (figures often >70% in surveys of residents and primary-care staff). This lack of training is repeatedly identified as a primary barrier (Dyer & Das, 2013).

- Research in diabetes clinics shows many patients with sexual problems are never asked about them: in some cohorts only ~10% had been asked by providers, despite a much higher prevalence of dysfunction. Clinician discomfort and lack of skills contribute strongly to this gap (Bilen et al., 2023).
- Reviews of sexual-health education programs show that targeted training (even short courses) improves clinician knowledge and self-rated competence—yet such programs are not routinely included in medical or nursing curricula (Bilen et al., 2023).

9.6.3 Absence of Routine Screening Protocols

Despite high prevalence, sexual dissatisfaction and dysfunction in people with T2D remain grossly under-detected in primary care. In a Netherlands-based study using the Brief Sexual Symptom Checklist (BSSC), 36.6% of the 786 patients screened reported sexual dissatisfaction, and 61.8% of those expressed a need for care yet such tools are rarely used in routine consultations (Bijlsma-Rutte et al., 2017).

In one study, over half of patients (53.8%) reported having sexual problems, but just 9.9% were ever asked by their physician. Only 6.3% of women and 15.3% of men volunteered the issue themselves. The absence of structured inquiry is a major barrier to care (Bilen et al., 2023).

The absence of systematic screening protocols combined with clinician discomfort and competing priorities—means SD and intimacy issues in diabetes often go undiagnosed and untreated. Routine, structured inquiry is both feasible (via tools like the BSSC) and necessary to improve patient quality of life and holistic healthcare.

9.6.4 Communication Challenges in Patient-Provider Interactions

Effective communication between patients and healthcare providers is crucial for diagnosing and treating SD and intimacy issues in individuals with diabetes. However, several communication challenges impede this process, leading to underdiagnosis and undertreatment.

- Research indicates that both patients and providers experience difficulties when discussing sexual problems in clinical practice (Barbagallo et al., 2020).
- Cultural taboos and societal stigma surrounding sexual health can further complicate communication.
- The absence of standardized screening protocols for SD in diabetes care contributes to communication challenges. Without routine inquiries, patients may not have the opportunity to disclose sexual health concerns, and providers may not recognize the need to address them.

Table 9.1 Some PDE5 inhibitors, their required time to response and sustainability

Drug	Initiation of response	Duration
Sildenafil	30–60 min	4–5 h
Tadalafil	30 min	Up to 36 h
Vardenafil	30–60 min	4–5 h
Avanafil	15–30 min	6 h

9.7 Medical and Therapeutic Interventions

9.7.1 Pharmacological Treatments

Pharmacological treatments is the first-line medical intervention to manage SD in diabetic individuals.

9.7.1.1 Phosphodiesterase Type 5 (PDE5) Inhibitor

This inhibitor is the primary pharmacological treatment for ED in diabetic men. Erectile function relies on the ability of penile smooth muscle to relax and allow the increase blood flow into the corpora cavernosa during sexual arousal. This process is procced by NO through cyclic guanosine monophosphate (cGMP) pathway. The operating principle of PDE5 inhibitor include; sexual arousal begins, activation of cGMP pathway, smooth muscles relaxation, erection termination by PDE5 enzyme, PDE5 inhibitor (e.g. Sildenafil, Tadalafil) block the PDE5 enzyme (Derosa et al., 2023) (Table 9.1).

9.7.1.2 Hormonal Replacement Therapy

Hormonal Replacement Therapy (HRT) is the way to provide hormones to replace or supplement the body's natural hormone levels at the time of deficiencies or imbalance, it helps to restore the normal hormone level and improve sexual health. There are various hormone replacement therapy, they are:

- **Testosterone Replacement Therapy (TRT);** men with T2D are at high risk of hypogonadism because of insulin resistance, obesity, and chronic inflammation. Reduced testosterone level can lead to low sexual desire, ED, fatigue and reduced muscle mass, depression. Therapeutic strategies include intramuscular injections, topical gels, subcutaneous pellets, oral formulation etc., that restore sexual desire, improves erectile quality many more.
- **Estrogen Therapy;** women with postmenopausal have suffer from estrogen deficiency that lead to vaginal dryness and atrophy, dyspareunia and decreased sexual desire and arousal. Medical intervention like local estrogen therapy (creams,

vaginal tablets), systemic estrogen therapy (oral or transdermal), that improve vaginal lubrication and elasticity, reduced pain, enhanced sexual satisfaction.

9.7.2 Managing Blood Glucose for Better Sexual Health

Managing glucose level in blood is fundamental ground for preventing and maintaining SD in diabetic individuals. Well maintained blood glucose level help to protect vascular integrity, hormonal imbalance, and nerve signal needed for arousal and orgasm and decreased libido in both male and female.

9.7.3 Physical Activity and Weight Management

Regular physical activity and weight management are important for maintaining SD in diabetic individuals. Exercise increase endothelial function and prompt NO production, which is important for penile erection in men and genital vasocongestion in women. Excess body weight basically central or visceral obesity enhance insulin resistance, systemic inflammation and oxidative stress which damaged vascular and hormonal health important for sexual response that caused decreased testosterone levels, erectile dysfunction, hormonal imbalance, lower libido etc. Also weight reduction decrease cardiovascular strain, that support better genital blood flow and sexual performance.

9.7.4 Role of Dietary Antioxidants and Nutraceuticals for Sexual Health Maintenance

Nutraceuticals are the food-derived bioactive compounds (e.g., omega-3 fatty acids, L-arginine) and anti-oxidants are the molecules that resist oxidation of other molecule by neutralizing free radicals, prevent cellular damage. These play important role in maintaining SD by minimizing oxidative stress, enhance NO accessibility, balancing hormone, improve vascular health, reduced inflammation many more (Table 9.2).

9.7.5 Alternative and Complementary Therapies

Alternation and complementary therapies have obtained a supportive strategies for maintaining SD through common strategy like herbal medicine, acupuncture, yoga, mindfulness meditation and pelvic floor exercises. Herbal remedies such as *Panax ginseng, Tribulus terrestris and Mucuna pruriens*, these are used to increase

Table 9.2 Nutraceuticals and antioxidants in maintaining sexual health (Beygi et al., 2021)

Nutraceuticals and antioxidants	Roles
L- arginine	Act as a forerunner to NO, improved penile blood flow and erectile rigidity in men and increase genital Vaso-congestion in women
Omega -3 fatty acids	Present in fish oil, flaxseeds and walnuts, helps to reduced systemic inflammation, improve endothelial health and supports in hormone production
Polyphenols (Resveratrol, Flavonoids)	Found in berries, grapes, green tea and cocoa, that improve vascular function, minimized oxidative stress and improve sexual desire and performance
Vitamins (E&C)	It is an antioxidants that protect vascular endothelium and nerve tissue from glycation and oxidative injury
Zinc and Selenium	These are the important minerals for synthesis of testosterone, sperm motility and antioxidant enzyme activity

libido, erectile function, sexual stamina etc. Acupuncture helps through regulating neuroendocrine pathway, reduce stress, improve pelvic blood flow etc. (Traish et al., 2011).

9.8 Psychosocial Support and Counselling

Erectile dysfunction is not only a biomedical condition but also a psychosocial challenge that profoundly impacts men and their partners. Beyond pharmacological or surgical approaches, psychosocial support and counselling play a vital role in restoring confidence, improving communication, and rebuilding intimacy. Psychosocial interventions address the emotional and relational aspects of ED, thereby complementing medical treatment and enhancing quality of life.

9.8.1 Importance of Couple-Based Interventions

Couple-based interventions play a crucial role in addressing SD, as the condition impacts both partners and the relationship itself. Men may struggle with guilt, shame, or fear of rejection, while partners often perceive the issue as diminished affection or mistrust. Joint therapy provides a supportive space for open communication, shared responsibility, and emotional understanding, reducing self- or partner-blame. Importantly, these approaches encourage couples to explore non-penetrative forms of intimacy, alleviating performance pressure. Evidence shows that couple-focused strategies enhance treatment satisfaction, strengthen trust, and promote healthier, more resilient relationships.

9.8.2 Sex Therapy and Psychosexual Counselling

Sex therapy and psychosexual counselling offer supportive, structured ways to manage the psychological side of ED. Beyond medical treatment, they address issues like performance anxiety, fear of failure, poor body image, or past negative experiences that may worsen ED. Therapists guide individuals and couples through techniques such as sensate focus or reframing unhelpful beliefs, helping them see intimacy as more than just penetration. This approach eases pressure, strengthens emotional closeness, and opens up healthier expressions of sexuality. By combining psychological support with medical care, therapy can improve both erectile function and overall relationship satisfaction.

9.8.3 Peer Support Groups and Online Forums

Living with ED can be an isolating experience. Peer support groups provide a safe and empathetic space where men and their partners can share experiences without fear of judgment. Such groups allow members to normalize their struggles, exchange coping strategies, and learn about available treatment options from peers who have undergone similar journeys. Online forums and virtual communities have further expanded access, offering anonymity for those uncomfortable with face-to-face discussions. Digital peer platforms are especially helpful in societies where discussing sexual health remains taboo. The sense of belonging and reassurance gained from peer networks reduces psychological distress and encourages men to pursue medical and psychosocial interventions more confidently. These communities thus serve as a bridge between self-isolation and active engagement with treatment.

9.8.4 Mindfulness, Cognitive Behavioral Therapy, and Stress Management

Mindfulness-based practices, including breathing exercises, meditation, and body awareness, help couples remain present during sexual activity rather than preoccupied with performance worries. Mindfulness reduces stress hormone levels, improves emotional regulation, and enhances physical relaxation—all of which contribute to improved erectile response. Cognitive Behavioral Therapy (CBT) addresses the negative thought cycles that accompany ED. By challenging irrational beliefs, CBT reshapes cognitive patterns that sustain anxiety. Stress management techniques, including relaxation training, exercise, and sleep hygiene, further support mental health and indirectly improve sexual functioning. Together, mindfulness and CBT offer men practical tools to break the cycle of fear and avoidance, creating a healthier psychological context for sexual intimacy.

9.8.5 Tele-counselling and Psychological Support

In the digital era, tele-counselling has emerged as a valuable tool for addressing the psychosocial dimensions of ED. Online platforms allow men to access therapy discreetly, without the stigma or inconvenience of in-person visits. For many, especially those living in rural or resource-limited settings, telehealth services provide the only feasible means of receiving professional psychological support. Tele-counselling maintains privacy and continuity of care, which are essential in managing sensitive conditions like ED. Virtual therapy sessions can deliver the same interventions as traditional counselling, including CBT, mindfulness coaching, and sex therapy, but with added flexibility and accessibility. Moreover, digital platforms often integrate educational resources, self-assessment tools, and chat-based peer support, creating a comprehensive support system. The COVID-19 pandemic accelerated the acceptance of online psychological support, demonstrating its effectiveness and convenience. Today, tele-counselling stands as a sustainable model for extending mental health and sexual health care to a wider population.

9.9 Creating A More Inclusive and Supportive Healthcare System

9.9.1 Integrating Sexual Health into Diabetes Management Plans

Integrating sexual health into diabetes management plan refers as the methodical involvement of sexual health assessment, counselling, and treatment as a routine and important part of diabetic management. This can be executed through several ways like:

Routine screening like applying validated questionnaires (e.g., Female Sexual Function Index, International Index of Erectile Function at the time of routine check-ups for identification of sexual problems.

By working with urologists, gynaecologists, endocrinologists, psychologists, and sex therapists to create a interrelated treatment plan to individuals. Educating patient by telling how diabetes affect sexual health, ensuring patient that these problems are common and treatable and guide them towards safe and evidence-based solutions.

Recognizing sexual well-being as a part of quality of life with controlled glycemic control, cardiovascular health and mental health.

9.9.2 Building Trust and Open Communication

Building trust and open communication refers to the creation of safe, respectful and nonjudgemental environment to feel comfortable about discussing in sensitive topics like SD and intimacy by active listening, empathy and validation, confidentiality assurance, non-stigmatizing languages etc. this helps patients to speak about their problem freely without hesitation.

9.9.3 Educating Healthcare Workers on Sensitive Topics

By educating doctors, nurses, diabetes educators and healthcare professionals with the knowledge, skills and confidence to addressing with patient about their sexual health or SD. Training should include medical knowledge, communication skills, cultural competence, ethics and confidentiality many more.

9.9.4 Policy Recommendations and Awareness Campaigns

Policy recommendations and awareness campaigns play important role in stigma around SD in people with diabetes and ensure appropriate care. This include an standardized screening protocols, ensuring that sexual health evaluation became a routine part of diabetes check-ups that extend upto SD.

Various policies include national health guidelines, training of healthcare professionals, multidisciplinary care inclusion etc. and awareness campaigns like mass media campaigns (using TV, radio or social media), community outreach (Organizing workshop in community center, workplace, school, office), use of testimonials, collaboration with NGOs and advocacy group.

9.10 Future Perspectives and Research Directions

9.10.1 Emerging Therapies and Innovations

Traditional therapies often target symptoms rather than the root molecular mechanisms of diabetic ED and FSD. Recent years have seen a shift toward regenerative and biologically driven treatments. Stem cell therapy and platelet-rich plasma injections show promise in restoring endothelial and neural function by enhancing angiogenesis and tissue repair. Similarly, low-intensity shockwave therapy has emerged as a non-invasive technique that stimulates neovascularization and improves penile blood flow. Gene-based therapies are also under investigation, aiming to upregulate eNOS or enhance vascular growth factors in cavernous tissue. Nanomedicine is another frontier, with nanoparticles designed to deliver NO donors or antioxidant molecules directly to penile tissues, potentially reducing systemic side effects. Advances in wearable health devices and digital health tools may also provide men with real-time monitoring of physiological parameters, enabling more responsive and adaptive care. While many of these innovations are still experimental, they represent a paradigm shift from symptomatic management to disease modification and functional restoration in diabetic ED and FSD.

9.10.2 Personalized Medicine in Diabetic Sexual Health

Not all men with diabetes respond equally to standard treatments, highlighting the need for personalized approaches. Personalized medicine may be based on genetic, metabolic, and psychosocial profiles. For instance, polymorphisms in genes regulating NO production or androgen receptor activity may influence both the risk of ED and treatment response. Pharmacogenomics could identify which patients are most likely to benefit from PDE5 inhibitors, while others may require alternative strategies such as hormonal therapy or regenerative interventions. Integration of biomarkers—including oxidative stress markers, inflammatory cytokines, and testosterone levels—can provide clinicians with a clearer picture of disease severity and prognosis. Beyond biology, personalization must also consider psychological and relational factors. Digital platforms can help capture lifestyle, stress, and mental health data, feeding into individualized treatment plans. Ultimately, precision sexual medicine offers the promise of moving away from "one-size-fits-all" therapy toward interventions that maximize efficacy and minimize adverse outcomes.

9.10.3 Addressing Gaps in Epidemiological and Clinical Research

Despite the high prevalence of ED among men with diabetes, significant research gaps remain. Epidemiological studies are often limited by underreporting, cultural stigma, and inconsistent diagnostic criteria. Many large-scale studies also fail to capture the psychosocial dimensions of ED and FSD, such as its impact on relationships, mental health, and quality of life. On the clinical side, most trials prioritize pharmacological therapies while overlooking psychosocial or lifestyle interventions. Longitudinal studies are needed to better understand how early metabolic control, lifestyle modification, or psychosocial support influence the natural course of ED in diabetes. Furthermore, clinical research should expand to diverse populations, as cultural norms, dietary patterns, and healthcare access significantly shape both prevalence and outcomes. Closing these gaps will require robust methodologies, community-based research, and integration of both biomedical and social sciences. By strengthening epidemiological and clinical evidence, future research can guide policies, improve awareness, and ensure more effective management strategies.

9.10.4 Need for Interdisciplinary Collaboration

Sexual dysfunction in diabetes cannot be fully addressed within the boundaries of a single discipline. Endocrinologists, urologists, cardiologists, psychologists, and sexual health specialists must work together to provide integrated care. For example, optimizing glycemic control through endocrinology, restoring vascular health through cardiology, and addressing emotional challenges through psychotherapy can produce synergistic benefits. Collaboration also extends to researchers in molecular biology, pharmacology, and biomedical engineering who are developing the next generation of therapies. Policy-makers and public health experts play a role in raising awareness, reducing stigma, and ensuring equitable access to emerging treatments. Furthermore, interdisciplinary education and training programs for healthcare providers can enhance sensitivity, communication skills, and overall patient management. In essence, interdisciplinary collaboration transforms this condition from a narrow biomedical model to a comprehensive, patient-centered approach that acknowledges the biological, psychological, and social dimensions of the condition.

9.11 Conclusion

Sexual dysfunction in diabetes represents a neglected but deeply significant complication that affects both physical and emotional well-being, often undermining self-esteem, intimacy, and the quality of relationships. Despite its prevalence, it remains shrouded in silence, largely due to stigma, embarrassment, and cultural taboos surrounding discussions of sexual health. This chapter highlighted that the roots of SD in diabetes are multifactorial, encompassing vascular impairment, neuropathy, oxidative stress, hormonal disturbances, and psychological burdens. Such complexities focus that sexual health must be regarded as an inseparable part of overall diabetes management rather than an optional concern. Effective strategies should combine medical therapies, glycemic control, lifestyle interventions, and nutraceutical support with counselling, open communication, and couple-focused care. Moreover, dismantling the stigma requires healthcare providers to approach the subject with sensitivity, ensuring that patients feel safe to disclose concerns without fear of judgment. Integrating sexual health into standard diabetes care, supported by education, awareness campaigns, and training of professionals, can help normalize these conversations and reduce hidden suffering. Future research must also bridge existing gaps by exploring gender differences, cultural variations, and psychosocial outcomes to provide more personalized solutions. Ultimately, breaking the silence around sexual health in diabetes is both a medical imperative and a social responsibility. By fostering trust, empathy, and inclusive healthcare, we can ensure that people living with diabetes are supported not only in prolonging life but also in preserving intimacy, dignity, and human connection, which remain essential for a meaningful and fulfilling life.

References

American Diabetes Association Professional Practice Committee. (2025). Comprehensive medical evaluation and assessment of comorbidities: Standards of care in diabetes. *Diabetes Care, 48*(Supplement_1), S59–85.

An, J., Xiang, B., Peng, J., & Li, D. (2025). Understanding the erectile dysfunction–cardiovascular disease connection: Clinical and pathophysiological insights. *Sexual Medicine Reviews, 13*, 406–422.

Augustovski, F., Colantonio, L. D., Galante, J., Bardach, A., Caporale, J. E., Zárate, V., Chuang, L. H., Pichon-Riviere, A., & Kind, P. (2017). Measuring the benefits of healthcare: DALYs and QALYs—Does the choice of measure matter? A case study of two preventive interventions. *International Journal of Health Policy and Management, 7*, 1–17.

Barbagallo, F., Mongioì, L. M., Cannarella, R., La Vignera, S., Condorelli, R. A., & Calogero, A. E. (2020). Sexual dysfunction in diabetic women: An update on current knowledge. *Diabetology, 1*, 11–21.

Begum, M., Choubey, M., Tirumalasetty, M. B., Arbee, S., Sadik, S., Mohib, M. M., Srivastava, S., Minhaz, N., Alam, R., & Mohiuddin, M. S. (2024). Exploring the molecular link between diabetes and erectile dysfunction through single-cell transcriptome analysis. *Genes, 15*, 1–18.

Beygi, Z., Forouhari, S., Mahmoudi, E., Hayat, S. M., & Nourimand, F. (2021). Role of oxidative stress and antioxidant supplementation in male fertility. *Current Molecular Medicine, 21*, 265–282.

Bijlsma-Rutte, A., Braamse, A. M., van Oppen, P., Snoek, F. J., Enzlin, P., Leusink, P., Nijpels, G., & Elders, P. J. (2017). Screening for sexual dissatisfaction among people with type 2 diabetes in primary care. *Journal of Diabetes and Its Complications, 31*, 1614–1619.

Bilen, H., Dayanan, R., Ciftel, E., Bilen, A., Ciftel, S., Mercantepe, F., & Capoglu, I. (2023). Do we care enough about the presence of sexual problems in diabetic patients? *International Journal of General Medicine, 31*, 5147–5156.

Derosa, G., Romano, D., D'Angelo, A., & Maffioli, P. (2023). Female sexual dysfunction in subjects with type 2 diabetes mellitus. *Sexuality and Disability, 41*, 221–233.

Dyer, K., & Das, N. R. (2013). Why don't healthcare professionals talk about sex? A systematic review of recent qualitative studies conducted in the United Kingdom. *The Journal of Sexual Medicine, 10*, 2658–2670.

Eberle, C., & Stichling, S. (2021). Clinical improvements by telemedicine interventions managing type 1 and type 2 diabetes: Systematic meta-review. *Journal of Medical Internet Research, 23*, 1–12.

Hoorsan, R., Lamyian, M., Ahmadi, F., Azin, S. A., & Rahimiforoushani, A. (2022). Exploring sexual life experiences and perceptions of women with diabetes: A qualitative study. *International Journal of Community Based Nursing and Midwifery, 10*, 1–11.

International Diabetes Federation (IDF). (2008). International Curriculum for Diabetes Health Professional Education. *Module III-9: diabetes and sexual health.* IDF. https://idf.org/media/uploads/2023/05/attachments-33.pdf

Isidro, M. L. (2012). Sexual dysfunction in men with type 2 diabetes. *Postgraduate Medical Journal, 88*, 152–159.

Kaiser, A., & Mehboob, N. (2020). Impact of diabetes distress on self-management, and self-esteem among diabetics. *Pakistan Journal of Medical Research, 59*, 51–54.

Kalra, S., Jena, B. N., & Yeravdekar, R. (2018). Emotional and psychological needs of people with diabetes. *Indian Journal of Endocrinology and Metabolism, 22*, 696–704.

Kato, A., Fujimaki, Y., Fujimori, S., Izumida, Y., Suzuki, R., Ueki, K., Kadowaki, T., & Hashimoto, H. (2016). A qualitative study on the impact of internalized stigma on type 2 diabetes self-management. *Patient Education and Counseling, 99*, 1233–1239.

Kitaw, T. A., Abate, B. B., Tilahun, B. D., Yilak, G., Rede, M. B., Getie, A., & Haile, R. N. (2024). The global burden of erectile dysfunction and its associated risk factors in diabetic patients: An umbrella reviews. *BMC Public Health, 24*, 1–12.

Kumar, R., Saha, P., Kumar, Y., Sahana, S., Dubey, A., & Prakash, O. (2020). A review on diabetes mellitus: Type1 & Type2. *World Journal of Pharmacy and Pharmaceutical Sciences, 9*, 838–850.

Langer, R., Sharma, E., Langer, B., Gupta, R. K., Kumari, R., & Majeed, M. (2019). Erectile dysfunction: Prevalence and determinants among T2DM men attending a tertiary care hospital in northern India. *International Surgery Journal, 6*, 1115–1119.

Lin, K., Wang, J., Bai, X., & Liu, Y. (2024). Social isolation in people with type 2 diabetes: A concept analysis. *Heliyon, 10*, 1–10.

Lin, M. H., Ou, H. Y., Wang, R. H., Lin, C. H., Liao, H. Y., & Chen, H. M. (2022). Glycaemic control mediates the relationships of employment status and self-stigma with self-care behaviours in young adults with type 2 diabetes. *Journal of Clinical Nursing, 31*, 582–591.

Meamar, F. Z., Dastjerdi, M. S., Salehi, P., Ghahramannejad, N., & Boromandfar, Z. (2025). Improving the sexual health of couples with diabetes: Study protocol of an action research study. *Reproductive Health, 22*, 1–13.

Morano, S. (2003). Pathophysiology of diabetic sexual dysfunction. *Journal of Endocrinological Investigation, 26*, 65–71.

Pal, D., Halder, S., Ghosh, D., & Jana, K. (2024). Role of apoptosis in male infertility: Therapeutic targets and strategies. In *Apoptosis and human health: Understanding mechanistic and therapeutic potential* (pp. 341–352). Springer Nature Singapore.

Penckofer, S., Ferrans, C. E., Velsor-Friedrich, B., & Savoy, S. (2007). The psychological impact of living with diabetes women's day-to-day experiences. *The Diabetes Educator, 33*, 680–690.

Rana, R. K., Barnwal, R. K., Sinha, A., & Sinha, R. (2025). Prevalence of erectile dysfunction among patients with type 2 diabetes mellitus in India: A meta-analysis. *Expert Review of Endocrinology & Metabolism*, 1–8.

Rogoznica, M., Perica, D., Borovac, B., Belančić, A., & Matovinović, M. (2023). Sexual dysfunction in female patients with type 2 diabetes mellitus—Sneak peek on an important quality of life determinant. *Diabetology, 4*, 527–536.

Sarkadi, A., & Rosenqvist, U. (2003). Intimacy and women with type 2 diabetes: An exploratory study using focus group interviews. *The Diabetes Educator, 29*, 641–652.

Schiavi, R. C., Stimmel, B. B., Mandeli, J., Schreiner-Engel, P., & Ghizzani, A. (1995). Diabetes, psychological function and male sexuality. *Journal of Psychosomatic Research, 39*, 305–314.

Singh, V. P., Bali, A., Singh, N., & Jaggi, A. S. (2014). Advanced glycation end products and diabetic complications. *The Korean Journal of Physiology & Pharmacology, 18*, 1–14.

Talwar, V., & Talwar, G. (2021, May 15). Prevalence of erectile dysfunction among the subjects with type 2 diabetes mellitus in the Indian state of Punjab. In *Endocrine abstracts* (Vol. 73). Bioscientifica.

Traish, A. M., Kang, H. P., Saad, F., & Guay, A. T. (2011). Dehydroepiandrosterone (DHEA)—A precursor steroid or an active hormone in human physiology (CME). *The Journal of Sexual Medicine, 8*, 2960–2982.

Yafi, F. A., Jenkins, L., Albersen, M., Corona, G., Isidori, A. M., Goldfarb, S., Maggi, M., Nelson, C. J., Parish, S., Salonia, A., & Tan, R. (2016). Erectile dysfunction. *Nature Reviews Disease Primers, 2*, 1–20.

Chapter 10
Food as Medicine: Therapeutic Nutrition for Healing and Function in Diabetic Patients

Dipankar Saha, Surajit Majumder, Nirmalya Kumar Sinha, Pradipta Banerjee, and Rajkumar Maiti

Abstract Diabetes is a metabolic disorder, very common in the adults in recent days and become epidemic throughout the globe. The major complain is the hyperglycemic condition of the body due to the insufficient production of the insulin. Persistent hyperglycemia further leads to other complications like cardiovascular disease, kidney disease, lower limb amputation, vision loss etc. Several medicines are available to treat diabetes, but all are having several side effects on the body and also not cost effective. The major culprit behind this devastating disease is the food and their respective glycemic index. Therefore, choosing the right food is very important for persons suffering from diabetes in order to control the hyperglycemia. In ancient India, it was traditional to use several foods, and food component to treat the diseases, a practice known as Ayurveda. As a result, the search for proper foods or their components from natural products—mainly herbal sources—has increased tremendously in recent decades. However, the selection of the herbs depends on the several factors like, stage of the diabetes, type of comorbidity arises, availability and affordability. The research has recognized several foods, food components and herbs that may use as the remedies to control the diabetes. This chapter mainly focused on the food and the other natural herbs that paly major role to control the diabetes and their underlying mechanism to control the hyperglycemia.

Keywords Food · Herbs · Herbal medicine · Glycemic index · Hyperglycemia

D. Saha · S. Majumder
Department of Zoology, Bankura Sammilani College, Kenduadihi, Bankura, India

N. K. Sinha
Department of Nutrition and Department of NSS & CESR, Raja Narendralal Khan Women's College (Autonomous), Midnapore, Paschim Medinipur, India

P. Banerjee
Department of Surgery, McGowan Institute for Regenerative Medicine, University of Pittsburgh, Pittsburgh, PA, USA

R. Maiti (✉)
Department of Physiology, Bankura Christian College, Bankura, India
e-mail: rajkumar@bankurachristiancollege.in

K. Adhikary et al. (eds.), *Healing Beyond Blood Sugar*,
https://doi.org/10.1007/978-981-95-8946-3_10

10.1 Introduction

Diabetes mellitus (DM) is one of the most common systematic metabolic diseases. It is characterized by hyperglycemia and causes by the reduced insulin secretion from pancreatic β cell or reduce the insulin action or both (Altan, 2003). There are different types of DM such as type-1, type-2, gestational diabetes and others (Adinortey, 2017). The disease is associated with the reduced quality of life and increased risk factors for mortality and morbidity. The uncontrolled hyperglycemia for prolonged period leads to manifest the several acute complications and in case of overlooked the symptoms it may results several chronic complications including hypertension, stroke, foot ulceration, retinopathy, nephropathy and many more life-threatening diseases (Adinorteyet al., 2011). In the current report provided by World Health Organization (WHO) in 2024 showed that the 14% of the adult population (18 years and above) were suffering from DM (WHO, 2024). In India almost 3.2 crore people were affected with the DM and leads the global list, and the number is continuously increasing day by day. The prediction shows the number will reach 7.94 crore by the end of 2030 (Ahmad & Joshi, 2023; Wild et al., 2004). Several survey reports shows that the distribution of the DM patients is high among the urban areas, up to 16% than the rural areas, which shows the affected persons near about 8% (Phillips, 2016). At macro level, the high burden of the DM has been attributed to urbanization and change in the work pattern and food pattern.

Lifestyle modification including dietary management may promote the insulin secretion that helpful to manage this metabolic disease through modulating blood glucose homeostasis (Shin et al., 2020). It has been reported that among the 45% of adult DM patients were not achieved the glycemic control (Wang et al., 2015).

10.1.1 The Food Sources for Hyperglycemia

Glucose is the most important energy sources for human body. It has a wide spectrum of the physiological effect in the body and proper regulation of the glucose metabolism can reduce the risk of disease. Glycemia represent the blood glucose concentration after combine effect of carbohydrate uptake. This is highly regulated by a homeostatic regulatory system (Jenkins et al., 2002). The intake of carbohydrate enriched diet can lead to increased blood glucose levels which results hyperglycemia. On the basis of metabolic effects and their potential to raise blood glucose levels, carbohydrates may be classified into different categories. However, glycemic index is varied in different carbohydrate-containing foods. For instance, whole-grain bread has potentially low glycemic index than the white bread. Usually, foods that are digested and absorbed more rapidly lead to a sharper increase in blood glucose level compared to those that are broken down more gradually.

Over the past few decades in developing countries, the number of fast-food restaurants has increased steadily. These foods are with a high calorie content, processed carbohydrates, processed meats, saturated and trans fats, and sugar-sweetened beverages—all these elements contribute to impaired metabolic function and greater susceptibility to type 2 diabetes (Ley et al., 2014).

10.1.2 Side Effect of the Medicines

Currently, there is no approved cure for DM, thus primary course of action is pharmacotherapy and nutritional therapy for successful disease management. Pharmacotherapy treatment depends on the type of DM diagnosed. As the injection insulin recommended for the treatment of type-1 DM patients (Shaikh et al., 2022). For type-2 DM patients, several oral medications are available, listed in Table 10.1. Sometimes type-2 DM patients were may also require insulin injection for proper management (Silver et al., 2018). The listed oral medications were used for the management of the DM, but often fail to completely control the management. Also, the continuous use of those medication leads the negative side-effect. Previous study reports that the use of metformin harm the patient's night sleep and lactic acidosis (Susilawati et al., 2023). It has also reported that sulfonylureas use results hypoglycemia among the elderly patients who have renal problem, hepatic problem, alcohol abuse and other disorder (Zaman et al., 2023). The use of thiazolidinedione's has been restricted due to the potential side effect of liver toxicity, cardiac failure and edema (Lebovitz, 2019). The common side effect of the meglitinides is dizziness, diarrhea, constipation, arthralgia, headache and cough (Black et al., 2007). The use of α-glucosidase inhibitors among the patients suffering from abdominal pain, diarrhea and also elevate the liver enzyme, which results the various liver disease (Corathers et al., 2013).

10.1.3 Importance of the Food and Food Product as a Medicine

As the synthetic oral medicines used for management of DM has a huge side effect, thus the WHO lists more than 400 plants and herbs for the treatment of DM. The plant products are cost effective, long lasting and limited side effect thus these are the valuable source of therapeutic agents (Kumar et al., 2021).

10.1.4 Scope and Purpose of the Chapter

This chapter aims to provide comprehensive overview of the common pharmacological medicine used for management of the DM and their potential side effect. It also emphasis on foods and herbs having potential antidiabetic properties that can

Table 10.1 Available oral drugs and their mode of action used for diabetes management

S. no.	Type of medicine	Available drug	Mode of action	References
1	Biguanides	Metformin	Alter the sensitivity of insulin in liver	Shaikh et al. (2022) and Padhi et al. (2020)
2	Sulfonylureas	Gliclazide, glimepiride, glipizide, and glibenclamide	Stimulates insulin secretion by β-cells of the pancreas,	Shaikh et al. (2022) and Padhi et al. (2020)
3	α-glucosidase inhibitors	Miglitol and acarbose	Inhibit α-glucosidase Enzyme within small intestine, thus delay the digestion and absorption of the carbohydrate	Shaikh et al. (2022) and Padhi et al. (2020)
4	Thiazolidinediones	Rosiglitazone and pioglitazone	Increase the insulin sensitivity among muscle tissue	Shaikh et al. (2022) and Padhi et al. (2020)
5	Meglitinides	Netaglinid and repaglinide	Increases insulin secretion by triggering pancreatic β-cells	Shaikh et al. (2022) and Padhi et al. (2020)
6	Sodium-glucose co-transporter 2 inhibitors	Canagliflozin, ipragliflozin, dapagliflozin, and empagliflozin	Prevent the glucose r absorption in kidneys and improve glucose excretion	Shaikh et al. (2022) and Padhi et al. (2020)
7	Dopamine D2 and its receptor agonist	Bromocriptine	Improve the insulin sensitivity	Shaikh et al. (2022) and Padhi et al. (2020)
8	Bile acid sequestrant	Colestimide and colesevelam	Develops glucose-lowering effect and improves glucose tolerance	Shaikh et al. (2022) and Padhi et al. (2020)

be used for the management of DM. The current evidence of antidiabetic effect of the human edible plants and discus their effects on glycemic control, insulin secretion and insulin sensitivity for the management of DM. This chapter also address the on limitations of the plant products for clinical validations. By combining the modern pharmacological and earlier traditional practices and their clinical insight, this chapter try to establish the role of the traditional herbal medicine as alternative therapeutics in diabetic management and facilitate the use of herbal medicine into evidence based medical practices.

10.2 Foods that Control the Hyperglycemia

10.2.1 Food and Glycemic Index

Glycemic control is referred to the blood sugar level of DM patients. Simple carbohydrate consumption influences the glycemia. The current World health Organization Guidelines for the carbohydrate intake for the children and adult does not recommend on the amount of carbohydrate, rather this are mainly focused on the types of carbohydrate should be intake (WHO 2023). The guideline recommends the carbohydrate intake should emphasis nutrient dense carbohydrate that are high in fiber and minimally processed. The carbohydrate quality was determined by evaluating the glycemic response of the carbohydrate through the glycemic index (GI) and glycemic load (GL) (Bhupathiraju et al., 2014). The several studies indicates that the two index is highly related to the risk of DM (Dong et al., 2011; Livesey et al., 2013). Not only the carbohydrate, protein intake also improves the insulin response in the body and help in the glycemic control (Khazrai et al., 2014).

The two strategies are proposed for the management of the DM, caloric restriction and reduce glycemic excursion.

10.2.2 Importance of Glycemic Index

Glycemic index represents the quality of the carbohydrate of food by assessing the timeline for impact on the blood glucose level. GI is calculated by calculating the ratio of glycemic response (postprandial changes in blood glucose level after consumption of food) of any food contain 50 g of carbohydrate, in respect to the glycemic response of 50 g of glucose. Food having the high GI undergoes fast digestion, absorption and metabolism. In contract the food takes much time to digest and slow in absorption and metabolism are categories as low GI food. The food were categories into two types based on the GI, i.e. high GI food and low GI food. Another important index is the GL, which reflects both the quality and quantity of the carbohydrate. It is determined by multiplying the GI by the total amount of carbohydrate present in specific amount of food (Augustin et al., 2015). Thus, for management of the DM patients, not only the GI of food is important, but the GL also play a very crucial role.

10.2.3 Role of Glycemic Index in the Diabetes

Diabetes patients were generally present with the high blood glucose level. As the GI and GL provides the duration of the increasing blood glucose level after taking the meal thus these are very much important for the management of the DM patients. The GI of food depends on several factors like, cooking and processing methods and also the micronutrients present in the food. The GI of the food taking in the meal regulates the overall glycemic control of the DM patients. The changes of the glycated hemoglobin level (HbA_{1c}) or fructosamine level are common parameters for measuring the glycemic control. Several meta-analysis and randomized controlled trials have been performed focused on the low GI diet and low GL diet on glycemic control among DM patients. The study results that, meal with low GI food create a good impact on the postprandial blood glucose excursion minimization and ultimately improved the glycemic control by subsequently lowering the HbA_{1c} level (Cox et al., 2020). Another random trial revels that a low GL meal for 20 to 40 weeks shows high impact on the glycemic control by reducing the HbA_{1c} level and also significantly reduces the body weight for overweight DM patients (Fabricatore et al., 2011). Study from Asian DM population indicates that taking low GI, GL meal continuously for 12 weeks helps in glycemic control by significantly lowering the HbA_{1c} level (BarakatunNisaket al., 2010; Yusof et al., 2009). Another study form the Latinos reports that the reduce GI/GL meal consumption significantly impact on HbA_{1c} level and glycemic control among the DM patients (Wang et al., 2015). Although few studies from different part of the world fail to establish the role of GI in glycemic control (Viseket al., 2014; Woleveret al., 2008). Despite of the absence on difference in HbA_{1c} level, low GI/GL diet is significantly reducing the blood glucose level. Thus, this is highly recommending to consumption of the low GI/GL diet for DM patients.

10.3 Diet for Diabetic Patients

The role of diet in the etiology of type-2 DM plays a major role. It has been observed that the intake of the carbohydrate and fats has direct association in the type-2 DM development (Corathers et al., 2013). Recent evidence suggests that the consumption of the soft drink highly associated with the obesity and diabetes (Khatib, 2004). Soft drink contains the glycated chemicals which also increases the insulin resistance (Nseir et al., 2010). Another study from Japan indicates that intake of the white rice also associated with the increased risk of the DM (Nanriet al., 2010). Whereas there was a negative correlation with consumption of the fruits and vegetables and development of the DM, as these are containing high amount of fiber and antioxidant which act as a protective barrier (Villegas et al., 2008). Thus, the diet is very important factors for the DM. The diet is not similar for the DM patients, rather it varies with the age group, metabolism rate, lifestyle, physical activity of the individuals.

10.3.1 Types of Diet

A variety of the diets are accepted for the management of the diabetes.

10.3.1.1 Mediterranean Diet

This are mainly based on the plant-based food, specifically fruits, vegetables, beans, nut and seeds and whole grains as the source of carbohydrate. Fish, and other see food as the principal sources of the protein, olive oil as the principal fat sources. Dairy products in low and moderate amount. This diet mainly calorie restricted diet pattern with low carbohydrate and low fat. These can restrict HbA1C and lower triglyceride among the DM patients and reduce the cardiovascular disease (Esposito et al., 2009).

10.3.1.2 Vegan Diet

Vegan diet emphasizes on the plant-based food such as fruits, vegetables, legumes, whole grains, cereal, tubers, roots, vegetable oils, nuts and seed oils instead of all flesh food and animal derived food, but includes egg and diary product. It has been observed that vegan diet can reduces the HbA1c level among the type-2 DM patients. It is also reported that vegan diet reduced weight, waist circumference, LDL-C, HDL-C, triglycerides and blood pressure (Viguiliouket al., 2019).

10.3.1.3 Low-Fat Diet

This diet pattern involves ingesting 25–30% fat within the total energy value. This includes consumption of fruits, vegetables, legumes, whole grains, fish, lean meats, skimmed dairy products, vegetable oils, nuts, avocados, eggs and seed oils, but without excess. Lowering total fat intake mostly related to weight loss, which reduced risk of diabetes (Davis et al., 2009).

10.3.1.4 Very Low-Fat Diet (Ornish/Pritikin Diet)

This diet emphasizes on high fiber rich diet, e.g. whole grains, nonfat diary product, fish, egg white. This diet comprises more than 70% carbohydrate, 20% protein and less than 10% fat of total energy value. The consumption of this very low-fat diet improves the glucose levels, weight, blood pressure (Barnardet al., 1983).

10.3.1.5 Low Carbohydrate Diet

Low carbohydrate diet promotes reducing the consumption of the ultra-processed food. This diet emphasizes 26–45% carbohydrate intake of total energy value mainly from vegetables low in carbohydrate; and protein in form of meat, poultry, fish, shellfish, egg, cheese, nuts including fruits; fat from animal foods, oils, butter and avocado. Low carbohydrate eating patterns have shown to reduce HbA1c level, lower triglycerides which reduce blood pressure and recommend for anti-hyperglycemic medications for type-2 DM patients (van Zuurenet al., 2018).

10.4 Selection of Herbal Food Ingredients for Diabetes Management

Herbal products are usually used for dietary use, such as food, nutrition etc. Food addition of the nutrition contains some specific ingredients, biologically active compound, which have potential body function and reduce the risk of disease, these are also known as functional food. Functional food concept revises the concept of food as not only used for basic nutrition but also used as a source of physical and mental well beings. Herbal medicine utilizes different part of plant such as flower, fruit, leaves, bark and root for medicinal purpose. The use of herbal product to treat the diseases start long ago around 5000 years (Petrovska, 2012). The use of medicinal plant continuing in modern era, as most of the modern-day medicines used worldwide were derived from plants. There are many plants used to treat diverse range of diseases including liver disorder, gastrointestinal disorder, inflammatory disorder, cardiovascular disorder including hypertension, dermatological infection, urinary tract infection and also for the diabetes.

10.4.1 Criteria for Selection of Plants

Uses of herbal medicine have been started for treatment of diabetes long ago, and the scientific publication regarding the use of herbal medicine in diabetes is gradually increasing. Numerous common herbs are claimed to reduce the blood glucose level, thus use of herbs as complementary and alternative therapy draw attention to many diabetic patients. Plant based drug are considered to be a less toxic and free from side effect than synthetic drugs. The selection of herbs for the management of diabetes might depend on several factors, like stage of progression of diabetes, comorbidity of the patients, availability, affordability and the toxic profile of the plants. Many plants that human consumes may be tarns into toxic due to the attack of pathogen, which results the production of the toxic chemicals in the plant body.

10.4.2 Herbal Food Ingredients Use for Diabetic Management

A number of plants have been described in the Ayurveda and other traditional medicine for treatment of the diabetes. Many medicinal plants have shown the experimental or clinical antidiabetic activity and those are used as traditional medicine. Several plants have shown diverse level of hypoglycemic activity (Fig. 10.1). There are several functional food ingredients are reported which are used in diabetic management.

10.4.2.1 Garlic

The bulbs of *Allium sativum* L., has a wide range of the effect in medicinal purpose, also used to reduce glucose metabolism. Intake of juice results better utilization of glucose and found effective in lowering serum glucose level in alloxan-induced diabetic mice. The reason behind the hypoglycaemic activity of garlic is either by the secretion of the insulin from the pancreatic beta cell or by releasing the cysteine bound ineffective insulin (Jain & Vyas, 1975).

10.4.2.2 Onion

The bulbs of *Allium cepa* L., has a long history of medicinal use. Many Asian and African countries this is used for treatment of diabetes. It helps to improve the metabolic condition among the diabetic patients, and reduce the diabetic associated nephropathy during hypoglycaemic condition (Baldé et al., 2006).

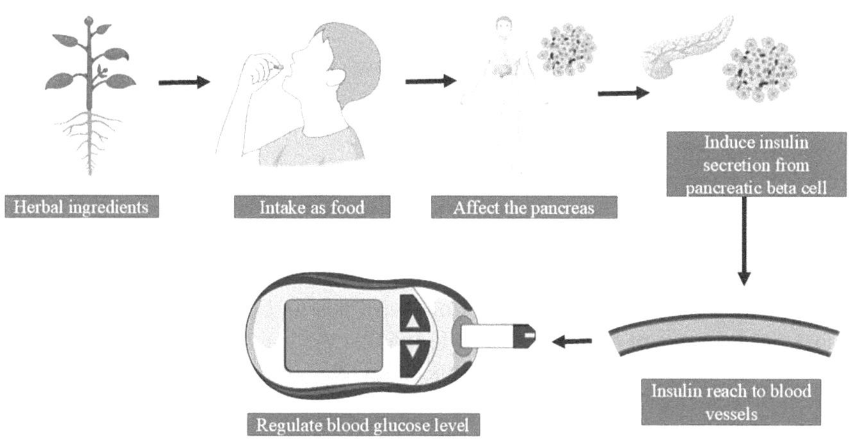

Fig. 10.1 Management of diabetes mellitus through herbal nutrition approach

10.4.2.3 Methi

The seed of *Trigonella foenum-graecum* L. has used as herbal medicine in many parts of the world. Several experimental study result indicates that the use of powder of the seed can lower the blood glucose level among diabetic persons. The high fibre content and other phytochemicals like saponins, amino acid plays the antidiabetic role (Gupta et al., 2001).

10.4.2.4 Cinnamon

The bark of the plant is traditionally used as a spice and flavored beverages. It is used as herbal medicine due to its anti-bacterial, anti-inflammatory and anti-diabetic properties. The anti-diabetic activity of cinnamon through various ways, by reducing the digestion of the carbohydrate, by modulating insulin sensitivity and also insulin secretory activity (Sahib, 2016).

10.4.2.5 Sweet Tulsi

This plant has used to treat diabetes for many years ago in China and other part of world. This plant contains stevioside sweeteners that reduces the postprandial blood glucose level among the tpe-2 DM and also help in glucose metabolism via induce of insulin secretion from pancreatic beta cells (Jeppesen et al., 2002).

10.5 Herbal Food Ingredients Use for Regulating Glucose Absorption

10.5.1 List of Plants Used for Glucose Regulation and Mode of Action

10.5.1.1 Guava

This tropical fruit contain high amount of dietary fibre and lots of natural antioxidant compounds like vitamin C, B1, B2, B6. Recently it has been observed from the clinical study, that the ripe fruit peel of guava has an anti-diabetic property as it contains high amount of Mg. It is also found that the leaves also help to reduce the plasma glucose level in the diabetic induced rat (Rai et al., 2007).

10.5.1.2 Karela

This is not only the vegetables but it is widely used as traditional medicine to treat DM. The fruit juice causes a significant reduction in the blood glucose level. The extract contains many phytochemicals, especially one poly peptide, named as plant insulin which shows the antidiabetic activity (Arulselvan et al., 2006).

10.5.1.3 Ginseng

This plat is originally found in china and the branched root has been used as herbal medicine in China for more than 5000 years. Several studies revealed the use of dried root for management of the diabetes. It improves the glucose metabolism and significant reduction of both the fasting and postprandial glucose level, and also lowering the HbA1c level among the treated patients. In some animal model, panaxadiol, results the dose dependent reduction of fasting glucose by increase of insulin sensitivity through the synthesis of the insulin receptors.

10.6 Herbal Food Ingredients Use for Insulin Regulation

10.6.1 Herbs Regulate Insulin Secretion

Defect of insulin secretion is a key cause of the DM. Prolonged use of the conventional insulin inducer, e.g. glibenclamide among diabetes patients tend to cause damage of pancreatic beta cells due to the overstimulation of the pancreatic islets. Thus, treatment can be switched to the use of herbs which can regulate insulin secretion. Recently numerous herbs have selected which can regulate the insulin secretion and shows the antidiabetic potential (Table 10.2).

10.6.2 Herbs Control Insulin Resistance

Insulin resistance is the most common character of type-2 DM, where muscle tissue, liver and fat tissue fail to respond efficiently to circulating insulin. This impairment leads to compensatory hyperinsulinemia and ultimately beta cell dysfunction. Although this insulin resistance is reversible and may be corrected through few pharmacological substances. Although the synthetic pharmacological product has some adverse effect, it is the most effective alternative is the herbal medicines.

Table 10.2 List of the plants and their effective part used for insulin secretion to regulate DM

S. no.	Botanical name	Common name	Part used	Effects	References
1	*Afzelia africana*	African mahogany	Stem bark	The blood glucose level was significantly reduced in a dose-dependent manner with the best result obtained at 200 mg kg^{-1} body weight per day,	Choudhury et al. (2017)
2	*Aloe vera*	Ghrit Kumari	Leaf	The leaf gel extract enhances the regeneration of the pancreatic beta cells and increase the insulin secretion at a dose of 300 mg/kg body weight	Noor et al. (2017)
3	*Anacardium occidentale*	Kaju	Leaf	Blood glucose was decreased 147.67 ± 6.09 mg dL^{-1} to 123.83 ± 2.87 mg dL^{-1} after 30 days' treatment with plant extract. At the same time, glycosylated haemoglobin level, FIRI and serum insulin level were decreased in treatment group	Choudhury et al. (2017)
4	*Azadirachta indica*	Neem	Leaves	The leaf extract paly crucial role in reducing the blood glucose by altered insulin level, insulin signalling molecule and also reduce the glucose absorption by altering the alpha-amylase and alpha-glucosidase	Choudhury et al. (2017)
5	*Brassica oleracea*	Cabbage	Leaves	Improves postprandial glucose level	Li et al. (2015)

(continued)

Table 10.2 (continued)

S. no.	Botanical name	Common name	Part used	Effects	References
6	*Chloroxylon swietenia*	Bhirra	Bark	Diabetic rats in treatment group showed moderate reduction in blood glucose and glycosylated haemoglobin levels, in addition, plasma insulin were elevated after intregastric intubation for 45 days	Jayaprasad et al. (2016)
7	*Cinnamomum verum*	Cinnamon	Dried bark	Increases the insulin sensitivity and the lowering the gluconeogenesis, also increase the glycogen synthesis	Sharma et al. (2020)
8	*Coccinia grandis*	Telakucha	Leaf	Significant reduction in plasma glucose level and increase in serum insulin level in a dose-dependent manner	Choudhury et al. (2017)
9	*Crocus sativus*	Saffron	Flower stigma	Help in the insulin resistance and glucose homeostasis	Behrouz et al. (2020)
10	*Cuminum cyminum*	Jeera	Seed	It increases the beta cell production. And the oil of cumin at dose of 25 μg/mL for 45 days increase the insulin secretion almost 3–fourfold	Patil et al. (2013)
11	*Forsythia suspensa*	Weeping Forsythia	Fruit	Blood glucose was significantly decreased; insulin secretion and glucose tolerance were significantly increased	Choudhury et al. (2017)
12	*Helicterus angustifolia*	Antamora	Root	The blood glucose, plasma insulin level and HOMA-IR were significantly reduced in treatment group	Choudhuryet al. (2017)
13	*Juglans regia*	Walnut	Husks, kernels	Lowering the blood glucose level and increase the insulin secretion	Liu et al. (2020)

(continued)

Table 10.2 (continued)

S. no.	Botanical name	Common name	Part used	Effects	References
14	*Nigella sativa*	Kalo-jeera	Seed	The extract of seed increased level o insulin and help to reduce the body weight	Hannan et al. (2019)
15	*Pleurotus ostreatus*	Oyster mushroom	–	Treatment group showed significant reduction in fasting blood glucose level, FINS and HOM-IR and increase in ISI and HOM- β in a dose-dependent manner	Choudhury et al. (2017)
16	*Prunella vulgaris*	Woundwort	Flowers	Repair beta cells of pancreatic islet to release insulin	Perera and Li (2012)
17	*Symplocos cochinchinensis*	Lodhra	Bark	Blood glucose level was significantly reduced at day 20 on diabetic induced insulin resistance rat	Choudhury et al. (2017)
18	*Urtica dioica*	Bichhu Buti	Leaf	The blood glucose and fasting insulin resistance index in hyperglycemic rats were reduced in a dose-dependent manner with the best result obtained at 200 mg kg^{-1} body weight/day. The plasma insulin level was also found to be reduced in treatment group	Choudhury et al. (2017)
19	*Uvaria chamae*	Finger root	Root	The treatment group showed significant blood glucose reduction with formation of regenerated islet of Langerhans shown in photomicrograph of pancreas	Choudhury et al. (2017)

(continued)

Table 10.2 (continued)

S. no.	Botanical name	Common name	Part used	Effects	References
20	*Uvaria chamae*	Finger root	Root	The treatment group showed significant blood glucose reduction with formation of regenerated islet of Langerhans shown in photomicrograph of pancreas	Choudhury et al. (2017)
21	*Vitis vinifera*	Blue berries	Dried fruits	Lower the glucose absorption and also control the blood glucose level	Olmo-Cunillera et al. (2020)

10.7 Herbal Food Ingredients in Clinical Trial for Managing Diabetes

Herbal medicines consist of multiple bioactive constituents, each with distinct pharmacological activities, and have been employed for centuries as part of traditional medical practices worldwide. Their therapeutic potential has contributed to their global acceptance and integration into complementary and alternative medicine. However, for most herbal medicinal products, comprehensive data on safety, efficacy, pharmacodynamics, pharmacokinetics, and clinical validation remain insufficient. This paucity of robust scientific evidence poses challenges in fulfilling regulatory requirements and hinders the standardization, quality control, and global harmonization of herbal drug development.

10.7.1 Successfully Clinical Trial

Extensive research on herbal medicines particularly the human edible plants for the management of DM has led to the development and commercialization of several antidiabetic formulations worldwide. These plants have also been used in the traditional medicine for the management of DM from the time of immemorial with no or limited side effects in some culture. The human edibility and wide availability of these plants make it promising alternative for developing safe, accessible, and cost-effective therapeutic or dietary interventions for diabetic management. Thus, some clinical trials / randomized controlled trials have been made to study the efficacy of these plants and some of this is presented in Table 10.3. The positive results of the clinical or randomized control trials showed that the food if properly consumed can protect the human beings from different diseases including DM.

10.7.2 Ongoing Clinical Trial

Several studies have been conducted among the diabetic patient with various herbal medicine and found positive response. A study with cinnamon supplementation over 60 days on insulin sensitivity among the insulin resistance diabetic patients. Result indicates there are marked reduction in the insulin resistance and remarkable increase of insulin sensitivity (Sengsuk et al., 2015). Another study with the extract of *Ficus racemose* in a group of diabetic patients along with the oral hypoglycemic. After taking the bark extract twice a day for 15 days results remarkable reduction in the blood glucose level (Gul-e-Rana et al., 2013). The antidiabetic potential of *Portulaca oleracea* L. seeds was evaluated in subjects with type 2 diabetes mellitus (T2DM), where administration of 5 g twice daily for two months was compared with a standard dose of metformin (1500 mg/day). Treatment with *P. oleracea* resulted in

Table 10.3 Randomized control trial of the various plant product and their effect in diabetes control

S. no.	Name of the plant	Common name	Edible part	Outcome	References
1	*Abelmoschus esculentus*	Lady's finger	Whole fruit	Lowering FBG and HbA1c	Saatchi et al (2022)
2	*Arachis hypogeal*	Peanut	Seed	Improving blood lipids and glycemic control	Wien et al. (2014)
3	*Fragaria × ananassa*	Strawberries	Whole fruit	Lowering plasma glucose and improve glycaemic profile	Törrönenet al. (2012)
4	*Momordica charantia*	Bitter gourd	Whole fruit	Lowering fasting plasma glucose	Krawinkelet al. (2018)
5	*Prunus dulcis*	Almond	Seed	Lowering HbA1c	Cohen and Johnston (2011)
6	*Psidium guajava*	Red guava	Whole fruit	Lowering FPG	Kumari et al. (2016)
7	*Punica granatum*	Pomegranate	Seed	Lowering FBG and HbA1c	Seyed Hashemi et al. (2021)
8	*Ribes nigrum*	Blackcurrants	Whole fruit	Lowering plasma glucose and improve glycaemic profile	Törrönenet al. (2012)
9	*Syzygium cumini*	Jammun	Seed	Lowering fasting plasma glucose and post-prandial plasma glucose and HbA1C	Sidana et al. (2017)
10	*Trigonella foenum-graecum*	Fenugreek Seed	Seed	Lowering fasting plasma glucose, and systolic blood pressure	Hadi et al, (2020)
11	*Vaccinium myrtillus*	Wild European blueberries	Whole fruit	Lowering plasma glucose and improve glycaemic profile	Törrönenet al. (2012)
12	*Vaccinium oxycoccos*	Cranberries	Whole fruit	Lowering plasma glucose and improve glycaemic profile	Törrönenet al. (2012)

(continued)

Table 10.3 (continued)

S. no.	Name of the plant	Common name	Edible part	Outcome	References
13	*Zingiber officinale*	Ginger	Rhizome	Lowering FBG and Total cholesterol level	Carvalho et al. (2020)
14	*Ziziphus vulgaris*	Chinese date	Dried fruit	Lowering homeostasis model assessment-insulin resistance [HOMA-IR] and increasing quantitative insulin check index [QUICKI]	Niri et al. (2021)

significant reductions in fasting and postprandial blood glucose, insulin levels, serum LDL cholesterol, triglycerides, total cholesterol, liver enzymes (ALT, AST, and γ-glutamyl transferase), bilirubin, body weight, and body mass index (BMI). Additionally, a significant increase in high-density lipoprotein cholesterol (HDL-C) and serum albumin was observed. In contrast, the metformin group did not demonstrate significant improvements across these parameters (El-Sayed, 2011). Clinical studies have demonstrated the potential of resveratrol in improving glycemic control in patients with diabetes. In one trial, administration of resveratrol as a dietary supplement (150 mg/day) to obese individuals for 30 days resulted in a significant suppression of postprandial glucagon responses, indicating its role in modulating glucose homeostasis (Knop et al., 2013). Another clinical trial conducted in mild to moderate type-2 DM patients with *Scoparia dulcis* leaf extract. The result shows significant reduction in the fasting blood glucose ad HaA1c level in the treated patients (Senadheeraet al., 2015).

10.8 Future Perspective

The origins of modern pharmacotherapy can be traced to plant-derived compounds, many of which continue to underpin contemporary drug development. Numerous medicinal plants have been reported to possess antidiabetic activities, acting through multiple mechanisms such as stimulation of pancreatic insulin secretion, enhancement of peripheral insulin sensitivity, modulation of intestinal glucose uptake, and regulation of carbohydrate metabolism. Beyond their hypoglycemic effects, several herbs also contribute to the management of diabetes-related comorbidities, particularly cardiovascular complications, by lowering serum triglycerides, cholesterol levels, and body mass index (BMI). The use of plants as therapeutic agents is one of the oldest traditions in human healthcare and continues to hold relevance in modern society. The ongoing interest in herbal medicines arises from the need to understand the mechanisms underlying their pharmacological actions, as well as to evaluate their therapeutic benefits and possible adverse effects. Today, herbal medicines are widely employed for the prevention, maintenance of well-being, and treatment of diabetes mellitus. Advances in laboratory research have facilitated the translation of herbal remedies into clinical applications, leading to an increasing number of clinical trials and marketed polyherbal formulations. Despite notable progress, the rapid expansion of the ethno pharmaceutical sector presents several critical challenges. Foremost among these is the urgent requirement for validated and standardized testing protocols to ensure consistency in herbal preparations. Rigorous qualitative and quantitative characterization of bioactive constituents in final formulations is indispensable for reproducibility and therapeutic reliability. In parallel, evidence from well-designed, large-scale randomized controlled clinical trials is necessary to establish the safety, efficacy, and clinical relevance of herbal interventions. Regulatory frameworks must also evolve to incorporate stringent guidelines for standardization, quality assurance, pharmacovigilance, and product certification. Such measures are essential to enhance scientific credibility, ensure consumer safety, and promote the integration of herbal medicines into evidence-based strategies for diabetes management.

10.9 Conclusion

Herbal medicine has been used for long time and served in traditional healthcare system. Herbal medicine is also playing vital role in management of DM. Several medicinal plant and polyherbal formulation have demonstrated antidiabetic effect through several mechanisms like, glucose metabolism alteration, enhancement of insulin secretion, alteration of the insulin resistance. However, significant challenges like, standardization of the dose, limited pharmacokinetics data, sufficient clinical data, and the other adverse effect of the plant-based product are also holding back the integration of the herbal product in regular evidence-based medicine. These gaps are address recently through the phyto chemical analysis, perform random control trial to established the safety, efficacy of the herbal medicine. With this proper knowledge offers a new era of pharmacotherapy on which herbal medicine contributes a significant, meaningful contribution in diabetic management.

References

Adinortey, M. B. (2017). Biochemicophysiological mechanisms underlying signs and symptoms associated with diabetes mellitus. *Advances in Biology Research, 11*(6), 382–390.

Adinortey, M. B., Gyan, B. E., Adjimani, J., Nyarko, P., Sarpong, C., Tsikata, F. Y., & Nyarko, A. K. (2011). Dyslipidaemia associated with type 2 diabetics with micro and macrovascular complications among Ghanaians. *Indian Journal of Clinical Biochemistry, 26*(3), 261–268. https://doi.org/10.1007/s12291-010-0101-3

Ahmad, F., & Joshi, S. H. (2023). Self-care practices and their role in the control of diabetes: A narrative review. *Cureus., 15*(7), Article e41409. https://doi.org/10.7759/cureus.41409.PMID: 37546053;PMCID:PMC10402910

Altan, V. M. (2003). The pharmacology of diabetic complications. *Current Medicinal Chemistry, 10*, 1317–1327.

Arulselvan, P., Senthilkumar, G. P., Sathish Kumar, D., & Subramanian, S. (2006). Anti-diabetic effect of Murrayakoenigii leaves on streptozotocin induced diabetic rats. *Die Pharmazie, 61*(10), 874–877.

Augustin, L. S. A., Kendall, C. W. C., Jenkins, D. J. A., et al. (2015). Glycemic index, glycemic load and glycemic response: An International Scientific Consensus Summit from the International Carbohydrate Quality Consortium (ICQC). *Nutrition, Metabolism and Cardiovascular Disease, 25*(9), 795–815. https://doi.org/10.1016/j.numecd.2015.05.005

Baldé, N. M., Youla, A., Baldé, M. D., et al. (2006). Herbal medicine and treatment of diabetes in Africa: An example from Guinea. *Diabetes & Metabolism, 32*(2), 171–175. https://doi.org/10.1016/s1262-3636(07)70265-3

BarakatunNisak, M. Y., Ruzita, A. T., Norimah, A. K., Gilbertson, H., & Nor Azmi, K. (2010). Improvement of dietary quality with the aid of a low glycemic index diet in Asian patients with type 2 diabetes mellitus. *Journal of the American College of Nutrition, 29*(3), 161–170. https://doi.org/10.1080/07315724.2010.10719830

Barnard, R. J., Massey, M. R., Cherny, S., O'Brien, L. T., & Pritikin, N. (1983). Long-term use of a high-complex-carbohydrate, high-fiber, low-fat diet and exercise in the treatment of NIDDM patients. *Diabetes Care, 6*(3), 268–273. https://doi.org/10.2337/diacare.6.3.268

Behrouz, V., Dastkhosh, A., Hedayati, M., Sedaghat, M., Sharafkhah, M., & Sohrab, G. (2020). The effect of crocin supplementation on lycemic control, insulin resistance and active AMPK levels in patients with type 2 diabetes: A pilot study. *Diabetology & Metabolic Syndrome, 12*, 59.https://doi.org/10.1186/s13098-020-00568-6

Bhupathiraju, S. N., Tobias, D. K., Malik, V. S., et al. (2014). Glycemic index, glycemic load, and risk of type 2 diabetes: Results from 3 large US cohorts and an updated meta-analysis. *American Journal of Clinical Nutrition, 100*(1), 218–232. https://doi.org/10.3945/ajcn.113.079533

Black, C., Donnelly, P., McIntyre, L., Royle, P. L., Shepherd, J. P., & Thomas, S. (2007). Meglitinide analogues for type 2 diabetes mellitus. *Cochrane Database of Systematic Reviews, 2*, CD004654. https://doi.org/10.1002/14651858.CD004654.pub2

Carvalho, G. C. N., Lira-Neto, J. C. G., Araújo, M. F. M., Freitas, R. W. J. F., Zanetti, M. L., & Damasceno, M. M. C. (2020). Effectiveness of ginger in reducing metabolic levels in people with diabetes: A randomized clinical trial. *Revista Latino-Americana De Enfermagem, 28*, Article e3369. https://doi.org/10.1590/1518-8345.3870.3369

Choudhury, H., Pandey, M., Hua, C. K., et al. (2017). An update on natural compounds in the remedy of diabetes mellitus: A systematic review. *Journal of Traditional & Complementary Medicine, 8*(3), 361–376. https://doi.org/10.1016/j.jtcme.2017.08.012

Cohen, A. E., & Johnston, C. S. (2011). Almond ingestion at mealtime reduces postprandial glycemia and chronic ingestion reduces hemoglobin A(1c) in individuals with well-controlled type 2 diabetes mellitus. *Metabolism, 60*(9), 1312–1317. https://doi.org/10.1016/j.metabol.2011.01.017

Corathers, S. D., Peavie, S., & Salehi, M. (2013). Complications of diabetes therapy. *Endocrinology and Metabolism Clinics of North America, 42*(4), 947–970. https://doi.org/10.1016/j.ecl.2013.06.005

Cox, D. J., Banton, T., Moncrief, M., et al. (2020). Glycemic excursion minimization in the management of type 2 diabetes: A novel intervention tested in a randomized clinical trial. *BMJ Open Diabetes Research & Care, 8*(2), Article e001795. https://doi.org/10.1136/bmjdrc-2020-001795

Davis, N. J., Tomuta, N., Schechter, C., et al. (2009). Comparative study of the effects of a 1-year dietary intervention of a low-carbohydrate diet versus a low-fat diet on weight and glycemic control in type 2 diabetes. *Diabetes Care, 32*(7), 1147–1152. https://doi.org/10.2337/dc08-2108

Dong, J. Y., Zhang, L., Zhang, Y. H., & Qin, L. Q. (2011). Dietary glycaemic index and glycaemic load in relation to the risk of type 2 diabetes: A meta-analysis of prospective cohort studies. *British Journal of Nutrition, 106*, 1649–1654. https://doi.org/10.1017/S000711451100540X

El-Sayed, M. I. (2011). Effects of Portulaca oleracea L. seeds in treatment of type-2 diabetes mellitus patients as adjunctive and alternative therapy. *Journal of Ethnopharmacology, 137*(1), 643–651. https://doi.org/10.1016/j.jep.2011.06.020

Esposito, K., Maiorino, M. I., Ciotola, M., et al. (2009). Effects of a Mediterranean-style diet on the need for antihyperglycemic drug therapy in patients with newly diagnosed type 2 diabetes: A randomized trial. *Annals of Internal Medicine, 151*(5), 306–314. https://doi.org/10.7326/0003-4819-151-5-200909010-00004

Fabricatore, A. N., Wadden, T. A., Ebbeling, C. B., et al. (2011). Targeting dietary fat or glycemic load in the treatment of obesity and type 2 diabetes: A randomized controlled trial. *Diabetes Research and Clinical Practice, 92*(1), 37–45. https://doi.org/10.1016/j.diabres.2010.12.016

Gul-e-Rana, K. S., Khurhsid, R., et al. (2013). Hypoglycemic activity of Ficus racemosa bark in combination with oral hypoglycemic drug in diabetic human. *Acta Poloniae Pharmaceutica, 70*(6), 1045–1049.

Gupta, A., Gupta, R., & Lal, B. (2001). Effect of *Trigonella foenum-graecum* (fenugreek) seeds on glycaemic control and insulin resistance in type 2 diabetes mellitus: A double blind placebo controlled study. *Journal of the Association of Physicians of India, 49*, 1057–1061.

Hadi, A., Arab, A., Hajianfar, H., Talaei, B., Miraghajani, M., Babajafari, S., Marx, W., & Tavakoly, R. (2020). The effect of fenugreek seed supplementation on serum irisin levels, blood pressure, and liver and kidney function in patients with type 2 diabetes mellitus: A parallel randomized clinical trial. *Complementary Therapies in Medicine, 49*, Article 102315. https://doi.org/10.1016/j.ctim.2020.102315

Hannan, J. M. A., Ansari, P., Haque, A., et al. (2019). Nigella sativa stimulates insulin secretion from isolated rat islets and inhibits the digestion and absorption of $(CH_2O)_n$ in the gut. *Bioscience Reports, 39*(8), BSR20190723. https://doi.org/10.1042/BSR20190723

Jain, R. C., & Vyas, C. R. (1975). Garlic in alloxan-induced diabetic rabbits. *American Journal of Clinical Nutrition, 28*(7), 684–685. https://doi.org/10.1093/ajcn/28.7.684

Jayaprasad, B., Sharavanan, P. S., & Sivaraj, R. (2016). Antidiabetic effect of *Chloroxylon swietenia* bark extracts on streptozotocin induced diabetic rats. *Beni-Suef University Journal of Basic and Applied Sciences, 5*(1), 1e9. https://doi.org/10.1016/j.bjbas.2016.01.004.

Jenkins, D. J., Kendall, C. W., Augustin, L. S., et al. (2002). Glycemic index: Overview of implications in health and disease. *American Journal of Clinical Nutrition, 76*(1), 266S-S273. https://doi.org/10.1093/ajcn/76/1.266S

Jeppesen, P. B., Gregersen, S., Alstrup, K. K., & Hermansen, K. (2002). Stevioside induces anti-hyperglycaemic, insulinotropic and glucagonostatic effects in vivo: Studies in the diabetic Goto-Kakizaki (GK) rats. *Phytomedicine, 9*(1), 9–14. https://doi.org/10.1078/0944-7113-00081

Khatib, O. (2004). Noncommunicable diseases: Risk factors and regional strategies for prevention and care. *Eastern Mediterranean Health Journal, 10*(6), 778–788.

Khazrai, Y. M., Defeudis, G., & Pozzilli, P. (2014). Effect of diet on type 2 diabetes mellitus: A review. *Diabetes/Metabolism Research and Reviews, 30*(Suppl. 1), 24–33.https://doi.org/10.1002/dmrr.2515

Knop, F. K., Konings, E., Timmers, S., Schrauwen, P., Holst, J. J., & Blaak, E. E. (2013). Thirty days of resveratrol supplementation does not affect postprandial incretin hormone responses, but suppresses postprandial glucagon in obese subjects. *Diabetic Medicine, 30*(10), 1214–1218. https://doi.org/10.1111/dme.12231

Krawinkel, M. B., Ludwig, C., Swai, M. E., Yang, R. Y., Chun, K. P., & Habicht, S. D. (2018). Bitter gourd reduces elevated fasting plasma glucose levels in an intervention study among prediabetics in Tanzania. *Journal of Ethnopharmacology, 216*, 1–7. https://doi.org/10.1016/j.jep.2018.01.016

Kumar, S., Mittal, A., Babu, D., & Mittal, A. (2021). Herbal medicines for diabetes management and its secondary complications. *Current Diabetes Review, 17*(4), 437–456. https://doi.org/10.2174/1573399816666201103143225

Kumari, S., Rakavi, R., & Mangaraj, M. (2016). Effect of Guava in blood glucose and lipid profile in healthy human subjects: A randomized controlled study. *Journal of Clinical and Diagnostic Research, 10*(9), BC04-BC07. https://doi.org/10.7860/JCDR/2016/21291.8425

Lebovitz, H. E. (2019). Thiazolidinediones: The forgotten diabetes medications. *Current Diabetes Reports, 19*, 151. https://doi.org/10.1007/s11892-019-1270-y

Ley, S. H., Hamdy, O., Mohan, V., & Hu, F. B. (2014). Prevention and management of type 2 diabetes: Dietary components and nutritional strategies. *Lancet, 383*(9933), 1999–2007. https://doi.org/10.1016/S0140-6736(14)60613-9

Li, D., Zhang, Y., Liu, Y., Sun, R., & Xia, M. (2015). Purified anthocyanin supplementation reduces dyslipidemia, enhances antioxidant capacity, and prevents insulin resistance in diabetic patients. *Journal of Nutrition, 145*, 742–748. https://doi.org/10.3945/jn.114.205674

Liu, R., Su, C., Xu, Y., Shang, K., Sun, K., Li, C., & Lu, J. (2020). Identifying potential active components of walnut leaf that action diabetes mellitus through integration of UHPLC-Q-Orbitrap HRMS and network pharmacology analysis. *Journal of Ethnopharmacology, 253*, Article 112659. https://doi.org/10.1016/j.jep.2020.112659

Livesey, G., Taylor, R., Livesey, H., & Liu, S. (2013) Is there a dose-response relation of dietary glycemic load to risk of type 2 diabetes? Meta-analysis of prospective cohort studies. *The American Journal of Clinical Nutrition, 97*, 584–596.https://doi.org/10.3945/ajcn.112.041467

Nanri, A., Mizoue, T., Noda, M., et al. (2010). Rice intake and type 2 diabetes in Japanese men and women: The Japan public health center-based prospective study. *American Journal of Clinical Nutrition, 92*(6), 1468–1477. https://doi.org/10.3945/ajcn.2010.29512

Niri, Z. I., Shidfar, F., Jabbari, M., Zarrati, M., Hosseini, A., Malek, M., & Dehnad, A. (2021). The effect of dried Ziziphus vulgaris on glycemic control, lipid profile, Apo-proteins and hs-CRP in patients with type 2 diabetes mellitus: A randomized controlled clinical trial. *Journal of Food Biochemistry, 45*(3), Article e13193. https://doi.org/10.1111/jfbc.13193

Noor, A., Gunasekaran, S., & Vijayalakshmi, M. A. (2017). Improvement of insulin secretion and pancreatic β-cell function in streptozotocin-induced diabetic rats treated with aloe vera extract. *Pharmacognosy Research, 9*(Suppl 1), S99–S104. https://doi.org/10.4103/pr.pr_75_17

Nseir, W., Nassar, F., & Assy, N. (2010). Soft drinks consumption and nonalcoholic fatty liver disease. *World Journal of Gastroenterology, 16*(21), 2579–2588. https://doi.org/10.3748/wjg.v16.i21.2579

Olmo-Cunillera, A., Escobar-Avello, D., Pérez, A. J., Marhuenda-Muñoz, M., Lamuela-Raventós, R. M., & Vallverdú-Queralt, A. (2020). Is eating raisins healthy? *Nutrients, 12*(1), 54.https://doi.org/10.3390/nu12010054

Padhi, S., Nayak, A. K., & Behera, A. (2020). Type II diabetes mellitus: A review on recent drug-based therapeutics. *Biomedicine & Pharmacotherapy, 131*, Article 110708. https://doi.org/10.1016/j.biopha.2020.110708

Patil, S. B., Takalikar, S. S., Joglekar, M. M., Haldavnekar, V. S., & Arvindekar, A. U. (2013). Insulinotropic and β-cell protective action of cuminaldehyde, cuminol and an inhibitor isolated from Cuminum cyminum in streptozotocin-induced diabetic rats. *British Journal of Nutrition, 110*(8), 1434–1443. https://doi.org/10.1017/S0007114513000627

Perera, P. K., & Li, Y. (2012). Functional herbal food ingredients used in type 2 diabetes mellitus. *Pharmacognosy Reviews, 6*(11), 37–45. https://doi.org/10.4103/0973-7847.95863

Petrovska, B. B. (2012). Historical review of medicinal plants' usage. *Pharmacognosy Reviews, 6*(11), 1–5. https://doi.org/10.4103/0973-7847.95849

Phillips, A. (2016). Improving self-management of type 1 and type 2 diabetes. *Nursing Standard, 30*(19), 52–60. https://doi.org/10.7748/ns.30.19.52.s44

Rai, P. K., Rai, N. K., Rai, A. K., & Watal, G. (2007). Role of LIBS in elemental analysis of P. guajava responsible for glycemic potential. *Instrumentation Science & Technology, 35*, 507–522.

Saatchi, A., Aghamohammadzadeh, N., Beheshtirouy, S., Javadzadeh, Y., Afshar, F. H., & Ghaffary, S. (2022). Anti-hyperglycemic effect of Abelmoschus culentesus (Okra) on patients with diabetes type 2: A randomized clinical trial. *Phytotherapy Research, 36*(4), 1644–1651. https://doi.org/10.1002/ptr.7341

Sahib, A. S. (2016). Anti-diabetic and antioxidant effect of cinnamon in poorly controlled type-2 diabetic Iraqi patients: A randomized, placebo-controlled clinical trial. *Journal of Intercultural Ethnopharmacology, 5*, 108–113.https://doi.org/10.5455/jice.20160217044511

Senadheera, S. P., Ekanayake, S., & Wanigatunge, C. (2015). Anti-hyperglycaemic effects of herbal porridge made of Scoparia dulcis leaf extract in diabetics—A randomized crossover clinical trial. *BMC Complementary and Alternative Medicine, 15*, 410. https://doi.org/10.1186/s12906-015-0935-6

Sengsuk, C., Sanguanwong, S., Tangvarasittichai, O., & Tangvarasittichai, S. (2015). Effect of cinnamon supplementation on glucose, lipids levels, glomerular filtration rate, and blood pressure of subjects with type 2 diabetes mellitus. *Diabetology International, 7*(2), 124–132. https://doi.org/10.1007/s13340-015-0218-y

Seyed Hashemi, M., Namiranian, N., Tavahen, H., Dehghanpour, A., Rad, M. H., Jam-Ashkezari, S., Emtiazy, M., & Hashempur, M. H. (2021). Efficacy of pomegranate seed powder on glucose and lipid metabolism in patients with type 2 diabetes: A prospective randomized double-blind placebo-controlled clinical trial. *Complement Med Res, 28*(3), 226–233. https://doi.org/10.1159/000510986

Shaikh, A. A., Kolhatkar, M. K., Sopane, D. R., & Thorve, A. N. (2022). Review on: Diabetes mellitus is a disease. *Int J Res Pharm Sci, 13*(1), 102–109.

Sharma, S., Mandal, A., Kant, R., Jachak, S., & Jagzape, M. (2020). Is cinnamon efficacious for glycaemic control in type-2 diabetes mellitus? *JPMA. Journal of the Pakistan Medical Association, 70*, 2065–2069.

Shin, S. W., Jung, S. J., Jung, E. S., Hwang, J. H., Kim, W. R., So, B. O., Park, B. H., Lee, S. O., Cho, B. H., Park, T. S., Kim, Y. G., & Chae, S. W. (2020). Effects of a lifestyle-modification program on blood-glucose regulation and health promotion in diabetic patients: A randomized controlled trial. *Journal of Lifestyle Medicine, 10*(2), 77–91. https://doi.org/10.15280/jlm.2020.10.2.77

Sidana, S., Singh, V. B., Meena, B. L., Beniwal, S., Singh, K., Kumar, D., & Singla, R. (2017). Effect of *Syzygiumcumini* (jamun) seed powder on glycemic control: A double-blind randomized controlled trial. *Journal of Medical Society, 31*(3), 185–189. https://doi.org/10.4103/jms.jms_62_16

Silver, B., Ramaiya, K., Andrew, S. B., et al. (2018). EADSG guidelines: Insulin therapy in diabetes. *Diabetes Therapy, 9*(2), 449–492. https://doi.org/10.1007/s13300-018-0384-6

Susilawati, E., Levita, J., Susilawati, Y., & Sumiwi, S. A. (2023). Review of the case reports on metformin, sulfonylurea, and thiazolidinedione therapies in type 2 diabetes mellitus patients. *Medical Science (Basel), 11*(3), 50. https://doi.org/10.3390/medsci11030050

Törrönen, R., Sarkkinen, E., Niskanen, T., Tapola, N., Kilpi, K., & Niskanen, L. (2012). Postprandial glucose, insulin and glucagon-like peptide 1 responses to sucrose ingested with berries in healthy subjects. *British Journal of Nutrition, 107*(10), 1445–1451. https://doi.org/10.1017/S0007114511004557

van Zuuren, E. J., Fedorowicz, Z., Kuijpers, T., & Pijl, H. (2018). Effects of low-carbohydrate-compared with low-fat-diet interventions on metabolic control in people with type 2 diabetes: A systematic review including GRADE assessments. *American Journal of Clinical Nutrition, 108*(2), 300–331. https://doi.org/10.1093/ajcn/nqy096

Viguiliouk, E., Kendall, C. W., Kahleová, H., et al. (2019). Effect of vegetarian dietary patterns on cardiometabolic risk factors in diabetes: A systematic review and meta-analysis of randomized controlled trials. *Clinical Nutrition, 38*(3), 1133–1145. https://doi.org/10.1016/j.clnu.2018.05.032

Villegas, R., Shu, X. O., Gao, Y. T., et al. (2008). Vegetable but not fruit consumption reduces the risk of type 2 diabetes in Chinese women. *Journal of Nutrition, 138*(3), 574–580. https://doi.org/10.1093/jn/138.3.574

Visek, J., Lacigova, S., Cechurova, D., & Rusavy, Z. (2014). Comparison of a low-glycemic index vs standard diabetic diet. *Biomedical Papers of the Medical Faculty of the University Palacky, Olomouc, Czech Republic, 158*(1), 112–116. https://doi.org/10.5507/bp.2012.103

Wang, M. L., Gellar, L., Nathanson, B. H., et al. (2015). Decrease in glycemic index associated with improved glycemic control among latinos with type 2 diabetes. *Journal of the Academy of Nutrition and Dietetics, 115*(6), 898–906. https://doi.org/10.1016/j.jand.2014.10.012

Wien, M., Oda, K., & Sabaté, J. (2014). A randomized controlled trial to evaluate the effect of incorporating peanuts into an American Diabetes Association meal plan on the nutrient profile of the total diet and cardiometabolic parameters of adults with type 2 diabetes. *Nutrition Journal, 13*, 10. https://doi.org/10.1186/1475-2891-13-10

Wild, S., Roglic, G., Green, A., Sicree, R., & King, H. (2004). Global prevalence of diabetes: Estimates for the year 2000 and projections for 2030. *Diabetes Care, 27*(5), 1047–1053. https://doi.org/10.2337/diacare.27.5.1047

Wolever, T. M., Gibbs, A. L., Mehling, C., et al. (2008). The Canadian Trial of Carbohydrates in Diabetes (CCD), a 1-y controlled trial of low-glycemic-index dietary carbohydrate in type 2 diabetes: No effect on glycated hemoglobin but reduction in C-reactive protein. *American Journal of Clinical Nutrition, 87*(1), 114–125. https://doi.org/10.1093/ajcn/87.1.114

World Health Organization. (2023). *Carbohydrate intake for adults and children: WHO guideline*. World Health Organization. https://www.who.int/publications/i/item/9789240073593

World Health Organization. (2024). *Diabetes*. World Health Organization. Retrieve on 14 November 2024 https://www.who.int/news-room/fact-sheets/detail/diabetes

Yusof, B. N., Talib, R. A., Kamaruddin, N. A., Karim, N. A., Chinna, K., & Gilbertson, H. (2009). A low-GI diet is associated with a short-term improvement of glycaemic control in Asian patients with type 2 diabetes. *Diabetes, Obesity, and Metabolism, 11*(4), 387–396. https://doi.org/10.1111/j.1463-1326.2008.00984.x

Zaman, M. S. Z., Hassan, P. H., Islam, S. M. S. I., Ullah, M. A. U., & Rabbani, M. G. R. (2023). Comparative efficacy of insulin, biguanides and sulfonylureas in the glycemic control of newly diagnosed diabetes mellitus patients in Rajshahi, Bangladesh. *Journal of Biosciences, 31*, 39–49. https://doi.org/10.3329/jbs.v31i1.69533

Chapter 11
Infection Control in Diabetes: The Role of Antibiotics and Antiseptics

Susmita Chakrabarty, Bangmayee Dash, Sunday Oyedemi, and Shasank Sekhar Swain

Abstract Diabetes mellitus (DM) significantly increases the risk of several infections in outpatient and hospitalized patients having weakened immune defences/being immunocompromised, abnormal microcirculation, and neuropathy. The most prevalent infections in diabetic patients are skin and soft tissue infections, urinary tract infections (UTIs), respiratory tract infections (RTIs), chronic diabetic ulcers, etc. Infection control in DM cases is an ideal strategy to avoid complications and achieve higher clinical success. This chapter emphasizes the importance of antiseptics and antibiotics, including empirical and culture-directed therapy, in managing infections and chronic wounds in diabetic patients, as well as addressing antibiotic therapy, antimicrobial resistance, and the pharmacodynamics of different classes of drugs. Further, the study assesses principal antiseptics, such as chlorhexidine, povidone-iodine, and silver-containing agents, emphasizing their modes of action, effectiveness, and cytotoxicity. Clinical evidence is compiled to guide optimal practices in wound management, the prevention of surgical site infections, and catheter-associated infections (CAI). Emerging trends are nano-based antiseptic technology and personalized medicine strategies, highlighting the importance of coordinated, evidence-based infection control in the management of diabetes.

Keywords Diabetes mellitus · Diabetic chronic wounds · Antimicrobial resistance · Catheter associated infections

---

S. Chakrabarty · B. Dash
School of Allied and Healthcare Sciences, DRIEMS University, Cuttack, India

S. Oyedemi
School of Science and Technology, Nottingham Trent University, Nottingham, UK

S. S. Swain (✉)
School of Biotechnology, Centurion University of Technology and Management, Bhubaneswar, India
e-mail: swain.shasanksekhar86@gmail.com

Research and Development Division, BRIC-Institute of Life Sciences Bioincubator, Niladri Vihar, Bhubaneswar, India

K. Adhikary et al. (eds.), *Healing Beyond Blood Sugar*,
https://doi.org/10.1007/978-981-95-8946-3_11

11.1 Introduction

Diabetes mellitus (DM) is acknowledged as a multifactorial immunocompromised condition characterized by chronic low-grade inflammation and impaired immune cell function, which elevates the higher risk of infections (Bodke et al., 2023; Abbas et al., 2025). This immunocompromised condition is classified with more mechanical understanding of the necessity of infection control strategies for diabetic patients as a secondary immune system impairment rather than a primary immunodeficiency (Akash et al., 2020). As a result, diabetic patients have greatly enhanced susceptibility to infection and create more complications for management (Akash et al., 2020; Abbas et al., 2025). The overall chapter highlights and gives a more mechanical understanding of the necessity of infection control strategies for diabetic patients (Akash et al., 2020; Zhou et al., 2024).

Metabolic complications and immunocompromised conditions, along with comorbidities, are challenging to the health outcomes and quality of life of diabetic patients (Bodke et al., 2023; Abbas et al., 2025). Chronic hyperglycemia, compromised immune responses, and vascular deficiencies altogether make more favorable conditions for pathogenic bacteria, which enhance the life-threatening conditions; therefore, infection prevention is an important therapeutic strategy in contemporary diabetes care (Akash et al., 2020; Abbas et al., 2025). The implementation and targeting context greatly revise the functions of antibiotics and antiseptics, particularly in DM cases. Precision antibiotic therapies, antimicrobial peptides (AMPs), emerging nano-based antiseptic agents, etc. are transforming infection control toward more extensive efficacy with lower resistance rates. Clinical evidence and practice guidelines further bolster these innovations, establishing successful infection control as a fundamental component in safeguarding diabetic patients, reducing complications, and promoting long-term health (Chávez-Reyes et al., 2021).

11.1.1 Background on Diabetes and Susceptibility to Infection

Diabetes mellitus (Fig. 11.1) is a common metabolic disorder in more than 11–14% of the world's population, with chronic hyperglycemia due to defects in insulin secretion, insulin action, or both (Dilworth et al., 2021; Hossain et al., 2024). Metabolic derangements in diabetes—most particularly persistent high glucose concentrations—have a striking impact on immune function by impairing neutrophil activity, blunting the antioxidant defense system, and modifying humoral and cellular immunity (Dilworth et al., 2021; Hossain et al., 2024). Consequently, individuals with diabetes are predisposed to bacterial, viral, and fungal infections and often exhibit a more severe disease progression compared to non-diabetic individuals (Holt et al., 2024; Dilworth et al., 2021; Zhou & Lansang, 2000).

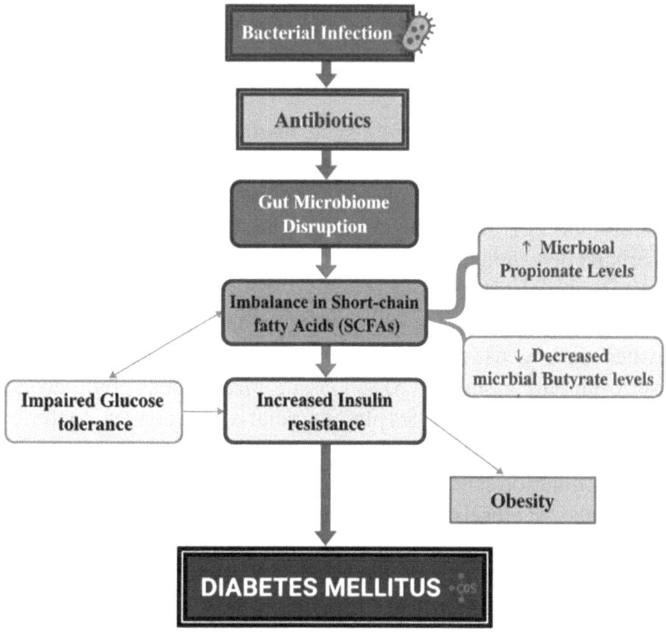

Fig. 11.1 Graphical illustration of bacterial infection in diabetes mellitus, starting from disrupting the gut microbiome to increasing insulin resistance and glucose tolerance, leading to obesity (Park et al., 2021)

Specific infections like pneumonia, urinary tract infections (UTIs), skin and soft tissue infections, and diabetic foot infections (DFIs) are especially common and severe in patients with diabetes (Dilworth et al., 2021; Kim & Choi, 2025). The hyperglycemic environment facilitates pathogen growth and impedes immunity, leading to higher hospitalization rates, longer stays, and higher complication risks. The complexity of infections is further compounded by vascular and neuropathic complications from diabetes, which facilitate impaired wound healing and further weaken host defenses (Carey et al., 2018; Zhou & Lansang, 2000; Dilworth et al., 2021).

Mechanistically, diabetes also impairs innate as well as adaptive immune systems. Research indicates abnormal neutrophil chemotaxis, compromised phagocytosis, and defective lymphocyte function in hyperglycemic environments (Bodke et al., 2023; Thimmappa et al., 2023). Epidemiological evidence associates diabetes with a heightened incidence of severe infections, such as COVID-19 and influenza, resulting in greater morbidity and mortality compared to non-diabetic individuals (Bodke et al., 2023; Abbas et al., 2025; Carey et al., 2018; Geerlings & Hoepelman, 1999).

11.1.2 Importance of Infection Control in Diabetic Populations

Infection control is of utmost significance in diabetic patients because of their increased susceptibility and the risk of quick deterioration after infection sets in (Akash et al., 2020; Abbas et al., 2025). Poor control of blood sugar predisposes to disease and aggravates the course of infectious diseases, and hence active control is a crucial determinant of healthier outcomes (Casqueiro et al., 2012; Akash et al., 2020; Abbas et al., 2025).

Preventive strategies, such as glycaemic optimization, prompt immunization against prevalent pathogens (e.g., influenza, pneumococcus, COVID-19), and regular clinical monitoring, are essential (Akash et al., 2020; Abbas et al., 2025). Pharmacists, clinicians, and health educators play a crucial role in conveying these measures, emphasizing stringent blood glucose management, adherence to therapy, dietary protocols, and vaccination schedules (Bodke et al., 2023; Abbas et al., 2025). Diabetic patients should also be closely monitored for early infections and should be treated promptly with evidence-based antimicrobial treatment and supportive care (Akash et al., 2020; Abbas et al., 2025).

Efforts to optimize glycaemic control have been demonstrated to augment immune status and mitigate the risk and severity of infection. In addition, education on a continuing basis about infection prevention, such as hygienic measures and wound care, constitutes a vital part of integrated diabetes care (Dilworth et al., 2021; Casqueiro et al., 2012).

11.1.3 Scope and Objectives of the Review

This chapter aims to highlight three primary objectives:

- To clarify the epidemiology and mechanisms through which diabetes enhances susceptibility and severity of infections in affected individuals.
- To examine the clinical consequences of infection in diabetic patients, emphasizing the necessity for targeted prevention and prompt, effective treatment.
- To provide an evidence-based analysis of current infection control practices, identify knowledge deficiencies, and suggest avenues for future research concerning infectious disease risks associated with diabetes (Casqueiro et al., 2012).

The scope includes both type 1 and type 2 diabetes, distinguishing the risk profiles where applicable, and examines the bidirectional association between uncontrolled glycemic levels and infection outcomes. Of particular attention are infections of public health importance such as respiratory tract infections, skin and soft tissue infections, and DFIs, as well as how recent progress in diabetes therapies and their effect on infection risk (Critchley et al., 2018; Zhou & Lansang, 2000).

The overall objectives are:

- To integrate existing knowledge of pathophysiological mechanisms of diabetes-related immune dysfunction.
- To summarize the most common and life-threatening infections in diabetic patients, with practical recommendations for prevention and management.
- To identify critical deficiencies and prospective trajectories, particularly regarding the influence of novel diabetes treatments and vaccines on the incidence and outcomes of infections.
- This chapter aims to advance understanding in the critical area of diabetes management with evidence from epidemiological, clinical, and mechanistic studies, thereby informing best practices to improve patient outcomes worldwide.
- This introduction provides a balanced, evidence-based overview for a 2000-word paper. It emphasizes the necessity to comprehend and mitigate the infection risk in individuals with diabetes (Banday et al., 2020).

11.2 Pathophysiology of Diabetes and Infection

Diabetes is a metabolic disorder that fundamentally modifies immune status and vascular well-being, augmenting susceptibility and severity of infections by virtue of both impaired host defense and numerous microvascular as well as neurological complications (Akash et al., 2020; Dilworth et al., 2021). This extensive chapter undertakes a detailed examination of these processes, incorporating relevant research and clinical observations characterized by hyperglycemia resulting from defective insulin secretion or action. This persistent hyperglycemia initiates a series of pathophysiological changes that impair immune system functionality and lead to complications, including microvascular damage and neuropathy (Daryabor et al., 2020).

11.2.1 Compromised Host Defenses and Immunity

Diabetic patients undergo dysfunction in both the innate and adaptive immunity systems. Chronic hyperglycemia creates a pro-inflammatory condition ("inflam-maging"), elevating plasma cytokines like tumour necrosis factor-alpha (TNF-α), interleukins, and reactive oxygen species (ROS) (Thimmappa et al., 2023; Caturano et al., 2023; Alexander et al., 2024). Such an environment hampers vital immune cell behaviour:

- Neutrophil Dysfunction: Diabetics show reduced neutrophil chemotaxis, phagocytosis, and killing ability, resulting in reduced pathogen clearance.
- Macrophage and Monocyte Dysfunction: Decreased expression of Fcγ receptors delays endocytosis and early immune response. Hyperglycemia modulates macrophage activation to preclude effective microbial defense.

- Natural Killer (NK) Cell Alteration: NK cells exhibit reduced receptor expression and activity, impairing monitoring for virally infected targets.
- T-Cell and B-Cell Changes: Both cellular and humoral arms of adaptive immunity are impaired. There are lower pathogen-specific T-helper (Th17) responses and a loss of regulatory T cells, which advance chronic inflammation and tissue damage (Caturano et al., 2023; Alexander et al., 2024).

These are exacerbated to more frequent and severe infections by defects, including bacterial, viral, and fungal infections like pneumonia, UTIs, and dermatitis (Abbas et al., 2025). Additionally, immune cell senescence, immunocyte acceleration of aging, blunts response to vaccines and enhances susceptibility to novel pathogens (Fu et al., 2025). Side effects of medications, such as some glucose-lowering drugs, also impair immune function (Caturano et al., 2023; Quiros-Roldan et al., 2024).

11.2.2 Microvascular and Neurological Problems

Microvascular diabetic complications target the small blood vessels and are caused by chronic hyperglycaemia and inflammation. They occur as:

- Retinopathy: Retinal blood vessel damage that predisposes to vision loss and eye infection.
- Nephropathy: Glomerular damage that exposes the patient to UTIs and compromises systemic immune function.
- Peripheral Vascular Disease: Endothelial dysfunction and decreased vascular density compromise tissue perfusion and healing.

Neuropathy, nerve injury associated with microvascular disease, undermines the body's mechanism for detecting injury, especially in the lower limbs (Yang et al., 2025). Delayed detection of wounds results in recurrent skin and soft tissue infections, such as diabetic foot ulcers (DFUs) (Wang et al., 2025). Impaired blood supply and immune compromise synergistically impair wound healing, usually requiring extended antimicrobial treatment and doubling amputation risk (Antar et al., 2023).

Hyperglycaemia also causes gut microbiota dysbiosis, enhancing intestinal permeability and systemic infection susceptibility (Yu et al., 2025). Chronic inflammation also disturbs bone marrow composition, shifting immune cell production towards myeloid lineages and away from lymphoid lineages, thus decreasing the adaptive immune capability of the body (Burak et al., 2024).

Molecular and Cellular Pathways: Sustained increases in blood glucose and free fatty acids activate transcription factors NF-κB and AP-1, which induce the generation of inflammatory mediators and enhance both pancreatic β-cell and immune cell apoptosis. Immunosuppression by these mediators over time impairs insulin release, worsens metabolic instability, and continues immune dysfunction (Berbudi et al., 2025).

Endoplasmic reticulum (ER) stress markers are increased in diabetes and lead to defective expression of NK cell receptors and reduced cellular immunity. Decreased cytokine signalling, compromised antigen presentation, and faulty leukocyte recruitment all contribute collectively to delaying the body's response to infection (Daryabor et al., 2020).

Clinical Consequences: The synergy of immune, vascular, and neurological derangement explains the increase in infection risk, severity, and complications that is seen in diabetic patients. Increased hospital stays; greater use of antibiotics, prolonged recovery, and a higher frequency of severe outcomes (such as sepsis and amputation) are the hallmarks of this group (Abbas et al., 2025).

Tight glycaemic control and targeted therapy, immunizations, wound care, and early antimicrobial therapy are key factors in preventing these risks and in enhancing outcomes. This chapter presents an in-depth, current review of the interactions among diabetes, immune dysfunction, and vascular complications that underpin holistic infection risk management within diabetic subjects (Daryabor et al., 2020; Fernandes et al., 2019).

11.3 Common Infections in Diabetes

Diabetes mellitus remarkably enhances the possibilities of different infections due to damaged immunity, neuropathy, hyperglycemia, and vascular insufficiency (Akash et al., 2020; Abbas et al., 2025). Chronic high blood glucose changes neutrophil function, decreases cytokine properties, and reduces blood flow, making it easier for pathogens to create an infection. Apart from this, glycosuria (sugar in urine) and tissue ischemia help environments that enhance bacterial and fungal growth. Below are the common infections related to diabetes in detail (Casqueiro et al., 2012; Akash et al., 2020; Wang et al., 2025).

11.3.1 Skin and Soft Tissue Infections

Skin and soft tissue infections are among the most common and major infections in diabetic patients. Increased glucose levels deactivate the skin barrier and destroy immune defenses, creating bacteria such as *Staphylococcus aureus* (including MRSA), *Streptococcus pyogenes*, and Gram-negative bacilli to occupy (Akash et al., 2020; Wang et al., 2025). Common indications include cellulitis, abscesses, folliculitis, and carbuncles. Neuropathy and decreased sensation in the extremities mean that even small injuries can become entry points for infection. In severe or poorly managed conditions, infections may enhance to necrotizing fasciitis, a rapidly spreading and life-threatening condition (Akash et al., 2020; Wang et al., 2025). Recurrent boils and chronic skin irritation are the main causes for Diabetics, which are indirectly associated with slowing down the process of wound healing and enhance the death rate. To decrease the recurrence and severity of these infections, the major factors include good glycemic control, personal hygiene, and prompt treatment with appropriate antibiotics (Akash et al., 2020; Cheng et al., 2024).

11.3.2 Urinary Tract Infections

As compared with normal people, sugar patients are five to six times for possibility to develop UTIs (Akash et al., 2020; Holt et al., 2024). Microorganisms can be easily used for glucosuria in their growth and development. However, in the case of autonomic neuropathy, it leads to incomplete bladder emptying and urinary stasis, which can result in bacterial colonization (Akash et al., 2020; Holt et al., 2024). The primary infections are caused by *Escherichia coli*, but *Klebsiella pneumoniae, Proteus mirabilis, Enterococcus spp.*, and *Candida spp.* are also common. Difficult conditions such as pyelonephritis, emphysematous cystitis, and emphysematous pyelonephritis are uniquely common with diabetes and can be very dangerous if not detected at the perfect timing (Akash et al., 2020; Holt et al., 2024). These severe infections are often associated with hospitalization, imaging studies, and aggressive therapy. In the case of asymptomatic bacteriuria is more common in diabetics, the importance of regular urine testing and monitoring in these patients (Akash et al., 2020; Berbudi et al., 2020).

11.3.3 Respiratory Tract Infections

Respiratory tract infections, which include pneumonia, bronchitis, and tuberculosis, are remarkably more important in persons with diabetes (Akash et al., 2020; Abbas et al., 2025). High blood sugar degrades neutrophil chemotaxis and phagocytosis, while microangiopathy reduces oxygen and nutrient delivery to the lungs, making them more vulnerable to pathogens. Common bacterial agents such as *Streptococcus pneumoniae* and *Haemophilus influenzae*, while viral infections like influenza and COVID-19 are more important in diabetics (Akash et al., 2020; Abbas et al., 2025).

Uncontrolled diabetes not only increases infection risk but also worsens clinical outcomes, resulting in higher rates of hospitalization and increased death rate. Tuberculosis is particularly concerning in regions with high prevalence, as diabetes enhances the risk of progression from latent to active disorder (Akash et al., 2020; Abbas et al., 2025). Vaccinations (influenza, pneumococcal, and COVID-19), coupled with good glycemic management, are major preventive measures (Sartelli et al., 2018; Akash et al., 2020; Abbas et al., 2025).

11.3.4 Diabetic Wounds and Ulcers (Including Foot Infections)

DFUs and chronic wounds are key causes of morbidity in diabetic patients (McDermott et al., 2023). Neuropathy results to loss of pain sensation, so small injuries may go unnoticed and become infected (McDermott et al., 2023; Yang et al., 2025). Poor circulation, ischemia, and impaired immune function further hinder healing. These infections are often polymicrobial, involving *S. aureus*, *Streptococcus spp.*, *Pseudomonas aeruginosa*, and anaerobes (Akash et al., 2020; Holt et al., 2024).

If untreated, infections can extend into deeper tissues, resulting in cellulitis, osteomyelitis, abscess formation, and eventually gangrene. DFIs are one of the major causes of non-traumatic lower limb amputations worldwide (Yang et al., 2025). Regular foot examination, patient education on proper footwear, early debridement, and effective antibiotic treatment are vital in decreasing complications and inhibiting amputations (Ahmed et al., 2023).

11.3.5 Fungal and Opportunistic Infections

Fungal infections are particularly common in diabetic patients due to high glucose levels create an ideal environment for fungal growth. *Candida albicans* causes oral candidiasis (thrush), vaginal infections, balanitis, and chronic onychomycosis (Shahabudin et al., 2024; Elizondo-Elizondo et al., 2026). Dermatophytes may also result to recurrent tinea infections. These infections are often in opposition to standard treatment of diabetes remains poorly controlled (Shahabudin et al., 2024; Elizondo-Elizondo et al., 2026).

Opportunistic infections such as mucormycosis, cryptococcosis, and aspergillosis can occur in uncontrolled diabetes or in those treated with corticosteroids. Mucormycosis (black fungus), which invades the sinuses, brain, and lungs, is particularly aggressive and has enhanced the death rate if untreated (Shahabudin et al., 2024; Elizondo-Elizondo et al., 2026). Early diagnosis, antifungal therapy (like amphotericin B), surgical debridement, and strict glucose management are crucial to survival (Al-Sayyar et al., 2022).

11.4 Antibiotics in Diabetic Infection Control

Infections in diabetic patients are often severe, recurrent, and complicated due to decreased immunity, delayed wound healing, and poor circulation (Akash et al., 2020; Wang et al., 2025). Antibiotics play an important role in controlling these infections, but their use must be guided by specific principles to avoid resistance and ensure effective outcomes (Holt et al., 2024; Kim & Choi, 2025).

11.4.1 Principles of Antibiotic Use

The first principle of antibiotic use in diabetes is to start therapy promptly, as infections can progress instantly and lead to severe complications such as sepsis or gangrene (Holt et al., 2024; Kim & Choi, 2025). Proper selection of antibiotics needs consideration of the site of infection, likely pathogens, and patient comorbidities (Bodke et al., 2023; Dilworth et al., 2021). Broad-spectrum antibiotics may be started first but treatment should be refined once microbiological data is available.

Equally important is ensuring adequate dosing and duration of therapy. Due to vascular insufficiency in diabetics, antibiotics may have decreased tissue penetration, so higher or prolonged doses may be required. Overuse or misuse of antibiotics can enhance resistance; hence, clinicians must balance aggressive infection control with judicious antibiotic stewardship (Yu et al., 2025; Murphy-Lavoie et al., 2025).

11.4.2 Empirical Versus Culture-Guided Therapy

Empirical antibiotic therapy is often initiated when immediate treatment is needed, especially in severe infections like DFUs or sepsis (Wang et al., 2025). The choice is commonly based on the most common pathogens, such as *S. aureus*, *Streptococcus spp.*, Gram-negative bacilli, and anaerobes (Akash et al., 2020; Holt et al., 2024). Empirical regimens typically include broad-spectrum antibiotics to cover multiple organisms until laboratory results are available (Holt et al., 2024; Kim & Choi, 2025).

Culture-guided treatment, on the other hand, is the gold standard. Once culture and sensitivity results are obtained, antibiotics can be tailored to target particular pathogens, enhancing efficacy while decreasing toxicity and resistance (Holt et al., 2024; Kim & Choi, 2025). This approach is particularly key in recurrent infections, polymicrobial wounds, or cases where MDR organisms are suspected (Mikkelsen et al., 2015; Wang et al., 2025).

11.4.3 Antibiotic Classes and Their Applications

Several antibiotic classes are particularly used in diabetic infections (Akash et al., 2020; Mougakou et al., 2023). Beta-lactams (e.g., penicillins, cephalosporins, carbapenems) are frequently used for skin, soft tissue, and urinary infections (Akash et al., 2020; Mougakou et al., 2023). Fluoroquinolones provide good coverage in opposition to Gram-negative bacteria and are often used in UTIs and RTIs. Clindamycin and metronidazole are valuable for anaerobic coverage, particularly in foot infections (Akash et al., 2020; Mougakou et al., 2023).

Apart from this, glycopeptides (vancomycin, teicoplanin) or newer agents like linezolid and daptomycin may be needed to combat MRSA and resistant Gram-positive infections (Akash et al., 2020; Mougakou et al., 2023; Holt et al., 2024; Kim & Choi, 2025). Combination therapy is often utilized in polymicrobial infections, ensuring broader coverage. Proper antibiotic choice is critical to decreasing complications and inhibiting long-term disability (Karlsson et al., 2013).

11.4.4 Challenges: Resistance, Biofilms, and Tissue Penetration

Antibiotic resistance is a creating challenge in managing diabetic infections (Akash et al., 2020; Mougakou et al., 2023; Holt et al., 2024). Repeated antibiotic exposure, coupled with impaired immune defenses, enhances the likelihood of infections caused by MDR organisms (MDROs). MRSA, extended-spectrum beta-lactamase (ESBL)-synthesizing bacteria, and carbapenem-resistant strains are commonly used in diabetic wounds and urinary infections (Akash et al., 2020; Mougakou et al., 2023; Holt et al., 2024).

Biofilm formation adds another layer of complexity. In DFUs and chronic wounds, bacteria created in biofilms are shielded from both antibiotics and host immune responses, making eradication difficult (Akash et al., 2020; Holt et al., 2024). Moreover, poor circulation in peripheral tissues decreases antibiotic delivery, resulting in suboptimal concentrations at the infection site (Akash et al., 2020; Mougakou et al., 2023; Holt et al., 2024). Overcoming these challenges requires integrated strategies, including surgical debridement, the use of combination therapy, and new drug delivery systems (Pouget et al., 2020).

11.5 Antiseptics in Diabetic Infection Control

Perhaps the most daunting diabetic care challenge is infection control, first and foremost, those resulting from chronic wounds and DFUs (Akash et al., 2020; Cwajda-Białasik et al., 2022). Diabetic wounds are long to heal because of microvascular compromise and immunocompromise, making them highly susceptible to serious morbidity and mortality. Antiseptics are used as part of multidimensional approaches to wound management as a routine means to inhibit microbial growth and facilitate tissue repair (Cwajda-Białasik et al., 2022). However, not all antiseptics are equal in either antimicrobial activity or cytotoxicity, and thus careful selection based on evidence is required (Ramirez-Acuña et al., 2019; Cwajda-Białasik et al., 2022).

11.5.1 Role and Mechanism of Antiseptics

a. **The Need for Antisepsis in Diabetic Wound Care**

Diabetic wounds create a conducive setting for opportunistic pathogens owing to hyperglycaemia-induced immunosuppression and dysfunctional leukocytes (Cwajda-Białasik et al., 2022; Wang et al., 2025). Biofilm formation also makes treatment more challenging, with embedded bacteria not being susceptible to conventional treatments. Antiseptics, by virtue of their definition, are agents that inhibit or destroy microorganisms on living tissue, thereby minimizing infection and lowering bioburden (Spampinato et al., 2020).

b. **Mechanistic Insights**

Antiseptics have different mechanisms of action:

- Protein Denaturation: Alcohol-based antiseptics such as isopropyl alcohol interfere with the structure of microbial proteins, making them ineffective.
- Cell Membrane Disruption: Agents like chlorhexidine and polyhexanide disrupt bacterial cell walls, leading to leakage of cellular material.
- Oxidative Damage: Hypochlorous acid and povidone-iodine produce reactive oxygen species (ROS) and free iodine, respectively, resulting in destruction of vital biomolecules in microbes.
- Enzyme Inhibition: Silver compounds disrupt enzymatic activity necessary for microbial reproduction.

These multifunctional activities render antiseptics a central part of wound irrigation, dressing, and cleansing, all for the aim of reducing the threat of infection and healing (McDonnell & Russell, 1999; Cwajda-Białasik et al., 2022; Wang et al., 2025).

11.5.2 Overview of Key Antiseptics

Chlorhexidine: Chlorhexidine is a cationic bisbiguanide antiseptic also a widely known for rapid and residual bactericidal action, for which it has particular utility in surgical site preparation (Cwajda-Białasik et al., 2022; Wang et al., 2025). Its mechanism involves the destruction of bacterial cell walls resulting in cytolysis and cell death, and it retains activity in the presence of organic load such as blood. Its persistent antibacterial activity and low skin staining have favoured widely used in clinical practice (Bai et al., 2024).

Povidone-Iodine: Povidone-iodine is a polymer carrier of iodine, an antiseptic which acts through the release of free iodine that inactivates microbial proteins (Lepelletier et al., 2020). It has wide-spectrum antimicrobial activity against bacteria, fungi, and viruses. Its effectiveness could be diminished under acidic or bloody environments, and long exposure can cause transient skin discoloration.

Hypochlorous Acid: Hypochlorous acid has significant microbicidal activity against various microbes, with the benefit of relatively low cytotoxicity under suitable concentrations and exposure durations (Souza et al., 2024). It naturally occurs in the human innate immune system and is appropriate for cleaning and decontamination purposes, particularly in wound therapy.

Silver-Based Compounds: Silver antiseptics such as mild silver protein and silver sulfadiazine act by interfering with microbial DNA and proteins, which results in inhibition and cell killing (Du et al., 2026). These drugs are commonly utilized in burn and wound care because they are active against bacterial pathogens, although at higher concentrations they can be cytotoxic.

Polyhexanide (Polyhexamethylene Biguanide): Polyhexanide is a biguanide polymer antiseptic with broad-spectrum microbicidal activity of low cytotoxicity and with a good biocompatibility index (Alparslan et al., 2025). It is used for irrigation in wound care and in the treatment of chronic wounds due to its balance of efficacy and tolerability.

Isopropyl Alcohol: Isopropyl alcohol is an alcoholic antiseptic that denatures cell membrane proteins, resulting in instantaneous microbial death. It is a rapid-acting solution and evaporates quickly, minimizing skin contamination but without residual activity after application. Its cytotoxicity is usually low but may induce skin dryness or irritation upon chronic use (Lepelletier et al., 2020).

11.5.3 Antimicrobial Efficacy Versus Cytotoxicity

The cytotoxicity of antiseptics usually correlates with their antimicrobial activity; very strong antiseptic solutions will compromise cell viability and inhibit healing of the tissue (Akash et al., 2020; Cwajda-Białasik et al., 2022). The biocompatibility index (BI), being the ratio of cytotoxic concentration to effective microbicidal concentration, is a useful measure of an antiseptic's efficacy and safety. Chlorhexidine, povidone-iodine, and polyhexanide have potent microbicidal activity but also higher cytotoxicity than milder compounds such as saline or some hypochlorous acid solutions (Lepelletier et al., 2020).

Experimental models demonstrate that such agents as chlorhexidine provide a dramatic reduction of pathogen load, but their cytotoxicity becomes systemic and endures long after use, possibly hindering wound healing. In contrast, agents with reduced cytotoxicity—such as certain hypochlorous acid preparations or polyhexanide—provide a more favorable profile at the cost of occasional compromise in speed of antimicrobial action (Damour et al., 1992).

11.5.4 *Guidelines and Best Practices for Antiseptic Use*

- Choose antiseptics depending on the clinical situation, seeking to balance quick antimicrobial activity with tissue compatibility.
- Preoperative skin preparation is best done with chlorhexidine because of its potent, persistent action and acceptability, apart from where there are contraindications.
- Povidone-iodine would be used when broad-spectrum action is required and blood or exudates are sparse.
- Silver-based products and polyhexanide can be used with chronic wounds or burns at concentrations that have minimal cytotoxicity but are not ineffective against microorganisms.
- Isopropyl alcohol works well for hand cleaning and rapid surface disinfection but has no residual action.
- Limit antiseptic duration of exposure and concentration to reduce cytotoxicity effects, particularly to open wounds or exposed tissues.
- Use local and international clinical guidelines, with antiseptic choice being modified according to patient-specific indications such as allergies, wound class, and anatomical site of application.
- This combined strategy provides effective infection prevention while ensuring maximum tissue healing and biocompatibility for each chosen antiseptic agent (Bai et al., 2024)

11.6 Evidence-Based Applications in Clinical Settings

11.6.1 *Surgical Site Infections (SSIs)*

- Diabetes patients are at risk of surgical site infections because they have immune dysfunction and hyperglycemia, which compromise wound healing (Wang et al., 2025).
- There is evidence that strict glycaemic control during the perioperative period (aiming at blood glucose levels less than 200 mg/dL) lowers the rates of surgical site infections, especially following cardiac and orthopaedic procedures.
- Prophylactic antibiotic and antiseptic practices, like chlorhexidine skin prep, are advocated to further minimize SSI risk (Cwajda-Białasik et al., 2022).
- Increased monitoring protocols and prompt identification of infection are essential, contributing to better patient outcomes and fewer complications at the time of surgery (Draznin et al., 2022).

11.6.2 Management of Diabetic Ulcer

- Diabetic foot infections (DFIs) are multifaceted and need a multi-dimensional, comprehensive approach comprising wound management, glycemic optimization, infection control, and patient education (Wang et al., 2025).
- Local microbial patterns dictate the use of empirical antibiotics, and therapy is customized after culture and sensitivity reports.
- Adjunctive therapies consist of advanced dressings, offloading, topical antiseptics, and innovation in diagnostic imaging (MRI, PET-CT) and molecular tests (PCR, NGS) for precise pathogen identification.
- Early surgery (e.g., debridement) can be required in the case of a severe or deep infection to reduce complications and avoid amputation (Senneville et al., 2024).

11.6.3 Catheter-Associated Infections

- Catheters and injection devices (such as insulin pumps) employed in diabetes management pose risk for device-associated infections through repeated puncture of the skin and possible contamination (Akash et al., 2020).
- Strict adherence to aseptic insertion methods, constant site monitoring, and prompt device replacement can have a marked reduction in infection rates.
- Barrier antiseptics and antimicrobial-coated catheters are increasingly favored in hospital practice.
- Health care providers, patients, and caregivers must be trained in identifying early warning signs of device infection (erythema, pain, discharge) and applying timely intervention (Patel & Priefer, 2021).

11.6.4 Traditional Remedies for Wound and Infection Care

- Some traditional medicines (e.g., honey, turmeric, neem, aloe vera) have been found to possess some antimicrobial and healing activities, especially in the treatment of diabetic patients with chronic wounds (Rayate et al., 2023).
- Preclinical and clinical evidence for these treatments is variable, but honey and some herbal extracts have been found to be inhibitory against prevalent wound pathogens in vitro and in small-scale clinical trials.
- Use of traditional remedies must always be under the control of a physician, as an adjunct not a substitute to established evidence-based treatments like antibiotics and antiseptics.
- There is a need for further research to determine the best use, safety profiles, and efficacy of traditional methods in the contemporary clinical environment (Aladejana et al., 2024; Nazari et al., 2025).

11.7 Comparative Efficacy: Antibiotics Versus Antiseptics

The comparative efficacy of antibiotics and antiseptics depends on their distinct yet complementary modes of action (Akash et al., 2020; Cwajda-Białasik et al., 2022). Antibiotics are systemic agents that particularly target bacterial growth and replication, creating them essential for treating deep-seated and systemic infections. Apart from this, antiseptics act locally on wounds, skin, and mucosal surfaces, resulting in broad-spectrum antimicrobial effects without entering the bloodstream (Akash et al., 2020; Cwajda-Białasik et al., 2022). While antibiotics can create challenges like resistance and side effects, antiseptics are less prone to resistance but may cause irritation or be less effective in various internal infections (Akash et al., 2020; Cwajda-Białasik et al., 2022). Together, they provide a balanced method- antibiotics creating internal pathogens and antiseptics decreasing surface microbial load, creating to better infection prevention and treatment outcomes when used judiciously (Nankervis et al., 2016).

11.7.1 Synergistic Use

The combination of antibiotics and antiseptics is often used in various clinical practices to increase antimicrobial efficacy (Ahmed et al., 2014; Hegazy et al., 2021; Kim & Choi, 2025). Antibiotics work systemically, reaching the bloodstream and tissues to kill bacteria from within, whereas antiseptics act locally by disinfecting wounds, mucosal surfaces, or surgical sites. When used together, they decrease the risk of infection more effectively than when used alone (Akash et al., 2020; Mougakou et al., 2023; Holt et al., 2024). For instance, applying an antiseptic to a surgical wound before administering prophylactic antibiotics creates a dual barrier, decreasing the chances of bacterial survival and biofilm formation.

Additionally, the synergistic effect can help reduce antibiotic resistance. By decreasing the bacterial load at the infection site through antiseptic application, the requirement for higher antibiotic doses is reduced, which lowers selective pressure on microorganisms. This combination strategy is especially valuable in high-risk environments such as intensive care units, surgical theaters, and diabetic wound management, where preventing infections is as critical as treating them (Carrillo-Larco et al., 2022).

11.7.2 Pros and Cons

Antibiotics and antiseptics each carry their advantages and limitations. Antibiotics provide targeted action in opposition to specific pathogens, making them highly effective for systemic infections (Singh & Gupta, 2017; Akash et al., 2020; Cwajda-Białasik et al., 2022). They can easily penetrate tissues and act internally, which antiseptics cannot achieve (Mougakou et al., 2023; Holt et al., 2024). On the other hand, antiseptics offer broad-spectrum antimicrobial properties with minimal systemic side effects, creating them ideal for immediate surface disinfection and wound care.

However, antibiotics are prone to misuse and overuse, which are associated with antimicrobial resistance, creating a global health crisis (Mougakou et al., 2023; Holt et al., 2024). Antiseptics, while useful, may be less effective in deep infections and can sometimes cause tissue irritation or delayed healing if applied excessively. Balancing these pros and cons is crucial in clinical decision-making, ensuring that each agent is used in the right context for maximum benefit and minimal harm (Kyu et al., 2018).

11.7.3 Clinical Outcomes and Case Studies

Clinical evidence highlights that combining antibiotics with antiseptics can remarkably improve patient outcomes (Mougakou et al., 2023; Holt et al., 2024). In surgical site infection prevention, for example, preoperative skin disinfection with antiseptics such as chlorhexidine, mixed with systemic antibiotic prophylaxis, has been shown to decrease postoperative infection rates compared to using either method alone (Akash et al., 2020; Mougakou et al., 2023; Holt et al., 2024). Similar benefits are seen in DFUs, where topical antiseptics decrease surface colonization while antibiotics address deep-seated infections.

In certain wound care cases, patients treated only with systemic antibiotics showed delayed healing due to persistent surface contamination (Akash et al., 2020; Holt et al., 2024). When antiseptics were integrated into treatment, healing was enhanced and recurrence rates dropped. These examples underscore the complementary roles of antibiotics and antiseptics, showing that clinical outcomes are optimized when both are used judiciously according to the infection site and severity (Gachet et al., 2025).

11.8 Antimicrobial Resistance in Diabetic Populations

Generally, diabetic populations have higher susceptibility to infections and develop resistance due to frequent exposure to antibiotics (Akash et al., 2020; Holt et al., 2024). Poor glycemic control, impaired immunity, and decreased circulation create a favorable environment for recurrent infections such as DFUs, UTIs, and RTIs, often requiring repeated or prolonged antibiotic use (Wang et al., 2025; Kim & Choi, 2025). This frequent exposure, combined with misutilization of broad-spectrum antibiotics and incomplete adherence to treatment, accelerates the emergence of resistant organisms like MRSA and MRD Gram-negative bacteria, which not only cause diabetic patients to face more severe and persistent infections but also contribute to the wider public health challenge of AMR, underscoring the need for careful antibiotic stewardship and targeted infection prevention methods in this vulnerable group (Abbas et al., 2025; Kim & Choi, 2025).

11.8.1 Factors Contributing to Resistance

Poor glycemic control increases chronic infections such as UTIs, DFUs, and RTIs that need long-term antibiotic treatments with a precise approach (Rather et al., 2017; Abbas et al., 2025; Kim & Choi, 2025). The misutilization of broad-spectrum antibiotics, self-medication, and incomplete adherence to prescribed regimens further fuel resistance, leading to treatment failures and increased healthcare costs (Dilworth et al., 2021; Bodke et al., 2023; Wang et al., 2025). Apart from that, decreased blood flow in diabetic patients hampers antibiotic penetration into infected tissues, forming an environment where resistant organisms can thrive (Dilworth et al., 2021; Bodke et al., 2023; Wang et al., 2025).

11.8.2 Observational Data and Tendencies

Recent studies indicate that individuals with diabetes have a higher prevalence of MDR organisms compared to those without diabetes (Dilworth et al., 2021; Bodke et al., 2023; Wang et al., 2025). DFUs and other infections frequently harbor resistant strains, and once infected with any MDR pathogens, need hospitalization and long-term therapy. Therefore, a diabetic is not only likely to acquire an infection but also a host where resistant organisms can thrive, which makes treatment harder and puts more stress on the healthcare system (Shook et al., 2025).

11.8.3 Strategies for Reduction AMR

To reduce antimicrobial resistance in diabetes, a multifaceted approach such as precise blood glucose monitoring and antibiotic administration is essential (Ahmed et al., 2014; Akash et al., 2020; Hegazy et al., 2021). Mainly, antibiotic stewardship programs emphasize that the correct medication, dosage, and treatment duration, along with efficient wound care and upholding hygiene, are critical strategies to avert the acquisition of resistant pathogens (Akash et al., 2020; Hegazy et al., 2021; Kim & Choi, 2025). Employing culture-guided treatment instead of administering broad-spectrum antibiotics without prior testing improves infection management and reduces the emergence of unnecessary resistance. Guiding patients to comply with prescribed medication protocols instead of self-medicating is essential for mitigating antimicrobial resistance over time (Akash et al., 2020; Kim & Choi, 2025; Nazari et al., 2025).

11.9 Future Perspectives and Innovations

Diabetic patients are more vulnerable to infections and need alternative antimicrobial strategies, including several newly proposed AMPs, nanomedicine, etc., showing promise (Sahoo et al., 2021; Swain et al., 2023; Sousa et al., 2025). Along with monitoring devices, advanced wound care, and personalized antibiotic-antiseptic medication are showing promise to improve the quality of life for individuals with diabetes (Kabra et al., 2025; Wassif et al., 2025). Overall, patient-specific and cutting-edge therapies could be a more effective strategy (Akash et al., 2020; Wassif et al., 2025).

11.9.1 Alternative Strategy of Antibiotics

Antibiotic resistance also makes a significant challenge in the management of diabetic infections, particularly in DFUs (McDermott et al., 2023; Wang et al., 2025). The emergence of MDR and biofilm-producing pathogens is gradually reducing the effectiveness of applied antibacterials. In this perspective, several AMPs reported from natural resources as well as synthesized in the laboratory condition are capable of breaking down bacterial membranes and biofilms, whereas nanomedicine-based approaches also show benefits through controlled drug release and active cell wall penetration (Sahoo et al., 2021; Sousa et al., 2025). Nisin and citropin, along with guanylated polymethacrylates and microporous technology, like Acapsil®, have sped up healing in clinical settings for DFUs (Sahoo et al., 2021; Sousa et al., 2025). Furthermore, the incorporation of natural product derivatives such as eugenol, curcumin, carvacrol, and neem in individual and nano-form possesses potent antimicrobial activities that are oftentimes potentiated with higher cell-membrane permeability. Antibiotic stewardship, expedited diagnostics, and personalized therapy increasingly enhance such alternatives, providing new hope against resistant and recurrent infection in diabetes (Sahoo et al., 2021; Moya-Salazar et al., 2023).

11.9.2 Nano-Based Antiseptic Solution Strategy

Nanotechnology has the potential to transform infection control in diabetics. Antiseptic solutions based on nanoparticles like silver, copper, or titanium dioxide at ultrasmall sizes cause damage to microbial cell walls, produce reactive oxygen species, and prevent biofilm formation, advantages crucial for chronic wound and ulcer management (Swain et al., 2023; Zhu et al., 2025; Du et al., 2026). Colloidal nano-silver solutions, benzalkonium chloride nano-spray solutions, and device coatings have residual antimicrobial effects against bacteria, fungi, and viruses, including drug-resistant strains like MRSA. These antiseptics are applied in wound irrigation, surface disinfection, and as protective coatings on medical devices. Clinical trials exhibit rapid inactivation of pathogens, improved tissue biocompatibility, and long-lasting protection (Zhu et al., 2025; Du et al., 2026). Regular monitoring of nanoparticle cytotoxicity and long-term safety is imperative. New developments in personalized nano-antiseptics via customized particle size and surface chemistry show enormous potential for tailoring therapies to individual diabetic patients prone to recurring infections (Kordestani et al., 2014; Zhu et al., 2025).

11.9.3 Infection Control Strategies and Personalized Medicine in Diabetes

Diabetes increases the risk of infection by causing immune dysfunction with hyperglycemia, defective wound healing, and enhanced susceptibility to drug-resistant pathogens (Akash et al., 2020; Holt et al., 2024; Wang et al., 2025). Current infection control practices now integrate strict glycemic control, specific vaccination, sophisticated wound management, and extensive education programs. Novelty comprises continuous glucose sensors, intelligent drug delivery systems, and integrative care teams (Holt et al., 2024; Zhu et al., 2025). The practice of personalized medicine is transforming diabetes management: genomics and proteomics direct patient-specific risk stratification, customize antimicrobial treatment, and facilitate the prediction of complications. Artificial intelligence and predictive analytics inform the creation of patient-specific infection prevention protocols, streamlined antibiotic selection, and early intervention strategies (Akash et al., 2020; Holt et al., 2024). By incorporating infection control with precision technology, personalized medicine improves treatment outcomes, reduces negative results, and empowers the patient for a lifetime of self-management through both technological advancement and evidence-based infection prevention (Sugandh et al., 2023; Holt et al., 2024; Zhu et al., 2025).

11.10 Conclusion

Generally, DM significantly elevates the risk of infection due to hyperglycemia-induced immune dysfunction, vascular insufficiency, and tissue damage. Effective infection control management is therefore critical for diabetic patients to reduce morbidity and mortality, necessitating strict targeted antimicrobial strategies and glycemic control. Advances in antimicrobial approaches, such as novel antibiotics and nanobased antiseptics, present promising directions toward resistance defeat and therapeutic improvement. Further, the incorporation of personalized medicine, with emphasis on patient-specific risk factors, is also another advanced strategy for infection-prognosis improvement in diabetes. Overall, multidisciplinary intervention, including active infection surveillance, utilizing appropriate antimicrobials, patient education, and personalized care plans, is essential to minimize the high risk of morbidity and mortality from infections in diabetes.

References

Abbas, U., Kumar, H., Hussain, N., Ahmed, I., Laghari, R. N., Tanveer, M., Hadif, M., Fatima, K., Khalid, M. U., Anwar, K., & Khan, M. (2025). Immune dysregulation in type 2 diabetes mellitus: Implications for tuberculosis, COVID-19, and HIV/AIDS. *Infectious Medicine (Beijing), 4*(4), 100211. https://doi.org/10.1016/j.imj.2025.100211

Ahmed, A., Azim, A., Gurjar, M., & Baronia, A. (2014). Current concepts in combination antibiotic therapy for critically ill patients. *Indian Journal of Critical Care Medicine, 18*(5), 310–314.

Ahmed, A. E., Abdelkarim, S., Zenida, M., Baiti, M. A. H., Alhazmi, A. A. Y., Alfaifi, B. A. H., et al. (2023). Prevalence and associated risk factors of urinary tract infection among diabetic patients: A cross-sectional study. *Healthcare (Basel), 11*(6), 861. https://doi.org/10.3390/healthcare11060861

Akash, M. S. H., Rehman, K., Fiayyaz, F., Sabir, S., & Khurshid, M. (2020). Diabetes-associated infections: Development of antimicrobial resistance and possible treatment strategies. *Archives of Microbiology, 202*(5), 953–965.

Aladejana, E. B., Adelabu, O. A., Aladejana, A. E., & Ndlovu, S. I. (2024). Antimicrobial properties of alternative medicines used in the management of infections in diabetic patients: A comprehensive review. *Pharmacological Research—Modern Chinese Medicine, 11*, Article 100432.

Alexander, M., Cho, E., Gliozheni, E., Salem, Y., Cheung, J., & Ichii, H. (2024). Pathology of diabetes-induced immune dysfunction. *International Journal of Molecular Sciences, 25*(13), 7105.

Alparslan, L., Torkay, G., Bal-Öztürk, A., Köksal Karayıldırım, Ç., & Özdemir, S. (2025). Smart thermoresponsive sol–gel formulation of polyhexanide for rapid and painless burn and wound management. *Polymers (Basel), 17*(15), 2079. https://doi.org/10.3390/polym17152079

Al-Sayyar, A., Hulme, K. D., Thibaut, R., Bayry, J., Sheedy, F. J., Short, K. R., et al. (2022). Respiratory tract infections in diabetes—Lessons from tuberculosis and influenza to guide understanding of COVID-19 severity. *Front Endocrinology (Lausanne), 13*, Article 919223.

Antar, S. A., Ashour, N. A., Sharaky, M., Khattab, M., Ashour, N. A., Zaid, R. T., et al. (2023). Diabetes mellitus: Classification, mediators, and complications; A gate to identify potential targets for the development of new effective treatments. *Biomedicine & Pharmacotherapy, 168*, Article 115734.

Bai, D., Zhou, F., & Wu, L. (2024). RETRACTED: Comparing the efficacy of chlorhexidine and povidone–iodine in preventing surgical site infections: A systematic review and meta-analysis. *International Wound Journal, 21*(2), Article e14463.

Banday, M. Z., Sameer, A. S., & Nissar, S. (2020). Pathophysiology of diabetes: An overview. *Avicenna Journal of Medicine, 10*(4), 174–188.

Berbudi, A., Rahmadika, N., Tjahjadi, A. I., & Ruslami, R. (2020). Type 2 DM and its impact on the immune system. *Current Diabetes Review, 16*(5), 442–449.

Berbudi, A., Khairani, S., & Tjahjadi, A. I. (2025). Interplay between insulin resistance and immune dysregulation in type 2 diabetes mellitus: Implications for therapeutic interventions. *Immuno Targets and Therapy, 14*, 359–382.

Bodke, H., Wagh, V., & Kakar, G. (2023). Diabetes mellitus and prevalence of other comorbid conditions: A systematic review. *Cureus,15*(11), e49374. https://doi.org/10.7759/cureus.49374.

Burak, M. F., Stanley, T. L., Lawson, E. A., Campbell, S. L., Lynch, L., Hasty, A. H., Domingos, A. I., Dixit, V. D., Hotamışlıgil, G. S., Sheedy, F. J., Dixon, A. E., Brinkley, T. E., Hill, J. A., Donath, M. Y., & Grinspoon, S. K. (2024). Adiposity, immunity, and inflammation: Interrelationships in health and disease: A report from 24th annual Harvard nutrition obesity symposium-2023. *The American Journal of Clinical Nutrition, 120*(1), 257–268.

Carey, I. M., Critchley, J. A., DeWilde, S., Harris, T., Hosking, F. J., & Cook, D. G. (2018). Risk of infection in type 1 and type 2 diabetes compared with the general population: A matched cohort study. *Diabetes Care, 41*(3), 513–521.

Carrillo-Larco, R. M., Anza-Ramírez, C., Saal-Zapata, G., Villarreal-Zegarra, D., Zafra-Tanaka, J. H., Ugarte-Gil, C., et al. (2022). Type 2 diabetes mellitus and antibiotic-resistant infections: A systematic review and meta-analysis. *Journal of Epidemiology and Community Health, 76*(1), 75–84.

Casqueiro, J., Casqueiro, J., & Alves, C. (2012). Infections in patients with diabetes mellitus: A review of pathogenesis. *Indian J Endocrinol Metabolism, 16*(Suppl1), S27-36.

Caturano, A., D'Angelo, M., Mormone, A., Russo, V., Mollica, M. P., Salvatore, T., Galiero, R., Rinaldi, L., Vetrano, E., Marfella, R., Monda, M., Giordano, A., & Sasso, F. C. (2023). Oxidative stress in type 2 diabetes: Impacts from pathogenesis to lifestyle modifications. *Current Issues in Molecular Biology, 45*(8), 6651–6666.

Chávez-Reyes, J., Escárcega-González, C. E., Chavira-Suárez, E., León-Buitimea, A., Vázquez-León, P., Morones-Ramírez, J. R., Villalón, C. M., Quintanar-Stephano, A., Marichal-Cancino, B. A. (2021). Susceptibility for some infectious diseases in patients with diabetes: The key role of glycemia. *Frontiers in Public Health, 9*, 559595. https://doi.org/10.3389/fpubh.2021.559595

Cheng, S., Poh, B. R. M., Tay, V. W. Y., et al. (2024). The interplay between diabetes mellitus and soft tissue infections in general surgical patients. *BMC Endocrine Disorders, 24*, 106.

Critchley, J. A., Carey, I. M., Harris, T., DeWilde, S., Hosking, F. J., & Cook, D. G. (2018). Glycemic control and risk of infections among people with type 1 or type 2 diabetes in a large primary care cohort study. *Diabetes Care, 41*(10), 2127–2135.

Cwajda-Białasik, J., Mościcka, P., & Szewczyk, M. T. (2022). Antiseptics and antimicrobials for the treatment and management of chronic wounds: A systematic review of clinical trials. *Postępy Dermatologii i Alergologii, 39*(1), 141–151.

Damour, O., Hua, S. Z., Lasne, F., Villain, M., Rousselle, P., & Collombel, C. (1992). Cytotoxicity evaluation of antiseptics and antibiotics on cultured human fibroblasts and keratinocytes. *Burns, 18*(6), 479–485.

Daryabor, G., Atashzar, M. R., Kabelitz, D., Meri, S., & Kalantar, K. (2020). The effects of type 2 diabetes mellitus on organ metabolism and the immune system. *Frontiers in Immunology, 11*, 1582.

Dilworth, L., Facey, A., & Omoruyi, F. (2021). Diabetes mellitus and its metabolic complications: The role of adipose tissues. *International Journal of Molecular Sciences, 22*(14), 7644. https://doi.org/10.3390/ijms22147644

Draznin, B., Aroda, V. R., Bakris, G., Benson, G., Brown, F. M., Freeman, R., et al. (2022). Diabetes care in the hospital: Standards of medical care in diabetes-2022. *Diabetes Care, 45*.

Du, Y., Lu, J., Guo, X., Xia, Z., & Ji, S. (2026). The role of silver and silver-based products in wound management: A review of advances and current landscape. *Journal of Functional Biomaterials, 17*(1), 27. https://doi.org/10.3390/jfb17010027

Elizondo-Elizondo, M., González-Silva, A., de Oca-Sánchez, G. M., Tirado-Sánchez, A., Frias-De-León, M. G., Diaz-Molina, V. L., Acosta-Altamirano, G., & Bonifaz, A. (2026). Superficial fungal infections in patients with diabetes. Is hyperglycemia the only associated factor? *Future Microbiology, 21*(1), 59–72.

Fernandes, R., Viana, S. D., Nunes, S., & Reis, F. (2019). Diabetic gut microbiota dysbiosis as an inflammaging and immunosenescence condition that fosters progression of retinopathy and nephropathy. *Biochimica Et Biophysica Acta, Molecular Basis of Disease, 1865*(7), 1876–1897.
Fu, Y., Wang, B., Alu, A., Hong, W., Lei, H., He, X., Shi, H., Cheng, P., & Yang, X. (2025). Immunosenescence: Signaling pathways, diseases and therapeutic targets. *Signal Transduction and Targeted Therapy, 10*(1), 250. https://doi.org/10.1038/s41392-025-02371-z
Gachet, B., Schechter, M. C., Armstrong, D. G., Robineau, O., & Senneville, E. (2025). Not all in vein: Oral antibiotics for diabetic foot osteomyelitis: A narrative review. *Journal of Clinical Medicine, 14*(5), 1405.
Geerlings, S. E., & Hoepelman, A. I. (1999). Immune dysfunction in patients with diabetes mellitus (DM). *FEMS Immunology and Medical Microbiology, 26*(3–4), 259–265.
Hegazy, W. A. H., Rajab, A. A. H., Lila, A. S. A., & Abbas, H. A. (2021). Anti-diabetics and antimicrobials: Harmony of mutual interplay. *World Journal of Diabetes, 12*(11), 1832–1855.
Holt, R. I. G., Cockram, C. S., Ma, R. C. W., & Luk, A. O. Y. (2024). Diabetes and infection: Review of the epidemiology, mechanisms and principles of treatment. *Diabetologia, 67*(7), 1168–1180.
Hossain, M. J., Al-Mamun, M., & Islam, M. R. (2024). Diabetes mellitus, the fastest growing global public health concern: Early detection should be focused. *Health Science Reports, 7*(3), e2004. https://doi.org/10.1002/hsr2.2004
Kabra, R., Poonia, N., Subudhi, R. N., Singh, T., Joshi, G., Sharma, R., & Arora, V. (2025). Innovative strategies for the management of diabetic wounds: A step toward faster recovery. *Journal of Drug Delivery Science and Technology*,107824. https://doi.org/10.1016/j.jddst.2025.107824
Karlsson, F. H., Tremaroli, V., Nookaew, I., et al. (2013). Gut metagenome in European women with normal, impaired and diabetic glucose control. *Nature, 498*(7452), 99–103.
Kim, T., & Choi, S. H. (2025). Diabetes mellitus and infectious diseases: Current evidence and clinical implications. *Diabetes & Metabolism Journal, 49*(5), 915–933.
Kordestani, S., NayebHabib, F., & Saadatjo, M. H. (2014). A novel wound rinsing solution based on nano colloidal silver. *Nanomedicine Research Journal, 1*(5), 315–323.
Kyu, H. H., Abate, D., Abate, K. H., et al. (2018). Global, regional, and national disability-adjusted life-years (DALYs) for 359 diseases and injuries and healthy life expectancy (HALE) for 195 countries and territories, 1990–2017: A systematic analysis for the global burden of disease study 2017. *Lancet, 392*(10159), 1859–1922. https://doi.org/10.1016/S0140-6736(18)32335-3
Lepelletier, D., Maillard, J. Y., Pozzetto, B., & Simon, A. (2020). Povidone iodine: Properties, mechanisms of action, and role in infection control and Staphylococcus aureus decolonization. *Antimicrobial Agents and Chemotherapy, 64*(9), e00682–20. https://doi.org/10.1128/AAC.00682-20
McDermott, K., Fang, M., Boulton, A. J., Selvin, E., & Hicks, C. W. (2023). Etiology, epidemiology, and disparities in the burden of diabetic foot ulcers. *Diabetes Care, 46*(1), 209–221.
McDonnell, G., & Russell, A. D. (1999). Antiseptics and disinfectants: Activity, action, and resistance. *Clinical Microbiology Reviews, 12*(1), 147–179.
Mikkelsen, K. H., Knop, F. K., Frost, M., Hallas, J., & Pottegård, A. (2015). Use of antibiotics and risk of type 2 diabetes: A population-based case-control study. *Journal of Clinical Endocrinology and Metabolism, 100*(10), 3633–3640. https://doi.org/10.1210/jc.2015-2696
Mougakou, E., Mastrogianni, E., Kyziroglou, M., & Tziomalos, K. (2023). The role of novel antibiotics in the management of diabetic foot infection. *Diabetes Therapy, 14*(2), 251–263.
Moya-Salazar, J., Chamana, J. M., Porras-Rivera, D., Goicochea-Palomino, E. A., Salazar, C. R., & Contreras-Pulache, H. (2023). Increase in antibiotic resistance in diabetic foot infections among Peruvian patients: A single-center cross-sectional study. *Front Endocrinology (Lausanne), 14*, 1267699.
Murphy-Lavoie, H. M., Ramsey, A., Nguyen, M., et al. (2025). Diabetic foot infections. In *StatPearls* [Internet]. StatPearls Publishing [updated 2025 Apr 11]
Nankervis, H., Thomas, K. S., Delamere, F. M., et al. (2016). Scoping systematic review of treatments for eczema. In: *Antimicrobials including antibiotics, antiseptics and antifungal agents.* NIHR Journals Library (Programme Grants for Applied Research, No. 4.7).

Nazari, M., Shokoohizadeh, L., & Taheri, M. (2025). Natural products in the treatment of diabetic foot infection. *European Journal of Medical Research, 30*(1), 8.

Park, S. J., Park, Y. J., Chang, J., et al. (2021). Association between antibiotics use and diabetes incidence in a nationally representative retrospective cohort among Koreans. *Science and Reports, 11*, 21681.

Patel, B., & Priefer, R. (2021). Infections associated with diabetic-care devices. *Diabetes and Metabolic Syndrome: Clinical Research and Reviews, 15*(2), 519–524.

Pouget, C., Dunyach-Remy, C., Pantel, A., Schuldiner, S., Sotto, A., & Lavigne, J. P. (2020). Biofilms in diabetic foot ulcers: Significance and clinical relevance. *Microorganisms, 8*(10), 1580. https://doi.org/10.3390/microorganisms8101580

Quiros-Roldan, E., Sottini, A., Natali, P. G., & Imberti, L. (2024). The impact of immune system aging on infectious diseases. *Microorganisms, 12*(4), 775.

Ramirez-Acuña, J. M., Cardenas-Cadena, S. A., Marquez-Salas, P. A., Garza-Veloz, I., Perez-Favila, A., Cid-Baez, M. A., et al. (2019). Diabetic foot ulcers: Current advances in antimicrobial therapies and emerging treatments. *Antibiotics, 8*(4), 193.

Rather, I. A., Ķim, B. C., Bajpai, V. K., & Park, Y. H. (2017). Self-medication and antibiotic resistance: Crisis, current challenges, and prevention. *Saudi Journal of Biological Sciences, 24*(4), 808–812.

Rayate, A. S., Nagoba, B. S., Mumbre, S. S., Mavani, H. B., Gavkare, A. M., & Deshpande, A. S. (2023). Current scenario of traditional medicines in management of diabetic foot ulcers: A review. *World Journal of Diabetes, 14*(1), 1–16.

Sahoo, A., Swain, S. S., Behera, A., Sahoo, G., Mahapatra, P. K., & Panda, S. K. (2021). Antimicrobial peptides derived from insects offer a novel therapeutic option to combat biofilm: A review. *Frontiers in Microbiology, 12*, 661195. https://doi.org/10.3389/fmicb.2021.661195

Sartelli, M., Guirao, X., Hardcastle, T. C., Kluger, Y., Boermeester, M., Raşa, K., et al. (2018). 2018 WSES consensus conference: Recommendations for the management of skin and soft-tissue infections. *World Journal of Emergency Surgery, 13*(1), 58.

Senneville, É., Albalawi, Z., Van Asten, S. A., Abbas, Z. G., Allison, G., Aragón-Sánchez, J., et al. (2024). IWGDF/IDSA guidelines on the diagnosis and treatment of diabetes-related foot infections (IWGDF/IDSA 2023). *Diabetes/metabolism Research and Reviews, 40*(3), Article e3687.

Shahabudin, S., Azmi, N. S., Lani, M. N., Mukhtar, M., & Hossain, M. S. (2024). Candida albicans skin infection in diabetic patients: An updated review of pathogenesis and management. *Mycoses, 67*(6), e13753. https://doi.org/10.1111/myc.13753

Shook, J. C., et al. (2025). Diabetes potentiates the emergence and expansion of antibiotic resistance. *Science Advances, 11*, eads1591.

Singh, S. K., & Gupta, B. (2017). Choices and challenges of antibiotics therapy in diabetic foot infection. *Indian Journal of Endocrinology and Metabolism, 21*(5), 647–648. https://doi.org/10.4103/ijem.IJEM_481_17

Sousa, C., Sahoo, A., Swain, S. S., Gupta, P., Silva, F., Azevedo, A. S., & Rodrigues, C. F. (2025). In Silico and in vitro potential antifungal insights of insect-derived peptides in the management of Candida sp. infections. *International Journal of Molecular Sciences, 26*(15), 7449. https://doi.org/10.3390/ijms26157449

Souza, M. A., Zanella, M. L., Vanin, G. N., Dallepiane, F. G., Pizzi, C. Y. M., Ferreira, E. R., Fuhr, M. C. S., Piccolo, N. M., Palhano, H. S., da Silva Koch, J., Souza, K. R., da Costa, U. M., Dos Santos, V. V., Steier, L., Bertol, C. D., & Figueiredo, J. A. P. (2024). Antimicrobial action and cytotoxicity of hypochlorous acid obtained from an innovative electrolytic device–An in vitro study. *Archives of Oral Biology, 163*, 105966. https://doi.org/10.1016/j.archoralbio.2024.105966

Spampinato, S. F., Caruso, G. I., De Pasquale, R., Sortino, M. A., & Merlo, S. (2020). The treatment of impaired wound healing in diabetes: Looking among old drugs. *Pharmaceuticals, 13*(4), 60.

Sugandh, F. N., Chandio, M., Raveena, F. N., Kumar, L., Karishma, F. N., Khuwaja, S., Memon, U. A., Bai, K., Kashif, M., Varrassi, G., & Khatri, M. (2023, August 18). Advances in the management of diabetes mellitus: A focus on personalized medicine. *Cureus, 15*(8).

Swain, S. S., Paidesetty, S. K., Padhy, R. N., & Hussain, T. (2023). Nano-technology platforms to increase the antibacterial drug suitability of essential oils: A drug prospective assessment. *OpenNano, 9*, 100115. https://doi.org/10.1016/j.onano.2022.100115

Thimmappa, P. Y., Vasishta, S., Ganesh, K., Nair, A. S., & Joshi, M. B. (2023). Neutrophil (dys) function due to altered immuno-metabolic axis in type 2 diabetes: Implications in combating infections. *Human Cell, 36*(4), 1265–1282.

Wang, Q., Liu, C., An, J., Liu, J., Wang, Y., & Cai, Y. (2025). Mechanisms of microbial infection and wound healing in diabetic foot ulcer: Pathogenicity in the inflammatory-proliferative phase, chronicity, and treatment strategies. *Frontiers in Endocrinology (Lausanne), 16*, 1657928. https://doi.org/10.3389/fendo.2025.1657928

Wassif, R. K., Shamma, R. N., El-Hoffy, N. M., & El-Kayal, M. (2025). Recent advances in the local drug delivery systems for diabetic wound healing: A comprehensive review. *AAPS PharmSciTech, 26*(6), 177. https://doi.org/10.1208/s12249-025-03172-x

Yang, Y., Zhao, B., Wang, Y., Lan, H., Liu, X., Hu, Y., & Cao, P. (2025). Diabetic neuropathy: Cutting-edge research and future directions. *Signal Transduction and Targeted Therapy, 10*(1), 132. https://doi.org/10.1038/s41392-025-02175-1

Yu, X., Li, M., & Li, H. (2025). The role of gut dysbiosis and mitochondrial dysfunction in type 2 diabetes: Insights on pathogenesis, intervention and future perspective. *Biomedicine & Pharmacotherapy, 193*, 118846. https://doi.org/10.1016/j.biopha.2025.118846

Zhou, K., & Lansang, M. C. (2000). Diabetes mellitus and infection [Internet]. In K. R. Feingold, S. F. Ahmed, B. Anawalt, et al. (Eds.), *Endotext*. MDText.com, Inc. [updated 2024 Jun 30; cited 2025 Sep 27]. https://www.ncbi.nlm.nih.gov/books/NBK569326/

Zhu, J., Xia, F., Wang, S., Guan, Y., Hu, F., & Yu, F. (2025). Recent advances in nanomaterials and their mechanisms for infected wounds management. *Materials Today Bio, 31*, 101553. https://doi.org/10.1016/j.mtbio.2025.101553

Chapter 12
Digital Healing for Diabetic Disabilities: Tools for Monitoring, Mobility, and Self-Management

Krishnendu Adhikary, Krishnendu Ganguly, Monalisha Maity, Priyanka Mahata, and Oyindamola John Samson

Abstract This chapter examines the transformative role of digital health technologies in managing diabetes-related disabilities, focusing on tools that enhance monitoring, mobility, and long- term functional independence. As diabetes remains a leading cause of chronic complications affecting nerve function, wound healing, and mobility, emerging digital solutions—such as continuous glucose monitors (CGMs), smart insoles, mobile health apps, and remote patient monitoring (RPM)—offer proactive, personalized approaches to care. Innovations in AI-powered analytics and telemedicine are enabling earlier detection of complications like diabetic foot ulcers and gait instability, while digital physiotherapy platforms support rehabilitation and physical activity. The integration of these tools into routine diabetes management has the potential to empower patients, reduce hospitalizations, and alleviate the overall healthcare burden. This chapter also explores practical challenges in implementation, including device accessibility, digital literacy, data security, and adherence. By bridging clinical care with technology and patient-centered design, digital interventions are reshaping the landscape of diabetes care—beyond blood sugar control—to address the full spectrum of diabetes-related disabilities.

Keywords Diabetes-related disabilities · Digital health technologies · Remote Patient Monitoring (RPM) · Mobility and rehabilitation · Continuous Glucose Monitoring (CGM)

K. Adhikary · K. Ganguly · M. Maity · P. Mahata
Department of Medical Laboratory Technology, Paramedical College Durgapur, Durgapur, India

K. Adhikary
Research and Development Cell, Lovely Professional University, Jalandhar, Phagwara, Punjab, India

O. J. Samson (✉)
Department of Microbiology, Olabisi Onabanjo University, Ago-Iwoye, Nigeria
e-mail: oyindamolasamson1997@gmail.com

K. Adhikary et al. (eds.), *Healing Beyond Blood Sugar*,
https://doi.org/10.1007/978-981-95-8946-3_12

12.1 Introduction

Diabetes mellitus poses a global health burden due to its increasing prevalence and associated long-term disabilities (Wang et al., 2022). Beyond cardiovascular and renal risks, patients frequently experience vision loss, neuropathic pain, impaired mobility, and cognitive decline, often leading to severe disability (Fung et al., 2022; Longendyke et al., 2024). These complications frequently co-occur, compounding their impact on quality of life. Families and healthcare systems share the burden through caregiving demands and rising long-term care costs (Tan & Wong, 2023). In low- and middle-income countries, limited access to care exacerbates socioeconomic inequities and work-related disability (Huang et al., 2022). Addressing this requires not only medical advances but integrated care systems prioritizing prevention, early detection, and sustained support (Cioana et al., 2023).

The rapid innovation of digital health technologies is transforming diabetes care by enabling continuous, individualized management beyond traditional face-to-face consultations (Li et al., 2023; Tang et al., 2023). Tools such as telemedicine, mobile apps, wearables, and continuous glucose monitors provide real-time data and support timely interventions (Al-Moussally et al., 2025). AI-driven systems further personalize care by predicting complications and optimizing treatments (Tang et al., 2023). These technologies also empower patients through self-management, adherence support, and interactive education, while mobile platforms expand access in low-resource settings (Li et al., 2023). Additionally, virtual peer networks help address emotional challenges. Despite concerns around privacy, interoperability, and equity, digital health is paving the way for proactive, person-centered, and sustainable chronic care (Sung et al., 2022).

12.2 Understanding Diabetes-Related Disabilities

12.2.1 Neuropathy and Mobility Loss

Peripheral neuropathy, affecting up to 50% of individuals with long-standing diabetes, is a common and disabling complication caused by chronic hyperglycemia-induced nerve damage (Jensen et al., 2022). It leads to sensory loss, burning pain, muscle weakness, and balance issues, increasing the risk of falls, fractures, and reduced autonomy. Motor dysfunction may result in foot deformities, gait changes, and impaired daily functioning. The emotional toll includes depression, anxiety, and social isolation due to physical limitations (Martins & Lee, 2023). In advanced stages, autonomic neuropathy can cause cardiovascular instability, gastrointestinal problems, and urinary incontinence, further reducing quality of life. Because neuropathy often progresses silently, early screening and intervention are critical. Preventive strategies—such as glycemic control, foot care education, and physical activity—are essential to preserve function and delay disability (Nguyen et al., 2024).

12.2.2 Diabetic Foot Ulcers and Wound Complications

Diabetic foot ulcers (DFUs), driven by neuropathy and vascular dysfunction, are among the most disabling complications of diabetes (Singh et al., 2023). Loss of protective sensation prevents early detection of injuries, while poor circulation impairs healing, increasing susceptibility to infection and chronic wounds. Severe cases can progress to osteomyelitis and often result in amputation—the leading cause of non-traumatic lower-limb loss worldwide (Mehta et al., 2022). Beyond physical disability, amputations cause emotional distress, caregiver dependence, and social stigma. Recurrence of ulcers is common, contributing to long-term disability and reduced quality of life (O'Brien & Tan, 2024). Preventive strategies—regular foot exams, patient education, protective footwear, and early referral to multidisciplinary care—are critical. Innovative therapies like bioengineered dressings, negative pressure therapy, and regenerative treatments show promise, though access remains limited globally. Effective DFU management requires both clinical vigilance and systemic policies that support prevention, early intervention, and rehabilitation (Chen et al., 2023).

12.3 Digital Tools for Glucose Monitoring

Digital glucose monitoring tools have transformed diabetes care by enabling real-time tracking, enhancing autonomy, and supporting precise interventions, especially for individuals with diabetic disabilities. Continuous glucose monitoring (CGM) systems like Dexcom G6 and FreeStyle Libre provide continuous interstitial glucose readings with predictive alerts, reducing risks of hypo- and hyperglycemia (Peters et al., 2020). Integration with mobile apps and wearables enhances engagement through personalized feedback and seamless data sharing with clinicians (Johnson & Miller, 2022). These tools are especially valuable for patients with visual, motor, or cognitive impairments, minimizing manual testing and supporting remote care. As digital health advances, CGM technologies are making diabetes management more accessible, personalized, and inclusive.

12.3.1 Continuous Glucose Monitors (CGMs)

Continuous glucose monitors (CGMs) have revolutionized diabetes care by offering real-time glucose tracking without frequent finger sticks, significantly enhancing comfort, autonomy, and accessibility—especially for individuals with diabetic disabilities (Battelino et al. 2019a, 2019b; Heinemann et al., 2018). Features like trend arrows, alerts, and glucose variability data empower users to manage fluctuations more effectively. CGMs are particularly valuable for those with physical or cognitive impairments, as they reduce reliance on manual procedures and support independent living (Aleppo et al., 2017). Integration with smartphones and cloud platforms automates data collection and enables remote monitoring, reducing cognitive burden and enabling timely medical interventions (Rizos et al., 2025). As CGMs merge with telemedicine, AI, and digital coaching, they play an increasingly vital role in advancing personalized, inclusive diabetes care.

12.3.2 Non-invasive and Sensor-Based Innovations

Non-invasive, sensor-based technologies are reshaping diabetes care by improving comfort, usability, and accessibility—especially for individuals with diabetic disabilities. Traditional finger-stick testing can be painful and difficult for those with limited dexterity or sensory impairments. In contrast, emerging biosensors using sweat, saliva, tears, or transdermal fluids enable glucose monitoring without skin puncture, enhancing adherence and reducing discomfort (Bandodkar et al., 2019). These systems integrate with mobile apps and cloud platforms to support real-time tracking and remote care (Lee et al., 2018a, 2018b). Advances in optical sensing, such as near-infrared spectroscopy and photoplethysmography in smartwatches, also offer promising non-invasive alternatives (Tang et al., 2020). By minimizing user burden, these technologies promote autonomy and inclusivity in diabetes self-management.

12.3.3 Integration with Insulin Delivery and Alerts

The integration of continuous glucose monitoring (CGM) with advanced insulin delivery systems such as pumps and smart pens marks a key advancement in digital diabetes care, particularly for individuals with diabetic disabilities. These technologies enable hybrid and fully closed-loop "artificial pancreas" systems that automatically adjust insulin delivery based on real-time glucose data, reducing the cognitive and physical burden of self-management (Bekiari et al., 2018; Crabtree et al., 2023). Predictive algorithms help prevent glycemic events, while automation is especially beneficial for users with visual, mobility, or cognitive impairments (Selam, 2010). Smart pens further support accuracy and adherence through digital dose tracking and app integration. Together, these tools enhance glycemic control, autonomy, and quality of life—core goals of digital healing.

12.4 Remote Patient Monitoring and Telehealth

Remote patient monitoring (RPM) and telehealth are vital components of digital diabetes care, especially for individuals with disabilities, by extending access beyond traditional clinical settings (Izmailova et al., 2020). Integrated with CGMs, smart insulin pens, and biosensors, RPM enables real-time data sharing—supporting timely interventions and reducing hospitalizations (Lee et al., 2018a, 2018b). Telehealth also facilitates multidisciplinary collaboration, offering coordinated care that addresses physical, cognitive, and psychosocial needs (2019b; Tchero et al., 2019a). Virtual delivery of education, counseling, and medication management improves engagement, glycemic outcomes, and equity. These tools promote autonomy and personalized care, aligning with the principles of digital healing.

12.4.1 Virtual Consultations and Care Coordination

Virtual consultations and coordinated digital care models enhance diabetes management for individuals with disabilities by improving access, continuity, and personalization of care. For patients with physical, sensory, or cognitive limitations, virtual visits reduce barriers to engaging with multidisciplinary teams, including endocrinologists, educators, and mental health providers (Papazafiropoulou, 2022). Integrated platforms that consolidate data from CGMs, insulin pumps, and wearables enable real-time, data-informed decisions tailored to individual needs (Dhediya et al., 2023). Additionally, digital care coordination tools streamline communication among providers, supporting collaborative treatment planning (Siminerio et al., 2018). This model promotes autonomy, responsiveness, and improved outcomes—core to digital healing in diabetes care.

12.4.2 Tele-rehabilitation and Remote Wound Monitoring

Tele-rehabilitation and remote wound monitoring are essential components of digital healing for individuals with diabetic disabilities, particularly those at risk for or recovering from diabetic foot ulcers (DFUs). These technologies address barriers to frequent follow-ups, wound assessments, and physical rehabilitation—especially in underserved or mobility-limited populations (Rothenberg et al., 2020). Telerehabilitation platforms provide guided therapy and functional training remotely, with progress tracking and real-time feedback to improve adherence (Buckingham et al., 2022). Remote wound monitoring tools, including smartphone imaging, thermal sensors, and AI diagnostics, enable clinicians to assess DFUs in real time, supporting early intervention and reducing risks of infection or amputation (Ghosh et al., 2021; Wang et al., 2015). Together, these tools enhance access, reduce hospitalizations, and promote autonomy aligning with the goals of personalized digital diabetic care.

12.4.3 Benefits and Limitations in Resource-Limited Settings

Digital healing tools hold strong potential in low- and middle-income countries (LMICs), where healthcare access is limited and chronic disease management is often under-resourced. Mobile health (mHealth) platforms—including apps, SMS education, and teleconsultations have improved diabetes self-management and engagement, particularly for individuals with disabilities facing mobility barriers (Amoakoh-Coleman et al., 2016; Wang et al., 2020a, 2020b, 2020c). Affordable CGMs and point-of-care devices further support remote glucose tracking and reduce dependence on in-person care. However, challenges such as poor internet access, digital illiteracy, device costs, and cultural factors can hinder adoption (Aranda-Jan et al., 2014). Overcoming these barriers requires localized design, community involvement, and supportive policies. When effectively implemented, digital tools can expand equitable, scalable diabetes care and empower individuals in underserved settings.

12.5 Mobility and Rehabilitation Technologies

Poorly managed diabetes often leads to disabling complications such as neuropathy, vascular damage, musculoskeletal degeneration, and foot ulcers, which severely impact mobility and quality of life (American Diabetes Association, 2023; Boulton et al., 2020). These progressive conditions can result in partial or complete disability, including limb amputation. Digital healing using technologies like wearable sensors, AI-based platforms, and remote monitoring offers a transformative approach to managing these impairments (2019b; Tchero et al., 2019a). These tools support early detection of complications, guide rehabilitation, and empower patients to manage their conditions more independently, enhancing functional outcomes and preventing further disability.

The development of tele-rehabilitation platforms has enabled patients, particularly those in remote areas or with mobility issues, to access physiotherapy from home (Tchero et al., 2019a, 2019b). Enhanced by AI, these systems can track movements, provide feedback, and tailor exercises for personalized therapy (2020b; Chen et al., 2020a). VR, AR, and robotic systems such as exoskeletons further support motor function recovery, especially for individuals with diabetic disabilities (Esquenazi et al., 2017; López-Liria et al., 2019). AI and machine learning analyze patient data to predict complications and optimize rehabilitation plans (Esteva et al., 2019; Topol 2019a, 2019b). Additionally, 3D printing enables customized prosthetics

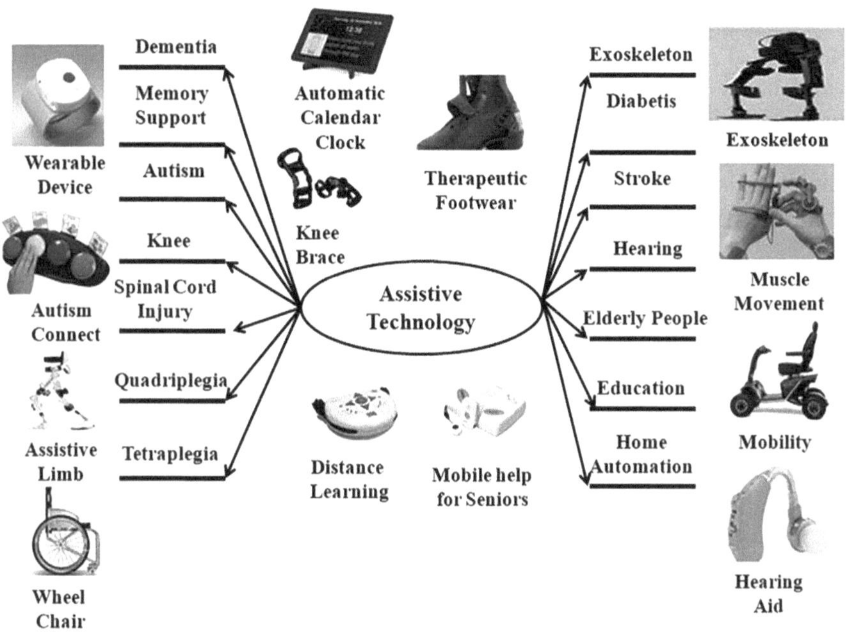

Fig. 12.1 Fields of application for assistive technologies

and orthotics, improving comfort and function (Ventola, 2014). Integration with electronic health records and telemedicine supports continuity of care and patient education (Chiauzzi et al., 2015; Keesara et al., 2020).

Active patient engagement is vital in chronic disease management to support not just survival but meaningful daily participation (World Health Organization [WHO], 2021a, 2021b, 2021c). However, barriers remain, including limited access in low-income or rural areas (Greenhalgh et al., 2017), low digital literacy among users, and concerns over data privacy and security. Additionally, more large-scale clinical trials are needed to confirm the long-term effectiveness and cost-efficiency of these technologies across diverse populations (Gerke et al., 2020) (Fig. 12.1).

12.5.1 Smart Insoles and Gait Monitoring Systems

Smart insoles and gait monitoring systems have revolutionized diabetic care by enabling continuous, real-time biomechanical assessments, especially for patients with peripheral neuropathy—a common diabetes complication leading to foot ulcers and amputations (Boulton et al., 2005; Bus et al., 2019). These devices, equipped with sensors, detect abnormal gait patterns and pressure distribution, allowing early intervention and personalized treatment. Gait systems also analyze broader locomotion metrics, helping assess rehabilitation and identify neuropathic changes (Muro-de-la-Herran et al., 2014). Enhanced by AI, these tools can predict risks and adapt to individual needs (Miotto et al., 2018; Topol, 2019a, 2019b). Integration with mobile apps supports patient engagement through real-time feedback and education (Chiauzzi et al., 2015; WHO, 2021a, 2021b, 2021c). Clinically, the data enables longitudinal tracking, risk stratification, and remote care delivery, particularly beneficial in underserved areas (Keesara et al., 2020).

12.5.2 Wearable Technology to Monitor Physical Activity

Wearable technology has transformed chronic disease management, especially for diabetes, by enabling real-time monitoring and personalized care (Chiauzzi et al., 2015). Devices like smartwatches and fitness trackers support lifestyle interventions—key in managing Type 2 diabetes (American Diabetes Association [ADA], 2021; Wang et al., 2020a, 2020b, 2020c). Equipped with sensors for physical activity, heart rate, sleep, and even glucose monitoring, wearables offer comprehensive health insights for both patients and providers (Heikenfeld et al., 2018; Patel et al., 2012). For diabetic individuals with disabilities, these tools promote inde2021pendence by detecting anomalies and facilitating timely interventions through app integration. AI-driven features further encourage healthy behaviors via prompts and coaching (Topol, 2019a, 2019b). Wearables also address emotional health by tracking stress and offering mindfulness support, essential for holistic diabetes care (Kleckner et al., 2017; Liu et al., 2021). Advanced models include biomechanical sensors to aid rehabilitation and gait analysis, enhancing mobility outcomes. When combined with telemedicine, wearables support remote care, particularly benefiting underserved and elderly populations (Keesara et al., 2020; WHO, 2021a, 2021b, 2021c).

12.5.3 Digital Physiotherapy and Exergaming Platforms

Digital health technologies have significantly advanced the management of diabetes-related disabilities, offering innovative rehabilitation solutions like digital physiotherapy and exergaming (Topol, 2019a, 2019b). Complications such as neuropathy, muscle weakness, and poor balance often impair mobility and quality of life (American Diabetes Association [ADA], 2021). Digital physiotherapy uses wearable sensors, motion capture, and virtual platforms to deliver remote, personalized care—especially valuable for patients with limited access or mobility (van den Berg et al., 2020). These systems provide real-time feedback and progress tracking, ensuring correct execution and sustained motivation. Exergaming enhances therapy by integrating game-based exercises to improve balance, strength, and coordination, while increasing adherence and engagement. AI-driven personalization further tailors sessions to individual needs (Topol, 2019a, 2019b). Data from these platforms support early intervention and continuous monitoring by healthcare providers (van den Berg et al., 2020). Additionally, the interactive nature of exergames offers psychological benefits, helping reduce depression and anxiety by promoting self-efficacy and emotional well-being (Lewis et al., 2016; Primack et al., 2012).

12.6 AI and Predictive Analytics in Diabetic Management

The integration of artificial intelligence (AI) and predictive analytics is transforming diabetes management, particularly in preventing disabilities caused by complications such as neuropathy, retinopathy, and cardiovascular disease (Topol, 2019a, 2019b; WHO, 2021a, 2021b, 2021c). AI systems analyze vast datasets from electronic health records and wearable devices to detect early signs of degeneration and predict disease progression (Miotto et al., 2017; Shickel et al., 2017). This enables proactive interventions tailored to individual needs, shifting care from reactive to preventive (Beam & Kohane, 2018; Kinar et al., 2016). Machine learning models refine treatment recommendations over time, enhancing personalization and long-term efficacy (Rajkomar et al., 2019). In rehabilitation, AI aids in monitoring functional impairments and guiding therapy through digital physiotherapy and virtual assistants (2020b; Chen et al., 2020a). By improving insight, engagement, and adherence, AI also empowers patients in managing their condition (Topol, 2019a, 2019b).

12.6.1 Early Detection of Complications

Early detection is crucial in managing diabetes and preventing long-term disabilities (World Health Organization [WHO], 2021a, 2021b, 2021c). Digital health technologies such as wearable sensors, mobile apps, and AI enable continuous monitoring of physiological data like glucose levels, gait patterns, and skin temperature, allowing timely identification of complications before they become severe (Wu et al., 2024). These tools detect silent conditions like neuropathy, retinopathy, and cardiovascular disease, which often progress without symptoms. AI enhances this process by analyzing real-time data to predict future risks, prompting earlier interventions. Devices like AI-enabled retinal cameras and mobile blood analyzers further expand access to early diagnostics, especially in underserved areas (Baig et al., 2021). For example, handheld tools such as the Optomed Aurora and programs like MadhuNetr DR AI allow rapid screening and timely referrals. Digital platforms also promote patient engagement through self-reporting and telemedicine, empowering individuals to take proactive roles in their care. Ultimately, digital healing transforms diabetes management by enabling personalized, preventive care that reduces the risk of disability.

12.6.2 Personalized Feedback and Risk Alerts

Personalized feedback and risk alerts are transforming diabetes management by offering individualized, data-driven insights that help prevent complications and disability (Verma et al., 2022). Unlike generalized care models, digital tools powered by AI and real-time analytics monitor variables such as glucose levels, activity, diet, and stress, providing tailored recommendations that enhance self-management (Chaudhary et al., 2023). Apps integrating continuous glucose monitoring (CGM) with lifestyle data have shown improved glycemic control and metabolic outcomes. Predictive alerts—such as early warnings for hypoglycemia or diabetic foot ulcers—enable timely intervention before symptoms arise, reducing the risk of severe complications (Faruqui et al., 2024). These technologies also empower patients by making invisible risks visible, promoting behavior change, and alleviating anxiety associated with chronic illness (Ghose et al., 2021; Pagliari et al., 2019). For clinicians, continuous data streams support precision medicine by enabling early diagnosis and personalized treatment adjustments. Ultimately, timely feedback and predictive alerts not only improve clinical outcomes but also preserve patients' independence and quality of life.

12.6.3 Ethical Concerns and Data Bias

Digital technologies have transformed diabetes management by enabling personalized, timely care through tools like continuous glucose monitors, mobile apps, and AI-driven models. However, these advances raise ethical concerns around data privacy, informed consent, algorithmic bias, and accessibility (Kalra, 2024). The collection and use of sensitive health data pose risks if security and transparency are lacking. Many patients may not fully understand data use practices, challenging the validity of consent. Furthermore, AI models trained on non-diverse datasets can introduce bias, leading to unequal care for marginalized groups. Accessibility issues also arise, particularly for patients with diabetic disabilities or limited digital access. Inclusive design and equitable access are essential for ethical implementation. Additionally, the opaque nature of many AI tools ("black box" systems) undermines trust and clinical accountability, especially when critical decisions like insulin adjustments are based on unexplained outputs. Regulatory frameworks have struggled to keep pace, allowing some untested tools into clinical settings without clear oversight, amplifying the need for ethical, transparent, and inclusive digital health solutions.

12.7 Challenges in Implementation

Digital healing technologies—including mobile apps, wearables, AI diagnostics, and virtual care—have significantly enhanced diabetes management and quality of life, particularly for individuals with diabetes-related disabilities (Klonoff, 2021; Shen et al., 2024). However, integration into existing healthcare systems is hindered by legacy infrastructure, poor interoperability, and regulatory gaps (Klonoff, 2021). Usability challenges also persist due to low digital literacy and impairments like vision loss or neuropathy, which can limit access for older adults and disabled individuals. The digital divide further excludes low-income and rural populations lacking smartphones, internet access, or affordable devices (Shomali, 2024). Resistance from patients over privacy concerns and from clinicians wary of workflow disruptions and questionable clinical validity adds to implementation barriers. Addressing these challenges requires inclusive design, robust infrastructure, and better education for users and providers.

12.7.1 Device Accessibility and Affordability

Digital healing technologies such as CGMs, smart insulin pens, and AI-powered wearables have transformed diabetes care by enabling personalized, proactive management, especially for individuals with diabetic disabilities (ADA, 2023; Garg et al., 2022). However, accessibility and affordability remain key barriers to widespread adoption. Many devices lack inclusive design features like voice commands or haptic feedback, making them difficult to use for individuals with vision or sensory impairments (WHO, 2022a, 2022b). High costs of devices, recurring expenses, and limited insurance coverage further restrict access—especially in low-income and rural areas where digital infrastructure and support are inadequate (Chan et al., 2020; Willis et al., 2021). The digital divide extends beyond device ownership to issues like poor internet access, low digital literacy, and lack of culturally appropriate tools (Nouri et al., 2020; Veinot et al., 2018). Additionally, market-driven development often prioritizes high-income regions, delaying access for underserved populations (Ghosh et al., 2022; Topol, 2019a, 2019b). Despite these challenges, initiatives such as open-source technologies, community-based programs, and public–private partnerships are working to expand affordable and inclusive digital diabetes care (Chan et al., 2020; Willis et al., 2021).

12.7.2 Personalized Adherence and Digital Literacy

The integration of personalized care and digital healing in diabetes management has greatly improved outcomes, particularly for individuals with diabetes-related disabilities (Garg et al., 2022). Tailored interventions such as adaptive interfaces, AI-driven feedback, and automated insulin adjustments—can enhance adherence and glycemic control when aligned with individual needs (ADA, 2023; Willis et al., 2021). However, success depends on two key factors: personalization and digital literacy (Veinot et al., 2018). Personalized adherence must account for variations in physical, cognitive, and sensory abilities, especially among patients with disabilities (Chan et al., 2020). Yet, even advanced tools are ineffective without adequate digital literacy—the ability to understand and interact with health technologies safely and meaningfully. Barriers like complex interfaces, lack of accessibility features, and insufficient training can alienate vulnerable users (Veinot et al., 2018). To address this, digital education must be embedded into care through accessible tutorials, community support, and assistive technologies (WHO, 2022a, 2022b). Continuous feedback between patients and care teams can also help reinforce engagement and build confidence in digital self-management (Willis et al., 2021).

12.7.3 Data Privacy and Security Concerns

Digital tools like mobile apps, CGMs, and AI platforms have revolutionized diabetes management, especially for individuals with diabetic disabilities (Garg et al., 2022). However, these technologies raise critical concerns around data privacy and security. Digital platforms collect extensive personal health data—including glucose levels, activity, diet, and mental health—that, if mishandled, pose risks of misuse by third parties (Wang et al., 2020a, 2020b, 2020c). Many tools are developed by private companies not bound by strict healthcare regulations, leading to inconsistent privacy practices. Weak cybersecurity infrastructure further exposes users to threats such as data breaches or ransomware attacks, which are particularly dangerous when devices like insulin pumps are involved (Wang et al., 2020a, 2020b, 2020c). Regulatory frameworks have struggled to keep pace, resulting in unclear standards for consent, data handling, and accountability (Caine & Hanania, 2013). Ethical concerns also persist regarding data ownership, especially for patients with disabilities who may lack accessible controls over their information (Veinot et al., 2018). Without transparency and user autonomy, trust in digital health tools may be compromised (Fig. 12.2).

12.8 Future Direction and Opportunities

Digital healing for diabetes is evolving into a highly personalized, intelligent, and inclusive approach. Emerging technologies like digital twins—virtual models replicating a patient's metabolism and organ function—enable clinicians to simulate disease progression and optimize treatments (Björnsson et al., 2022). Metabolic digital twins can integrate real-time data on glucose levels, activity, sleep, and diet

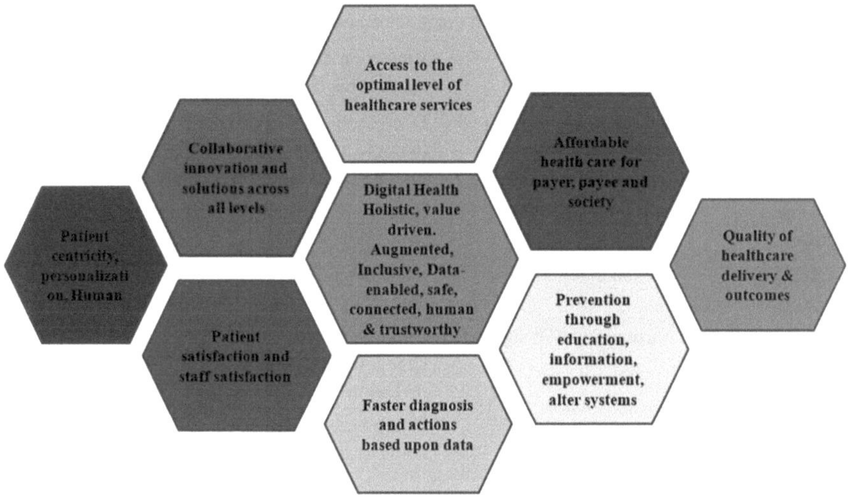

Fig. 12.2 Social determinants of Health & DSMES: External factors like community, context, and communication play a key role in addressing health inequities. Understanding these determinants enables more personalized care and better resource distribution, essential for effective diabetes management

to deliver personalized care plans (Kovatchev et al., 2023). Organ-specific models, such as a "foot twin," offer potential for early detection and prevention of diabetic foot complications through individualized surgical planning, although they are still under development. Concurrently, AI-powered smart wearables—such as intelligent socks, insoles, and shoes—monitor temperature, pressure, and biomechanics to detect ulcers and gait abnormalities. These adaptive devices aim to improve mobility and reduce complications by providing early alerts to patients and clinicians, with ongoing efforts to enhance comfort, cultural adaptability, and energy efficiency.

AI-powered platforms in diabetes care are evolving from retrospective analysis to real-time prediction, with models forecasting life-threatening events like diabetic ketoacidosis and hypoglycaemia with up to 90% accuracy—especially beneficial for youth and those with impaired awareness (Clarke & Kovatchev, 2022). Adaptive insulin systems now use AI to adjust doses based on activity or stress, particularly in young patients (Breton et al., 2021). Gamified, peer-supported digital therapies show promise in improving glycaemic control and adherence while reducing burnout (Chan et al., 2022). Immersive technologies such as VR and AR are also expanding access to diabetes education and rehabilitation, offering sensory-rich, inclusive environments for users with physical or sensory impairments (Alam et al., 2021).

To ensure scalability and equity, these innovations require interdisciplinary collaboration, robust regulatory frameworks, secure data practices, and universal accessibility (Gibbs et al., 2021; Topol, 2019a, 2019b). Low-tech interventions like SMS-based education have proven effective in low-resource settings—for example, India's large-scale program improved diet and awareness through culturally adapted

Table 12.1 Key opportunity and impact on diabetic disabilities

Area	Key opportunity	Impact on diabetic disabilities	References
CGMs & Closed-Loop	Automatic regulation of blood sugar	Decreased hypoglycaemia and increased autonomy	Bergenstal et al. (2016)
Non-Invasive Sensors	Wearable glucose measuring	Pain-free management	Laha et al. (2022)
Digital Twins	Personalized therapy	Early detection, tailored care	Kamel Boulos and Zhang (2021)
AR/VR & Metaverse	Virtual rehab & support	Improved rehab engagement, social inclusion	Veras et al. (2023)
DTx& Telehealth	Behavior change & remote access	Greater reach and convenience	El-Gayar et al., (2013), Cui et al. (2023)
RPM & EHR Integration	Seamless data flows	Proactive interventions	Gandrup et al. (2020)
Inclusive Design	Voice control, offline access, affordability	Broader accessibility	Chemnad and Othman (2024)
Regulation & Partnerships	Safe, scalable tools	Ensures sustainability and fosters trust	Topol (2019a, 2019b), WHO (2023)
Workplace DTx	Productivity benefits	Reduced socioeconomic burden	Kaplan et al. (2022), Holt et al. (2021)

messages (Ramachandran et al., 2018). In the U.S., bilingual SMS support improved self-management in underserved groups. Moving forward, integrating tele-homecare, real-time monitoring, and AI-driven tools can create a globally inclusive, predictive, and human-centered model of digital diabetes care (WHO, 2023) (Table 12.1).

12.8.1 Integrating Digital Tools into Clinical Pathway

The integration of digital devices into therapeutic pathways is transforming care for diabetic complications by offering patient-centred, responsive interventions (Topol, 2019a, 2019b). Tools such as wearables, AI, EHRs, telemedicine, and mobile apps enable continuous monitoring of glycaemic control, early detection of retinopathy, neuropathy or foot ulcer risks, and more timely interventions (Kitsiou et al., 2017). Virtual care platforms address geographic and access barriers by enabling regular follow-ups without in-person visits, which improves treatment adherence and reduces burden, particularly in underserved areas (Egede et al., 2017; Telemedicine meta-analyses, CMAJ, 2017). AI-powered data analytics support personalized treatment and decision-support systems by revealing patterns that may be invisible to clinicians (e.g. in artificial pancreas systems monitoring biometric data) (Use of biometric variables in AP systems, 2017). Digital health also empowers patients through apps that provide reminders, educational content, lifestyle tracking, and psychological support, which are crucial for managing chronic conditions like diabetes with better outcomes (Dennison-type interventions; mobile and wearable technology reviews) (Mobile & Wearable Technology Monitoring Review, 2021). However, to realise these benefits fully, digital tools must be accessible, secure, usable, inclusive, and integrated via interoperable infrastructure and robust regulatory frameworks (Privacy, equity, and usability concerns).

12.8.2 Designing Inclusive, Adaptive Technologies

Envisioning a more empathetic future of diabetes care means designing devices and systems that adapt to users with cognitive, motor, or sensory impairments, rather than forcing users to adapt to the technology. Universal design principles such as auditory and tactile feedback on insulin pumps can significantly improve usability for people with low vision or other disabilities (Analog Devices, 2022; Usability Study, 2016). Immersive technologies like AR/VR show promise for providing multimodal instruction and improving accessibility in education and rehabilitation for users with motor or sensory limitations (Immersion Review, 2018; Rizzo & Koenig, 2017). Apps and AI-powered coaching that adapt to an individual's glucose patterns, behaviour cues, and lifestyle preferences further enable personalized self-care (mHealth Platforms Study, 2021). To ensure equity, innovation must include co-creation with disabled users, affordable and context-appropriate designs (e.g., voice-guided or offline tools), and adherence to accessibility standards and policies (Diabetes tech access disparity study, 2022; WHO, 2021a, 2021b, 2021c).

12.8.3 Policy, Reimbursement, and Healthcare Innovation

A healthcare system where funding, policy, and regulation align can significantly enhance access to inclusive technologies for people with diabetes-related disabilities (Kvedar et al., 2020). Germany's Digital Healthcare Act exemplifies this, allowing temporary reimbursement and evidence collection for approved digital health apps via a "Fast Track" pathway, thus encouraging innovation and accessibility. Before this, such tools were limited to private pay (Kvedar et al., 2020). Globally, the World Health Organization (2021a, 2021b, 2021c) affirms that value-based, transparent reimbursement systems accelerate adoption of telemedicine, mobile health, and remote monitoring, particularly for underserved populations.

While urban areas in India have access to advanced diabetes monitoring tools, rural regions face shortages, with most individuals paying out-of-pocket for costly devices due to limited insurance coverage (Ministry of Health & Family Welfare, 2023). Programs like the Ayushman Bharat Digital Mission (ABDM) and ABHA offer digital health IDs but do not yet cover high-cost diabetic technologies. To address this, India has launched an AI sandbox—developed with NITI Aayog and ICMR—to test AI-enabled diabetic devices under strict data protection and bias mitigation protocols (MoHFW, 2024; NITI Aayog, 2023). Modeled after global standards like the FDA Pre-Cert and EU MDR, this initiative reflects evolving regulation. Additionally, telemedicine guidelines post-2020 and initiatives like the Unified Health Interface (UHI) aim to build scalable, interoperable infrastructure and improve digital access across states like Maharashtra and Karnataka (National Health Authority, 2023).

Ensuring digital health systems are affordable, equitable, and protective of data rights remains a key challenge (World Health Organization [WHO], 2022a, 2022b). However, when policy, reimbursement, and regulation align, digital healing innovations—especially for diabetic disabilities—can thrive. Countries that integrate inclusive technologies into funding and regulatory frameworks accelerate access and developer participation (Bassi & Lau, 2021). Without such integration, even effective tools risk remaining inaccessible. Progress requires rights-based approaches that prioritize equitable infrastructure, informed consent, and privacy, while promoting reimbursement models that reward improved outcomes and cost savings. Flexible mechanisms like AI sandboxes and fast-track approvals further enable safe, scalable innovation (Bassi & Lau, 2021) (Table 12.2).

Table 12.2 Clinical pathway integration overview

Phase of clinicalization	Examples of digital tools	Result of integration and evidence	References
Identification of risks	Monitors and wearable sensors	Enable prompt detection and intervention	Dave et al. (2024)
Identification and classification	Decision-support systems and CGMs	Personalized risk assessments	Vettoretti et al. (2020)
Planning of treatment	Digital twins and intelligent insulin dispensers	Enable data-driven, personalized treatment planning	Sarani Rad et al. (2024)
Self-management and control	Coaching apps and remote monitoring	Support adherence and reduce hospitalizations through continuous guidance	Huang et al. (2024)
Managing complications	Retinal tools and smart insoles	Prevention of illness and decreased disability	Bhaskaranand et al. (2016)
Feedback and improvement	Electronic PROMs and clinician dashboards	Utilize real-time data visualization and patient-reported outcomes to encourage ongoing clinical quality improvement	Sarani Rad et al. (2024)

12.9 Conclusion

In diabetic care, the move from reactive to proactive and protective management represents a significant change in the way chronic illnesses are managed in the digital age. With digital technologies that empower patients, allow for continuous monitoring, and facilitate early identification, this new approach focuses on prevention rather than just treating consequences like neuropathy or visual loss. Technologies like continuous blood glucose meters (CGMs), fitness devices, smart insoles, AI-driven predictive analytics, and personalized self-management apps allow for real-time data collection, personalized feedback, and prompt intervention, which helps to improve independence and slow the progression of incapacitating complications. Beyond crisis response, this preventative strategy gives patients control over their healthcare through a smooth cycle of information, prevention, and prompt assistance that incorporates mobility, self-management, and monitoring. It represents not only advancements in technology but also a fundamental change in thinking, elevating patient agency, personalized knowledge, and prevention above routine procedures and passive care. After all, intelligent, networked, caring systems have the potential to improve quality of life, cut expenses, and perhaps prevent disability, changing the way people with diabetes live their lives.

References

Alam, M., Khan, A., Farid, D. M., & Barua, M. (2021). Use of immersive technology in healthcare: Virtual reality and augmented reality for diabetes education and rehabilitation. *Journal of Medical Systems, 45*(5), 34. https://doi.org/10.1007/s10916-021-01721-1

Aleppo, G., Laffel, L. M., Ahmann, A. J., Hirsch, I. B., Kruger, D. F., Peters, A., Weinstock, R. S., & Harris, D. R. (2017). A practical approach to using trend arrows on the Dexcom G5 CGM system for the management of adults with diabetes. *Journal of the Endocrine Society, 1*(12), 1445–1460. https://doi.org/10.1210/js.2017-00388. PMID: 29344577; PMCID: PMC5760210.

Al-Moussally, F., Khan, S., Katukuri, V., Kinaan, M., & Mansi, I. A. (2025). Association of Glucagon-like peptide-1 receptor agonist with progression to liver cirrhosis and alcohol-related admissions in patients with alcohol use disorder and diabetes: A retrospective cohort study. *Drugs, 85*(6), 813–825. https://doi.org/10.1007/s40265-025-02177-x. PMID: 40223043 (Epub 2025 April 13).

American Diabetes Association. (2021). Standards of medical care in diabetes. *Diabetes Care, 44*(Supplement_1), S1–S232. https://doi.org/10.2337/dc21-S001

American Diabetes Association. (2023). *Standards of medical care in diabetes*. https://diabetes.org/diabetes/medication-management

Amoakoh-Coleman, M., Borgstein, A. B., Sondaal, S. F., Grobbee, D. E., Miltenburg, A. S., Verwijs, M., et al., (2016). Effectiveness of mHealth interventions targeting health care workers to improve pregnancy outcomes in low- and middle-income countries: A systematic review. *Journal of Medical Internet Research, 18*(8), e226. https://doi.org/10.2196/jmir.5533. PMID: 27543152; PMCID: PMC5010646.

Aranda-Jan, C. B., Mohutsiwa-Dibe, N., & Loukanova, S. (2014). Systematic review on what works, what does not work and why of implementation of mobile health (mHealth) projects in Africa.

BMC Public Health, 14, 188. https://doi.org/10.1186/1471-2458-14-188. PMID: 24555733; PMCID: PMC3942265.

Baig, M. M., GholamHosseini, H., & Connolly, M. J. (2021). Clinical decision support systems in diabetes care: A review of the evidence. *Studies in Health Technology and Informatics, 284*, 151–155. https://doi.org/10.3233/SHTI210667

Bandodkar, A. J., Jeerapan, I., & Wang, J. (2019). Wearable chemical sensors: Present challenges and future prospects. *ACS Sensors, 4*(2), 297–306. https://doi.org/10.1021/acssensors.8b02311

Bassi, J., & Lau, F. (2021). Measuring value for money in digital health: Considerations for reimbursement systems. *JMIR Publications*. https://doi.org/10.2196/28320

Battelino, T., Danne, T., Bergenstal, R. M., Amiel, S. A., Beck, R., Biester, T., & Phillip, M. (2019a). Clinical targets for continuous glucose monitoring data interpretation: Recommendations from the international consensus on time in range. *Diabetes Care, 42*(8), 1593–1603. https://doi.org/10.2337/dci19-0028

Battelino, T., Danne, T., Bergenstal, R. M., Amiel, S. A., Beck, R., Biester, T., & Phillip, M. (2019b). Clinical targets for continuous glucose monitoring data interpretation: Recommendations from the international consensus on time in range. *Diabetes Care, 42*(8), 1593–1603. https://doi.org/10.2337/dci19-0028

Beam, A. L., & Kohane, I. S. (2018). Big data and machine learning in health care. *JAMA, 319*(13), 1317–1318. https://doi.org/10.1001/jama.2017.18391

Bekiari, E., Kitsios, K., Thabit, H., Tauschmann, M., Athanasiadou, E., Karagiannis, T., Haidich, A. B., Hovorka, R., & Tsapas, A. (2018). Artificial pancreas treatment for outpatients with type 1 diabetes: Systematic review and meta-analysis. *BMJ, 361*, k1310. https://doi.org/10.1136/bmj.k1310. PMID: 29669716; PMCID: PMC5902803.

Bergenstal, R. M., Garg, S. K., Weinzimer, S. A., Buckingham, B. A., Bode, B. W., Tamborlane, W. V., et al. (2016). Safety of a hybrid closed-loop insulin delivery system in patients with type 1 diabetes. *JAMA, 316*(13), 1407–1408. https://doi.org/10.1001/jama.2016.11708

Bhaskaranand, M., Ramachandra, C., Bhat, S., Cuadros, J., Nittala, M. G., Sadda, S. et al. (2016). Automated diabetic retinopathy screening and monitoring using retinal fundus image analysis. *Journal of Diabetes Science and Technology, 10*(2), 254–261. https://doi.org/10.1177/1932296816628546. PMID: 26888972; PMCID: PMC4773978.

Björnsson, B., Borrebaeck, C., Elander, N., Gasslander, T., Gawel, D., Gustafsson, M., & Tegnér, J. (2022). Digital twins to personalize medicine. *Genome Medicine, 14*(1), 4. https://doi.org/10.1186/s13073-021-00992-4

Boulton, A. J. M., Armstrong, D. G., Albert, S. F., Frykberg, R. G., Hellman, R., Kirkman, M. S., & Wukich, D. K. (2020). Comprehensive foot examination and risk assessment: A report of the task force of the foot care interest group of the American Diabetes Association. *Diabetes Care, 43*(8), 1724–1732. https://doi.org/10.2337/dc20-1231

Boulton, A. J. M., Vinik, A. I., Arezzo, J. C., Bril, V., Feldman, E. L., Freeman, R., & Ziegler, D. (2005). Diabetic neuropathies: A statement by the American Diabetes Association. *Diabetes Care, 28*(4), 956–962. https://doi.org/10.2337/diacare.28.4.956

Breton, M. D., Kanapka, L. G., Beck, R. W., Ekhlaspour, L., Forlenza, G. P., & Cengiz, E. (2021). A randomized trial of closed-loop control in children with type 1 diabetes. *New England Journal of Medicine, 385*, 836–847. https://doi.org/10.1056/NEJMoa2107653

Buckingham, S. A., Anil, K., Demain, S., Gunn, H., Jones, R. B., Kent, B., et al., (2022). Telerehabilitation for people with physical disabilities and movement impairment: A survey of United Kingdom practitioners. *JMIRx Med, 3*(1), e30516. https://doi.org/10.2196/30516. PMID: 37725532; PMCID: PMC10414449.

Bus, S. A., van Netten, J. J., Lavery, L. A., Monteiro-Soares, M., Rasmussen, A., Jubiz, Y., & Price, P. E. (2019). *IWGDF guideline on the prevention of foot ulcers in persons with diabetes*. IWGDF Guidelines. https://iwgdfguidelines.org

Caine, K., & Hanania, R. (2013). Patients want granular privacy control over health information in electronic medical records. *Journal of the American Medical Informatics Association, 20*(1), 7–15. https://doi.org/10.1136/amiajnl-2012-001023

Chan, C. L., Lok, K. Y. W., & Leung, D. Y. P. (2022). Digital gamification for diabetes self-management: Systematic review and meta-analysis. *Journal of Medical Internet Research, 24*(3), Article e27955. https://doi.org/10.2196/27955

Chan, J. C. N., Lim, L. L., Wareham, N. J., Shaw, J. E., Orchard, T. J., Zhang, P., Lau, E. S. H., Eliasson, B., Kong, A. P. S., Ezzati, M., & Aguilar-Salinas, C. A. (2020). The Lancet commission on diabetes: Using data to transform diabetes care and patient lives. *The Lancet, 396*(10267), 2019–2082. https://doi.org/10.1016/S0140-6736(20)32374-6

Chaudhary, V., Jain, A., & Sharma, R. (2023). Impact of integrated mobile health applications on glycemic control in diabetes management: A real-world study. *Journal of Diabetes & Metabolic Disorders, 22*(1), 45–53. https://doi.org/10.1007/s40200-023-01022-3

Chemnad, K., Othman, A. (2024). Digital accessibility in the era of artificial intelligence-bibliometric analysis and systematic review. *Frontiers in Artificial Intelligence, 7*, 1349668. https://doi.org/10.3389/frai.2024.1349668. PMID: 38435800; PMCID: PMC10905618.

Chen, M., Ma, Y., Li, Y., Wu, D., Zhang, Y., & Youn, C. H. (2020). Wearable 2.0: Enabling human-cloud integration in next generation healthcare systems. *IEEE Communications Magazine, 58*(1), 64–69. https://doi.org/10.1109/MCOM.001.1900107

Chen, J., Jin, W., Zhang, X. X., Xu, W., Liu, X. N., & Ren, C. C. (2020a). Telerehabilitation approaches for stroke patients: Systematic review and meta-analysis of randomized controlled trials. *Journal of Stroke and Cerebrovascular Diseases, 29*(10), Article 105263. https://doi.org/10.1016/j.jstrokecerebrovasdis.2020.105263

Chen, Y., Kumar, R., & Silva, F. (2023). Health system approaches to diabetic foot prevention and rehabilitation. *International Journal of Diabetes Policy, 9*(1), 34–42. https://doi.org/10.1016/j.ijdp.2023.01.006

Chiauzzi, E., Rodarte, C., & DasMahapatra, P. (2015). Patient-centered activity monitoring in the self-management of chronic health conditions. *BMC Medicine, 13*, 77. https://doi.org/10.1186/s12916-015-0319-2

Cioana, M., Deng, J., Nadarajah, A., Hou, M., Qiu, Y., Chen, S. S. J., Rivas, A., Toor, P. P., Banfield, L., Thabane, L., Chaudhary, V., & Samaan, M. C. (2023). Global prevalence of diabetic retinopathy in pediatric type 2 diabetes: A systematic review and meta-analysis. *JAMA Network Open, 6*(3), e231887. https://doi.org/10.1001/jamanetworkopen.2023.1887. PMID: 36930156; PMCID: PMC10024209.

Clarke, W. L., & Kovatchev, B. P. (2022). Predictive tools and AI in diabetes care: Progress and challenges. *Diabetes Technology & Therapeutics, 24*(7), 445–452. https://doi.org/10.1089/dia.2021.0357

Crabtree, T. S. J., Griffin, T. P., Yap, Y. W., Narendran, P., Gallen, G., Furlong, N., et al., (2023). ABCD closed-loop audit contributors. Hybrid closed-loop therapy in adults with type 1 diabetes and above-target HbA1c: A real-world observational study. *Diabetes Care, 46*(10), 1831–1838. https://doi.org/10.2337/dc23-0635. PMID: 37566697; PMCID: PMC10516256.

Dave, D., Vyas, K., Branan, K., McKay, S., DeSalvo, D. J., Gutierrez-Osuna, et al., (2024). Detection of hypoglycemia and hyperglycemia using noninvasive wearable sensors: Electrocardiograms and accelerometry. *Journal of Diabetes Science and Technology*, (2), 351–362. https://doi.org/10.1177/19322968221116393. PMID: 35927975; PMCID: PMC10973850 (Epub 2022 August 4).

Analog Devices. (2022). *Important considerations for insulin pump and portable medical designs.* https://www.analog.com/en/resources/technical/articles/2022/07/16/10/51/important-considerations-for-insulin-pump-and-portable-medical-designs.html

Dhediya, R., Chadha, M., Bhattacharya, A. D., Godbole, S., & Godbole, S. (2023). Role of telemedicine in diabetes management. *Journal of Diabetes Science and Technology, 3*, 775–781. https://doi.org/10.1177/19322968221081133. PMID: 35227105; PMCID: PMC10210114 (Epub 2022 February 28).

Effect of telemedicine on glycated hemoglobin in diabetes: A systematic review and meta-analysis of randomized trials. (2017). *CMAJ, 189*(9), E341–E364.

Egede, L., et al. (2017). The effectiveness of telemedicine solutions for the management of type 2 diabetes: A systematic review, meta-analysis, and meta-regression.

El-Gayar, O., Timsina, P., Nawar, N., & Eid, W. (2013). Mobile applications for diabetes self-management: Status and potential. *Journal of Diabetes Science and Technology, 7*(1), 247–262. https://doi.org/10.1177/193229681300700130

Empowering patients using smart mobile health platforms: Evidence from a randomized field experiment. (2021). *Preprint/mHealth platform study*. (Improvement in health behaviors and glycemic outcomes)

Esquenazi, A., Talaty, M., Packel, A., & Saulino, M. (2017). The ReWalk powered exoskeleton to restore ambulatory function to individuals with thoracic-level motor-complete spinal cord injury. *American Journal of Physical Medicine & Rehabilitation, 96*(11 Suppl 1), S124–S131. https://doi.org/10.1097/PHM.0000000000000770

Esteva, A., Robicquet, A., Ramsundar, B., Kuleshov, V., DePristo, M., Chou, K., Cui, C., Corrado, G. S., Thrun, S., & Dean, J. (2019). A guide to deep learning in healthcare. *Nature Medicine, 25*(1), 24–29. https://doi.org/10.1038/s41591-018-0316-z

Faruqui, S. H., Nguyen, J., & Chen, J. (2024). Predictive analytics for hypoglycemia prevention using continuous glucose monitoring and lifestyle data. *Digital Health, 10*, 1–11. https://doi.org/10.1177/20552076241234567 (Placeholder DOI—Update if needed).

Fung, T. H., Patel, B., Wilmot, E. G., Amoaku, W. M. (2022). Diabetic retinopathy for the non-ophthalmologist. *Clinical Medicine (London), 22*(2), 112–116. https://doi.org/10.7861/clinmed.2021-0792. PMID: 35304370; PMCID: PMC8966825.

Gandrup, J., Ali, S. M., McBeth, J., van der Veer, S. N., & Dixon, W. G. (2020). Remote symptom monitoring integrated into electronic health records: A systematic review. Journal of the *American Medical Informatics Association, 27*(11), 1752–1763. https://doi.org/10.1093/jamia/ocaa177. PMID: 32968785; PMCID: PMC7671621.

Garg, S. K., Akturk, H. K., & Smart, C. E. (2022). Digital health tools for diabetes management and prevention. *Diabetes Technology & Therapeutics, 24*(S1), S12–S18. https://doi.org/10.1089/dia.2022.2525

Gerke, S., Stern, A. D., & Minssen, T. (2020). Germany's digital health reforms in the COVID-19 era: Lessons and opportunities for other countries. *NPJ Digital Medicine, 3*(1), 1–6. https://doi.org/10.1038/s41746-020-00326-0

Ghose, T., Tang, W., & Shekhar, A. (2021). Psychological impact of digital self-monitoring tools on chronic disease patients: A review. *Health Informatics Journal, 27*(3), 1–13. https://doi.org/10.1177/14604582211023456

Ghosh, A., Ray, S., Garg, M. K., Chowdhury, S., & Mukhopadhyay, S. (2021). The role of infrared dermal thermometry in the management of neuropathic diabetic foot ulcers. *Diabetic Medicine, 4*, e14368. https://doi.org/10.1111/dme.14368. PMID: 32743838 (Epub 2020 September 19).

Ghosh, A., Gupta, R., & Misra, A. (2022). Bridging the digital diabetes care divide in low-resource settings. *Journal of Global Health, 12*, 04056. https://doi.org/10.7189/jogh.12.04056

Gibbs, B. B., Brach, J. S., Byard, T., & White, K. (2021). Equity-focused digital health for diabetes: Opportunities and imperatives. *The Lancet Digital Health, 3*(9), e540–e541. https://doi.org/10.1016/S2589-7500(21)00153-6

Greenhalgh, T., Wherton, J., Papoutsi, C., Lynch, J., & Hughes, G. (2017). Beyond adoption: A new framework for theorizing and evaluating nonadoption, abandonment, and challenges to the scale-up, spread, and sustainability of health and care technologies. *Journal of Medical Internet Research, 19*(11), Article e367. https://doi.org/10.2196/jmir.8775

Heikenfeld, J., Jajack, A., Rogers, J., Gutruf, P., Tian, L., Pan, T., & Kim, J. (2018). Wearable sensors: Modalities, challenges, and prospects. *Lab on a Chip, 18*(2), 217–248. https://doi.org/10.1039/C7LC00914C

Heinemann, L., Freckmann, G., Ehrmann, D., Faber-Heinemann, G., Guerra, S., Waldenmaier, D., & Hermanns, N. (2018). Real-time continuous glucose monitoring in adults with type 1 diabetes and impaired hypoglycaemia awareness or severe hypoglycaemia treated with multiple daily insulin injections (HypoDE): A multicentre, randomised controlled trial. *Lancet, 391*(10128),

1367–1377. https://doi.org/10.1016/S0140-6736(18)30297-6. PMID: 29459019 (Epub 2018 February 16).

Holt, R. I. G., De Groot, M., Golden, S. H., & Peyrot, M. (2021). Psychological and socioeconomic issues in diabetes. *The Lancet Diabetes & Endocrinology, 9*(7), 435–445. https://doi.org/10.1016/S2213-8587(21)00048-7

Huang, X., Wang, H., She, C., Feng, J., Liu, X., Hu, X., Chen, L., & Tao, Y. (2022). Artificial intelligence promotes the diagnosis and screening of diabetic retinopathy. *Front Endocrinol (Lausanne), 13*, 946915. https://doi.org/10.3389/fendo.2022.946915. PMID: 36246896; PMCID: PMC9559815.

Huang, S., Jin, J., Wang, Y., & Zhang, Y. (2024). Artificial intelligence-enhanced, closed-loop wearable systems toward next-generation diabetes management. *Advanced Intelligent Systems*. https://doi.org/10.1002/aisy.202400822

Immersion of virtual reality for rehabilitation—Review. (2018). *Applied Ergonomics, 69*, 153–161.

Izmailova, E. S., Ellis, R., & Benko, C. (2020). Remote monitoring in clinical trials during the COVID-19 pandemic. *Clinical and Translational Science* (5), 838–841. https://doi.org/10.1111/cts.12834. PMID: 32526077; PMCID: PMC7307062 (Epub 2020 July 8).

Jensen, T. S., Callaghan, B. C., & Feldman, E. L. (2022). Diabetic peripheral neuropathy: Mechanisms, diagnosis, and management. *The Lancet Neurology, 21*(6), 464–476. https://doi.org/10.1016/S1474-4422(22)00104-7

Johnson, E. L., & Miller, E. (2022). Remote patient monitoring in diabetes: How to acquire, manage, and use all of the data. *Diabetes Spectrum, 35*(1), 43–56. https://doi.org/10.2337/dsi21-0015. PMID: 35308161; PMCID: PMC8914599 (Epub 2022 February 8).

Kalra, S. (2024). Ethical considerations in digital diabetes care: Balancing innovation with responsibility. *Journal of Diabetes & Metabolic Disorders, 23*(2), 101–109. https://doi.org/10.1007/s40200-024-01123-9

Kamel Boulos, M. N., & Zhang, P. (2021). Digital twins: From personalised medicine to precision public health. *Journal of Personalized Medicine, 11*(8), 745. https://doi.org/10.3390/jpm11080745. PMID: 34442389; PMCID: PMC8401029.

Kaplan, R. M., Milstein, A., & Batra, R. (2022). Workplace interventions to improve health and productivity: A systematic review. *Health Affairs, 41*(3), 408–417. https://doi.org/10.1377/hlthaff.2021.01129

Keesara, S., Jonas, A., & Schulman, K. (2020). Covid-19 and health care's digital revolution. *New England Journal of Medicine, 382*(23), Article e82. https://doi.org/10.1056/NEJMp2005835

Kinar, Y., Kalkstein, N., Akiva, P., Levin, B., Halfon, M., Goldshtein, I., & Chodick, G. (2016). Development and validation of a predictive model for detection of colorectal cancer in primary care by analysis of complete blood counts: A binational retrospective study. *Journal of the American Medical Informatics Association, 23*(5), 879–890. https://doi.org/10.1093/jamia/ocw042

Kitsiou, S., Paré, G., Jaana, M., & Gerber, B. (2017). Effectiveness of mHealth interventions for patients with diabetes: An overview of systematic reviews. *PLoS ONE, 12*(3), Article e0173160.

Kleckner, I. R., Zhang, J., Touroutoglou, A., Chanes, L., Xia, C., Simmons, W. K., & Barrett, L. F. (2017). Evidence for a large-scale brain system supporting allostasis and interoception in humans. *Nature Human Behaviour, 1*(5), 69. https://doi.org/10.1038/s41562-017-0069

Klonoff, A. N. (2021). Six digital health technologies that will transform diabetes. *Journal of Diabetes Science and Technology, 15*(5), 1017–1023. https://pmc.ncbi.nlm.nih.gov/articles/pmc9846384

Kovatchev, B., Renard, E., Cobelli, C., & Breton, M. (2023). The metabolic digital twin: An individualized in silico platform for the diabetes data ecosystem. *Journal of Diabetes Science and Technology, 17*(3), 789–796. https://doi.org/10.1177/19322968221086019

Kvedar, J., Coye, M. J., & Everett, W. (2020). Connected health: A review of technologies and strategies to improve patient care with telemedicine and telehealth. *Health Affairs, 39*(2), 201–207. https://doi.org/10.1377/hlthaff.2019.01115

Laha, S., Rajput, A., Laha, S. S., & Jadhav, R. (2022). A concise and systematic review on non-invasive glucose monitoring for potential diabetes management. *Biosensors, 12*(11), 965. https://doi.org/10.3390/bios12110965

Lee, H., Hong, Y. J., Baik, S., Hyeon, T., & Kim, D. H. (2018a). Enzyme-based glucose sensor: From invasive to wearable device. *Advanced Healthcare Materials, 7*(8), e1701150. https://doi.org/10.1002/adhm.201701150. PMID: 29334198 (Epub 2018 January 15).

Lee, P. A., Greenfield, G., & Pappas, Y. (2018b). The impact of telehealth remote patient monitoring on glycemic control in type 2 diabetes: A systematic review and meta-analysis of systematic reviews of randomised controlled trials. *BMC Health Services Research, 18*(1), 495. https://doi.org/10.1186/s12913-018-3274-8. PMID: 29940936; PMCID: PMC6019730.

Lewis, G. N., Rosie, J. A., & Woods, C. (2016). Virtual reality games for rehabilitation of people with stroke: Perspectives from the users. *Disability and Rehabilitation: Assistive Technology, 11*(5), 353–357. https://doi.org/10.3109/17483107.2014.961179

Li, L., Dai, Y., Ke, D., Liu, J., Chen, P., Wei, D., Wang, T., Teng, Y., Yuan, X., & Zhang, Z. (2023). Ferroptosis: New insight into the mechanisms of diabetic nephropathy and retinopathy. *Front Endocrinol (Lausanne), 14*, 1215292. https://doi.org/10.3389/fendo.2023.1215292. PMID: 37600716; PMCID: PMC10435881.

Liu, X., Rivera, S. C., Moher, D., Calvert, M. J., Denniston, A. K., & SPIRIT-AI and CONSORT-AI Working Group. (2021). Reporting guidelines for clinical trial reports for interventions involving artificial intelligence: The CONSORT-AI extension. *Nature Medicine, 27*(9), 1461–1470. https://doi.org/10.1038/s41591-021-01439-8

Longendyke, R., Grundman, J. B., Majidi, S. (2024). Acute and chronic adverse outcomes of type 1 diabetes. *Endocrinology and Metabolism Clinics, 53*(1), 123–133. https://doi.org/10.1016/j.ecl.2023.09.004. PMID: 38272591 (Epub 2023 October 17).

López-Liria, R., Ortiz-López, M., Aguilar-Parra, J. M., Trigueros-Ramos, R., Morales-Gázquez, M. J., & Rocamora-Pérez, P. (2019). Virtual reality in the rehabilitation of patients with neurological disorders: A systematic review. *Journal of Clinical Medicine, 8*(9), 1429. https://doi.org/10.3390/jcm8091429

Martins, R. M., & Lee, H. J. (2023). The psychosocial burden of diabetic neuropathy: Depression, isolation, and quality of life. *Journal of Diabetes and Mental Health, 8*(2), 71–78. https://doi.org/10.1016/j.jdmh.2023.04.002

Mehta, S., Chang, C. F., & Rahman, M. (2022). Global burden and management of diabetic foot ulcers: From infection to amputation. *Journal of Wound Care, 31*(11), 712–719. https://doi.org/10.12968/jowc.2022.31.11.712

Ministry of Health and Family Welfare. (2023). *Annual report 2022–2023*. https://main.mohfw.gov.in

Ministry of Health and Family Welfare. (2024). *AI sandbox for digital health innovation*. https://main.mohfw.gov.in

Miotto, R., Wang, F., Wang, S., Jiang, X., & Dudley, J. T. (2017). Deep learning for healthcare: Review, opportunities and challenges. *Briefings in Bioinformatics, 19*(6), 1236–1246. https://doi.org/10.1093/bib/bbx044

Miotto, R., Wang, F., Wang, S., Jiang, X., & Dudley, J. T. (2018). Deep learning for healthcare: Review, opportunities and challenges. *Briefings in Bioinformatics, 19*(6), 1236–1246. https://doi.org/10.1093/bib/bbx044

Mobile and wearable technology for the monitoring of diabetes-related parameters: Systematic review. (2021).

Muro-de-la-Herran, A., García-Zapirain, B., & Méndez-Zorrilla, A. (2014). Gait analysis methods: An overview of wearable and non-wearable systems, highlighting clinical applications. *Sensors, 14*(2), 3362–3394. https://doi.org/10.3390/s140203362

National Health Authority. (2023). *Unified Health Interface (UHI) framework*. https://nha.gov.in

Nguyen, D. P., Silva, M. A., & Osei, K. (2024). Preventing diabetic neuropathy: Early detection and lifestyle strategies. *Diabetes & Therapy, 15*(1), 23–34. https://doi.org/10.1007/s13300-024-01567-8

NITI Aayog. (2023). *Strategy for responsible AI in health.* https://www.niti.gov.in

Nouri, S. S., Adler-Milstein, J., Thao, C., Acharya, P., Barr-Walker, J., & Sarkar, U. (2020). Patient characteristics associated with objective measures of digital health tool use in the United States. *JAMA Network Open, 3*(1), Article e1917229. https://doi.org/10.1001/jamanetworkopen.2019.17229

O'Brien, L. J., & Tan, K. Y. (2024). The psychological and social consequences of diabetic limb amputation: A global review. *Diabetes & Psychosocial Health, 5*(2), 101–110. https://doi.org/10.1016/j.dph.2024.03.009

Pagliari, C., Detmer, D., & Singleton, P. (2019). Potential psychological impact of health information technologies. *BMJ Health & Care Informatics, 26*(1), Article e100012. https://doi.org/10.1136/bmjhci-2019-100012

Papazafiropoulou, A. (2022). Telemedicine and diabetes during the COVID-19 era. *Archives of Medical Sciences. Atherosclerotic Diseases, 7*, e131–e135. https://doi.org/10.5114/amsad/150506.PMID:36158062;PMCID:PMC9487796

Patel, M. S., Asch, D. A., & Volpp, K. G. (2012). Wearable devices as facilitators, not drivers, of health behavior change. *JAMA, 313*(5), 459–460. https://doi.org/10.1001/jama.2014.14781

Peters, A. L., Ahmann, A. J., Battelino, T., Evert, A., Hirsch, I. B., Murad, M. H., & Winter, W. E. (2020). Diabetes technology—Continuous subcutaneous insulin infusion therapy and continuous glucose monitoring in adults: An endocrine society clinical practice guideline. *The Journal of Clinical Endocrinology & Metabolism, 105*(5), 1351–1378. https://doi.org/10.1210/clinem/dgaa051

Primack, B. A., Carroll, M. V., McNamara, M., Klem, M. L., King, B., Rich, M., & Nayak, S. (2012). Role of video games in improving health-related outcomes: A systematic review. *American Journal of Preventive Medicine, 42*(6), 630–638. https://doi.org/10.1016/j.amepre.2012.02.023

Rajkomar, A., Dean, J., & Kohane, I. (2019). Machine learning in medicine. *New England Journal of Medicine, 380*(14), 1347–1358. https://doi.org/10.1056/NEJMra1814259

Ramachandran, A., Snehalatha, C., Ram, J., Selvam, S., Simon, M., Nanditha, A., & Johnston, D. G. (2018). Effectiveness of mobile phone messaging in preventing type 2 diabetes by lifestyle modification in men in India: A prospective, parallel-group, randomized controlled trial. *The Lancet Diabetes & Endocrinology, 6*(3), 191–198. https://doi.org/10.1016/S2213-8587(18)30039-7

Real-world diabetes technology: What do we have? Who are we missing? (2022). *Diabetes Technology & Therapeutics* (Study on SES disparities in tech access and HbA1c).

Rizos, E. C., Markozannes, G., Charitakis, N., Filis, P., Stoimeni, A. E., Nørgaard, K., Ntzani, E. E., & Tsilidis, K. K. (2025). Continuous glucose monitoring in type 1 diabetes, type 2 diabetes, and diabetes during pregnancy: A systematic review with meta-analysis of randomized controlled trials. *Diabetes Technology & Therapeutics, 27*(7), 537–552. https://doi.org/10.1089/dia.2024.0599. PMID: 40049630 (Epub 2025 March 6).

Rizzo, A. S., & Koenig, S. T. (2017). Is clinical virtual reality ready for primetime? *Neuropsychology, 31*(8), 877–899.

Rothenberg, G. M., Page, J., Stuck, R., Spencer, C., Kaplan, L., Gordon, I. (2020). Remote temperature monitoring of the diabetic foot: From research to practice. *Federal Practitioner, 3*, 114–124. PMID: 32317847; PMCID: PMC7170172.

Sarani Rad, F., Hendawi, R., Yang, X., & Li, J. (2024). Personalized diabetes management with digital twins: A patient-centric knowledge graph approach. *Journal of Personalized Medicine, 14*(4), 359. https://doi.org/10.3390/jpm14040359. PMID: 38672986; PMCID: PMC11051158.

Selam, J. L. (2010). Evolution of diabetes insulin delivery devices. *Journal of Diabetes Science and Technology, 4*(3), 505–513. https://doi.org/10.1177/193229681000400302. PMID: 20513314; PMCID: PMC2901025.

Shen, Y., Zou, X., & Hu, G. (2024). Digital technology in the management and prevention of diabetes. *Frontiers in endocrinology* [Editorial]. https://pmc.ncbi.nlm.nih.gov/articles/pmc11540762

Shickel, B., Tighe, P. J., Bihorac, A., & Rashidi, P. (2017). Deep EHR: A survey of recent advances in deep learning techniques for electronic health record (EHR) analysis. *IEEE Journal of Biomedical and Health Informatics, 22*(5), 1589–1604. https://doi.org/10.1109/JBHI.2017.2767063

Shomali, M. (2024). Equity in digital diabetes care: Overcoming socioeconomic and geographic barriers. *Journal of Diabetes & Metabolic Disorders, 23*(1), 12–19. https://doi.org/10.1007/s40200-024-01112-0

Siminerio, L. M., Albright, A., Fradkin, J., Gallivan, J., McDivitt, J., Rodríguez, B., et al., (2018). The national diabetes education program at 20 years: Lessons learned and plans for the future. *Diabetes Care, 2*, 209–218. https://doi.org/10.2337/dc17-0976. Erratum in: Diabetes Care. 2018 May;41(5):1116. https://doi.org/10.2337/dc18-er05b. PMID: 29358463; PMCID: PMC5780052.

Singh, N., Armstrong, D. G., & Lipsky, B. A. (2023). Preventing diabetic foot ulcers: Risk factors, strategies, and innovations. *The Lancet Diabetes & Endocrinology, 11*(2), 95–104. https://doi.org/10.1016/S2213-8587(23)00011-3

Sung, C., Chung, C. H., Lin, F. H., Chien, W. C., Sun, C. A., Tsao, C. H., & Weng, C. E. (2022). Risk of cardiovascular disease in patients with alcohol use disorder: A population-based retrospective cohort study. *PLoS ONE, 17*(10), Article e0276690. https://doi.org/10.1371/journal.pone.0276690.PMID:36282879;PMCID:PMC9595521

Tan, T. E., Wong, T. Y. Diabetic retinopathy: Looking forward to 2030. *Front Endocrinol (Lausanne), 13*, 1077669. https://doi.org/10.3389/fendo.2022.1077669. PMID: 36699020; PMCID: PMC9868457.

Tang, Y., Shi, Y., Fan, Z. (2023). The mechanism and therapeutic strategies for neovascular glaucoma secondary to diabetic retinopathy. *Front Endocrinol (Lausanne), 14*, 1102361. https://doi.org/10.3389/fendo.2023.1102361. PMID: 36755912; PMCID: PMC9900735.

Tang, L., Chang, S. J., Chen, C.-J., & Liu, J.-T. (2020). Non-Invasive blood glucose monitoring technology: A review. *Sensors, 20*(23), 6925. https://doi.org/10.3390/s20236925

Tchero, H., Kangambega, P., Briatte, C., Brunet-Houdard, S., Retali, G. R., & Rusch, E. (2019a). Clinical effectiveness of telemedicine in diabetes mellitus: A meta-analysis of 42 randomized controlled trials. *Telemedicine Journal and E-Health, 7*, 569–583. https://doi.org/10.1089/tmj.2018.0128. PMID: 30124394 (Epub 2018 August 20).

Tchero, H., Kangambega, P., Lin, L., Mukisi-Mukaza, M., Brunet-Houdard, S., Retali, G. R., & Rusch, E. (2019b). Clinical effectiveness of telemedicine in diabetes foot care: A systematic review and meta-analysis. *BMJ Open Diabetes Research and Care, 7*(1), Article e000565. https://doi.org/10.1136/bmjdrc-2018-000565

Topol, E. (2019a). *Deep medicine: How artificial intelligence can make healthcare human again.* Basic Books.

Topol, E. J. (2019b). High-performance medicine: The convergence of human and artificial intelligence. *Nature Medicine, 25*(1), 44–56. https://doi.org/10.1038/s41591-018-0300-7

Usability of medical devices for patients with diabetes who are visually impaired or blind. (2016). *Journal/Report, Issue* (Study showing insulin pumps with audio, tactile feedback etc.).

van den Berg, M., Sherrington, C., Killington, M., Smith, S. T., & Bongers, B. (2020). Digital physiotherapy: Technologies for rehabilitation and improved movement analysis. *Physical Therapy Reviews, 25*(1), 26–32. https://doi.org/10.1080/10833196.2020.1720113

Veinot, T. C., Mitchell, H., & Ancker, J. S. (2018). Good intentions are not enough: How informatics interventions can worsen inequality. *Journal of the American Medical Informatics Association, 25*(8), 1080–1088. https://doi.org/10.1093/jamia/ocy052

Ventola, C. L. (2014). Medical applications for 3D printing: Current and projected uses. *Pharmacy and Therapeutics, 39*(10), 704–711. https://www.ncbi.nlm.nih.gov/pmc/articles/PMC4189697/

Veras, M., Labbé, D. R., Furlano, J., Zakus, D., Rutherford, D., Pendergast, B., et al. (2023). A framework for equitable virtual rehabilitation in the metaverse era: Challenges and opportunities. *Front RehabilSci., 4*, 1241020. https://doi.org/10.3389/fresc.2023.1241020.PMID:37691912; PMCID:PMC10488814

Verma, N., Mehta, R., & Kapoor, D. (2022). Role of artificial intelligence in personalized diabetes management. *Frontiers in Endocrinology, 13*, Article 857940. https://doi.org/10.3389/fendo.2022.857940

Vettoretti, M., Cappon, G., Facchinetti, A., Sparacino, G. (2020). Advanced diabetes management using artificial intelligence and continuous glucose monitoring sensors. *Sensors (Basel), 20*(14), 3870. https://doi.org/10.3390/s20143870. PMID: 32664432; PMCID: PMC7412387.

Wang, L., Pedersen, P. C., Strong, D. M., Tulu, B., Agu, E., & Ignotz, R. (2015). Smartphone-based wound assessment system for patients with diabetes. *IEEE Transactions on Biomedical Engineering, 2*, 477–488. https://doi.org/10.1109/TBME.2014.2358632. PMID: 25248175 (Epub 2014 September 17).

Wang, Y., Min, J., Khuri, J., Xue, H., Xie, B, Kaminsky, A. L., & Cheskin L. J. (2020). Effectiveness of mobile health interventions on diabetes and obesity treatment and management: systematic review of systematic reviews. *JMIR Mhealth Uhealth 8*(4):e15400. https://doi.org/10.2196/15400. PMID: 32343253; PMCID: PMC7218595.

Wang, F., Mao, Y., Wang, H., Liu, Y., & Huang, P. (2022). Semaglutide and diabetic retinopathy risk in patients with type 2 diabetes mellitus: A meta-analysis of randomized controlled trials. *Clinical Drug Investigation, 42*(1), 17–28. https://doi.org/10.1007/s40261-021-01110-w. PMID: 34894326 (Epub 2021 December 11).

Wang, E., Zhu, H., Liu, R., Liu, Y., & Liu, J. (2020b). Application of wearable technology in clinical healthcare: A systematic review. *BMC Medical Informatics and Decision Making, 20*, 112. https://doi.org/10.1186/s12911-020-01100-6

Wang, Y., Kung, L., & Byrd, T. A. (2020c). Big data analytics: Understanding its capabilities and potential benefits for healthcare organizations. *Technological Forecasting and Social Change, 126*, 3–13. https://doi.org/10.1016/j.techfore.2015.12.019

Willis, M., Riley-Doucet, C., & Ferguson, C. (2021). Barriers to digital health adoption among people with diabetes: A qualitative study. *Journal of Diabetes Science and Technology, 15*(3), 662–669. https://doi.org/10.1177/1932296820951049

World Health Organization. (2021a). *Diabetes*. https://www.who.int/news-room/fact-sheets/detail/diabetes

World Health Organization. (2021b). *Global report/guidelines on diabetes care and digital health.*

World Health Organization. (2021c). Global strategy on digital health 2020–2025. https://www.who.int/publications/i/item/9789240020924

World Health Organization. (2022a). *Global report on diabetes*. https://www.who.int/publications/i/item/9789241565257

World Health Organization. (2022b). *Global strategy on digital health 2020–2025*. https://www.who.int/publications/i/item/9789240020924

World Health Organization (WHO). (2023). *Global strategy on digital health 2020–2025*. https://www.who.int/publications/i/item/9789240020924

Wu, Y., Zhang, X., Lin, Z., & Liu, Y. (2024). Smart wearable technologies for diabetic foot monitoring: A systematic review. *Sensors, 24*(3), 842. https://doi.org/10.3390/s24030842

Chapter 13
Assisted Devices and Daily Life Adaptations in Diabetes

Ushasi Das, Dhiman Roy, Sudarshan Singh, and Sanchita Mandal

Abstract Diabetes mellitus (DM) comes with an inability to bear significant economic burden of health care. It is a fast-growing outbreak that covers 537 million individuals all over the globe aged between 20 and 79. The prevention of complications is based on early detection, timely treatment, and continued management. Lifestyle changes (self-monitoring, frequent exercise, weight loss, smoking rate, nutrition education, and mental support) were among the core strategies. The innovative technology insulin pumps, continuous glucose monitors, smart insulin pens allow the patients to manage their illness more precisely and stay independent. These tools, along with wearables and Smartphone applications, will help in the ease of gathering data and increase security, which will help reduce anxiety and increase the quality of life. The developments transform care at a personal level but there is still a challenge—the devices fail, cost is high, and people are not as digital as they should be. Discussed in this chapter, artificial intelligence has a potential of proactive and customized interventions in eight fields: diagnostic imaging, health monitoring, predictive modeling, public health, lifestyle management, clinical decision support, diabetes treatment, and patient engagement. AI results in the provision of specific care that positively impacts the outcome and the quality of life.

Keywords Diabetes · Assisted devices · AI · Lifestyle management · Individualized treatment

U. Das · D. Roy · S. Mandal (✉)
Department of Pharmaceutical Technology, Jadavpur University, Jadavpur, India
e-mail: smandal.pharmacy@jadavpuruniversity.in

S. Singh
Office of Research Administration, Chiang Mai University, Chiang Mai, Thailand

Faculty of Pharmacy, Chiang Mai University, Chiang Mai, Thailand

K. Adhikary et al. (eds.), *Healing Beyond Blood Sugar*,
https://doi.org/10.1007/978-981-95-8946-3_13

13.1 Introduction

Diabetes mellitus is a chronic metabolic disease that is characterized by persistent elevation of blood glucose due to insulin deficiency (lack of insulin production), insulin resistance or both. These are Type 1 diabetes mellitus (T1DM) (DiMeglio et al. 2018) and Type 2 diabetes mellitus (T2DM) (Kahn, 2003) that differ in etiology and pathophysiology. T1DM is an autoimmune disorder that kills the insulin and this leads to the complete deficiency of insulin (Foster et al., 2019). T2DM as a rule is a result of the interaction of insulin resistance and insufficient insulin secretion, and is frequently associated with obesity, age, and lifestyle choices.

Research progress has been directed towards biological and technological therapies until the year 2025. Advancements involve artificial pancreas systems, beta-cell regeneration therapy, and superior devices of insulin delivery including new pumps and continuous glucose monitor systems (CGMs) (Domingo-Lopez et al., 2022). Recent breakthrough therapies are under clinical trial, such as islet-cell therapies like Lantidra, stem-cell-based insulin-producing cell infusions (such as that of Vertex, Zimislecel), and CRISPR-edited stem-cell therapies (such as that of CRISPR Therapeutics, VCTX-211), engineered to avoid immune response. These treatments intend to incorporate the insulin production of the body and minimize or remove the external insulin need. Hybrid closed loop systems, which have automation of insulin delivery on a real time basis based on the glucose reading, have been found to significantly improve glycemic control and quality of life of the patient. Empirical research also comprises of the use of GLP-1 receptor agonists in combination with immune-regulation methodology using regulatory T cells, which have the potential to alter diabetes-treatment trajectories. Diabetes is a significant health concern across the world, which is accompanied by neuropathy, nephropathy, cardiovascular disease, and visual impairment. Inclusively performed management of glucose, medication, lifestyle change, meticulous glucose monitoring, and cutting-edge technology have been seen to effectively maximize the glucose management with minimal complications (Barmanray et al., 2022; Domingo-Lopez et al., 2022; Mandloi et al., 2025).

Effective diabetes care also depends on the use of assistive devices and daily adaptations, which significantly increase the capacity of patients to monitor and manage blood glucose and insulin administration, as well as the overall health level, which consequently leads to the improvement of quality of life (ElSayed et al., 2024a; Grunberger et al., 2021). The most important tools are the continuous glucose monitors (CGMs), insulin pumps, smart insulin pens, blood-glucose meters, and diabetes-management apps (Ambalavanan et al., 2024). Data on real-time glucose is delivered by CGM, which overcomes finger-stick testing and makes the decision in time using subcutaneous sensors. Hybrid closed-loop pumps that have been approved by FDA utilize the CGM data and algorithms to automate the delivery of insulin and obtain optimal glucose levels (Gonzales et al., 2019; Peters et al., 2016). Smart pens are precise dose calculators that take into account carbohydrate consumption and current glucose levels and can be linked to a smartphone application and AI-based wearables which combine data-feed on glucose, insulin, diet, activity, and sleep (Alzghaibi, 2025).

Daily life adaptations are equally crucial to diabetes self-care, addressing the condition's impact on physical and psychosocial functioning. This includes using assistive mobility devices and customized footwear for diabetic neuropathy to minimize foot ulcers and enhance adherence to preventative care. Educational and motivational strategies integrated into care models empower patients in adhering to their treatment regimens effectively (Hernandez-Tejada et al., 2012; Istek & Karakurt, 2016; Shrivastava et al., 2013). Remote monitoring and telehealth can also be used to have 24 h of care by enabling therapists to modify the therapy real time which is especially significant in patients with low mobility or in the remote regions (Benziger et al., 2021). The combination of assisted devices and lifestyle adaptations is vital for effective disease management and prevention of complications in diabetes care. These innovations enable patients to better incorporate treatments into their daily lives, alleviating both physical and emotional strains while promoting autonomy and sustained self-care (Mandloi et al., 2025; Taylor et al., 2023).

Diabetes management will not only involve medicine but also a major change in lifestyles and also through the use of assistive devices. The major changes in the lifestyle consist of healthy food, frequent physical activity, healthy weight, and non-consumption of tobacco, which enhance the quality of life and glycemic control. Glucose spikes may be smoothed by changing meal composition and doing after-meal activities. When used in conjunction with lifestyle changes, assistive devices, like blood-glucose meters, insulin-pumps and AI-created wearables, can offer people real-time feedback and help make informed decisions. Such an interactive practice allows patients to gain power, promote self-management, and collaborate with medical personnel to enhance their health results.

13.2 Overview of Diabetes and the Need for Daily Life Adaptations

Diabetes mellitus type 1 (T1DM) is an autoimmune pancreatic disease that is characterized by the destruction of insulin-producing beta cells. Diabetes is acutely hyperglycemic because of the loss of insulin. T1DM is most commonly diagnosed in children and young adults although it equally affects very young kids and ancient people. The signs that are typical include insatiable thirst, excessive urination, hunger, skin loss, tiredness and blurred vision (ElSayed et al., 2024b). Such symptoms may be severe; therefore the medical staff must address them as soon as possible to avoid such complications as diabetic ketoacidosis. The therapy of T1DM is a life-long dedication and involves replacement of insulin, restricted diet, as well as physical exercise. These measures normalize metabolism and prevent acute and chronic problems. Since T1DM is a complicated condition, the use of daily tools and support appliances is crucial in the effective management of the disease (ElSayed et al., 2024b; Foster et al., 2025). Whereas type 2 diabetes mellitus (T2DM) is a long-term condition where the body fails to use the insulin well, leading to having high blood sugar. It usually arises from resistance to insulin and the inability of the pancreas to produce enough insulin. The disease is common in adults but is being seen more in younger people. Management consists of lifestyle changes and medication to maintain blood sugar levels (Das et al., 2025; Dey et al., 2002 Feb; Galicia-Garcia et al., 2020). Figure 13.1 illustrates the pathophysiology of diabetes mellitus.

Technology has changed the way that DM is treated, deliveries of precise, customizable insulin amounts similar to a pancreas to achieve better blood glucose levels and a reduced risk of low glucose levels. Continuous glucose monitors (CGMs) can deliver real time glucose information, allowing the patient to immediately make adjustments to insulin, diet and activity. These devices are coupled with smartphone apps and other digital tools that support patients to make informed self-management

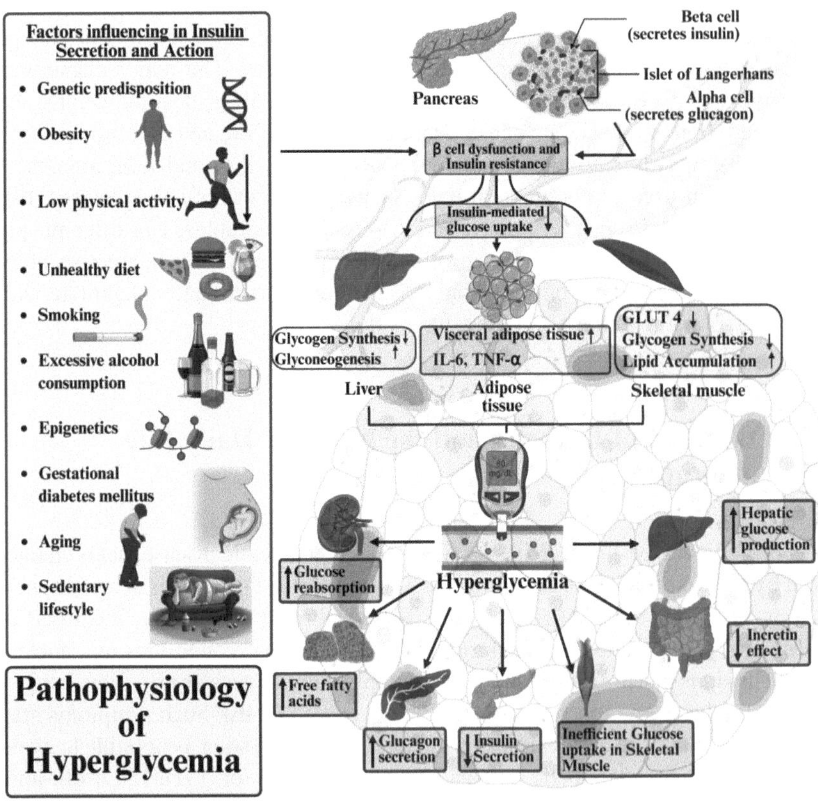

Fig. 13.1 Pathophysiology of diabetes mellitus

choices, maintain treatment adherence and improve quality of life. Additional daily adjustments including carbohydrate counting, individualized exercise, stress management, regular medical visits are important in the glucose control and minimization of complications. Education and psychosocial therapy allow patients to cope with their emotional distress and practice optimal self-care. The combination of technology to assist in managing one's own diabetes and lifestyle modifications form the basis of management of DM which focuses on individual approach to achieve steady glycemic management and overall well-being (Elian et al., 2023; Jacobsen et al., 2023).

13.3 Categories of Assisted Devices in Diabetes

In order to categorize technology in diabetes, devices have been divided into the following broad classes—blood glucose meters, CGM systems, insulin delivery devices, automated insulin delivery (AID) systems, and wearable digital health technologies (Fig. 13.2). Table 13.1 depicts currently used assisted devices for diabetes management. Blood glucose meters are portable devices capable of doing fast spot checks using a sample fingerstick, are available. CGM systems provide a helpful 'review', through a subcutaneous sensor, which shows continuous real time systems that provide trend data and low/high level glucose alarms. Insulin delivery devices such as syringes, pens, insulin pumps and patch pumps are available to allow precise and convenient administration of insulin based on individual needs. Insulin pumps deliver the insulin on a continuous basis very similar to the natural release (Dermawan & Purbayanto, 2022; Elian et al., 2023). Automated Open-Loop to Fully Closed-Loop AID Systems Automated insulin dosing takes user burden out of the loop with CGM-based automated insulin delivery systems using algorithms for dosing, ranging from hybrid systems that still require some user intervention to fully closed-loop systems that are run independently. Designed with the release of smart insulin pens, smartphone applications, and linked devices, wearable and digital health tech improve the data management, dosage calculation, reminder setup, and remote monitoring, making the user more in-control of their condition. These types of devices will enhance precision, convenience, and personalization of diabetes management support (Alzghaibi, 2025; Domingo-Lopez et al., 2022).

13.3.1 Blood Glucose Meters and Monitoring

Blood glucose meters (BGMs) are objects that are an indispensable part of everyday control. These standards state that 95% of BGM results should be within $\pm$ 15% of laboratory value for glucose levels greater than 100 mg/dL, and within $\pm$ 15 mg/dL for glucose levels less than 100 mg/dL. With such accuracy, patients can rely on the measurements to inform insulin dosing and lifestyle choices (Freckmann et al.,

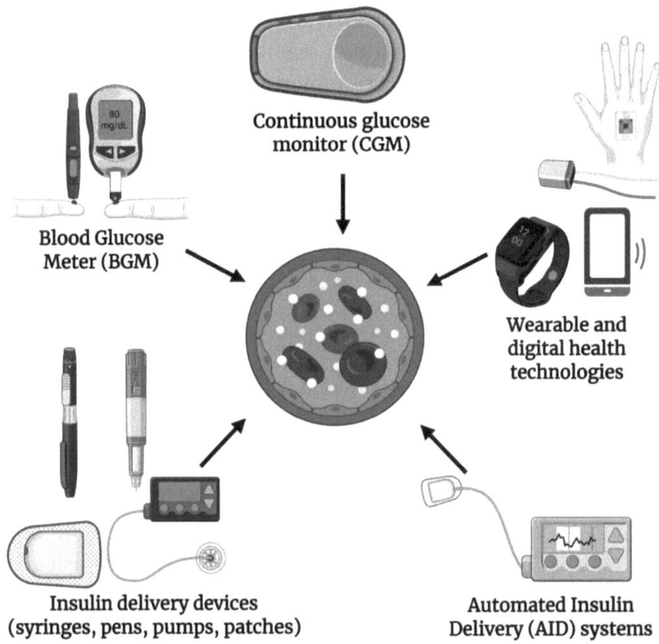

Fig. 13.2 Assisted devices in diabetes

2019b). Modern BGMs are able to give results in seconds with a small sample of blood so that it can be checked frequently. Depending on the device, the best types of meter have an accuracy of 90–98% in the proper range. They have become useful and indispensable due to their ease of use, ease of portability and low cost in situations where CGMs are not available to perform Daphnia bioassay. Regular calibration and careful usage of BGMs help in preventing of low or high blood sugars with the help of reliable information for taking an informed decision (Parkes et al., 2013; Tonyushkina & Nichols, 2009).

13.3.2 Continuous Glucose Monitoring (CGM) Systems

Real-time, continuous glucose monitoring systems measure the glucose concentration in interstitial fluid via body sensors (glucose biosensors). They provide improved trends, hypoglycemia and hyperglycemia alerts, and decrease the frequency of fingerstick glucose testing. FDA guidelines require that CGM results be within $\pm$ 20% of laboratory values for at least 87% of the results, and for greater than 85% of the results to be within $\pm$ 15% of the laboratory results for values $\leq$ 70 mg/dL. The mean of

Table 13.1 Assisted devices used for diabetes management

Category	Description	Performance standards	Clinical / Functional Evaluation	References
Blood glucose meters (BGMs)	Portable electronic devices for spot-checking blood glucose using capillary samples from fingerstick	• Accuracy: 95% of results within ± 15% for > 100 mg/dL and ± 15 mg/dL for < 100 mg/dL • Best devices: 90–98% accuracy • Provide results within seconds with small blood samples	• Quick and reliable self-testing • Supports insulin dosing and dietary adjustments • High portability and low cost • Essential for daily glucose management	Freckmann et al. (2019b) and Tonyushkina and Nichols (2009)
Continuous glucose monitoring (CGM) systems	Real-time systems using subcutaneous/ integrated biosensors to measure interstitial glucose continuously	• FDA standard: 87% readings within ± 20% of lab values; > 85% within ± 15% for ≤ 70 mg/dL • MARD: 9–13% • 88–96% readings in acceptable error grids	• Continuous glucose trend data -Hypo-/ hyperglycemia alerts • Reduced fingerstick testing • Integration with insulin pumps improves glycemic control and quality of life	Freckmann et al. (2019b) and Klonoff et al. (2025)
Insulin delivery devices (syringes, pens, pumps, patches)	Devices for administering insulin accurately and conveniently based on dosage needs	• Syringes and pens: Common for subcutaneous delivery • Pens: High-dose accuracy and user-friendly • Pumps (CSII): ± 5% bolus accuracy; > 95% within ± 15% target -Patches: Non-invasive, adhesive insulin delivery	• Controlled, consistent insulin release • Mimics physiological insulin profile • Enhances flexibility, reduces hypoglycemia. • When integrated with CGM/AID, improves glycemic control	Yang et al. (2025), Freckmann et al. (2019a), and Borot et al. (2014)

(continued)

Table 13.1 (continued)

Category	Description	Performance standards	Clinical / Functional Evaluation	References
Automated insulin delivery (AID) systems	Closed-loop or hybrid-loop systems linking CGM, insulin pump, and algorithm-based dosing	• Algorithms: "Treat-to-target" (100–120 mg/dL) or "treat-to-range" (112.5–160 mg/dL). • Adjusts basal rate every 5–10 min. • Safety thresholds to prevent overdosing	• Reduces hypo-/hyperglycemia events • Increases "time-in-range." -Personalizable parameters (e.g., insulin-to-carb ratio) • Reduces user burden and enhances life quality	Lakshman et al. (2023) and Sherr et al. (2022)
Wearable and digital health technologies	Smart digital and sensor-based technologies (smartwatches, trackers, smartphone apps) for real-time monitoring and data analytics	• Include sensors for glucose, heart rate, and activity • Noninvasive CGMs: MARD ~ 9–13% • Digital platforms for reminders, remote alerts, and telemedicine connections	-Data-driven personalization • Improved medication adherence and self-management • Real-time health analytics and remote monitoring -Support comprehensive diabetes and lifestyle management	Alzghaibi (2025), Reiterer et al. (2016), and Conway and Kelechi (2017)

the relative differences (MARD), one of the most important precision measures, is found to usually be between 9 and 13%. Clinical studies show 88–96% of the sensor readings fall within acceptable error grids which assess both numeric and clinical accuracy (Freckmann et al., 2019b; Klonoff et al., 2025). Although there exist a physiological delay between blood and interstitial glucose, CGMs deliver very valuable dynamic information that contribute to prompt treatment decision. When used with insulin pumps or automated delivery systems, CGMs have revolutionized the way diabetes is managed in terms of metabolic control and quality of life (Cho et al., 2023).

13.3.3 Insulin Delivery Devices (Syringes, Pens, Pumps, Patches)

Insulin delivery devices are necessity to diabetics as they provide accurate insulin delivery to keep the blood sugar levels in perfect. These medical devices include syringes, insulin pumps, insulin pens, and patch pumps. The most common ways that subcutaneous injections are given include pen and syringe injections. Pens—A greater number of pens are used because they offer greater convenience with dosage accuracy, especially among people with limited dexterity (Yang et al., 2025). Continual subcutaneous insulin (CSII) is an insulin pump. They allow a basal insulin background and the ability to program for the bolus dosing closely mimicking the natural insulin secretion. Studies have demonstrated pump bolus accuracy of ± 5% target doses with more than 95% boluses within ± 15% target doses. The timing of the bolus will change depending on the model, but once the device parameters are selected, it will be consistent (Freckmann et al., 2019a). Patch pumps provide another non-invasive alternative where insulin is delivered through disposable patches applied to the skin. Although there are no regulatory standards for accuracy when dealing with pumps, the performance data indicate a high level of accuracy that is compatible with other systems. Newer insulin regimen delivery systems have provided more flexibility for treatment, better glycemic control and reduced hypoglycemia. Integrating such devices with continuous glucose monitors and automated insulin delivery systems further integrates and improves management so patients can achieve more aggressive glucose goals and have an improved quality of life (Borot et al., 2014; Lingen et al. 2023).

13.3.4 Automated Insulin Delivery (AID) Systems

Automated Insulin Delivery (AID) systems are a combination of continuous glucose monitoring (CGM) with insulin pumps and smart algorithms that will automatically adjust insulin. Their goal is to maintain blood glucose within the target range reducing both glucose high and glucose low events. The common treatments available in an AID system are the treat-to-target algorithm that targets blood glucose levels around 100–120 mg/dl (5.6–6.7 mmol/L), and the treat-to-range algorithm that targets blood glucose levels between 112.5–160 mg/dl (6.3–8.9 mmol/L). The algorithms spend as much time as possible in range. The system adjusts basal insulin at 5–10 min intervals based on real-time CGM readings and/or may give automated correction boluses if it is anticipated that the glucose level will rise above certain thresholds such as 180 mg/dL (10.0 mmol/L) (Lakshman et al., 2023; Sherr et al., 2022). Safety threshold restricts the minimum basal and bolus doses to avoid overdosing. These include clinical studies that demonstrate AID systems enhance glycemic control, increase time in range and reduce hypoglycemia. Users can individualize parameters such as insulin to carbohydrate ratio and active insulin time according to user needs. While AID technology has lots of advantages, it requires proper configuration and the involvement of the end user. Physicians need to be aware of device settings in order to aid patients in optimizing therapy and improving outcomes. AID systems make significant progress in terms of improving the quality of life and glucose control in diabetes patients (Expert et al., 2023).

13.3.5 Wearable and Digital Health Technologies

Digital and wearable health technologies are increasingly becoming a growing group of assistive devices used to enhance the accuracy, convenience, and patient participation in the care of diabetes. These are, of course, wearables such as smart watches, fitness trackers, smartphone-connected devices that take an average of their data and analyse them in real time. Especially non-invasive wearable glucose sensors are of high importance. Current CGMs have MARD of 9–13%, which is clinically acceptable (Domingo-Lopez et al., 2022; Reiterer et al., 2016). Other sensors monitor heart rate, activity, and other critical health metrics, though, provide a comprehensive picture of health for the management of diabetes. While the only smartwatches or rings with glucose sensors that are currently available are those that do not get into the fasting glucose category as they are solely for activity and wellness analysis, there are many options out there for those that are looking for digital activity and wellness information. Over four in five users judge the data to be trustworthy and certain about its data's accuracy. Many of these devices are accompanied by a digital platform, which provides dose-calculation tools, reminders, current event notifications, telemedicine tools, etc. Digital data from these devices thus helps to improve medication compliance and individualized treatment. Some new non-intrusive techniques are still affected by calibration and accuracy problems. Overall, digital and wearable health technologies are essential in terms of continuous monitoring, timely action, and a better glucose control to support a better quality of life (Alzghaibi, 2025; Conway & Kelechi, 2017).

13.4 Machine Learning and Artificial Intelligence for Diabetes

Machine learning (ML) and artificial intelligence (AI) is changing how we care for people with diabetes by offering personalized data driven solutions. Machine Learning (ML) algorithms comb through intricate mountain ranges of data held from electronic health records, continuous glucose monitors (CGMs), wearable and patient histories to look for patterns, forecast potential-risk, and personalize treatment. Typical age-based models such as logistic regression and random forests calculate the risk of diabetes with a body mass index, fasting glucose, and family history, which allow early disease recognition (Luo et al., 2025; Tahir et al., 2025). Further, deep learning is used to improve CGM accuracy by predicting glucose concentration several hours in advance, well in time for a closed-loop control. Recent work on automated insulin delivery systems (AIS) that integrates decellularized data from continuous glucose monitoring (CGM) with pumps using convolutional neural networks has caused a decrease in HbA1c and hypoglycemia (Ellahham, 2020). Further, AI does a fine job at diagnosing diabetic retinopathy with retinal image analysis being comparable to ophthalmologists, particularly in under-privileged regions. With respect to prediction tasks, BERT-style transformer models are used to predict the risk of cardiovascular and neuropathy by pooling together the wearable data and clinical data. Technology is also used to ration resources by predicting risk of hospitalization and targeting high-risk patients. However, challenges still need to be addressed, such as the general ability of the model, privacy concerns, as well as the integration of AI in the clinical workflow. Nevertheless, ML and AI constitute a paradigm shift within the diabetes treatment, providing predictive information, automatic complicated processes, and providing direction to individual medicine to enhance the quality of life and reduce complications (Table 13.2). With more being done to improve these tools, these all promise management of Diabetes to be more accessible, efficient, and effective across the world (Adetunji & Evah 2022; Rigla et al., 2018).

13.5 Psychosocial and Quality-Of-Life Aspects

A vital part of comprehensive care, the psychosocial and quality-of-life aspects of diabetes management have a substantial impact on treatment results and emotional well-being. Significant psychological costs, such as emotional anguish, worry, and despair, are brought on by having diabetes and can impede treatment compliance and glucose control. Significant psychological anguish affects around 40% of diabetics, which makes managing their condition more difficult (Vlahovic et al., 2025). Due to difficulties and psychosocial pressures, emotional well-being and social functioning are two aspects of quality of life that are frequently poorer in people with diabetes than in healthy people. In order to meet these demands, foster resilience, and enhance health outcomes in diabetes care, multidisciplinary approaches—such as psychological therapy and regular evaluations for psychological distress—are crucial (Table 13.3) (Davies, 2022).

Table 13.2 List of AI/ML based models used to detect, predict, treat and mange diabetes and its complications

Model type	Application	Dataset used	Performance metrics	Notable techniques/ notes	References
Support Vector Machine (SVM), K-Nearest Neighbors (KNN), Decision Tree (DT)	Diabetes prediction and classification	Pima Indian dataset, LMCH dataset	Accuracy ~ 0.79 to 0.97; RMSE for regression tasks	Hyper parameter tuning, polynomial regression preprocessing, ensemble approaches	Peerbashab et al. (2023) and Feng et al. (2023)
Extreme Gradient Boosting (XGBoost), Random Forest (RF)	Diabetes risk prediction and classification	Pima Indian dataset, RTML dataset	Validation accuracy 0.85–0.87, AUC ~ 0.92–0.94	Grid search optimization, ADASYN for imbalanced data	Breiman (2001) and Sabejon et al. (2023)
Logistic Regression (LR), Bernoulli Naïve Bayes (BNB)	Early detection and classification of Type 2 Diabetes	Clinical datasets	Accuracy: KNN 79.6%, BNB 77.2%	Promising results for early detection	Emon et al. (2021), Joshi and Dhakal (2021), and Peretz et al. (2024)
Multi-layer Perceptron (MLP), Deep Neural Networks (DNN), Convolutional Neural Networks (CNN), Transformer	Diabetic foot risk prediction, insulin dependency prediction	Varied clinical and private datasets	Accuracy range: MLP (0.74–0.92), DNN and CNN ~ 0.70–0.74; AUC max 0.94 for stacking models	Ensemble stacking improves performance, deep learning for image/data analysis	Dayal et al. (2023), El-Bashbishy and El-Bakry (2024), Bmk et al. (2020), Al Sadi and Balachandran (2023); and Bian et al. (2024)
Stacking Ensemble (KNN, Logistic Regression, Decision Tree)	Risk prediction of diabetic complications	Training, validation, test datasets	Accuracy ~ 0.87; AUC ~ 0.94; balanced precision/recall/F1	Strong generalization, well-calibrated models	Attipoe et al. (2025) and Daza et al. (2024)
LightGBM	Prediction of insulin dependency	Clinical datasets (Chinese and others)	High accuracy and clinical applicability	Effective gradient boosting for complex diabetes data	Althobaiti et al. (2024), Rufo et al. (2021), and Wang and Wang (2020)

Table 13.3 Detailed description of psychological factors, social support, quality of life, behavioral aspects for the treatment and management of Diabetes

Aspect category	Specific factors	Description	Impact on diabetes management	Intervention/support approaches	References
Psychological factors	Depression	Common in diabetes, linked to poor glycemic control, increased complications, decreased QoL	Impairs medication adherence, coping, and self-care	Psychological support, counseling, antidepressants	Young-Hyman et al. (2016) and Chen et al. (2024a)
	Anxiety and diabetes distress	Emotional response to diabetes-related challenges: fear, worry, frustration, burnout	Increases emotional burden, negatively affects self-management	Cognitive behavioral therapy (CBT), education, social support	Rechenberg et al. (2017)
	Cognitive dysfunction	Subtle to severe cognitive impairment affecting management	Reduces treatment adherence and self-care capacity	Screening and tailored care strategies	Beverly et al. (2016)
Social support	Family intimacy and adaptability	Quality of family relationships impacts diabetes control and emotional well-being	Positive family support improves outcomes and adherence	Family education, involving family in care plans	Chen et al. (2024)
	Social relationships	Social isolation and reduced social skills affect well-being	Lack of support worsens psychological distress and QoL	Social engagement programs, peer support groups	Liu (2023)
Quality of life domains	Physical functioning	Diabetes leads to reduced physical capacity and complications	Poor physical health decreases overall QoL	Physical therapy, exercise programs	Aarthy et al. (2021)
	Emotional well-being	Diabetes-related stress and emotional instability	Lowered self-esteem, increased depression and anxiety	Mental health interventions, psychoeducation	Kalra et al. (2018)

(continued)

Table 13.3 (continued)

Aspect category	Specific factors	Description	Impact on diabetes management	Intervention/support approaches	References
	Social and occupational impact	Restrictions from diabetes affect social life and work	Financial burden, limited mobility, reduced social participation	Vocational counseling, financial support services	Bhat et al. (2020)
Behavioral aspects	Medical coping strategies	Strategies like confrontation, submission, and avoidance influence psychological adjustment	Negative coping linked with worse depression and QoL	Coping skills training, motivational interviewing	Chen et al. (2024)
Psychological interventions	Psychotherapy and education	Addressing psychological needs to improve adherence and well-being	Improves metabolic control and quality of life	Psychotherapy (CBT, family therapy), diabetes self-management education	Liu (2023) and Kalra et al. (2018)

13.5.1 Impact on Various Populations (Children, Elderly, Pregnancy, Psychiatric Conditions)

Psychosocial factors and quality of life issues contribute significantly to the management of diabetes in all age groups from children and teens, to older adults, to pregnant women and those with mental health conditions. Young patients are known to experience greater distress, anxiety and emotional burden linked to diabetes than adults and parent rates of anxiety can be as high as 23–55. Managing diabetes on a day-to-day basis is challenging to this age group and may take a toll on family relationship, school performance, and social life. In the aged population, there are physical comorbidities, cognitive impairment, and social isolation contributing to psychological stress, and it is becoming more difficult to self-care and monitor blood sugar levels (Young-Hyman et al., 2016). Pregnant women have unique concerns about their baby's health with strict glucose monitoring that has been shown to increase anxiety and decrease the quality of life (Association AD, 2018). People with psychiatric disorders such as depression, anxiety or schizophrenia are more likely to have diabetes, while their mental health issues often result in lack of adherence to self-management and they are likely to have poorer glycemic control (Rechenberg et al., 2017). Diabetes distress including emotional strain, regimen troubles, social pressures, and strained health-care relationships is common and associated with increased HbA1c level, cardiovascular risk and mortality. Quality of life is also determined by age, gender, education, social support, and co-morbidity. Particularly women have reported more emotional stress and depression associated with diabetes. Cognitive-behavioral therapy, stress management, motivational interviewing and family support can help to enhance mental health, adherence and clinical outcomes. Routinely screening for psychological distress and including mental healthcare services in diabetes management is essential to full management. Taking care of these psychosocial aspects will make not only better blood-sugar control but also better well-being, drawn attention to the need of patient-centered multidisciplinary care that is tailored to the diversity of the demands of individuals with diabetes (Beverly et al., 2016; Park et al., 2024).

13.5.2 Device Satisfaction and Barriers to Technology Use

Device satisfaction and technology barriers exert a large influence on the quality of life of people with diabetes. While there is state-of-the-art devices that can improve glucose control, such as CGM and insulin pump with automated delivery systems, people are not pleased with them depending on the complication, size, and ease of use of the device. Satisfaction is increased for integrated, automated systems, and many of them report easier daily living and more engagement in self-care. Clear health literacy and good patient education are the keys to good technology experiences; otherwise, frustration can result in device abandonment (Tanenbaum et al., 2017; Young-Hyman et al., 2016). Barriers are present at various levels. Sensors can potentially cause distress through skin irritation, alarm fatigue and the psychological burden of living with this amount of data that seems never-ending. Walking into a school cafeteria or mall, and seeing children at different ages eating will show that younger kids far more meaningfully than their original counterparts that have trouble with all the devices that children prefer. Technical restrictions like signal loss, calibration and maintenance are also a problem here and systemic barriers, such as inequitable access to care, and inconsistent coverage of insurance. Surveys indicate moderate levels of distress with every type of device, and it can be seen that technology does not ease or aggravate emotional burden—but positive attitudes increase device usage. Importantly, it is suggested that even moderate distress may increase HbA1c by about 0.5 standard deviations, and, thus, is clinically meaningful. Tackling these psychosocial and practical barriers with targeted education, continuing support, improved device design, and equitable access to devices is important to ensuring that the benefits of technology are maximized, satisfaction is increased, and clinical outcomes and quality of life for people with diabetes are improved (Hackett & Steptoe, 2016; Villaécija et al., 2023).

13.6 Daily Life Adaptations and Self-Management Strategies

Daily life adaptations and self management strategies are the key to a successful diabetes control and overall well being. Main habits like a balanced diet where blood glucose is regulated moderate amounts of carbohydrate meals, consumption of high amounts of vegetables, lean protein and low amounts of sugars, saturated fats. Exercising, a moderate level of exercise (such as walking) for 30 min most days of the week, lowers serum glucose, improves sensitivity to insulin, reduces cardiovascular risk and will elevate mood (Ahmad & Joshi, 2023; Bus et al. 2024). Early detection of high blood glucose level by using monitoring devices or CGMs leads to frequent decision-making and proper tools can be used to make a change in this decision. Violating the medication and insulin regimens metabolic stability is maintained through taking medications and insulin as prescribed. Additionally, reducing stress, sleeping a good amount of hours, and taking breaks while sitting for long periods of time also aid in promoting good health. High-quality care includes consulting providers and attending to doctor appointments that can be individualized. However, information on signs, symptoms and proper foot care practices go a long way toward prevention. Connection and support from a diabetes community offer resilience and motivation. These self-care and lifestyle behaviors enable people to take control of diabetes, improve outcomes, avoid complications and to be happier with their lives (Table 13.4) (Ahmad & Joshi, 2023; Wu et al., 2023).

Table 13.4 Detailed daily life adaptations and self management strategies for the treatment and management of Diabetes

Adaptation/ strategy	Description	Benefits	Examples/actions	References
Healthy diet	Consuming balanced meals, control carbohydrate intake, eating fiber-rich and low-fat foods	Helps control blood glucose, manage weight, reduce risk	Low-carb meals, balanced macros, meal timing	Reynolds and Mitri (2000)
Physical activity	Regular exercise tailored to individual capability	Lowers blood sugar, improves insulin sensitivity, reduces cardiovascular risk	30 min walking, strength training twice a week	Syeda et al. (2023) and Zahalka et al. (2000)
Medication adherence	Taking prescribed medications or insulin as directed	Maintains blood glucose within target range	Following regimen strictly, timing medications	Gow et al. (2024) and Sahoo et al. (2022)
Foot care	Daily inspection and care to prevent infections and ulcers	Prevents complications like foot ulcers and amputations	Clean and moisturize feet, check for wounds	Boulton et al. (2018) and Kumbhar and Bhatia (2024)
Stress management	Techniques to reduce stress	Reduces impact of stress-induced blood sugar spikes	Mindfulness, therapy, adequate rest	Zamani-Alavijeh et al. (2018) and Sharma et al. (2022)
Meal timing and sequencing	Eating carbs earlier in the day, sequencing protein/ vegetables before carbs	Improves glycemic control, reduces blood sugar spikes	Balanced breakfast, postmeal walks	Okami et al. (2022) and Yabe et al. (2019)
Postmeal exercise	Physical activity shortly after meals	Blunts glucose peaks, improves glucose use	30–45 min walk 30 min after eating	Chacko and Signore (2020)
Weight management	Maintaining a healthy weight through diet and exercise	Improves insulin sensitivity and overall glucose control	Calorie control, regular physical activity	Hamdy et al. (2018) and Kurtzhals et al. (2023)
Risk reduction behaviors	Avoiding smoking, limiting alcohol, and other behaviors	Reduces complications and comorbidities	No smoking, moderate alcohol intake	Ahmad and Joshi (2023)

13.6.1 Diet and Physical Activity Adaptations

Adaptation and self-management are necessary to achieve optimal diabetes control and high quality of life. The basis for this is an individual diet and exercise program. The overall standard is a consistent intake of carbohydrates with an emphasis on complex carbs from whole grains, vegetables and legumes along with less simple sugars, processed foods and saturated fat. Medical nutrition therapy often uses carb counting and portion sizes in order to maintain stable glucose levels. Regular physical activity at least 150 min (or 2.5 h) per week of moderate aerobic activity, e.g. walking, cycling, swimming, etc. increases insulin sensitivity, eases weight control, and reduces cardiovascular risks. Resistance training twice weekly is advised to increase muscle mass and uptake of glucose. Despite our inactive (sedentary) lifestyle, spreading small bursts of activity throughout the day—walking breaks, standing desks boosts the health of metabolism and reduces the effects of sedentary lifestyle (Alliston et al., 2024; Bronczek et al., 2021; Yamauchi et al., 2020). Routine blood glucose monitoring is a key component to allow real time changes in diet and exercise. Stress management techniques, stress causes instability in the sugar levels, so mindfulness, meditation, and proper sleep are all beneficial. Alcohol intake needs to be controlled and smoking cessation is highly recommended due to the detrimental effects it has on the vascular system. Foot care, keeping hydrated and regular health checkup are helpful in preventing complications. Understanding the symptoms of hypo- and hyperglycemia makes it possible to act in time. Motivation and adherence are being enhanced by psychological strength, and the support of family, friends and diabetes communities. When a team approach including medical therapy is employed, it provides the most comprehensive approach which is necessary to control blood sugar, prevent complications, and allow one to lead a full and active life (Walker et al., 2020; Weinstock et al., 2020).

13.6.2 Medication Adherence Tools

Self-management and modifications of the daily lifestyle are ways that people with diabetes manage the disease, prevent complications, and improve the quality of life associated with diabetes. A important facet of this effort is medication adherence; lack of adherence increases the risk of hyperglycemia, inpatient admission, and death. Tools and strategies to encourage consistent usage of prescribed oral hypoglycemics and insulin assist the patient in reaching this goal. A major tool is the employment of organized medicine regimens and pointers. The ability to schedule doses to meals, sleep and day activities help to reduce the likelihood of missing doses. Monitoring has been enhanced with the use of digital technology. Smartphone apps provide reminders, dose keeping and refill reminders Research shows that frequent reminders improve adherence levels by 20–30% (Alwatify & Radhi, 2025; Huang et al., 2021; Wabe et al., 2011). Some of the apps use AI to analyze the patterns and provide personalized motivational messages and education to create a behavioral change. Electronic medication dispensers organize doses physically by time and day and provide alerts if the patient misses a dose. They help in timely administration especially for elderly patients or those who have cognitive problems. Studies report effect on adherence as 15–25% and a reduction of medication error. Recorded history of U-200 insulin administration and calculation of U-200 insulin dosage based on glucose and carbohydrate levels so adherence is improved through smart insulin pens. When connected to continuous glucose monitoring (CGM) devices, they transmit information as it happens via providers. These tools have reduced hypoglycemia and glycemic control. Automated insulin delivery systems are a combination of CGM and pumps and provide semi- or fully automated dosing, reducing the burden of injections and specifying the insulin timing with more precision (Wabe et al., 2011). Education is critical in achieving good adherence. Structured diabetes self-management education (DSME) programs teach the patient how medications work, possible side effects and the importance of sticking to the plan. A change of HbA1c of about 0.6 to 1.2% is associated with these programmes (Ahmad & Joshi, 2023; Huang et al., 2021). Motivational counseling and interviewing help patients address issues such as injection anxiety, complicated delivery systems, and depression. The assistance from family, peers, or online communities can help in increasing motivation and accountability and significantly contribute to adherence. Providers can also use telemedicine to monitor patients at home, provide feedback, and intervene when adherence falters quickly, thanks to recent advances in mobile-health. Obstacles to adherence include: poor memory, complicated regimens, side effects, cost, distress or depression associated with diabetes, low health literacy, etc. These need to be treated multi-disciplinarily, specifically. Using validated measurement tools, tools like the Morisky Medication Adherence Scale and store pharmacy refill research can help identify problems before they occur (Moon et al., 2017).

13.6.3 School and Workplace Support (Including Legal and Practical Considerations)

Beyond our health rituals, there are also ways in which we adapt our daily lives, and there are ways in which we manage our own diabetes. They provide critical support structures in the school and employment settings. In such cases, help is needed for arrangements that ensure safety, the best possible control of blood sugar levels and greater quality of life, especially for children, adolescents, and working adults. Children and adolescents with diabetes require individualised health routines in school that allow for easy blood glucose monitoring, insulin administration, dietary management, and management of hypoglycaemic events to take place. Under the Americans with Disabilities Act (ADA) and the Individuals with Disabilities Education Act (IDEA), schools are mandated to accommodate students by making provisions such as access to materials, special places to check blood sugar and give injections, and being able to snack on demand. About 20–25% of diabetic students report intolerance in the form of stigma, bullying, or untrained personnel which has a negative impact on their academic performance and mental health. Thorough training of staff on diabetes care and emergency departments has decreased reports and contributes to inclusivity in the classrooms. Peer education also promotes acceptance and close to prevention of marginalization (Butler et al., 2014; March et al., 2020). The ADA requires such accommodations as time for glucose monitoring, private facilities for urine testing or blood glucose monitoring, flexible scheduling for illness or appointment schedules, and freedom from discrimination in hiring or promotions. One study indicates that around 35% of adult diabetics spend time away from work as a result of either high or low levels of blood glucose, which is why support mechanisms are so important. Diabetes and stress management programs based on wellness and healthy living as well as positive lifestyle changes improve employee health and reduce absenteeism. Stealthy glucose monitors, insulin pumps and other items allow workers to manage their condition without interrupting their work (Arent, 2003). Mental health support is also vital because of the association between workplace stress levels and glycaemic variability. Optimization behaviors that most individuals can adopt are disclosing diabetes needs to supervisors and human resources personnel, asserting one's legal right to accommodations, and using health programmes available through the employer. Flexible work arrangements and remote-work opportunities (those that might have been an important dynamic after pandemic shocks) to provide more opportunities for self-care and decrease exposure to stressors (Wyckoff et al., 2015). Maintaining privacy and confidentiality builds trust and helps to encourage people to disclose their diabetes status without any fear of stigma. And although legal protections vary from one region to the next, they all require non-discrimination and accommodation. Even where there are no laws in place, campaigning for change is needed. Teaching and employer/workplace training programs will promote awareness and understanding, reduce misconceptions and allow supportive action to take place. An integrated care team processed by medical providers, diabetes educator, educators, and occupational health specialists develops effective individualized support plans for all diabetics (Butler et al., 2014; McCarthy et al., 2021).

13.7 Education and Support for Device Use

Educating and supporting the use of diabetic devices is important to good management and optimal outcome for patients. Online courses, webinars, hands-on workshops and other comprehensive training programs enable patients and healthcare providers to confidently use continuous glucose monitors, insulin pumps and smart pens. Studies have determined that structured education increases device adherence, decreases errors, and increases glycemic control. Since diabetes technology changes quickly, sustained learning enables patients to take advantage of the technology for each device and, ultimately, enhance quality of life and clinical outcomes (Akturk & Bindal, 2024; Yoo & Kim, 2023).

13.7.1 Training for Users and Caregivers

Patient education and assistance for diabetes device use are critical for improving patient outcomes and effective self-management. Nkechi Okoye-Metcalf, Ph.D., and endocrinologist Katrina Prosniak at Baylor College of Medicine's Texas Medical Center believe that no device is effective without personalized education, training and support. Programs are interactive and cover various learning styles. They fuse an in-person contact with online tutorials, video conferencing and virtual chat. They also recognize the problems of complicated technology (Akturk & Bindal, 2024). Training programs on specification-based exercise including step by step commissioning, calibration, trouble shooting, alarm management and data interpretation Caregiver training—the parents, family members and school staff are also of vital importance specially the children or the elderly who may require immediate help in times like hypoglycemia. Research has demonstrated that a comprehensive and individualized education increases device adherence, decreases errors and decreases HbA1c by up to 1.1% (Agarwal et al., 2022). The ADA "Making Diabetes Technology Work" program is a continuing education program for healthcare professionals. This training will enable providers to better support their patients using new technologies. Continuing follow-up meant to address changing challenges, reinforce skills and to maximize devices by empowering the patients and caregivers with focused education and resources, diabetes care teams can significantly increase the efficiency of diabetes management, reduce diabetes complications, and improve the quality of life for those affected by diabetes (Agarwal et al., 2022; Kulzer et al., 2018).

13.7.2 Health Care Professional Roles

Healthcare professionals (HCPs) have a key role to play in education and support of diabetes device use in order to bridge the technological and patient self-management aspects of diabetes, to further the goal of better diabetes control. Certified Diabetes Care and Education Specialists (CDCES) and other trained providers are highly important to teaching patients and caregivers how to use CGMs, insulin pumps and smart pens. They provide full training on equipment set-up, calibration, troubleshooting and data interpretation, so that they comfortably manage their technology. HCPs tailor based on individual needs including barriers such as dexterity, health literacy and psychosocial factors (The Role of the Diabetes Care and Education Specialist in the Hospital Setting, 2022). The regular follow-up by diabetes educators is important in sustaining use of the devices, maintaining adherence to therapy, and adjusting therapy in a timely manner. Teams also interface with patients to integrate technology in the daily living and clinical care plans. In hospitals, diabetes care specialists monitor the effective use of these devices and train other staff to help patients effectively. Professionals keep up to date with new devices and guidelines by implementing evidence-based practice. Their role supports patient empowerment supporting them through reducing diabetes distress and quality of life achieved through personalised education and collaborative care. This on-going partnership between HCPs and patients is very important in achieving maximum benefits to diabetes technology and improving clinical outcomes (Hackett & Steptoe, 2016; The Role of the Diabetes Care and Education Specialist in the Hospital Setting, 2022).

13.8 Future Prospective and Conclusion

The use of cutting-edge technology and lifestyle modifications is set to revolutionize the treatment of diabetes in the future. Important advancements include better real-time data analysis and therapy modification, as well as improved customized management using artificial intelligence. Given the growing level of interconnectedness and convenient gadgets, the world is becoming accessible to people and well-monitored. Wearables facilitate ongoing monitoring of the essential metrics, and remote monitoring facilitates proactive healthcare. The other way technology promotes lifestyle transformation is through the provision of digital tools which support and adhere to community. Justice in the accessibility of care by either marginalized group on diabetes care will continue to be a priority. The aim of integrating the state-of-the-art technology and holistic lifestyle modification is to enable patients and enhance health results in most spheres.

New innovative technologies, including automated insulin delivery, AID, systems, continuous glucose monitoring, CGM, smart insulin pens, and wearable devices have revolutionized glucose management. These tools enhance better glycemic control, diminish risk of hypoglycemia and make the management of the disease easier to enable a personalized and responsive therapy. The lifestyle changes, such as improved nutrition and physical activity, and psychosocial interventions, are still imperative in the condition of diabetes management. Their effects are better glycemic control, reduction in cardiovascular and general health and quality of life. Collectively, the strategies would provide the patients with the resources to manage their condition and decrease the potential complications.

References

Aarthy, R., Mikocka-Walus, A., Pradeepa, R., Anjana, R. M., Mohan, V., & Aston-Mourney, K. (2021, September). Quality of life and diabetes in India: A scoping review. *Indian Journal of Endocrinology and Metabolism [Internet], 25*(5), 365–380 [cited 2025 Nov 10]. https://doi.org/10.4103/ijem.ijem_336_21

Adetunji, O., & Evah, P. T. (2022). Developing personalized diabetes management plans using artificial intelligence and machine learning. *World Journal of Advanced Research and Reviews, 27*, 605–624.

Agarwal, S., Simmonds, I., & Myers, A. K. (2022). The use of diabetes technology to address inequity in health outcomes: Limitations and opportunities. *Current Diabetes Reports, 22*(7), 275–281.

Ahmad, F., & Joshi, S. H. (2023, July 5). Self-care practices and their role in the control of diabetes: A narrative review. *Cureus* [Internet], *15*(7), e41409 [cited 2025 Nov 10]. https://www.cureus.com/articles/116262-self-care-practices-and-their-role-in-the-control-of-diabetes-a-narrative-review

Akturk, H. K., & Bindal, A. (2024, October). Advances in diabetes technology within the digital diabetes ecosystem. *JMCP, 30*(10-b Suppl), S7–20.

Al Sadi, K., & Balachandran, W. (2023, December 14). Revolutionizing early disease detection: A high-accuracy 4D CNN model for type 2 diabetes screening in Oman. *Bioengineering* [Internet],*10*(12), 1420 [cited 2025 Nov 10]. https://www.mdpi.com/2306-5354/10/12/1420

Alliston, P., Jovkovic, M., Khalid, S., Fitzpatrick-Lewis, D., Ali, M. U., & Sherifali, D. (2024, June 17). The effects of diabetes self-management programs on clinical and patient reported outcomes in older adults: A systematic review and meta-analysis. *Frontiers in Clinical Diabetes and Healthcare* [Internet], *5* [cited 2025 Nov 9]. https://doi.org/10.3389/fcdhc.2024.1348104/full

Althobaiti, T., Althobaiti, S., & Selim, M. M. (2024, May). An optimized diabetes mellitus detection model for improved prediction of accuracy and clinical decision-making. *Alexandria Engineering Journal* [Internet], *94*, 311–324 [cited 2025 Nov 10]. https://linkinghub.elsevier.com/retrieve/pii/S1110016824002904

Alwatify, S. S. D., & Radhi, M. M. (2025). Diabetes self-management and its association with medication adherence in diabetic patients. *Iranian Journal of War and Public Health, 17*(1), 17–22.

Alzghaibi, H. (2025b). Perspectives of people with diabetes on AI-integrated wearable devices: Perceived benefits, barriers, and opportunities for self-management. *Frontiers in Medicine., 12*, 1563003. https://doi.org/10.3389/fmed.2025.1563003/full

Ambalavanan, J., Isaacs, D., & Lansang, M. C. (2024, June). Diabetes technology: A primer for clinicians. *CCJM* [Internet], *91*(6), 353–360 [cited 2025 Nov 8]. https://doi.org/10.3949/ccjm.91a.23073

Arent, S. (2003). The role of health care professionals in diabetes discrimination issues at work and school. *Clinical Diabetes, 21*(4), 163–168.

Association AD. (2018). 13. Management of diabetes in pregnancy: Standards of medical care in diabetes—2018. *Diabetes Care, 41*(Supplement_1), S137–143.

Attipoe, E. K., Yussiff, A. S., Asante-Mensah, M. G., Tetteh, E. D., & Turkson, R. E. (2025, July 1). An ensemble learning approach for diabetes prediction using the stacking method. *Computer Science and Information Technology* [Internet], *6*(2), 102–111. https://iaesprime.com/index.php/csit/article/view/482

Barmanray, R. D., Kyi, M., & Fourlanos, S. (2022, May 2). Assistive technology for diabetes management: A toolkit. *British Journal of Healthcare Management* [Internet] [cited 2025 Nov 9], *28*(5), 118–121. https://doi.org/10.12968/bjhc.2022.0057

Benziger, C. P., Huffman, M. D., Sweis, R. N., & Stone, N. J. (2021, January 1). The telehealth ten: A guide for a patient-assisted virtual physical examination. *The American Journal of Medicine* [Internet], *134*(1), 48–51 [cited 2025 Nov 7]. https://doi.org/10.1016/j.amjmed.2020.06.015

Beverly, E. A., Ritholz, M. D., Shepherd, C., & Weinger, K. (2016). The psychosocial challenges and care of older adults with diabetes: "Can't do what I used to do; can't be who I once was." *Current Diabetes Reports, 16*(6), 48.

Bhat, N. A., Muliyala, K. P., & Chaturvedi, S. K. (2020, November 10). Psychological aspects of diabetes. *EMJ Diabetics* [Internet], 90–98 [cited 2025 Nov 10]. https://www.emjreviews.com/diabetes/article/psychological-aspects-of-diabetes/

Bian, Q., As'arry, A., Cong, X., Rezali, K. A. B. M., & Ahmad, R. M K. B. (2024, September 11). A hybrid transformer-LSTM model apply to glucose prediction. PLoS ONE [Internet], *19*(9), e0310084 [cited 2025 Nov 10,Kaiser, M. S. (Ed.)]. https://doi.org/10.1371/journal.pone.0310084

Borot, S., Franc, S., Cristante, J., Penfornis, A., Benhamou, P. Y., Guerci, B., et al. (2014). Accuracy of a new patch pump based on a microelectromechanical system (MEMS) compared to other commercially available insulin pumps: Results of the first in vitro and in vivo studies. *Journal of Diabetes Science and Technology, 8*(6), 1133–1141.

Boulton, A., Armstrong, D., Krisner, R., Attinger, C., Lavery, L., Lipsky, B., et al. (2018, October). Diagnosis and management of diabetic foot complications. *Compendia* [Internet], *2*, 1–20 [cited 2025 Nov 11]. https://doi.org/10.2337/db20182-1/144937/Diagnosis-and-Management-of-Diabetic-Foot

Breiman, L. (2001, October). Random forests. *Machine Learning* [Internet], *45*(1), 5–32 [cited 2025 Nov 10]. https://doi.org/10.1023/A:1010933404324

Bronczek, G. A., Soares, G. M., de Barros, J. F., Vettorazzi, J. F., Kurauti, M. A., Marconato-Júnior, E., et al. (2021). Resistance exercise training improves glucose homeostasis by enhancing insulin secretion in C57BL/6 mice. *Science and Reports, 11*(1), 8574.

Bus, S. A., Sacco, I. C. N., Monteiro-Soares, M., Raspovic, A., Paton, J., Rasmussen, A., et al. (2024). Guidelines on the prevention of foot ulcers in persons with diabetes (IWGDF 2023 update). *Diabetes/metabolism Research and Reviews, 40*(3), Article e3651.

Butler, K., Schatz, D., & Hathaway, K. (2014). Workplace checkup: Keeping patients with diabetes employed and safe on the job. *Clinical Diabetes, 32*(1), 44–48.

Chacko, E., & Signore, C. (2020). Five evidence-based lifestyle habits people with diabetes can use. *Clinical Diabetes* [Internet], *38*(3), 273–284 [cited 2025 Nov 10]. https://diabetesjournals.org/clinical/article/38/3/273/32294/Five-Evidence-Based-Lifestyle-Habits-People-With

Chen, L., Li, L., Qiao, K., Qiao, Z., Xiang, Y., Zhou, J., et al. (2024, November 18). Exploring factors influencing the quality of life in diabetes: a network analysis-based study. *Front Psychiatry,* [Internet], *15*, 1431772 [cited 2025 Nov 10]. https://doi.org/10.3389/fpsyt.2024.1431772/full

Chen, W., Cai, P., Zou, W., & Fu, Z. (2024a). Psychiatric adverse events associated with GLP-1 receptor agonists: A real-world pharmacovigilance study based on the FDA Adverse Event Reporting System database. *Frontiers in Endocrinology., 15*, 1330936.

Cho, S. H., Kim, S., Lee, Y. B., Jin, S. M., Hur, K. Y., Kim, G., et al. (2023). Impact of continuous glucose monitoring on glycemic control and its derived metrics in type 1 diabetes: A longitudinal study. *Frontiers in Endocrinology, 14*, 1165471.

Conway, C. M., & Kelechi, T. J. (2017). Digital health for medication adherence in adult diabetes or hypertension: An integrative review. *JMIR Diabetes, 2*(2), Article e20.

Das, U., Mali, S. N., & Mandal, S. (2025, June). Unveiling the ameliorative effects of phyto-selenium nanoparticles (PSeNPs) on anti-hyperglycemic activity and hyperglycemia irradiated complications. *BioNanoScience* [Internet], *15*(2), 231[cited 2025 May 8]. https://doi.org/10.1007/s12668-025-01830-9

Davies, M. (2022, November). Psychological aspects of diabetes management. *Medicine* [Internet], *50*(11), 749–751 [cited 2025 Nov 12]. https://linkinghub.elsevier.com/retrieve/pii/S1357303922002171

Dayal, K., Shukla, M., & Mahapatra, S. (2023, September 20). Disease prediction using a modified multi-layer perceptron algorithm in diabetes. In *EAI endorsed transactions on pervasive health and technology*.

Daza, A., Sánchez, C. F. P., Apaza-Perez, G., Pinto, J., & Ramos, K. Z. (2024). Stacking ensemble approach to diagnosing the disease of diabetes. *Informatics in Medicine Unlocked* [Internet], *44*, 101427 [cited 2025 Nov 10]. https://linkinghub.elsevier.com/retrieve/pii/S2352914823002733

Dermawan, D., & Kenichi Purbayanto, M. A. (2022). An overview of advancements in closed-loop artificial pancreas system. *Heliyon, 8*(11), Article e11648.

Dey, L., Attele, A. S., & Yuan, C. S. (2002). Alternative therapies for type 2 diabetes. *Alternative Medicine Review, 7*(1), 45–58.

DiMeglio, L. A., Evans-Molina, C., & Oram, R. A. (2018, June). Type 1 diabetes. *The Lancet* [Internet],. *391*(10138), 2449–2462 [cited 2025 Nov 9]. https://linkinghub.elsevier.com/retrieve/pii/S0140673618313205

Domingo-Lopez, D. A., Lattanzi, G. H. J., Schreiber, L., Wallace, E. J., Wylie, R., O'Sullivan, J., et al. (2022, June). Medical devices, smart drug delivery, wearables and technology for the treatment of Diabetes Mellitus. *Advanced Drug Delivery Reviews* [Internet], *185*, 114280 [cited 2025 Nov 9]. https://linkinghub.elsevier.com/retrieve/pii/S0169409X22001703

El-Bashbishy, A. E. S., & El-Bakry, H. M. (2024, February 20). Pediatric diabetes prediction using deep learning. *Scientific Reports* [Internet], *14*(1), 4206 [cited 2025 Nov 10]. https://www.nature.com/articles/s41598-024-51438-4

Elian, V., Popovici, V., Ozon, E. A., Musuc, A. M., Fița, A. C., Rusu, E., et al. (2023). Current technologies for managing type 1 diabetes mellitus and their impact on quality of life—a narrative review. *Life, 13*(8), 1663.

Ellahham, S. (2020). Artificial intelligence: The future for diabetes care. *The American Journal of Medicine, 133*(8), 895–900.

ElSayed, N. A., Aleppo, G., Bannuru, R. R., Bruemmer, D., Collins, B. S., Ekhlaspour, L., et al. (2024a, January 1). Diabetes technology: *Standards of care in diabetes—2024. Diabetes Care* [Internet], *47*(Supplement_1), S126–244[cited 2025 Nov 8]. https://diabetesjournals.org/care/article/47/Supplement_1/S126/153939/7-Diabetes-Technology-Standards-of-Care-in

ElSayed, N. A., Aleppo, G., Bannuru, R. R., Bruemmer, D., Collins, B. S., Ekhlaspour, L., et al. (2024b). 2. Diagnosis and classification of diabetes: Standards of care in diabetes—2024. *Diabetes Care* [Internet], *47* [cited 2025 Nov 8]. https://search.ebscohost.com/login.aspx?direct=true&profile=ehost&scope=site&authtype=crawler&jrnl=01495992&AN=174272903&h=RzQY%2BWzXZjsQO08OfJn8jWL9KpJNNCk50nQIi9myXCJ50utkgPSzGQTlCLmrWXbiPLXbpPeQBxyzruIujerXYQ%3D%3D&crl=c

Emon, M. U., Keya, M. S., Kaiser, Md. S., Islam, Md. A., Tanha, T., & Zulfiker, Md. S. (2021). *Primary stage of diabetes prediction using machine learning approaches*. 2021 International Conference on Artificial Intelligence and Smart Systems (ICAIS) [Internet]. Coimbatore, India: IEEE [cited 2025 Nov 10]. pp. 364–367. https://ieeexplore.ieee.org/document/9395968/

Expert, D. C. C. P. G., Chambers, A., Mackay, D., Farnsworth, K., Morrison, A. E., Witteman, H. O., et al. (2023). Do-it-yourself automated insulin delivery: a health-care practitioner user's guide. *Canadian Journal of Diabetes, 47*(5), 389–397.

Feng, C., Zhao, B., Zhou, X., Ding, X., & Shan, Z. (2023, January 8). An enhanced quantum k-nearest neighbor classification algorithm based on polar distance. *Entropy* [Internet], *25*(1), 127 [cited 2025 Nov 10]. https://www.mdpi.com/1099-4300/25/1/127

Foster, T. P., Bruggeman, B. S., & Haller, M. J. (2025). Emerging immunotherapies for disease modification of type 1 diabetes. *Drugs, 85*(4), 457–473.

Foster, N. C., Beck, R. W., Miller, K. M., Clements, M. A., Rickels, M. R., DiMeglio, L. A., et al. (2019, February). State of type 1 diabetes management and outcomes from the T1D exchange in 2016–2018. *Diabetes Technology & Therapeutics* [Internet], *21*(2), 66–72 [cited 2025 Nov 9]. https://doi.org/10.1089/dia.2018.0384

Freckmann, G., Kamecke, U., Waldenmaier, D., Haug, C., & Ziegler, R. (2019a). Accuracy of bolus and basal rate delivery of different insulin pump systems. *Diabetes Technology & Therapeutics, 21*(4), 201–208.

Freckmann, G., Pleus, S., Grady, M., Setford, S., & Levy, B. (2019b). Measures of accuracy for continuous glucose monitoring and blood glucose monitoring devices. *Journal of Diabetes Science and Technology, 13*(3), 575–583.

Galicia-Garcia, U., Benito-Vicente, A., Jebari, S., Larrea-Sebal, A., Siddiqi, H., Uribe, K. B., et al. (2020, August 30). Pathophysiology of type 2 diabetes mellitus. *IJMS* [Internet], *21* (17), 6275 [cited 2024 Jan 22]. https://www.mdpi.com/1422-0067/21/17/6275

Gow, K., Rashidi, A., & Whithead, L. (2024, February). Factors influencing medication adherence among adults living with diabetes and comorbidities: A qualitative systematic review. *Current Diabetes Reports* [Internet], *24*(2), 19–25 [cited 2025 Nov 11]. https://doi.org/10.1007/s11892-023-01532-0

Grunberger, G., Sherr, J., Allende, M., Blevins, T., Bode, B., Handelsman, Y, et al. (2021, June). American Association of clinical endocrinology clinical practice guideline: The use of advanced technology in the management of persons with diabetes mellitus. *Endocrine Practice* [Internet], *27*(6), 505–537 [cited 2025 Nov 8]. https://linkinghub.elsevier.com/retrieve/pii/S1530891X21001658

Gonzales, W. V., Mobashsher, A., & Abbosh, A. (2019, February 15). The progress of glucose monitoring—A review of invasive to minimally and non-invasive techniques, devices and sensors. *Sensors* [Internet], *19*(4), 800 [cited 2025 Nov 8]. https://www.mdpi.com/1424-8220/19/4/800

Hackett, R. A., & Steptoe, A. (2016). Psychosocial factors in diabetes and cardiovascular risk. *Current Cardiology Reports, 18*(10), 95.

Hamdy, O., Ashrafzadeh, S., & Mottalib, A. (2018). Weight management in patients with type 2 diabetes: A multidisciplinary real-world approach. *Current Diabetes Reports* [Internet], *18*(9), 66 [cited 2025 Nov 11]. https://doi.org/10.1007/s11892-018-1030-4

Hernandez-Tejada, M. A., Campbell, J. A., Walker, R. J., Smalls, B. L., Davis, K. S., & Egede, L. E. (2012, July). Diabetes empowerment, medication adherence and self-care behaviors in adults with type 2 diabetes. *Diabetes Technology & Therapeutics* [Internet], *14*(7), 630–634 [cited 2025 Nov 8]. https://doi.org/10.1089/dia.2011.0287

Huang, J., Ding, S., Xiong, S., & Liu, Z. (2021, November 4). Medication adherence and associated factors in patients with type 2 diabetes: A structural equation model. *Frontiers in Public Health* [Internet], *9* [cited 2025 Nov 9]. https://doi.org/10.3389/fpubh.2021.730845/full

Istek, N., & Karakurt, P. (2016). Effect of activities of daily living on self-care agency in individuals with type 2 diabetes. *JDM* [Internet], *6*(4), 247–262 [cited 2025 Nov 8]. https://doi.org/10.4236/jdm.2016.64026

Jacobsen, L. M., Sherr, J. L., Considine, E., Chen, A., Peeling, S. M., Hulsmans, M., et al. (2023). Utility and precision evidence of technology in the treatment of type 1 diabetes: A systematic review. *Communications Medicine, 3*(1), 132.

Joshi, R. D., & Dhakal, C. K. (2021). Predicting type 2 diabetes using logistic regression and machine learning approaches. *International Journal of Environmental Research and Public Health, 18*(14), 7346.

Kahn, S. E. (2003, January). The relative contributions of insulin resistance and beta-cell dysfunction to the pathophysiology of type 2 diabetes. *Diabetologia* [Internet], *46*(1), 3–19 [cited 2025 Nov 9]. https://doi.org/10.1007/s00125-002-1009-0

Kalra, S., Jena, B., & Yeravdekar, R. (2018). Emotional and psychological needs of people with diabetes. Indian Journal of Endocrine Metabolism [Internet], *22*(5), 696 [cited 2025 Nov 10]. https://doi.org/10.4103/ijem.IJEM_579_17

Klonoff, D. C., Gabbay, M., Moon, S. J., & Wilmot, E. G. (2025). Importance of FDA-integrated continuous glucose monitors to ensure accuracy of continuous glucose monitoring. *Journal of Diabetes Science and Technology, 19*(5), 1392–1399.

Kulzer, B., Daenschel, W., Daenschel, I., Schramm, W., Messinger, D., Weissmann, J., et al. (2018). Integrated personalized diabetes management improves glycemic control in patients with insulin-treated type 2 diabetes: Results of the PDM-ProValue study program. *Diabetes Research and Clinical Practice, 1*(144), 200–212.

Kumar, PBM, Perumal, R. S., Nadesh, & Arivuselvan, K. (2020, June). Type 2: Diabetes mellitus prediction using Deep Neural Networks classifier. *International Journal of Cognitive Computing in Engineering* [Internet], *1*, 55–61. https://linkinghub.elsevier.com/retrieve/pii/S2666307420300073

Kumbhar, S., & Bhatia, M. (2024, November). Advancements and best practices in diabetic foot Care: A comprehensive review of global progress. *Diabetes Research and Clinical Practice* [Internet], *217*, 111845 [cited 2025 Nov 11]. https://linkinghub.elsevier.com/retrieve/pii/S0168822724007551

Kurtzhals, P., Kreiner, F., & Bindra, R. S. (2023, September). The role of weight control in the management of type 2 diabetes mellitus: Perspectives on semaglutide. *Diabetes Research and Clinical Practice* [Internet], *203*, 110881 [cited 2025 Nov 11]. https://linkinghub.elsevier.com/retrieve/pii/S0168822723006447

Lakshman, R., Boughton, C., & Hovorka, R. (2023). The changing landscape of automated insulin delivery in the management of type 1 diabetes. *Endocrine Connections* [Internet], *12*(8) [cited 2025 Nov 8]. https://ec.bioscientifica.com/view/journals/ec/12/8/EC-23-0132.xml

Lingen, K., Pikounis, T., Bellini, N., & Isaacs, D. (2023). Advantages and disadvantages of connected insulin pens in diabetes management. *Endocrine Connections* [Internet], *12*(11) [cited 2025 Nov 8]. https://ec.bioscientifica.com/view/journals/ec/12/11/EC-23-0108.xml

Liu, X. (2023, December). Advances in psychological and social aetiology of patients with diabetes. *DMSO* [Internet], *16*, 4187–4194 [cited 2025 Nov 10]. https://www.dovepress.com/advances-in-psychological-and-social-aetiology-of-patients-with-diabet-peer-reviewed-fulltext-article-DMSO

Luo, J., Kumbara, A., Shomali, M., Han, R., Iyer, A., Aleppo, G., et al. (2025). A large sensor foundation model pretrained on continuous glucose monitor data for diabetes management. *NPJ Health Systems, 2*(1), 35.

Mandloi, A., Bisani, K. G., & Verma, R. (2025, February 14). Impact of lifestyle modification on type 2 diabetes outcomes. *Future Health* [Internet], *2*, 184–188 [cited 2025 Nov 9]. https://futurehealthjournal.com/impact-of-lifestyle-modification-on-type-2-diabetes-outcomes/

March, C. A., Nanni, M., Kazmerski, T. M., Siminerio, L. M., Miller, E., & Libman, I. M. (2020). Modern diabetes devices in the school setting: Perspectives from school nurses. *Pediatric Diabetes, 21*(5), 832–840.

McCarthy, M., Vorderstrasse, A., Yan, J., Portillo, A., & Dickson, V. V. (2021). Managing diabetes in the workplace. *Workplace Health Safety, 69*(5), 216–223.

Moon, S. J., Lee, W. Y., Hwang, J. S., Hong, Y. P., & Morisky, D. E. (2017). Accuracy of a screening tool for medication adherence: A systematic review and meta-analysis of the Morisky Medication Adherence Scale-8. *PLoS One, 12*(11), Article e0187139.

Okami, Y., Tsunoda, H., Watanabe, J., & Kataoka, Y. (2022, February). Efficacy of a meal sequence in patients with type 2 diabetes: A systematic review and meta-analysis. *BMJ Open Diabetes Research & Care* [Internet], *10*(1), e002534 [cited 2025 Nov 11]. https://doi.org/10.1136/bmjdrc-2021-002534

Park, H. S., Cho, Y., Seo, D. H., Ahn, S. H., Hong, S., Suh, Y. J., et al. (2024). Impact of diabetes distress on glycemic control and diabetic complications in type 2 diabetes mellitus. *Science and Reports, 6*(14), 5568.

Parkes, J. L., Harrison, B., & Pardo, S. (2013). Are blood glucose meters for home use acceptable for making appropriate diabetes management decisions? *Diabetes Management, 3*(1), 5–9.

Peerbashab, S., Iqbal, Y. M., Praveen, K. P, Surputheen, M. M., & Raja, A. S. (2023, July 24). Diabetes prediction using decision tree, random forest, support vector machine, k-nearest neighbors, logistic regression classifiers. *JOAASR* [Internet], *5*(4), 42–54 [cited 2025 Nov 10]. http://www.joaasr.com/index.php/joaasr/article/view/680

Peretz, O., Koren, M., & Koren, O. (2024, October). Naive Bayes classifier—An ensemble procedure for recall and precision enrichment. *Engineering Applications of Artificial Intelligence* [Internet], *136*, 108972 [cited 2025 Nov 10]. https://linkinghub.elsevier.com/retrieve/pii/S0952197624011308

Peters, A. L., Ahmann, A. J., Battelino, T., Evert, A., Hirsch, I. B., Murad, M. H., et al. (2016, November). Diabetes technology—Continuous subcutaneous insulin infusion therapy and continuous glucose monitoring in adults: An endocrine society clinical practice guideline. *The Journal of Clinical Endocrinology & Metabolism* [Internet], *101*(11), 3922–3937 [cited 2025 Nov 8]. https://doi.org/10.1210/jc.2016-2534

Rechenberg, K., Whittemore, R., & Grey, M. (2017). Anxiety in youth with type 1 diabetes. *Journal of Pediatric Nursing, 32*, 64–71.

Reiterer, F., Polterauer, P., Schoemaker, M., Schmelzeisen-Redecker, G., Freckmann, G., Heinemann, L., et al. (2016). Significance and reliability of MARD for the accuracy of CGM systems. *Journal of Diabetes Science and Technology, 11*(1), 59–67.

Reynolds, A., & Mitri, J. (2000). Dietary advice for individuals with diabetes. In K. R. Feingold, S. F. Ahmed, B. Anawalt, M. R. Blackman, A. Boyce, G. Chrousos, et al. (Eds.), *Endotext* [Internet]. MDText.com, Inc. [cited 2025 Nov 10]. http://www.ncbi.nlm.nih.gov/books/NBK279012/

Rigla, M., García-Sáez, G., Pons, B., & Hernando, M. E. (2018). Artificial intelligence methodologies and their application to diabetes. *Journal of Diabetes Science and Technology, 12*(2), 303–310.

Rufo, D. D., Debelee, T. G., Ibenthal, A., & Negera, W. G. (2021, September 19). Diagnosis of diabetes mellitus using gradient boosting machine (LightGBM). *Diagnostics* [Internet], *11*(9), 1714 [cited 2025 Nov 10]. https://www.mdpi.com/2075-4418/11/9/1714

Sabejon, J. A., Rejas, J. B., Lumacad, G. S., Zarate, R. L., Mendez, E. A. D., & Tinoy, F. M. L. O. (2023). *XGBoost–based analysis of the early–stage diabetes risk dataset*. 2023 International Conference in Advances in Power, Signal, and Information Technology (APSIT) [Internet]. Bhubaneswar, India: IEEE, pp. 19–24 [cited 2025 Nov 10]. https://ieeexplore.ieee.org/document/10201658/

Sahoo, J., Mohanty, S., Kundu, A., & Epari, V. (2022, December 29). Medication adherence among patients of type II diabetes mellitus and its associated risk factors: A cross-sectional study in a tertiary care hospital of Eastern India. *Cureus* [Internet] [cited 2025 Nov 11]. https://www.cureus.com/articles/128559-medication-adherence-among-patients-of-type-ii-diabetes-mellitus-and-its-associated-risk-factors-a-cross-sectional-study-in-a-tertiary-care-hospital-of-eastern-india

Sharma, K., Akre, S., Chakole, S., & Wanjari, M. B. (2022, September 13). Stress-induced diabetes: A review. *Cureus* [Internet] [cited 2025 Nov 11]. https://www.cureus.com/articles/112924-stress-induced-diabetes-a-review

Sherr, J. L., Heinemann, L., Fleming, G. A., Bergenstal, R. M., Bruttomesso, D., Hanaire, H., et al. (2022). Automated insulin delivery: benefits, challenges, and recommendations. A Consensus Report of the joint diabetes technology working group of the European Association for the study of diabetes and the American diabetes association. *Diabetes Care, 45*(12), 3058–3074.

Shrivastava, S. R., Shrivastava, P. S., & Ramasamy, J. (2013, March 5). Role of self-care in management of diabetes mellitus. *Journal of Diabetes Metabolism Disorder* [Internet], *12*(1), 14 [cited 2025 Nov 8]. https://doi.org/10.1186/2251-6581-12-14

Syeda, U. S. A., Battillo, D., Visaria, A., & Malin, S. K. (2023, June). The importance of exercise for glycemic control in type 2 diabetes. *American Journal of Medicine Open* [Internet], *9*, 100031 [cited 2025 Nov 10]. https://linkinghub.elsevier.com/retrieve/pii/S2667036423000018

Tahir, H. N., Ullah, N., Tahir, M., Domnic, I. S., Prabhakar, R., Meerasa, S. S., et al. (2025). Artificial intelligence versus manual screening for the detection of diabetic retinopathy: A comparative systematic review and meta-analysis. *Frontiers in Medicine, 12*, 1519768.

Tanenbaum, M. L., Adams, R. N., Hanes, S. J., Barley, R. C., Miller, K. M., Mulvaney, S. A., et al. (2017). Optimal use of diabetes devices: Clinician perspectives on barriers and adherence to device use. *Journal of Diabetes Science and Technology, 11*(3), 484–492.

Taylor, P. J., Thompson, C. H., Wycherley, T. P., & Brinkworth, G. D. (2023, June). A primary care delivered, technology supported lifestyle program for Type 2 Diabetes Management: An evaluation of changes in metabolic health, feasibility, and acceptability—A pilot interventional study protocol. *Contemporary Clinical Trials Communications* [Internet], *33*, 101152 [cited 2025 Nov 9]. https://linkinghub.elsevier.com/retrieve/pii/S2451865423000984

The Role of the Diabetes Care and Education Specialist in the Hospital Setting. (2022, June 1). *The Science of Diabetes Self-Management and Care, 48*(3), 184–191.

Tonyushkina, K., & Nichols, J. H. (2009). Glucose meters: A review of technical challenges to obtaining accurate results. *Journal of Diabetes Science and Technology, 3*(4), 971–980.

Villaécija, J., Luque, B., Castillo-Mayén, R., Farhane-Medina, N. Z., & Tabernero, C. (2023). Influence of family social support and diabetes self-efficacy on the emotional wellbeing of children and adolescents with type 1 diabetes: A longitudinal study. *Children, 10*(7), 1196.

Vlahovic, B., Jha, V., Stojanovic, V., Vojinovic, T., Dutta, A., Dutta, P., et al. (2025, March 11). Enhancing patient-centered care: Evaluating quality of life in type 2 diabetes management. *PLoS One* [Internet], *20*(3), e0319369 [cited 2025 Nov 12]. https://doi.org/10.1371/journal.pone.0319369

Wabe, N. T., Angamo, M. T., & Hussein, S. (2011). Medication adherence in diabetes mellitus and self management practices among type-2 diabetics in Ethiopia. *North American Journal of Medical Sciences, 3*(9), 418–423.

Walker, R. J., Garacci, E., Campbell, J. A., & Egede, L. E. (2020). The influence of daily stress on glycemic control and mortality in adults with diabetes. *Journal of Behavioral Medicine, 43*(5), 723–731.

Wang, Y., & Wang, T. (2020, May 6). Application of improved LightGBM model in blood glucose prediction. *Applied Sciences* [Internet], *10*(9), 3227. https://www.mdpi.com/2076-3417/10/9/3227

Weinstock, R. S., Aleppo, G., Bailey, T. S., Bergenstal, R. M., Fisher, W. A., Greenwood, D. A., et al. (2020). *The role of blood glucose monitoring in diabetes management* [Internet]. American Diabetes Association (ADA Clinical Compendia Series) [cited 2025 Nov 9]. http://www.ncbi.nlm.nih.gov/books/NBK566165/

Wu, M., Xu, X., Zhao, R., Bai, X., Zhu, B., & Zhao, Z. (2023). Effect of pharmacist-led interventions on medication Adherence and glycemic control in type 2 diabetic patients: A study from the Chinese population. *PPA, 11*(17), 119–129.

Wyckoff, L., Hanchon, T., & Gregg, S. R. (2015). Psychological, behavioral, and educational considerations for children with classified disabilities and diabetes within the school setting. *Psychology in the Schools, 52*(7), 672–682.

Yabe, D., Kuwata, H., Fujiwara, Y., Sakaguchi, M., Moyama, S., Makabe, N., et al. (2019, December). Dietary instructions focusing on meal-sequence and nutritional balance for prediabetes subjects: An exploratory, cluster-randomized, prospective, open-label, clinical trial. *Journal of Diabetes and its Complications* [Internet], *33*(12), 107450 [cited 2025 Nov 11]. https://linkinghub.elsevier.com/retrieve/pii/S105687271930621X

Yamauchi, T., Kamiya, H., Utsunomiya, K., Watada, H., Kawanami, D., Sato, J., et al. (2020). Medical nutrition therapy and dietary counseling for patients with diabetes-energy, carbohydrates, protein intake and dietary counseling. *Diabetology International, 11*(3), 224–239.

Yang, R., Yang, Z., Chi, J., & Zhu, Y. (2025). Insulin delivery devices in diabetes management: Applications and advancements. *Intelligent Pharmacy* [Internet] [cited 2025 Nov 8]. https://www.sciencedirect.com/science/article/pii/S2949866X25000139

Yoo, J. H., & Kim, J. H. (2023). Advances in continuous glucose monitoring and integrated devices for management of diabetes with insulin-based therapy: Improvement in glycemic control. *Diabetes and Metabolism Journal, 47*(1), 27–41.

Young-Hyman, D., de Groot, M., Hill-Briggs, F., Gonzalez, J. S., Hood, K., & Peyrot, M. (2016). Psychosocial care for people with diabetes: A position statement of the American Diabetes Association. *Diabetes Care, 39*(12), 2126–2140.

Zahalka, S. J., Abushamat, L. A., Scalzo, R. L., & Reusch, J. E. B. (2000). The role of exercise in diabetes. In K. R. Feingold, S. F. Ahmed, B. Anawalt, M. R. Blackman, A. Boyce, G. Chrousos et al. (Eds.). *Endotext* [Internet]. MDText.com, Inc. [cited 2025 Nov 10]. http://www.ncbi.nlm.nih.gov/books/NBK549946/

Zamani-Alavijeh F, Araban M, Koohestani HR, Karimy M. The effectiveness of stress management training on blood glucose control in patients with type 2 diabetes. Diabetol Metab Syndr [Internet]. 2018 Dec [cited 2025 Nov 11];10(1):39. Available from: https://dmsjournal.biomedcentral.com/articles/https://doi.org/10.1186/s13098-018-0342-5

Chapter 14
The Psychological and Social Impact of Diabetes on Patients' Lives

Md Abubakar, Ritu Dahiya, Kanika Goyal, Nitesh Kumar, Irshad Khan, Krishna Murti, and Amita Rai

Abstract Diabetes imposes substantial psychological and social burdens that significantly influence patients' overall health outcomes and quality of life. Research consistently demonstrates that the chronic nature of diabetes, coupled with its demanding self-management requirements, contributes to elevated levels of emotional distress, anxiety, and depressive symptoms. Persistent glycemic monitoring, dietary restrictions, and fear of complications often intensify psychological strain, while stigma and reduced social participation further disrupt well-being. Social determinants—including family dynamics, socioeconomic status, workplace pressures, and cultural expectations—play a critical role in shaping patients' coping capacity and treatment adherence. Studies have highlighted that limited social support and perceived isolation are strongly associated with poor metabolic control and an increased risk of burnout. Conversely, structured education programs, peer-support networks, and psychosocial interventions have been shown to enhance

Md Abubakar, Ritu Dahiya, Kanika Goyal—These authors are equally contributed.
Nitesh Kumar, Irshad Khan, Krishna Murti—Second position in contribution.

M. Abubakar · N. Kumar
Department of Pharmacology and Toxicology, National Institute of Pharmaceutical Education and Research, Hajipur, India

R. Dahiya
School of Pharmacy, Lingaya's Vidyapeeth (Deemed to Be University), Faridabad, India

K. Goyal
Ganpati Group of Institutions, Bilaspur, India

I. Khan · K. Murti
Department of Pharmacy Practice, National Institute of Pharmaceutical Education and Research, Hajipur, India

A. Rai (✉)
Department of Pharmaceutical Analysis, National Institute of Pharmaceutical Education and Research, Hajipur, India
e-mail: dramita.rai@niperhajipur.ac.in

K. Adhikary et al. (eds.), *Healing Beyond Blood Sugar*,
https://doi.org/10.1007/978-981-95-8946-3_14

resilience, improve self-efficacy, and promote long-term engagement with treatment plans. Overall, the psychological and social dimensions of diabetes represent central components of disease burden, underscoring the need for integrated care strategies that address emotional health, social context, and clinical management simultaneously.

Keywords Anxiety · Diabetes · Dietary · Insulin and psychosocial

14.1 Introduction

Diabetes mellitus is a chronic metabolic disorder that profoundly influences not only physiological functioning but also the psychological and social dimensions of patients' daily lives. As global prevalence continues to rise, scientific literature increasingly emphasizes that the burden of diabetes extends far beyond glycemic regulation. Studies consistently illustrate that individuals living with diabetes must engage in a demanding and uninterrupted cycle of self-management, including blood glucose monitoring, medication adherence, meal planning, and regular physical activity (Adjaye-Gbewonyo et al., 2025). These daily responsibilities accumulate into a significant cognitive load, contributing to persistent feelings of stress, emotional fatigue, and burnout in self-management. Such psychological strain is now recognized as a central component of the overall disease burden, often influencing clinical outcomes as strongly as biological factors. The emotional consequences of diabetes are multifaceted. Research frequently reports elevated rates of anxiety, depressive symptoms, and diabetes distress among patients across age groups and disease types (Agarwal et al., 2023). These psychological conditions arise from continuous fear of hypoglycaemia, uncertainties regarding long-term complications, and the overwhelming need for strict lifestyle modification. Importantly, empirical evidence highlights a bidirectional relationship between psychological well-being and metabolic stability: poor mental health negatively impacts self-care behaviours, while unstable glycemic patterns can intensify emotional distress. This interplay underscores the importance of routinely assessing mental health as part of comprehensive diabetes care, as untreated psychological challenges may accelerate disease progression and impair long-term quality of life (Alshaikhi et al., 2025).

In addition to emotional strain, diabetes influences multiple aspects of patients' social environments. Family dynamics, peer relationships, work-related pressures, and societal perceptions all play substantial roles in shaping disease experiences. Research indicates that supportive family and community networks can enhance treatment adherence and provide emotional support. In contrast, environments characterized by stigma, misunderstanding, or excessive pressure can heighten stress and reduce confidence in self-management abilities. Socioeconomic circumstances further compound these social challenges; limited financial resources, inadequate access to healthcare, and varying levels of health literacy may restrict an individual's capacity to manage their condition (Ashraf et al., 2024) effectively. These psychosocial inequities contribute to disparities in both mental well-being and metabolic outcomes.

The social burden of diabetes extends into educational and occupational domains as well. Many individuals face difficulties balancing the complex needs of diabetes management with academic expectations or workplace responsibilities. Concerns about discrimination, privacy, and the feasibility of routine glucose monitoring in professional settings may lead to emotional withdrawal or reduced participation in daily activities (Augustin et al., 2022). Over time, these challenges can erode social integration, limit mobility, and diminish overall quality of life. Scholarly work emphasizes that addressing these environmental and social pressures is crucial for optimizing both psychological resilience and metabolic control.

Given these wide-ranging implications, contemporary diabetes care frameworks increasingly advocate for a more holistic approach—one that integrates psychological support, social assessment, and patient-centred communication with traditional biomedical management. The literature underscores the value of cognitive-behavioural interventions, peer support programs, digital mental health tools, and structured education models in mitigating psychological distress and improving social adaptation (Bellass et al., 2021). These multidisciplinary strategies address the emotional, behavioural, and environmental factors that shape patient experiences and play a crucial role in sustaining long-term engagement with therapeutic goals.

This chapter, therefore, aims to comprehensively explore the psychological and social impact of diabetes on individuals' lives, drawing on primary research directions identified in Google Scholar literature. By examining the emotional burden, social determinants, coping mechanisms, and evidence-based psychosocial interventions, the chapter seeks to underscore the need for integrated care models that address the full spectrum of challenges faced by people living with diabetes (Borbjerg et al., 2025). Ultimately, understanding these interconnected dimensions is crucial for enhancing patient well-being, improving treatment effectiveness, and promoting long-term metabolic stability.

14.2 Psychological Impact of Diabetes

Diabetes is not only a physiologic disorder of glucose metabolism but also a chronic condition with profound psychological and social consequences. The ongoing demands of self-management, fear of complications, and the daily presence of symptoms can create sustained emotional strain (Ciarambino et al., 2022). These mental-health challenges both result from and influence diabetes management, producing a reciprocal relationship between psychological state and physical outcomes.

Epidemiology—how common are psychological problems in diabetes?

Extensive reviews and meta-analyses report that mental-health problems are substantially more common among people with diabetes than in the general population. Depression affects a considerable proportion of people with diabetes, with pooled estimates indicating prevalence rates well above community averages (Cicek et al., 2021). Diabetes-specific distress—emotional burden related directly to living with diabetes—is also highly prevalent; systematic reviews find that roughly one-third of patients can experience clinically significant distress, although prevalence varies widely across settings and studies.

14.2.1 Continuous Self-Management Creates Persistent Emotional Strain

Living with diabetes requires daily attention to blood glucose levels, diet, medications, and physical activity, creating a continuous mental workload. Research highlights that the relentless need for self-regulation can lead to emotional exhaustion, frustration, and a sense of being constantly preoccupied with the disease (Dumitrescu et al., 2025). This emotional burden increases during periods of unstable glycemic control or when patients struggle to meet recommended targets.

14.2.2 Elevated Rates of Depression Due to Chronic Disease Stressors

Google Scholar studies consistently show that people with diabetes are significantly more likely to develop depressive symptoms than the general population. The chronic nature of the disease, fear of complications, and limitations imposed on lifestyle contribute to feelings of sadness, hopelessness, and reduced motivation. Depression further complicates diabetes management by impairing decision-making, lowering treatment adherence, and worsening glycemic outcomes (Esubalew et al., 2024).

14.2.3 Diabetes Distress as a Core Psychological Challenge

Diabetes distress is widely recognized in academic literature as a distinct condition that captures the emotional burden related explicitly to managing diabetes. It includes feelings of being overwhelmed by daily tasks, fear of long-term health consequences, and frustration when glycemic targets are not achieved (Flint et al., 2025). This form of distress is highly prevalent and strongly predicts poor self-care behaviours, reduced engagement with treatment, and fluctuating glucose levels.

14.2.4 Anxiety and Fear of Hypoglycaemia Affect Daily Living and Confidence

Research shows that individuals with diabetes often experience heightened anxiety, especially related to unpredictable blood sugar drops. Fear of hypoglycaemia influences daily decisions such as food intake, activity level, travel, and sleep (Hecker et al., 2022). This anxiety may lead to avoidance of exercise, unnecessary overeating, or maintaining higher glucose levels for safety, which undermines long-term metabolic control and affects overall quality of life.

14.2.5 Cognitive and Emotional Fatigue Resulting in Diabetes Burnout

The mental effort required to monitor symptoms, track glucose, and adjust behaviours can lead to cognitive overload and emotional fatigue. Scholarly literature describes "diabetes burnout" as a state where individuals feel detached, tired, and unable to sustain the demands of self-management (Hermanns et al., 2024). This burnout can result in reduced treatment adherence, inconsistent monitoring, and a loss of confidence in disease management.

14.2.6 Stress-Induced Behavioural Changes that Negatively Affect Health

Stress experienced by individuals with diabetes often results in changes in eating habits, sleep patterns, and physical activity levels. Research indicates that stress can trigger emotional eating, sedentary behaviour, irritability, and difficulty following treatment plans. Physiologically, chronic stress elevates cortisol levels, which contributes to insulin resistance and worsens glycemic control, reinforcing the psychological–metabolic cycle (Jafari et al., 2024a).

14.2.7 Body Image Issues and Disordered Eating Risks, Especially in Youth

Google Scholar studies reveal that adolescents and young adults with diabetes, particularly type 1 diabetes, may develop body-image concerns and disordered eating behaviours. Some individuals misuse insulin as a weight-control method, posing severe medical risks (Jafari et al., 2024b). Emotional stress around body weight, food restrictions, and social pressure contributes to these harmful patterns and increases the likelihood of complications.

14.2.8 Reduced Quality of Life Due to Emotional, Physical, and Social Limitations

Diabetes affects multiple aspects of daily life, including work, relationships, physical activity, and leisure. Psychological difficulties such as depression, anxiety, and chronic stress amplify the perception of burden (Jassim et al., 2024). Research shows that many patients feel restricted by dietary rules, fear unpredictable glucose fluctuations, and face worry about long-term health outcomes, all of which diminish their perceived quality of life.

14.2.9 Influence of Social Determinants on Psychological Well-Being

Studies highlight that psychological outcomes in diabetes are strongly shaped by social and environmental factors such as financial strain, limited access to healthcare, family conflict, and lack of social support. Individuals with lower socioeconomic status face additional stress related to medication costs, food insecurity, and restricted access to glucose-monitoring technologies (Javed et al., 2025). These factors intensify emotional distress and hinder effective self-care.

14.2.10 Bidirectional Relationship Between Psychological State and Diabetes Outcomes

Evidence from scholarly literature shows that psychological problems such as depression, distress, and anxiety directly impair glycemic control, while poor metabolic outcomes further worsen mental health. This bidirectional relationship establishes a cycle where emotional difficulties increase the risk of complications, and health complications increase psychological burden (Karakolias & Iliopoulou, 2025). Breaking this cycle requires integrated care that addresses both mental and physical health (Fig. 14.1).

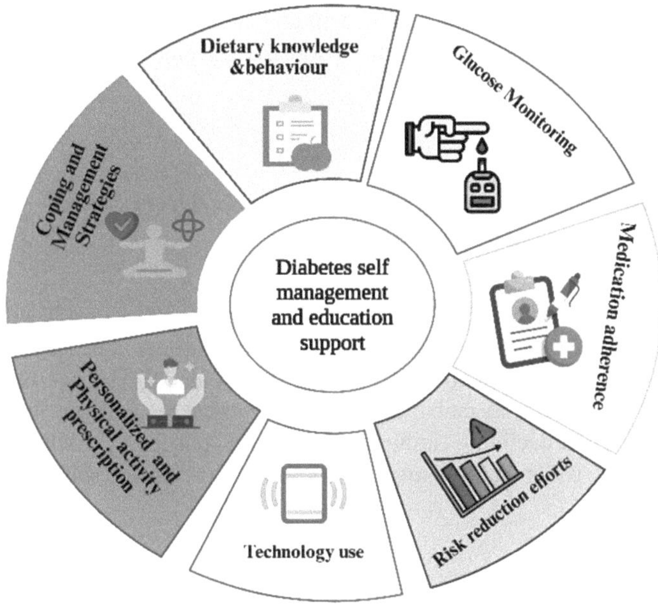

Fig. 14.1 Key components of diabetes self-management and education support in enhancing patient well-being

14.3 Social Impact of Diabetes

Living with diabetes extends far beyond medical management; it shapes how individuals interact with their families, workplaces, communities, and social environments. Studies across public-health, psychology, and social-sciences literature highlight that diabetes significantly influences social functioning, social roles, and overall quality of life (Kelly et al., 2024). Before highlighting the principal dimensions, it is essential to understand that the social burden of diabetes arises from the continuous need for self-care, lifestyle adjustments, dependency on healthcare systems, and the stigma often associated with chronic illness (Vlahovic et al., 2025).

14.3.1 Disruption of Daily Routines and Lifestyle Activities

Diabetes significantly alters how individuals structure their daily lives, as regular blood glucose monitoring, planned meals, and medication schedules must be integrated into every aspect of their routine (Kolarić et al., 2022). Research shows that these demands can limit spontaneity, reduce participation in social gatherings that revolve around food, and make leisure activities more stressful or restrictive. Over time, this disruption can lead to reduced social engagement and feelings of being different from peers.

14.3.2 Social Stigma and Misconceptions Affect Social Identity and Confidence

Studies on the social dimensions of chronic illness highlight that people with diabetes often encounter stigma, including blame, assumptions about unhealthy behaviours, and a lack of understanding about the disease (Liu et al., 2025). This stigma affects social identity, leading to embarrassment when checking glucose levels, taking insulin in public, or declining certain foods. Stigma contributes to withdrawal from social situations, which in turn harms emotional well-being and self-esteem.

14.3.3 Impact on Family Dynamics and Relationships

Diabetes influences family roles, expectations, and communication. Research indicates that families often oscillate between being overprotective and emotionally distant, which can create tension for the patient (Williams et al., 2022). Parents of children with diabetes may experience anxiety and hypervigilance, while partners may feel burdened by caregiving responsibilities. Such shifts in roles can strain relationships, reduce emotional closeness, and cause misunderstandings within the household (Madroumi et al., 2024).

14.3.4 Economic Burden Creates Stress and Social Limitations

The financial cost of diabetes management—including medications, glucose monitoring devices, clinical follow-ups, and healthy food choices—places considerable pressure on individuals and families (Mangoulia et al., 2024). Google Scholar literature frequently emphasizes that financial strain reduces access to advanced treatment options and limits engagement in social activities. Economic hardship can lead to job instability or decreased productivity, contributing to broader social inequality.

14.3.5 Work-Life Challenges and Reduced Professional Opportunities

Individuals with diabetes often face difficulties in workplace settings due to the need for flexible schedules, breaks for glucose monitoring, and potential sick days related to complications. Some studies report subtle discrimination, reduced career advancement, and misunderstandings about the nature of diabetes among employers and colleagues (Moghadam et al., 2025). The pressure to hide symptoms or avoid discussing health needs can lead to stress, decreased job satisfaction, and reduced participation in professional networks.

14.3.6 Limitations in Social Participation Due to Fear and Physical Symptoms

Fear of hypoglycemia, unpredictable energy levels, or diabetes-related complications can restrict participation in sports, travel, or community events. Research shows that patients often avoid distant trips, strenuous activities, or situations where medical support is not readily available (Montali et al., 2022). This limitation reduces quality of life, restricts recreation opportunities, and contributes to social isolation.

14.3.7 Cultural and Community Factors Shaping Social Experiences

Cultural norms surrounding food, family expectations, and community practices significantly influence how individuals with diabetes navigate their social lives (Zehe-Lindau et al., 2025). In many cultures, refusing traditional foods may be perceived as disrespectful, creating social tension for patients who are trying to manage their diet. Scholars note that cultural misconceptions about diabetes can shape beliefs about treatment, generating guilt, denial, or social discomfort when discussing the condition openly.

14.3.8 Caregiver Burden and Its Influence on Social Relationships

Diabetes not only affects the patient but also places emotional and practical burdens on caregivers. Studies show that caregivers often experience stress, fatigue, and reduced social activities due to their responsibilities (Moradi et al., 2021). This shared burden can shape family relationships, sometimes strengthening bonds but often leading to conflict, emotional strain, or a reduction in quality time with loved ones.

14.3.9 Inequities in Access to Healthcare and Social Support Systems

People living in rural areas, low-income communities, or minority populations often face barriers to healthcare access and diabetes education programs. These inequities, exacerbated by social determinants—such as access to transportation, literacy levels, and community infrastructure—negatively impact disease management and social participation (Mubayrik et al., 2024). Limited access to community support groups also deepens isolation and reduces opportunities for shared coping.

14.3.9.1 Overall Reduction in Social Quality of Life

The cumulative effects of stigma, lifestyle limitations, financial strain, and disrupted relationships contribute to a measurable decline in social quality of life. Research widely reports that individuals with diabetes often feel socially restricted, less confident in group interactions, and anxious about disclosing their condition (Noto, 2023). These social challenges interact with psychological issues, creating a complex burden that affects overall well-being.

14.4 Psychosocial Interventions and Support Strategies

Effective management of diabetes requires not only clinical treatment but also structured psychosocial interventions that address emotional distress, behavioural challenges, and social barriers. Research across psychology, behavioural medicine, and public health consistently emphasizes that psychosocial support improves self-care behaviours, glycemic control, and long-term quality of life (Oluchi et al., 2021). The points given below describe key interventions and strategies used to support individuals living with diabetes.

14.4.1 Diabetes Self-Management Education and Support (DSMES)

DSMES is one of the most widely recognized psychosocial interventions for people with diabetes. It equips individuals with the skills necessary to understand their condition, regulate blood glucose levels, adopt healthy lifestyle habits, and manage emotional stressors (Onu et al., 2025). Studies highlight that DSMES programs improve self-efficacy, reduce diabetes-related distress, and enhance long-term adherence to treatment. Structured education, delivered through group sessions, digital platforms, or individualized coaching, helps patients develop confidence in navigating daily decision-making related to diet, medication, physical activity, and symptom management (Pahn et al., 2025).

14.4.2 Cognitive Behavioural Therapy (CBT) for Emotional Well-Being

CBT is frequently recommended for patients experiencing depression, anxiety, or diabetes-related distress (Fu & Retnakaran, 2022). Literature suggests that CBT helps individuals reframe negative thoughts, develop healthier coping mechanisms, and manage emotional triggers that interfere with self-care. By addressing cognitive distortions and behavioural avoidance, CBT contributes to improved problem-solving, reduced emotional burden, and better glycemic outcomes (Panahi et al., 2024). Programs explicitly tailored to diabetes incorporate education about disease-related stress and strategies for integrating self-care routines into daily life.

14.4.3 Motivational Interviewing to Support Behavioural Change

Motivational interviewing (MI) is an evidence-based counselling approach that enhances motivation and commitment to diabetes self-management. MI helps patients resolve ambivalence toward lifestyle modifications by encouraging them to articulate personal goals and recognize barriers (Poole & Hackett, 2024). Research indicates that MI interventions lead to improved medication adherence, healthier dietary choices, consistent physical activity, and lower levels of diabetes-related distress. It is particularly effective for individuals who struggle with long-term behavioural change or feel overwhelmed by the demands of chronic illness.

14.4.4 Mindfulness-Based Interventions for Stress Reduction

Mindfulness practices—including meditation, breathing exercises, and mindful eating—are increasingly supported in literature for reducing stress and emotional burnout among people with diabetes. These interventions help individuals become more aware of their internal experiences, reduce reactivity to stressors, and cultivate acceptance of their condition. Studies indicate that mindfulness training can lower perceived stress, improve emotional regulation, and support better metabolic control by reducing stress-induced fluctuations in blood glucose (Pyatak et al., 2025).

14.4.5 Family-Focused Interventions

Family involvement plays a central role in sustaining behavioural change and emotional stability in individuals with diabetes. Interventions that educate families about disease management, communication strategies, and supportive behaviours have been shown to strengthen patient motivation and reduce conflict (Religioni et al., 2025). Research highlights that families who understand the emotional and physical demands of diabetes contribute positively to adherence and mental well-being. Such programs are beneficial for children, adolescents, and older adults who rely heavily on family support.

14.4.6 Peer Support Networks and Community-Based Programs

Peer support is a vital component of psychosocial care, providing individuals with an opportunity to share experiences, strategies, and challenges with others facing similar circumstances. Community-based programs run by trained peer mentors or patient advocacy groups provide emotional encouragement, reduce feelings of isolation, and foster a sense of empowerment (Reznik et al., 2024). Literature emphasizes that peer interactions enhance self-esteem, help normalise the diabetic experience, and promote long-term engagement in self-care practices.

14.4.7 Technology-Based Psychosocial Support

Digital tools such as mobile apps, telehealth counselling, online support groups, and virtual coaching have expanded access to psychosocial care (Sadeghi et al., 2024). Studies in digital health demonstrate that remote interventions can effectively reduce diabetes distress, enhance self-efficacy, and provide real-time educational guidance

(Rodriguez et al., 2022). Technology-based strategies are particularly valuable for individuals living in remote areas or those who face barriers to regular in-person consultations (Table 14.1).

Table 14.1 Key psychological and social impacts of diabetes on patients' lives

Domain	Key impacts	Description
Diabetes-related distress	Overwhelm, frustration with disease demands	Patients often experience burden from constant monitoring, dietary restrictions, and treatment adjustments, resulting in exhaustion and reduced motivation for self-care
Psychological distress	Emotional burden, anxiety, depression	Diabetes imposes continuous self-management demands that heighten emotional strain, leading to persistent worry about complications, fluctuating mood states, and feelings of helplessness
Social isolation	Withdrawal from social events	Dietary restrictions, embarrassment about checking glucose or injecting insulin in public, and fear of judgment often cause patients to avoid social gatherings
Stigma and misconceptions	Blame, judgment, discrimination	Public misunderstanding about diabetes origins and management leads to stigmatizing attitudes, which may discourage disclosure and increase psychological distress
Healthcare access barriers	Inequitable support, limited psychosocial services	Differences in socioeconomic status, location, and health literacy reduce access to diabetes education, mental health care, and community support programs
Financial stress	Economic burden of treatment	Costs related to medications, monitoring devices, and clinic visits can strain personal finances and restrict participation in social activities or quality-of-life experiences
Impact on self-identity	Altered self-perception, reduced confidence	Many individuals report feeling different from their peers or perceiving themselves as "ill," which can weaken self-esteem and influence social behaviour
Cognitive and behavioural challenges	Reduced concentration, decision fatigue	The need to make repeated health-related decisions each day contributes to cognitive overload and difficulty maintaining consistent behaviour over time
Interpersonal strain	Family conflict, caregiver stress	Family involvement in diabetes care may lead to tension, especially when expectations around diet, routine, or monitoring are not aligned among family members

14.5 Future Directions

Future directions in the study of the psychological and social impact of diabetes emphasize the need for more holistic, multidisciplinary, and culturally adaptable models of care that recognize the central role of emotional and social well-being in long-term disease management (Saleh et al., 2000). Emerging research suggests that integrating routine mental-health screening into diabetes care could significantly improve early detection of psychological distress, allowing timely intervention before it undermines self-management (Semerci Çakmak et al., 2025). There is increasing momentum toward developing personalized psychosocial interventions that consider individual coping styles, socioeconomic conditions, and cultural beliefs to improve engagement and treatment adherence (Shah et al., 2025). The rapid advancement of digital health—such as telemedicine counseling, mobile psychological support applications, and AI-enabled self-management tools—is expected to expand access to continuous psychosocial monitoring, particularly among rural, remote, and resource-limited populations (Shattnawi & Mahassneh, 2025). Future work also emphasizes the importance of strengthening family-centred and community-based support structures, as these environments significantly impact patients' motivation, emotional resilience, and social functioning. In addition, addressing persistent stigma, workplace discrimination, and health-literacy gaps remains essential to improving overall quality of life (Slowik et al., 2025). Researchers are also calling for policies that reduce socioeconomic barriers to mental health services, peer-support programs, and social care resources (Sułkowski et al., 2024). Collectively, these future directions advocate for a more equitable and integrated psychosocial care framework that positions psychological and social health as core components of comprehensive diabetes management (Ting et al., 2025).

14.6 Conclusion

In conclusion, the psychological and social impact of diabetes represents a critical dimension of chronic disease management, shaping how individuals cope with the daily demands of self-care and influencing their overall quality of life. Evidence from diverse studies highlights that diabetes extends far beyond its physiological manifestations, affecting emotional stability, cognitive functioning, family relationships, social participation, and economic well-being. Persistent stress, anxiety, and diabetes-related distress often intersect with social barriers such as stigma, limited support networks, workplace challenges, and disparities in access to healthcare resources. These multidimensional burdens underscore the need to integrate psychological assessment, personalized counseling, and community-based support into routine diabetes care. Strengthening family involvement, enhancing health literacy, and expanding digital and peer-support interventions can significantly improve emotional resilience and self-management outcomes. As healthcare systems shift toward more patient-centred models, recognizing the interconnected nature of psychological and social determinants will be crucial for promoting long-term well-being and alleviating the burden of diabetes on individuals and communities. Ultimately, addressing these psychosocial factors is not only fundamental to improving metabolic control but also to enabling patients to live fuller, healthier, and more empowered lives with diabetes.

Acknowledgements The images were created using www.Biorander.com and www.Grammarly.com to correct the grammar of this manuscript.

Author Contributions **Md Abubakar, Ritu Dahiya, and Kanika Goyal** was involved in the conceptualization, writing of the original draft, mechanistic insight, input on critical points, editing; **Nitesh Kumar, Irshad Khan, and Krishna Murti** contributed to the manuscript editing; **Amita Rai** was involved in the conceptualization, manuscript writing, reviewing, conceptualization of figures and approved the version to be published.

Funding None.

Availability of Data None.

Conflict of Interest None.

References

Adjaye-Gbewonyo, K., Kretchy, I. A., Baatiema, L., Grijalva-Eternod, C. S., Sanuade, O. A., Amon, S., et al. (2025). Non-communicable diseases, psychosocial wellbeing, and quality of life in Ga Mashie, Accra, Ghana: Analysis from a community-based cross-sectional study. *BMC Public Health, 25*(1), 1059.

Agarwal, S., Wade, A. N., Mbanya, J. C., Yajnik, C., Thomas, N., Egede, L. E., et al. (2023). The role of structural racism and geographical inequity in diabetes outcomes. *Lancet, 402*(10397), 235–249.

Alshaikhi, S. A., Alfaqih, F. H., Alrashdi, A. K., Alamri, F. A., Alzubaidi, A. S., Alnashri, A. I., et al. (2025). Assessment of self-efficacy, quality of life, and well-being of patients with diabetes mellitus in Alqunfudah, Saudi Arabia. *BMC Endocrine Disorders, 25*(1), 91.

Ashraf, M. N., Cheng, A. Y. Y., & Robinson, D. J. (2024). Emotional, psychological, and social well-being experience of long-term living with type 1 diabetes mellitus: A patient–psychiatrist–endocrinologist perspective. *Diabetes Therapy, 15*(2), 317–323.

Augustin, M., Misery, L., Von Kobyletzki, L., Armario-Hita, J. C., Mealing, S., & Redding, M. (2022). Unveiling the true costs and societal impacts of moderate-to-severe atopic dermatitis in Europe. *Journal of the European Academy of Dermatology and Venereology, 36*, 3–16.

Bellass, S., Lister, J., Kitchen, C. E. W., Kramer, L., Alderson, S. L., Doran, T., et al. (2021). Living with diabetes alongside a severe mental illness: A qualitative exploration with people with severe mental illness, family members and healthcare staff. *Diabetic Medicine, 38*(7), Article e14562.

Borbjerg, M. K., Wegeberg, A. M., Nikontovic, A., Mørch, C. D., Arendt-Nielsen, L., Ejskjaer, N., et al. (2025). Understanding the impact of diabetic peripheral neuropathy and neuropathic pain on quality of life and mental health in 6,960 people with diabetes. *Diabetes Care, 48*(4), 588–595.

Ciarambino, T., Crispino, P., Leto, G., Mastrolorenzo, E., Para, O., & Giordano, M. (2022). Influence of gender in diabetes mellitus and its complication. *International Journal of Molecular Sciences, 23*(16), 8850.

Cicek, M., Buckley, J., Pearson-Stuttard, J., & Gregg, E. W. (2021). Characterizing multimorbidity from type 2 diabetes: Insights from clustering approaches. *Endocrinology and Metabolism Clinics of North America, 50*(3), 531–558.

Dumitrescu, R., Bolchis, V., Popescu, S., Ivanescu, A., Bolos, A., Jumanca, D., et al. (2025). Oral health and quality of life in type 2 diabetic patients: Key findings from a Romanian study. *Journal of Clinical Medicine, 14*(2), 400.

Esubalew, H., Belachew, A., Seid, Y., Wondmagegn, H., Temesgen, K., & Ayele, T. (2024). Health-related quality of life among type 2 diabetes mellitus patients using the 36-item short form health survey (SF-36) in Central Ethiopia: A multicenter study. *Diabetes, Metab Syndr Obes,* 1039–1049.

Flint, S. W., Vázquez-Velázquez, V., Le Brocq, S., & Brown, A. (2025). The real-life experiences of people living with overweight and obesity: A psychosocial perspective. *Diabetes, Obesity & Metabolism, 27*, 35–47.

Fu, J., & Retnakaran, R. (2022). The life course perspective of gestational diabetes: An opportunity for the prevention of diabetes and heart disease in women. *EClinicalMedicine*, 45.

Hecker, J., Freijer, K., Hiligsmann, M., & Evers, S. (2022). Burden of disease study of overweight and obesity; the societal impact in terms of cost-of-illness and health-related quality of life. *BMC Public Health, 22*(1), 46.

Hermanns, N., Kulzer, B., & Ehrmann, D. (2024). Person-reported outcomes in diabetes care: What are they and why are they so important? *Diabetes, Obesity & Metabolism, 26*, 30–45.

Jafari, A., Naddafi^, F., Gholian-Aval, M., & Tehrani, H. (2024b). Relationship between diabetes health literacy, distress, burnout, social support, complications, self-care behaviors, and quality of life among patients with type 2 diabetes: A path analysis study. *Diabetology & Metabolic Syndrome, 16*(1), 150.

Jafari, A., Moshki, M., Ghelichi-Ghojogh, M., & Nejatian, M. (2024a). Role of diabetes health literacy, psychological status, self-care behaviors, and life satisfaction in predicting quality of life in type 2 diabetes. *Science and Reports, 14*(1), 1635.

Jassim, S. K., Abbass, Z., & Tiryag, A. M. (2024). A study of diabetes correlated emotional distress among patients with type 2 diabetes mellitus: A cross sectional study. *Academia Open, 9*(2), 10–21070.

Javed, S., Mohamed, M., Altaf, B., & Ghazali, W. S. W. (2025). The human cost of type-2 diabetes mellitus: Uncovering the hidden burden on quality of life. *Pakistan Journal of Medical Sciences, 41*(3), 712.

Karakolias, S., & Iliopoulou, A. (2025). Health-related quality of life and psychological burden among and beyond children and adolescents with type 1 diabetes: A family perspective. *Cureus, 17*(4), Article e81744.

Kelly, R. C., Holt, R. I. G., Desborough, L., Majidi, S., Town, M., Naranjo, D., et al. (2024). The psychosocial burdens of living with diabetes. *Diabetic Medicine, 41*(3), Article e15219.

Kolarić, V., Svirčević, V., Bijuk, R., & Zupančič, V. (2022). Chronic complications of diabetes and quality of life. *Acta Clinica Croatica, 61*(3), 520.

Liu, J., Li, J., Li, L., & Zeng, K. (2025). Impact of family environment on mental disorders and quality of life in children with type 1 diabetes mellitus: A cross-sectional study and intervention policy analysis. *Frontiers in Pediatrics, 13*, 1516411.

Madroumi, R., Newson, L., Umeh, F. K., Poole, H., & Jones, A. (2024). Identifying the key components of social support for patients living with type 2 diabetes: A protocol for a systematic review and meta-analysis of type 2 diabetes social support interventions. *PLoS ONE, 19*(8), Article e0306709.

Mangoulia, P., Milionis, C., Vlachou, E., & Ilias, I. (2024). The interrelationship between diabetes mellitus and emotional well-being: Current concepts and future prospects. In *Healthcare* (p. 1457). MDPI.

Moghadam, F. D., Rahami, Z., Ahmadi, S. A., Reisi, S., & Ahmadi, S. M. (2025). Predicting quality of life and self-care behaviors in patients with painful diabetic neuropathy based on psychological factors. *Science and Reports, 15*(1), 6431.

Montali, L., Zulato, E., Cornara, M., Ausili, D., & Luciani, M. (2022). Barriers and facilitators of type 1 diabetes self-care in adolescents and young adults. *Journal of Pediatric Nursing, 62*, 136–143.

Moradi, F., Tourani, S., Ziapour, A., Abbas, J., Hematti, M., Moghadam, E. J., et al. (2021). Emotional intelligence and quality of life in elderly diabetic patients. *International Quarterly of Community Health Education, 42*(1), 15–20.

Mubayrik, A. F. B., Alhoqail, R. I., Alhoqail, R. I., & Dous, R. A. B. (2024). Oral health-related quality of life among diabetic patients: A cross-sectional controlled study. *Journal of Family Medicine and Primary Care, 13*(2), 619–626.

Noto, S. (2023). Perspectives on aging and quality of life. In *Healthcare* (p. 2131). MDPI.

Oluchi, S. E., Manaf, R. A., Ismail, S., Kadir Shahar, H., Mahmud, A., & Udeani, T. K. (2021). Health related quality of life measurements for diabetes: A systematic review. *International Journal of Environmental Research and Public Health, 18*(17), 9245.

Onu, D. U., Obi-keguna, C. N., Oguguam, O. N., Ajaero, C. K., & Igwe, E. J. (2025). Social support may buffer, to an extent, the impact of stigma on health-related quality of life among type 2 diabetes mellitus patients. *Discover Public Health, 22*(1), 29.

Pahn, J., Yang, Y., & Kim, S. H. (2025). Factors influencing self-management and health-related quality of life in low-income patients with diabetes: a predictive model. *International Journal of Nursing Studies Advances*, 100349.

Panahi, N., Ahmadi, M., Hosseinpour, M., Sedokani, A., Sanjari, M., Khalagi, K., et al. (2024). The association between quality of life and diabetes: The Bushehr Elderly Health Program. *BMC Geriatrics, 24*(1), 267.

Poole, L., & Hackett, R. A. (2024). Diabetes distress: The psychological burden of living with diabetes. *The Lancet Diabetes and Endocrinology, 12*(7), 439–441.

Pyatak, E. A., Lee, P. J., Nnoli, N. D., Mo, Y., Khurana, A., Ali, A., et al. (2025). Telehealth occupational therapy improves psychosocial well-being but not glycemia among young adults with type 1 diabetes: The Resilient, Empowered, Active Living-Telehealth (REAL-T) randomized controlled trial. *Diabetes Research and Clinical Practice, 221*, Article 112005.

Religioni, U., Barrios-Rodríguez, R., Requena, P., Borowska, M., & Ostrowski, J. (2025). Enhancing therapy adherence: Impact on clinical outcomes, healthcare costs, and patient quality of life. *Medicina (b Aires), 61*(1), 153.

Reznik, Y., Bonnemaison, E., Fagherazzi, G., Renard, E., Hanaire, H., Schaepelynck, P., et al. (2024). The use of an automated insulin delivery system is associated with a reduction in diabetes distress and improvement in quality of life in people with type 1 diabetes. *Diabetes, Obesity & Metabolism, 26*(5), 1962–1966.

Rodriguez, K., Ryan, D., Dickinson, J. K., & Phan, V. (2022). Improving quality outcomes: The value of diabetes care and education specialists. *Clin Diabetes, 40*(3), 356–365.

Sadeghi, D., Motlagh, M. K., Darvish, A., Daryaafzoon, M., Mohamadnejad, E., Molaei, A., et al. (2024). Comparative effect of physical health training and psychological training of the theory of reasoned action (TRA) model on the life quality of patients with diabetes in Tehran, Iran: Utilization of message texting. *BMC Endocrine Disorders, 24*(1), 69.

Saleh, M. H. A., Dias, D. R., & Kumar, P. (2000). The economic and societal impact of periodontal and peri-implant diseases. *Periodontology 2000.*

Semerci, V., Sönmez Sari, E., & Çetinkaya, Ö. S. (2025). Experiences of adults with type 2 diabetes mellitus with low socioeconomic status: A qualitative study. *BMC Public Health, 25*(1), 381.

Shah, R., Finlay, A. Y., Ali, F. M., Otwombe, K., Nixon, S. J., George, L., et al. (2025). Comparison of the impact of type 1 and type 2 diabetes on quality of life of families of patients: A UK cross-sectional study. *Diabetes, Obesity & Metabolism, 27*(2), 652–662.

Shattnawi, K. K., & Mahassneh, S. M. (2025). Balancing life with type 1 diabetes mellitus: A qualitative study of Jordanian adolescents. *Journal of Pediatric Nursing, 80*, e40–e47.

Slowik, J., Kaczynski, L., Kaczor, M., & Wnuk, M. (2025). Oral health-related quality of life in patients with type II diabetes mellitus: A systematic review and meta-analysis. *BMC Oral Health, 25*(1), 485.

Sułkowski, L., Matyja, A., & Matyja, M. (2024). Social support and quality of life in hemodialysis patients: A comparative study with healthy controls. *Medicina (b Aires)., 60*(11), 1732.

Ting, Z., Huicai, W., Kudelati, Z., Yongkang, G., Alimu, A., Xiaotian, Z., et al. (2025). Exploring the dynamics of self-efficacy, resilience, and self-management on quality of life in type 2 diabetes patients: A moderated mediation approach from a positive psychology perspective. *PLoS ONE, 20*(1), Article e0317753.

Vlahovic, B., Jha, V., Stojanovic, V., Vojinovic, T., Dutta, A., Dutta, P., et al. (2025). Enhancing patient-centered care: Evaluating quality of life in type 2 diabetes management. *PLoS ONE, 20*(3), Article e0319369.

Williams, D. M., Jones, H., & Stephens, J. W. (2022). Personalized type 2 diabetes management: an update on recent advances and recommendations. *Diabetes, Metabolic Syndrome and Obesity: Targets and Therapy*, 281–295.

Zehe-Lindau, N., Lindau, B., Stöhr, H., Weber, B. H. F., Spital, G., & Kellner, U. (2025). Patient-reported social impact of molecularly confirmed retinitis pigmentosa. *Journal of Clinical Medicine, 14*(9), 3229.

Chapter 15
Sustained Approaches to Prevent Recurrence and Support Ongoing Diabetes Health

Abhishek Ambawatiya, Kanika Goyal, Ritu Dahiya, Zeeshan Hyderi, Lalit Kumar Singh, Jayahari Srivastava, Nitesh Kumar, and Md Abubakar

Abstract Sustaining long-term glycaemic control in individuals with diabetes requires comprehensive strategies that address both the biological progression of the disease and the behavioural factors contributing to relapse. Evidence from contemporary clinical studies suggests that the recurrence of hyperglycemia is often associated with declining β-cell function, persistent insulin resistance (IR), and inconsistent adherence to treatment and lifestyle recommendations. Consequently, durable diabetes management increasingly emphasizes multimodal interventions that extend beyond short-term metabolic correction. Pharmacological approaches, including incretin-based therapies, SGLT2 inhibitors, and advanced insulin analogues, have demonstrated long-term benefits in stabilizing glycaemic patterns and reducing cardiometabolic risk. Parallel findings from lifestyle intervention trials suggest that

Abhishek Ambawatiya, Kanika Goyal, and Ritu Dahiya—These authors are equally contributed.
Zeeshan Hyderi, Lalit Kumar Singh, and Jayahari Srivastava—Second position in contribution.

A. Ambawatiya · N. Kumar (✉) · M. Abubakar (✉)
Department of Pharmacology and Toxicology, Export Promotions Industrial Park (EPIP) Campus, National Institute of Pharmaceutical Education and Research, Hajipur, India
e-mail: nitesh.kumar04@niperhajipur.ac.in

M. Abubakar
e-mail: mdabuabakr731@gmail.com

K. Goyal
Ganpati Group of Institutions, Bilaspur, Yamuna Nagar, India

R. Dahiya
School of Pharmacy, Lingaya's Vidyapeeth (Deemed to be University), Faridabad, India

Z. Hyderi
Department of Biotechnology, Alagappa University, Karaikudi, India

L. K. Singh
Department of Biochemistry, University of Allahabad, Prayagraj, India

J. Srivastava
SMD University, Hitanu, Uttarkashi, India

K. Adhikary et al. (eds.), *Healing Beyond Blood Sugar*,
https://doi.org/10.1007/978-981-95-8946-3_15

structured nutritional counselling, weight-management programs, and consistent physical activity have sustained effects on insulin sensitivity and inflammatory pathways, thereby reducing the risk of recurrence. Digital health tools—particularly continuous glucose monitoring, mobile-based self-management platforms, and automated insulin delivery systems—enhance early detection of deglycation and support individualized decision-making. Integrated care models, which involve coordinated follow-up between primary care teams, endocrinologists, diabetes educators, and mental health professionals, further contribute to long-term success by improving adherence, addressing psychological barriers, and facilitating timely adjustments to therapy. Emerging evidence underscores the importance of precision-based approaches that incorporate metabolic profiles, comorbidities, and patient preferences to tailor long-term interventions. Collectively, these sustained strategies form a robust framework that not only reduces the likelihood of recurrence but also promotes continuous metabolic health and reduces the burden of long-term complications in individuals living with diabetes.

Keywords Deglycation · Diabetes · Glucose monitoring · Hyperglycemia · Insulin resistance · β-cell

15.1 Introduction

Diabetes mellitus is a chronic, progressive metabolic disorder characterized by persistent dysregulation of glucose homeostasis, progressive β-cell dysfunction, and systemic insulin resistance (IR). Although short-term improvements in glycemia can be achieved with pharmacotherapy and lifestyle modification, maintaining durable glycaemic control is challenging: many individuals experience recurrent deterioration in metabolic control (relapse) that increases the risk of micro- and macrovascular complications and contributes substantially to morbidity and health-care burden (Summary of revisions: Standards of Care in Diabetes, 2025). These patterns reflect the multifactorial nature of diabetes, in which biological deterioration (β-cell exhaustion, lipotoxicity, and inflammation), behavioural factors (medication nonadherence and lifestyle lapses), and health-system limitations (fragmented care and insufficient long-term follow-up) interact to undermine sustained success. Evidence demonstrates that intensive, structured lifestyle interventions can produce durable reductions in incident diabetes and sustained metabolic benefits; however, the magnitude and persistence of these effects depend on program intensity, duration of follow-up, and adherence support (Glycemic goals and hypoglycemia: Standards of Care in Diabetes, 2025). Landmark prevention trials and their long-term follow-up studies demonstrate that weight loss, improved dietary quality, and increased physical activity lead to significant, sustained reductions in diabetes incidence and related cardiometabolic risks when reinforcement and maintenance strategies are integrated into care pathways. These studies provide proof of concept that relapse is modifiable, but also underscore the need for long-term systems to preserve behavioural change.

Recent work on metabolic remission has demonstrated that profound, sustained caloric restriction and structured weight-loss programs can induce durable glycemic remission in subsets of individuals with type 2 diabetes (T2DM), revealing that targeted, intensive interventions may alter the disease trajectory when accompanied by long-term maintenance strategies (Abu Dabrh et al., 2025). Nonetheless, relapse remains a risk if weight regain or metabolic stressors recur, highlighting the imperative for integrated maintenance frameworks after initial remission.

Health-system approaches that coordinate multidisciplinary teams, integrate specialist input with primary and community care, and deliver continuous follow-up have been associated with improved intermediate outcomes (e.g., HbA1c, blood pressure, lipid control) and enhanced self-management capacity. Integrated care models and chronic care frameworks provide structural mechanisms to deliver sustained, proactive management rather than episodic, reactive care—an essential shift to prevent recurrence in chronic diabetes management (Aidoo, 2025).

Finally, digital technologies—most notably continuous glucose monitoring (CGM), automated insulin delivery, and telehealth platforms—have significantly enhanced the capacity to detect early glycemic deterioration, personalize treatment adjustments, and sustain patient engagement. Emerging evidence suggests that the use of CGM and remote monitoring improves glycemic metrics and facilitates timely therapeutic adjustments, making these tools central to contemporary sustained-care strategies (Alenazi & Khan, 2025). However, equitable access, cost, and long-term implementation remain practical challenges that must be addressed to translate technological promise into population-level reductions in recurrence. Taken together, these lines of evidence suggest a multi-layered paradigm for preventing recurrence and supporting ongoing diabetic health, one that combines durable lifestyle and weight-management strategies, optimized pharmacotherapy, multidisciplinary integrated care, and digital surveillance to detect and address early signs of relapse (Almuntashiri et al., 2025). Additionally, this chapter examines the mechanistic rationale, evidence base, and practical implementation considerations for each pillar of this sustained-care framework.

15.2 Pathophysiological Basis of Recurrence in Diabetes

Recurrence of hyperglycemia after an interval of improved glycemic control or remission reflects progression of the same pathophysiological processes that caused diabetes initially—principally inadequate insulin secretion relative to demand (β-cell dysfunction and loss of functional reserve) together with peripheral and hepatic IR (Aragón-Sánchez et al., 2025). Remission, therefore, is better viewed as a transient restoration of metabolic balance rather than a permanent cure; recurrence occurs when either insulin demand increases or β-cell capacity declines further. These interacting processes are dynamic and time-dependent: early in the disease, they may be reversible with intensive metabolic interventions, but with persistent metabolic stress, they become progressively fixed and harder to reverse (Association AD, 2023).

(15.2.1) **Progressive β-cell dysfunction mechanisms that enable relapse**

The β-cell dysfunction is the primary determinant of recurrence, as it limits the ability to match insulin secretion to prevailing IR. Chronic exposure to elevated glucose (glucotoxicity) and elevated circulating free fatty acids (lipotoxicity) impairs insulin gene expression, disturbs stimulus–secretion coupling, and provokes endoplasmic reticulum (ER) stress and mitochondrial dysfunction (Balakrishnan et al., 2025). These results increase production of reactive oxygen species (ROS), activate stress kinases and unfolded protein responses, and promote β-cell apoptosis or dedifferentiation (loss of β-cell identity markers). Although β-cells possess some capacity for recovery (functional rest, redifferentiation) if metabolic stress is removed early, sustained glucolipotoxicity stress leads to a progressive loss of β-cell mass and secretory reserve, setting the stage for recurrence even after an initial remission.

(15.2.2) **IR and tissue-level drivers of relapse**

The IR in skeletal muscle, adipose tissue, and liver increases the required insulin output from β-cells. Factors that re-establish IR after remission—weight regain, increased visceral adiposity, reduced physical activity, and adverse adipokine profiles—therefore precipitate relapse (Baris & Tabit, 2025). At the hepatic level, accumulation of diacylglycerols and other lipid metabolites perturbs insulin signaling and increases hepatic glucose production even when systemic circulating free fatty acids are not markedly elevated; this hepatic IR is a common pathway linking weight gain and ectopic fat accumulation to recurrent hyperglycemia (Fig. 15.1).

(15.2.3) **Ectopic fat: pancreas and liver as relapse reservoirs**

Ectopic lipid deposition—particularly intrahepatic and intra-pancreatic fat—plays a fundamental role in both the development and the recurrence of T2DM. Excess liver fat drives very-low-density lipoprotein (VLDL) overproduction and systemic lipid fluxes that promote fat accumulation in the pancreas. Pancreatic steatosis has been associated with impaired insulin secretory responses, and reductions in both liver and pancreatic fat accompany diet- or surgery-induced remissions (Brunner et al., 2025). In contrast, the accumulation of ectopic fat following weight regain is linked to a loss of remission. This means that ectopic fat serves as both a modifiable factor contributing to metabolic stress and a reservoir that can trigger β-cell dysfunction when energy balance worsens.

(15.2.4) **Inflammation, innate immunity, and programmed cell death**

Chronic low-grade inflammation originating from adipose tissue (adipocyte dysfunction, macrophage infiltration), islet-resident immune activation, and inflammasome signalling accelerate both IR and β-cell injury. Metabolic stress (glucolipotoxicity, oxidized lipids) activates NF-κB and the NLRP3 inflammasome in metabolic tissues and islets, increasing IL-1β and related cytokines that impair insulin secretion, promote β-cell apoptosis and can trigger pyroptotic cell death (Bus et al., 2024). Ageing, the gut microbiome, and environmental factors further modulate inflammasome activity. Targeting IL-1β–NLRP3 axes has therefore been explored as a strategy to reduce progression and potentially delay recurrence.

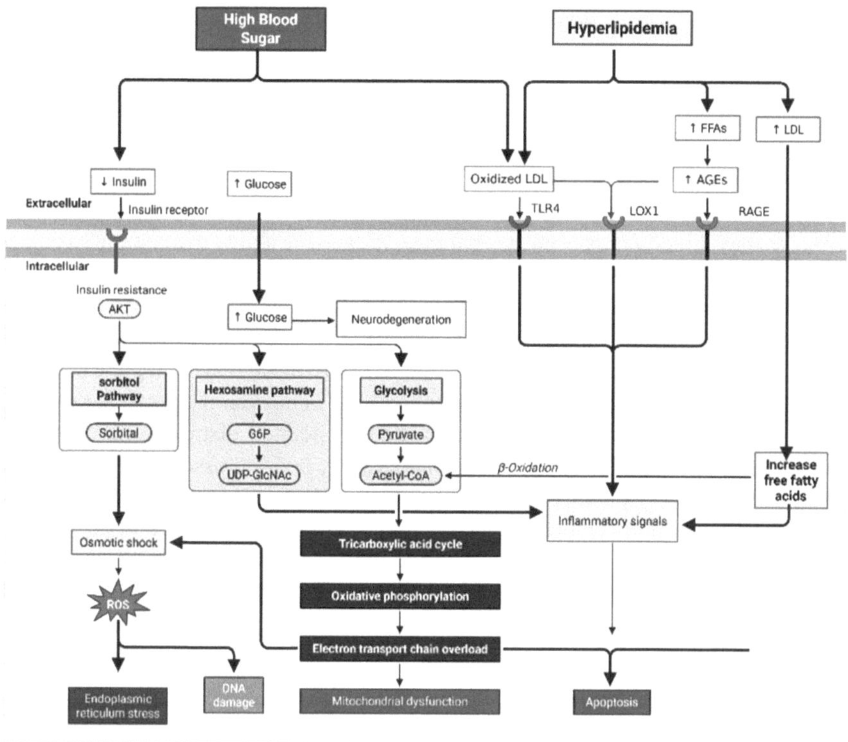

Fig. 15.1 Pathogenesis of diabetes

(15.2.5) **Oxidative stress and organelle dysfunction**

The pancreatic β-cells are relatively susceptible to oxidative stress due to their low intrinsic antioxidant capacity. ROS generation—driven by mitochondrial overload, ER stress, and chronic hyperglycemia—damages DNA, proteins, and membranes, dysregulates calcium handling, and triggers pro-apoptotic signalling (Care, 2025). Accumulation of oxidative damage over time reduces β-cell functional reserve and predisposes to relapse once compensatory mechanisms are exhausted. Antioxidant and organelle-protective interventions are biologically plausible approaches for preserving β-cell mass, although their clinical translation remains under investigation.

(15.2.6) **Incretin axis, gut–islet crosstalk, and hormonal modulators**

The incretin hormones glucagon-like peptide-1 (GLP-1) and glucose-dependent insulinotropic polypeptide (GIP) enhance glucose-stimulated insulin secretion and suppress the release of inappropriate glucagon. In T2DM, the insulinotropic effect of GIP is markedly blunted, and although GLP-1 secretion is sometimes preserved, its action is reduced due to receptor downregulation and chronic hyperglycemia (Chao et al., 2025). These impairments diminish the postprandial insulin response, making individuals more susceptible to hyperglycaemic relapse after periods of remission. Pharmacologic incretin mimetics (GLP-1 receptor agonists, dual agonists) can reproduce some of these hormonal benefits and are being evaluated for durable prevention of recurrence.

(15.2.7) **Behavioural and Psychosocial Factors**

Behavioural determinants are significant, modifiable factors that drive diabetes recurrence, as they directly impact energy balance, IR, and the ability to maintain sustained self-care (Ying et al., 2025). Poor adherence to pharmacotherapy, inconsistent dietary patterns, reduced physical activity, and failure to maintain weight loss rapidly re-establish metabolic stress (ectopic fat, and IR) that overwhelms remaining β-cell reserve and precipitates relapse (Committee ADAPP, 2023). Psychological disorders and chronic stress have independent biological and behavioural effects that increase relapse risk. Major depression and high diabetes-related distress reduce motivation and executive function needed for adherence, and are associated with worse glycaemic control. Concurrently, chronic stress, HPA-axis dysregulation (altered cortisol rhythms), and sympathetic activation raise hepatic glucose output, promote visceral adiposity, and impair insulin action—physiological pathways that compound behavioural lapses to accelerate metabolic deterioration (Cusi et al., 2025). Routine screening and treatment of depression and stress, therefore, constitute essential components of relapse prevention.

15.3 Lifestyle and Nutritional Interventions for Long-Term Maintenance

Sustained lifestyle modification remains the cornerstone for preventing recurrence of hyperglycemia after initial improvement or remission of T2DM. Durable maintenance requires not only an initial therapeutic perturbation (e.g., very-low-energy diet or intensive behavioural programme) that reduces adiposity and ectopic fat, but also structured, long-term strategies to preserve weight loss, reduce IR, and maintain β-cell "rest." Long-term follow-up studies indicate that the degree and persistence of weight loss are the strongest determinants of prolonged glycemic remission and reduced cardiometabolic events (Denby, 2025).

15.3.1 Dietary Strategies

15.3.1.1 High Fiber Consumption

Dietary fiber, especially soluble fiber from legumes, whole grains, and vegetables, enhances insulin sensitivity and slows gastric emptying (Desouter et al., 2025). Studies indicate that fibre-rich diets modulate gut microbiota composition, decrease systemic inflammation, and improve incretin hormone signaling, thereby contributing to more stable long-term glycemic outcomes.

15.3.1.2 Controlled Carbohydrate Intake

Moderating total carbohydrate intake—particularly refined starches—reduces the metabolic burden on pancreatic β-cells. Evidence from clinical studies suggests that carbohydrate-restricted diets can improve fasting glucose levels, reduce hepatic gluconeogenesis, and support remission maintenance in individuals with T2DM (DuBois et al., 2025).

15.3.1.3 Micronutrient-Rich Food Intake

Foods rich in magnesium, chromium, omega-3 fatty acids, and antioxidants support enzymatic pathways involved in glucose regulation (ElSayed et al., 2025). Adequate intake of micronutrients reduces oxidative stress and enhances metabolic adaptability, thereby lowering the risk of recurrence.

15.3.1.4 Calorie-Conscious Eating

Maintaining modest caloric deficits over the long term aids in fat loss and reduces metabolic strain. Studies indicate that even a 5–10% reduction in body weight can restore insulin sensitivity and improve β-cell responsiveness, helping prevent relapse after initial glycemic improvement (Fanelli et al., 2025).

15.3.1.5 Low-Glycemic Load

Research consistently shows that diets with a low glycaemic load attenuate postprandial glucose spike and reduce overall glycaemic variability (Ghanem et al., 2024). By slowing carbohydrate digestion and absorption, these diets help maintain steady insulin responses, thereby reducing the metabolic fluctuations that often precede the recurrence of diabetes.

15.3.2 *Physical Activity and Exercise Prescription*

15.3.2.1 Improvement of Mitochondrial Function and Metabolic Flexibility

Aerobic exercise stimulates mitochondrial biogenesis and improves oxidative capacity. This enhances metabolic flexibility, enabling better switching between lipid and glucose utilization, which is crucial for long-term glycemic stability (Grattoni et al., 2025).

15.3.2.2 Aerobic Training for Glycaemic Stability

Moderate to vigorous aerobic exercise, such as brisk walking, cycling, or swimming, improves cardiovascular fitness and reduces both fasting and postprandial blood glucose levels (Gregg et al., 2024). Studies indicate that 150–300 min per week of aerobic activity significantly supports long-term metabolic control.

15.3.2.3 Role of Regular Physical Activity

Evidence suggests that consistent physical activity enhances peripheral glucose uptake by increasing the translocation of GLUT4 in skeletal muscle. Even moderate-intensity exercise significantly improves insulin sensitivity, thereby reducing the risk of recurrent hyperglycemia (Herold et al., 2024).

15.3.2.4 Anti-inflammatory and Vascular Effects

Regular physical activity lowers systemic inflammatory markers (e.g., CRP, TNF-α), improves endothelial function and blood flow to metabolic tissues—favourable for long-term glycaemic stability (Watts et al., 2025).

15.3.3 *Behavioural Interventions*

15.3.3.1 Goal Setting and Action Planning

Explicit, measurable goals (e.g., weekly minutes of activity; grams of carbohydrate; target weight ranges) with written action plans increase behavioural enactment and provide objective anchors for monitoring (Velayutham et al., 2025).

15.3.3.2 Self-Monitoring and Feedback

Regular self-measurement (weight, steps, food logs, home glucose) combined with timely feedback (automated or clinician) is a consistent predictor of sustained behaviour change and early detection of relapse. Digital tools and wearables amplify adherence to self-monitoring protocols (Hilbrands & Gillard, 2025).

15.3.3.3 Treatment of Depression and Diabetes Distress

Screening and evidence-based therapies for depression (CBT, pharmacotherapy where indicated) reduce behavioural barriers to self-care and are associated with improved glycaemic trajectories; addressing diabetes-specific distress improves adherence and may lower relapse risk (Templer et al., 2024).

15.3.3.4 Stress-Reduction and Resilience Training

Mindfulness-based stress reduction, stress-management skills, and cognitive restructuring reduce HPA-axis activation and maladaptive eating behaviours—mechanisms relevant to preventing metabolic relapse (Huang et al., 2025). Evidence for a long-term glycaemic impact is emerging, but it is promising.

15.3.3.5 Combine Behavioural with Medical/weight-Loss Strategies

Behavioural support enhances retention and effectiveness of very-low-energy diets, pharmacotherapy (e.g., GLP-1 receptor agonists), and structured exercise programmes; combined approaches reduce weight regain and extend remission duration (Spanakis et al., 2022).

15.4 Digital Health and Continuous Monitoring Technologies

Digital technologies convert diabetes management from episodic clinic encounters into continuous, data-driven surveillance. By continuously capturing physiologic (glucose, heart rate), behavioural (activity, sleep), and contextual (meal timing, medication adherence) signals, these systems detect small but clinically meaningful deviations (e.g., rising post-prandial excursions, falling time-in-range, declining daily steps) that commonly precede biochemical relapse (Hussain et al., 2025). Early detection enables prompt, targeted responses (behavioural coaching, dietary re-induction, medication adjustment) that can interrupt the trajectory toward sustained hyperglycemia.

15.4.1 Continuous Glucose Monitoring (CGM)

CGM provides high-resolution interstitial glucose data and derived metrics (time-in-range [TIR], time above range, glycaemic variability), which are more responsive to short-term metabolic change than HbA1c. Randomized trials and meta-analyses in adults with T2DM show that CGM use improves TIR and reduces prolonged hyperglycemia and glycaemic excursions, and that CGM-guided behavioural feedback helps patients modify meal composition/timing and medication behaviours (Jacobsen et al., 2025). For persons in remission, intermittent or continuous CGM surveillance can therefore identify pattern changes (e.g., progressive post-prandial peaks) that warrant early intervention.

15.4.2 Wearables and Behavioural Sensors

Wearable accelerometers and multisensory devices objectively track daily steps, sedentary bouts, sleep quality, and heart-rate dynamics. Studies indicate that wearable-assisted programmes increase daily steps and can produce modest improvements in metabolic risk factors when coupled with behavioural coaching (Jiakponna et al., 2024). Because declines in activity and worsening sleep commonly precede weight regain and IR, continuous activity monitoring provides complementary early warning signals that enhance the predictive value of glucose surveillance alone.

15.4.3 Mobile Apps, Digital Therapeutics, and Remote Patient Monitoring (RPM)

The mHealth platforms and prescription digital therapeutics bundle self-management tools (food logs, medication reminders), behaviour-change techniques (goal setting, self-monitoring, feedback), and human or automated coaching. RPM platforms aggregate CGM, weight, and activity data into clinician dashboards and automated risk-stratification pipelines that trigger stepped escalation (teleconsultation, intensified coaching, short re-induction diets, or medication adjustment) (Klonoff et al. xxxx). Recent programmatic reports and pragmatic studies demonstrate that RPM models can substantially reduce HbA1c and facilitate rapid clinical responses that avert prolonged metabolic deterioration.

15.4.4 Automated Insulin Delivery

Automated insulin delivery systems represent a significant advancement in diabetes management by integrating continuous glucose sensing technologies with algorithm-driven insulin dosing. These systems function by linking a Continuous Glucose Monitor (CGM), which provides near real-time glucose values, to an insulin pump capable of delivering basal and corrective insulin doses. A predictive control algorithm processes the glucose data and trends to autonomously adjust insulin delivery autonomously, aiming to maintain glucose levels within a target range with minimal user intervention (Kosaji et al., 2025). Modern AID systems operate on a closed-loop feedback mechanism, where insulin infusion is modulated based on dynamic glucose fluctuations rather than fixed programmed doses. Adaptive algorithms, including proportional–integral–derivative (PID), model predictive control (MPC), or hybrid control models, forecast future glucose changes and titrate insulin accordingly. This approach helps mitigate postprandial hyperglycemia, nocturnal hypoglycemia, and glycemic variability—challenges often inadequately addressed by conventional insulin therapy (Kulzer et al., 2024). As technology evolves, next-generation AID systems are integrating adaptive learning algorithms, multi-hormone delivery (e.g., glucagon co-administration), and interoperability with digital health platforms, representing a transformative step toward durable, personalized glycaemic control.

15.5 Management of Comorbidities and Complications

Long-term diabetes management requires a comprehensive approach that extends beyond glycaemic control. Multiple comorbidities—such as hypertension, dyslipidaemia, obesity, fatty liver disease, chronic kidney disease, neuropathy, retinopathy, and cardiovascular dysfunction—interact synergistically with hyper glycemia. These interconnected metabolic burdens increase the risk of relapse, accelerate disease progression, and reduce treatment responsiveness (Lean et al., 2024). Therefore, sustained diabetic health must involve early detection, risk modification, and systematic management of these comorbidities.

Metabolic comorbidities, including obesity and non-alcoholic fatty liver disease (NAFLD), contribute significantly to IR. Structured weight management, calorie reduction, increased physical activity, and use of incretin-based pharmacotherapies reduce hepatic fat accumulation and improve insulin signalling (Lemos & Skyler, 2025). Microvascular complications such as neuropathy and retinopathy require annual screening and timely intervention to prevent progression and support functional health. Psychological and behavioural conditions—including depression, stress, and sleep disturbances—also affect metabolic stability and adherence; therefore, integrating mental-health evaluation improves long-term outcomes (Fig. 15.2).

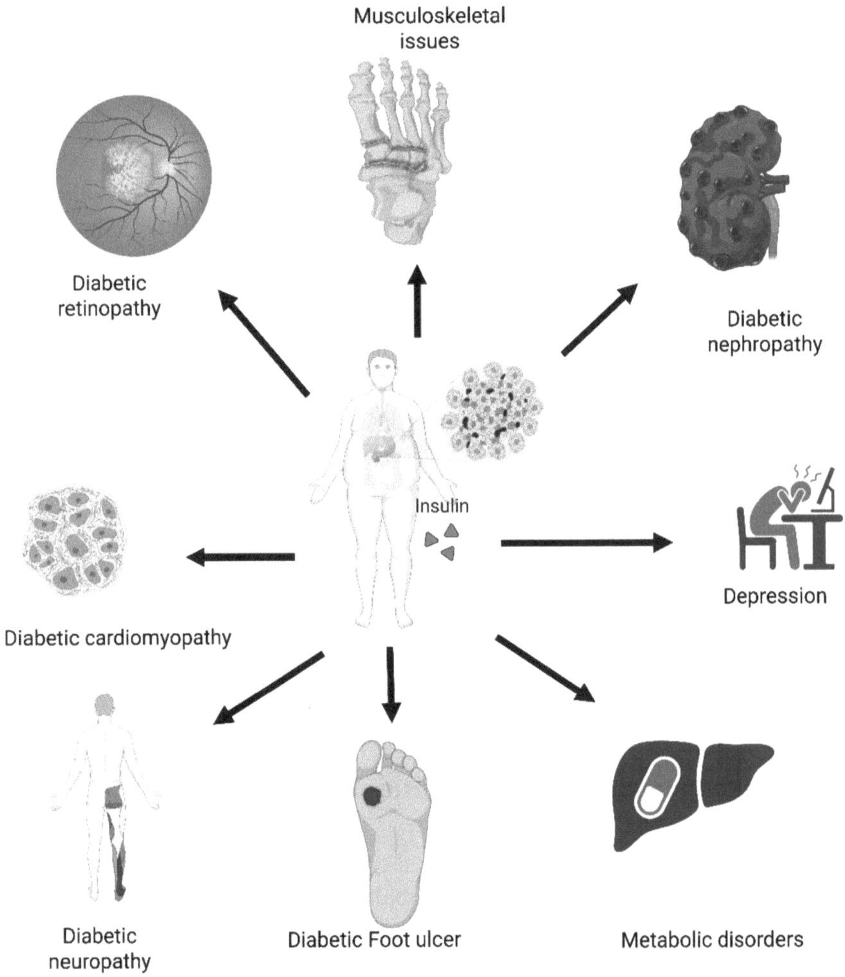

Fig. 15.2 Holistic management of diabetic comorbidities to support lifelong health

15.5.1 Cardiovascular Risk Management

Contemporary literature highlights that CVD remains the leading cause of morbidity in individuals with diabetes due to persistent endothelial dysfunction and chronic inflammatory signaling. Early identification of atherogenic risk through blood pressure monitoring, lipid profiling, and assessment of arterial stiffness is essential (Yousuff et al., 2024). Antihypertensive therapy—particularly ACE inhibitors, ARBs, and calcium channel blockers—has been shown to provide dual benefits in lowering cardiovascular events and preserving renal function. Statins remain the cornerstone of lipid management, while newer agents such as PCSK9 inhibitors are recommended for individuals with persistent dyslipidaemia despite maximal therapy.

Multimodal interventions that combine anti-inflammatory diets, supervised exercise, and cardioprotective medications demonstrate the most significant long-term benefits in preventing relapse and vascular complications (Mphasha & Mothiba, 2025).

15.5.2 Renal Protection and CKD Prevention

Renal impairment often precedes clinical diabetes relapse. Annual evaluation of albuminuria and estimated glomerular filtration rate (eGFR) is strongly supported by prospective cohort studies. SGLT2 inhibitors and GLP-1 receptor agonists have demonstrated renoprotective effects that are independent of glycemia, including reductions in intraglomerular pressure, albumin excretion, and inflammatory markers. Dietary sodium restriction, blood-pressure optimization, and weight management further enhance renal resilience (Munshi et al. 2025). Continuous monitoring is critical because recurrent hyperglycemia accelerates nephron loss, making proactive kidney protection a foundational component of sustained metabolic health.

15.5.3 Obesity, Fatty Liver Disease, and Metabolic Overload

Non-alcoholic fatty liver disease (NAFLD) is highly prevalent in diabetes and acts as a metabolic amplifier by contributing to hepatic IR (Odom & Goldstein, 2025). A weight reduction of 7–10%, achieved through calorie-controlled diets, structured physical activity, or pharmacological therapies (e.g., GLP-1 agonists, dual incretin agonists), has been shown to regress steatosis and lower the risk of relapse significantly. Addressing visceral adiposity is critical, as adipose-derived cytokines and lipotoxic intermediates accelerate β-cell dysfunction.

15.5.4 Mental Health and Psychosocial Comorbidities

Depression, chronic stress, diabetes distress, and sleep disorders are often under-recognized yet play substantial roles in metabolic instability. Evidence from behavioural medicine research indicates that patients with untreated psychological comorbidities experience poorer adherence, greater glycemic fluctuation, and higher relapse rates (Olsen et al., 2025). Regular screening using validated tools, integration of cognitive–behavioural therapy, sleep hygiene interventions, and stress-reduction strategies (such as mindfulness and breathing exercises) can significantly improve metabolic outcomes by enhancing self-regulation and reducing cortisol-related IR.

15.5.5 Infection Susceptibility and Inflammatory Burden

Chronic hyperglycemia impairs neutrophil function and elevates systemic inflammatory markers, thereby increasing susceptibility to infections, which in turn exacerbate IR. Vaccination (influenza, pneumococcal), periodontal care, and early treatment of diseases are recommended in many clinical reviews (Sindhwani et al., 2025). Studies show improved glycaemic stability in individuals receiving routine dental prophylaxis, underscoring the role of oral inflammation in metabolic decline.

15.5.6 Neuropathy, Retinopathy, and Microvascular Surveillance

Longitudinal studies underscore that microvascular complications often manifest silently before overt relapse occurs. Annual retinal imaging, monofilament testing, vibration perception threshold tests, and assessment of autonomic neuropathy support early detection. CGM-derived metrics such as glycaemic variability have been linked with microvascular progression, suggesting that stable glucose patterns may offer protective benefits (Rayala et al., 2025). Lifestyle interventions, combined with agents such as ACE inhibitors and antioxidants, may help decelerate microvascular decline by enhancing endothelial repair and reducing oxidative stress.

15.5.7 Polypharmacy and Medication Optimization

For patients with multiple comorbidities, inappropriate polypharmacy can increase hypoglycemia risk, promote weight gain, or create adherence barriers. Evidence-based medication reviews, conducted every 6–12 months, help eliminate redundant therapies and streamline regimens. Prioritizing agents with cardiometabolic benefits—such as SGLT2 inhibitors, GLP-1 agonists, ACE inhibitors, and statins—provides both therapeutic simplicity and improved long-term outcomes (Retnakaran et al., 2024). Deprescribing strategies are particularly relevant for older adults to reduce adverse drug interactions (Table 15.1).

15.6 Future Perspectives

Future perspectives on sustaining long-term diabetic health emphasise the transition toward more personalized, technology-enabled, and biologically informed care strategies. Emerging evidence from recent scientific literature suggests that integrating advanced digital tools—such as AI-assisted glucose analytics, adaptive

Table 15.1 Integrated strategies for managing diabetic comorbidities and long-term complications

Complication	Pathophysiological link to recurrence	Approaches to diabetes screening and surveillance	Evidence-based interventions	Long-term benefits for sustained diabetic health
Cardiovascular disease	Chronic inflammation and autonomic dysfunction	ECG annually; echocardiography for high-risk cases	Cardio-protective drugs, smoking cessation,	Better endothelial function and reduced mortality risk
Peripheral neuropathy	Impaired nerve function alters activity levels and increases fall risk	Monofilament and vibration testing are performed annually	Glycaemic control, foot care, pain-modulating agents	Prevents ulceration, improves mobility
Retinopathy	Microvascular stress increases oxidative burden	Annual retinal imaging	Laser therapy, anti-VEGF agents, BP/lipid control	Prevents vision loss and improves functional independence
Dyslipidaemia	Elevated LDL/TG promotes atherosclerosis and metabolic inflammation	Lipid profile every 6–12 months	Statins, ezetimibe, PCSK9 inhibitors; Mediterranean diet; omega-3 intake	Lower CVD risk and reduced inflammation
Hypertension	Increases vascular stiffness and IR; accelerates endothelial dysfunction	BP monitoring	ACEIs/ARBs, calcium channel blockers, sodium restriction, aerobic exercise	Reduced CV risk, improved renal outcomes, and better glycaemic stability
Chronic Kidney Disease (CKD)	Hyperfiltration and albuminuria predict future relapse	eGFR and albuminuria yearly	SGLT2 inhibitors, GLP-1 RAs, BP control, low-sodium diet	Delayed CKD progression, lower systemic inflammation
NAFLD / Hepatic steatosis	Fatty liver amplifies hepatic IR	Liver enzymes, ultrasound, fibrosis scores	Weight loss, aerobic training, and incretin-based therapy	Reversal of steatosis and improved hepatic metabolism
Infections and inflammatory burden	Acute inflammation worsens insulin sensitivity	Dental checkups, vaccination status, and annual review	Vaccinations, periodontal therapy, and early infection treatment	Lower inflammatory load and fewer metabolic disruptions

(continued)

Table 15.1 (continued)

Complication	Pathophysiological link to recurrence	Approaches to diabetes screening and surveillance	Evidence-based interventions	Long-term benefits for sustained diabetic health
Psychological comorbidities (depression, distress, anxiety)	Affects adherence, increases cortisol, worsens glucose control	Screening	CBT, stress reduction, sleep hygiene, pharmacotherapy	Better adherence and reduced glycaemic variability
Autonomic neuropathy	Disturbs glucose counter-regulation, heart rate variability	Cardiovascular reflex	Lifestyle management, glucose stabilization	Reduces hypoglycemia risk and improves heart function

insulin delivery systems, and remote monitoring platforms—can markedly improve early detection of metabolic instability and support timely intervention (Rosenfeld et al., 2025). Research also indicates growing interest in multi-omics profiling, including genomics, metabolomics, and microbiome analysis, to better characterize individual risk trajectories and guide precision lifestyle or pharmacological therapies (Zhang et al., 2022). Furthermore, novel therapies aimed at mitigating chronic inflammation, improving β-cell durability, and modulating gut-hormone pathways hold promise for reducing relapse in glycaemic control. Sustainable behavioural support, enhanced through digital coaching and tailored psychosocial frameworks, is expected to strengthen long-term adherence (Shastry & Shastry, 2023). Together, these advancements point toward a more integrated, proactive, and individualized model of diabetes maintenance that targets both metabolic and behavioural determinants of recurrence.

15.7 Conclusion

Sustained prevention of diabetes recurrence requires a multidimensional and forward-looking approach that extends beyond short-term glycaemic correction. Evidence across clinical and translational research demonstrates that relapse is strongly influenced by persistent metabolic stress, progressive β-cell vulnerability, and long-standing behavioural and environmental determinants. Thus, long-term diabetic health is best supported when therapeutic strategies are designed to stabilize these underlying biological and lifestyle-related drivers factors, rather than focusing solely on immediate glucose normalization. Integrating structured lifestyle modification with personalized pharmacotherapy, continuous monitoring technologies, and patient-centred education has shown consistent benefit in reducing relapse risk across diverse populations. Advances in automated insulin delivery systems, digital health platforms, and biomarker-driven risk assessment further enhance the capacity to detect early deviations from glycaemic stability and intervene proactively. At the same time, evidence highlights the need for sustained support mechanisms—such as regular counselling, nutritional guidance, and adherence-focused follow-up—to reinforce long-term behavioural resilience.

A comprehensive, sustained framework also acknowledges the importance of psychosocial well-being and socio-environmental factors, which substantially influence adherence and metabolic outcomes. Strategies that engage patients in shared decision-making and empower them to manage their condition autonomously contribute significantly to durable metabolic control. Overall, preventing recurrence and supporting ongoing diabetic health requires the coordinated application of biological, technological, and behavioural interventions. By addressing diabetes as a chronic, dynamic condition rather than a static metabolic disorder, healthcare systems can move toward truly sustainable management models that preserve β-cell function, minimize metabolic variability, and promote long-term health stability.

Acknowledgements We would like to acknowledge the infrastructure and fellowship support provided to Abhishek Ambawatiya extended thanks to the Department of Pharmaceuticals, Ministry of Chemicals and Fertilizers, Government of India, and NIPER Hajipur, as well as Md Abubakar and Dr. Nitesh Kumar, for their support and guidance in executing this work plan. The images were created using www.Biorander.com and www.Grammarly.com to paraphrasing and correct the grammar of this manuscript.

Author Contributions **Abhishek Ambawatiya, Kanika Goyal, and Ritu Dahiya** was involved in the conceptualization, writing of the original draft, mechanistic insight, input on critical points, editing; **Zeeshan Hyderi, Lalit Kumar Singh, and Jayahari Srivastava** contributed to the manuscript writing and editing; **Md Abubakar and Nitesh Kumar** was involved in the conceptualization, manuscript writing, reviewing, conceptualization of figures and approved the version to be published.

Funding None.

Availability of Data None.

Conflict of Interest None.

References

Abu Dabrh, A. M., Reddy, K., Beech, B. M., & Moore, M. (2025). Health & wellness coaching services: Making the case for reimbursement. *American Journal of Lifestyle Medicine, 19*(6), 800–813.

Aidoo, E. M. (2025). Advancing precision medicine and health education for chronic disease prevention in vulnerable maternal and child populations. *World Journal of Advanced Research and Reviews, 25*(2), 2355–2376.

Alenazi, F., & Khan, M. S. (2025). Novel antimicrobial strategies for diabetic foot infections: Addressing challenges and resistance. *Acta Diabetologica, 62*(3), 303–321.

Almuntashiri, S. A., Alsubaie, F. F., & Alotaybi, M. (2025). Plant-based diets and their role in preventive medicine: A systematic review of evidence-based insights for reducing disease risk. *Cureus, 17*(2).

Aragón-Sánchez, J., Víquez-Molina, G., Uçkay, I., Rojas-Bonilla, J. M., & Lipsky, B. A. (2025). A research-based, current approach to diabetes-related acute foot infections and chronic osteomyelitis. *Expert Review of Endocrinology & Metabolism*, 1–15.

Association, A. D. (2023). Standards of care in diabetes—2023 abridged for primary care providers. *Clinical Diabetes, 41*(1), 4–31.

Balakrishnan, K. R., Raj, D. R. S., Ghosh, S., & Robertson, G. A. J. (2025). Diabetic foot attack: Managing severe sepsis in the diabetic patient. *World Journal of Critical Care Medicine, 14*(1), 98419.

Baris, R. O., & Tabit, C. E. (2025). Heart failure readmission prevention strategies—A comparative review of medications, devices, and other interventions. *Journal of Clinical Medicine, 14*(16), 5894.

Brunner, K., Linder, T., Klaritsch, P., Tura, A., Windsperger, K., & Göbl, C. (2025). The impact of overweight and obesity on pregnancy: A narrative review of physiological consequences, risks and challenges in prenatal care, and early intervention strategies. *Current Diabetes Reports, 25*(1), 30.

Bus, S. A., Sacco, I. C. N., Monteiro-Soares, M., Raspovic, A., Paton, J., Rasmussen, A., et al. (2024). Guidelines on the prevention of foot ulcers in persons with diabetes (IWGDF 2023 update). *Diabetes/metabolism Research and Reviews, 40*(3), Article e3651.

Care D. (2025). 16. Diabetes care in the hospital: Standards of care in diabetes—2025. *Diabetes Care, 48*, S321.

Chao, A. M., Moore, M., & Wadden, T. A. (2025). The past, present, and future of behavioral obesity treatment. *International Journal of Obesity, 49*(2), 196–205.

Committee ADAPP. (2023). Glycemic goals and hypoglycemia: standards of care in diabetes—2024. *Diabetes Care, 47*(Suppl 1), S111.

Cusi, K., Abdelmalek, M. F., Apovian, C. M., Balapattabi, K., Bannuru, R. R., Barb, D., et al. (2025). Metabolic dysfunction–Associated steatotic liver disease (MASLD) in people with diabetes: The need for screening and early intervention. A consensus report of the American Diabetes Association. *Diabetes Care, 48*(7), 1057–1082.

Denby, N. (2025). Weight loss and prevention of weight gain in menopause. *Post Reproductive Health, 31*(2), 115–121.

Desouter, A. K., Keymeulen, B., Van de Velde, U., Van Dalem, A., Lapauw, B., De Block, C., et al. (2025). Repeated OGTT versus continuous glucose monitoring for predicting development of stage 3 type 1 diabetes: A longitudinal analysis. *Diabetes Care, 48*(4), 528–536.

DuBois, K. E., Delgado-Díaz, D. C., McGrievy, M., Valafar, H., Monroe, C., Wilcox, S., et al. (2025). The Mobile lifestyle intervention for food and exercise (mLife) study: Protocol of a remote behavioral weight loss randomized clinical trial for type 2 diabetes prevention. *Contemporary Clinical Trials, 148*, Article 107735.

ElSayed, N. A., McCoy, R. G., Aleppo, G., Balapattabi, K., Beverly, E. A., Briggs, Early, K., et al. (2025). 8. Obesity and weight management for the prevention and treatment of type 2 diabetes: Standards of care in diabetes–2025. *Diabetes Care, 48.*

Fanelli, G., Raschi, E., Hafez, G., Matura, S., Schiweck, C., Poluzzi, E., et al. (2025). The interface of depression and diabetes: Treatment considerations. *Translational Psychiatry, 15*(1), 22.

Ghanem, O. M., Abi Mosleh, K., Kerbage, A., Lu, L., Hage, K., & Dayyeh, B. K. A. (2024). Continued diabetes remission despite weight recurrence: Gastric bypass long-term metabolic benefit. *Journal of the American College of Surgeons, 238*(5), 862–871.

Glycemic goals and hypoglycemia: Standards of Care in Diabetes. (2025). *Diabetes Care, 48*(Supplement_1), S128–145.

Grattoni, A., Korbutt, G., Tomei, A. A., García, A. J., Pepper, A. R., Stabler, C., et al. (2025). Harnessing cellular therapeutics for type 1 diabetes mellitus: Progress, challenges, and the road ahead. *Nature Reviews Endocrinology, 21*(1), 14–30.

Gregg, E. W., Chen, H., Bancks, M. P., Manalac, R., Maruthur, N., Munshi, M., et al. (2024). Impact of remission from type 2 diabetes on long-term health outcomes: Findings from the Look AHEAD study. *Diabetologia, 67*(3), 459–469.

Herold, K. C., Delong, T., Perdigoto, A. L., Biru, N., Brusko, T. M., & Walker, L. S. K. (2024). The immunology of type 1 diabetes. *Nature Reviews Immunology, 24*(6), 435–451.

Hilbrands, R., & Gillard, P. (2025). Finding stability for unstable glucose. *Diabetes Care, 48*(5).

Huang, T. S., Chao, J. Y., Chang, H. H., Lin, W. R., & Lin, W. H. (2025). COVID-19 and diabetes: Persistent cardiovascular and renal risks in the post-pandemic landscape. *Life, 15*(5), 726.

Hussain, S., Irfan, M., Khan, M., Khan, M. K., Awan, S. K., Raza, S. S., et al. (2025). From glycemia to grip: A comprehensive review of musculoskeletal complications in diabetic patients. *Cureus, 17*(8).

Jacobsen, L. M., Felton, J. L., Nathan, B. M., Speake, C., Krischer, J., & Herold, K. C. (2025). Type 1 Diabetes TrialNet: Leading the charge in disease prediction, prevention, and immunotherapeutic mechanistic understanding. *Diabetes Care, 48*(7), 1112–1124.

Jiakponna, E. C., Agbomola, J. O., Ipede, O., Karakitie, L., Ogunsina, A. J., Adebayo, K. T., et al. (2024). Psychosocial factors in chronic disease management: Implications for health psychology. *International Journal of Science and Research Archive, 12*(2), 117–128.

Klonoff DC, Bergenstal RM, Cengiz E, Clements MA, Espes D, Espinoza J, et al. Continuous Glucose Monitoring Data Analysis 2.0: Functional Data Pattern Recognition and Artificial Intelligence Applications. J Diabetes Sci Technol. 2025;19(6):1515–27.

Kosaji, D., Awad, M. I., Katmah, R., Jelinek, H. F., Domingues, M. F., Baguneid, M., et al. (2025). Diabetic foot prevention, assessment, and management using innovative smart wearable technology: A systematic review. *Journal of Neuroengineering and Rehabilitation, 22*(1), 168.

Kulzer, B., Freckmann, G., Ziegler, R., Schnell, O., Glatzer, T., & Heinemann, L. (2024). Nocturnal hypoglycemia in the era of continuous glucose monitoring. *Journal of Diabetes Science and Technology, 18*(5), 1052–1060.

Lean, M. E. J., Leslie, W. S., Barnes, A. C., Brosnahan, N., Thom, G., McCombie, L., et al. (2024). 5-year follow-up of the randomised Diabetes Remission Clinical Trial (DiRECT) of continued support for weight loss maintenance in the UK: An extension study. *The Lancet Diabetes and Endocrinology, 12*(4), 233–246.

Lemos, J., & Skyler, J. S. (2025). Challenges in beta cell replacement for type 1 diabetes. *Hormone Research in Pædiatrics, 98*(4), 435–449.

Mphasha, M., & Mothiba, T. (2025). Personalised nutrition approaches in the prevention and management of type 2 diabetes: A narrative review of evidence and practice. *International Journal of Environmental Research and Public Health, 22*(7), 1047.

Munshi, M., Kahkoska, A. R., Neumiller, J. J., Alexopoulos, A. S., Allen, N. A., Cukierman-Yaffe, T., et al. (2025). Realigning diabetes regimens in older adults: A 4S Pathway to guide simplification and deprescribing strategies. *The Lancet Diabetes and Endocrinology, 13*(5), 427–437.

Odom, J., & Goldstein, R. (2025). Inpatient hypoglycemic rate reduction through the implementation of prescriber targeted decision support tools. *Current Diabetes Reports, 25*(1), 15.

Olsen, M. T., Klarskov, C. K., Jensen, S. H., Rasmussen, L. M., Lindegaard, B., Andersen, J. A., et al. (2025). In-Hospital diabetes management by a diabetes team and insulin titration algorithms based on continuous glucose monitoring or point-of-care glucose testing in patients with type 2 diabetes (DIATEC): A randomized controlled trial. *Diabetes Care, 48*(4), 569–578.

Rayala, R. V., Cheekati, S., Ruzieva, M., Vasudevan, V., Borra, C. R., & Sultanov, R. (2025). *Optimized deep learning for diabetes detection: A BGRU-based approach with SA-GSO hyperparameter tuning.* 2025 International Conference on Innovations in Intelligent Systems: Advancements in Computing, Communication, and Cybersecurity (ISAC3). IEEE. pp. 1–6.

Retnakaran, R., Kashyap, S. R., Gerstein, H. C., & Aroda, V. R. (2024). Contemporary clinical perspectives on targeting remission of type 2 diabetes. *Journal of Clinical Endocrinology and Metabolism, 109*(5), 1179–1188.

Rosenfeld, R. M., Grega, M. L., Karlsen, M. C., Abu Dabrh, A. M., Aurora, R. N., Bonnet, J. P., et al. (2025). Executive summary of lifestyle interventions for treatment and remission of type 2 diabetes and prediabetes in adults: a clinical practice guideline from the American college of lifestyle medicine. *American Journal of Lifestyle Medicine, 19*(2_suppl), 132S–154S.

Shastry, K. A., & Shastry, A. (2023). An integrated deep learning and natural language processing approach for continuous remote monitoring in digital health. *Decision Analytics Journal, 8*, Article 100301.

Sindhwani, R., Bora, K. S., & Hazra, S. (2025). The dual challenge of diabesity: Pathophysiology, management, and future directions. *Naunyn-Schmiedeberg's Archives of Pharmacology, 398*(5), 4891–4912.

Spanakis, E. K., Urrutia, A., Galindo, R. J., Vellanki, P., Migdal, A. L., Davis, G., et al. (2022). Continuous glucose monitoring–guided insulin administration in hospitalized patients with diabetes: A randomized clinical trial. *Diabetes Care, 45*(10), 2369–2375.

Summary of revisions: Standards of Care in Diabetes. (2025). *Diabetes Care, 48*(Supplement_1), S6–13.

Templer, S., Abdo, S., & Wong, T. (2024). Preventing diabetes complications. *Internal Medicine Journal, 54*(8), 1264–1274.

Velayutham, K., Panneerselvam, G., & Ramanathan, B. (2025). Understanding diabetes remission. *Apollo Medicine, 22*(3), 184–191.

Watts, G. F., Rosenson, R. S., Hegele, R. A., Goldberg, I. J., Gallo, A., Mertens, A., et al. (2025). Plozasiran for managing persistent chylomicronemia and pancreatitis risk. *New England Journal of Medicine, 392*(2), 127–137.

Ying, L. P., Yin, O. X., Quan, O. W., Jain, N., Mayuren, J., Pandey, M., et al. (2025). Continuous glucose monitoring data for artificial intelligence-based predictive glycemic event: A potential aspect for diabetic care. *International Journal of Diabetes in Developing Countries, 45*(2), 272–287.

Yousuff, A. R. M., Zainulabedin Hasan, M., Anand, R., & Rajasekhara, B. M. (2024). Leveraging deep learning models for continuous glucose monitoring and prediction in diabetes management: Towards enhanced blood sugar control. *International Journal of Systems Assurance Engineering and Management, 15*(6), 2077–2084.

Zhang, X., Wang, H., Du, C., Fan, X., Cui, L., Chen, H., et al. (2022). Custom-molded offloading footwear effectively prevents recurrence and amputation, and lowers mortality rates in high-risk diabetic foot patients: A multicenter, prospective observational study. *Diabetes, Metabolic Syndrome and Obesity: Targets and Therapy*, 103–109.

MIX
Papier aus verantwortungsvollen Quellen
Paper from responsible sources
FSC® C105338

If you have any concerns about our products,
you can contact us on
ProductSafety@springernature.com

In case Publisher is established outside the EU,
the EU authorized representative is:
Springer Nature Customer Service Center GmbH
Europaplatz 3, 69115 Heidelberg, Germany

Printed by Libri Plureos GmbH
in Hamburg, Germany